Advances in Treatments for Aortic Valve and Root Diseases

Khalil Fattouch • Patrizio Lancellotti
Mani A.Vannan • Giuseppe Speziale
Editors

Advances in Treatments for Aortic Valve and Root Diseases

Springer

Editors
Khalil Fattouch
Department of Cardiothoracic
and Vascular Surgery
GVM Care and Research, MEH
University of Palermo
Palermo
Italy

Mani A. Vannan
Marcus Heart Valve Center
Piedmont Heart Institute
Atlanta, Georgia
USA

Patrizio Lancellotti
Department of Cardiology
University of Liège
Liège
Belgium

Gruppo Villa Maria Care and Research
Anthea Hospital
Bari
Italy

Giuseppe Speziale
Cardiovascular Surgery Department
GVM Care & Research
Anthea Hospital
Bari
Italy

ISBN 978-3-030-09773-8 ISBN 978-3-319-66483-5 (eBook)
https://doi.org/10.1007/978-3-319-66483-5

Printed on acid-free paper

This Springer imprint is published by the registered company Springer International Publishing AG part of Springer Nature
The registered company address is: Gewerbestrasse 11, 6330 Cham, Switzerland

Contents

Part I

Anatomy

The Clinical Anatomy of the Aortic Root

1

Robert H. Anderson, Diane E. Spicer, and Shumpei Mori

1.1 Introduction

The definitive outflow tracts in the postnatal hearts possess three components. These are the intrapericardial arterial trunks, the arterial roots, and the subvalvar ventricular outflow tracts. The distal boundary of the aortic root with the intrapericardial component of the ascending aorta is clearly marked by the sinutubular junction. The proximal boundary, in contrast, has no direct anatomic substrate. It is represented by the virtual plane that can be created by joining together the basal attachments of the moving components of the root. As we will see, the virtual nature of this entrance to the root creates problems in defining the so-called valvar "annulus". This is the more so, since many surgeons consider the semilunar hinges of the moving components to represent the "annulus" [1]. This is but one of the issues with nomenclature which plague the search for consensus when describing the components of the aortic root. As was emphasised by the study group of German cardiac surgeons, the current situation can be considered as a modern-day "tower of Babel" [1]. In this chapter, as we describe the anatomical feature of the root, we also seek to provide solutions to the terminological problems. We emphasise the importance, if we are to

R.H. Anderson (✉)
Institute of Genetic Medicine, Newcastle University, Newcastle-upon-Tyne, UK

60 Earlsfield Road, London SW18 3DN, UK
e-mail: sejjran@ucl.ac.uk

D.E. Spicer
Department of Pediatric Cardiology, University of Florida, Gainesville, FL, USA

Johns Hopkins All Children's Heart Institute, St Petersburg, FL, USA

S. Mori
Division of Cardiovascular Medicine, Department of Internal Medicine,
Kobe University Graduate School of Medicine, Kobe, Japan

K. Fattouch et al. (eds.), *Advances in Treatments for Aortic Valve and Root Diseases*, https://doi.org/10.1007/978-3-319-66483-5_1

achive maximal clinical traction, of describing the components in attitudinally appropriate fashion [2]. With this in mind, we show how the availability of datasets obtained using computed tomography now permits the heart to be viewed with as much, or even more, accuracy during life as when the organ is held in one's hands in the autopsy room [3]. To start, we explain the reasons underscoring our choice of the terms used to describe the components of the root. Thereafter, we describe its central position within the heart. We then concentrate on those anatomical features that are of particular interest to the diagnostician, the surgeon, and the catheter interventionist.

1.2 Naming the Components of the Root

The words we use to describe the parts of the aortic root are equally applicable to the pulmonary root. They can, by and large, also be used to describe the components of the atrioventricular valves. This comparison serves also to emphasise some of the current difficulties. Thus, there are some who seek to differentiate the moving components of the atrioventricular valves as the leaflets, but to describe the moving parts of the arterial valves as the cusps. There are multiple reasons why this approach is less than satisfactory. In the first place, the right-sided atrioventricular valve is universally called the tricuspid valve, showing that, at some time previously, the moving parts of this valve, and the mitral valve, with its alternative title of the bicuspid valve, were also considered to be "cusps". This likely reflects the similarity to the surfaces of the molar and premolar teeth to the surfaces of the closed valves when viewed from their atrial aspect. The closed surfaces of the arterial valves also present a similar appearance when viewed from their ventricular aspect (Fig. 1.1a). It is very unusual nowadays, however, for the arterial valves to be assessed from this aspect. The surgeon tends to view the valves from the arterial aspect. For morphologists, they are typically viewed, and interrogated, in opened fashion (Fig. 1.1b). Assessment from the opened viewpoint then emphasises the inadequacy of using the word "cusp" to describe the moving components. When defined literally, a "cusp" is a point or elevation, or the crossing point of two curves. As is seen in Fig. 1.1b, the hinges of the curved moving components cross at the sinutubular junction. If defined literally, therefore, this crossing point should be recognised as the "cusp". Instead, these distal attachments of the moving components at the sinutubular junction are universally described as the valvar commissures (Fig. 1.1b).

This usage then creates still further problems in terms of naming, since for anatomists a "commissure" is the line of union of adjacent structures, as seen in the lips or the eyelids. If defined in anatomical fashion, therefore, it would be the zones of apposition of the moving components between their peripheral attachments at the sinutubular junction and the centroid of the valvar orifice which would be called the commissures (Fig. 1.2). It is most unlikely that clinicians will ever desist from naming the peripheral attachments as the commissures, so we follow this conventional

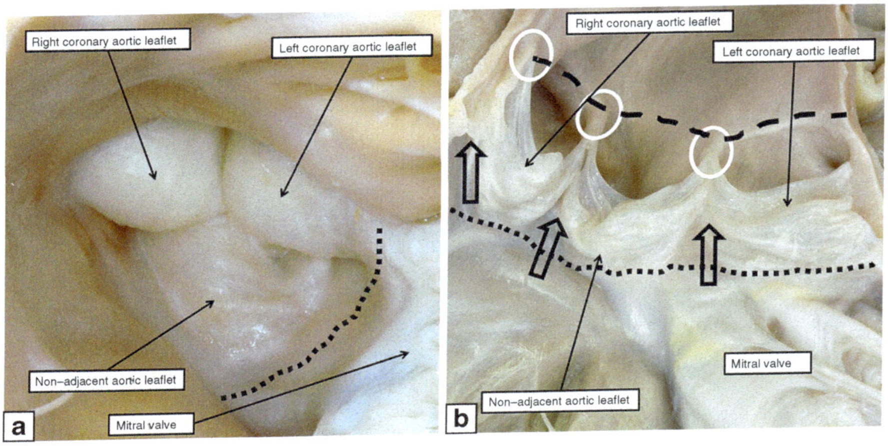

Fig. 1.1 The images show the problems with the use of "cusp" to describe the moving parts of the aortic root. If defined literally, a cusp is a point or elevation, or the crossing point of two curves. When seen in closed position (Panel **a**), there is a resemblance between the ventricular margins of the moving parts and the surface of a molar or premolar tooth, these surfaces also described as cusps. When seen in the open position, however, (Panel **b**), there is no resemblance of the moving parts to the surfaces of the teeth. Instead, the crossing points of their semilunar hinges become evident at the sinutubular junction (*white ovals* on broad dashed *black line*). These points, however, are traditionally described as the valvar commissures (see Fig. 1.2). Note the area of fibrous continuity between the moving components of the aortic and mitral valves, shown as a *black dotted line* in panel **a**, and the virtual nature of the entrance to the root shown as the *black dotted line* in Panel **b**. Note also the fibrous triangles separating the ventricular aspects of the semilunar moving components (*black arrows* in panel **b**). The authors retain their intellectual copyright in the images from which these figures were prepared

usage in this chapter. It is necessary, however, also to recognise the importance of the zones of apposition between the moving components. It is the snug closure along these areas (Fig. 1.2) that ensures valvar competence. That leaves us with the problem of how properly to describe the moving components themselves. We prefer to name these parts as the leaflets, thus avoiding the need to use "cusp". We have a further reason underscording this approach. This is because "cusp" is also seemingly used by some investigators, particularly electrophysiologists [4], to describe the pockets of the aortic root which support the leaflets in semilunar fashion. The components of the root that support the leaflets are the sinuses of Valsalva. They should not be labelled as "cusps".

The anatomy of the sinuses of Valsalva, furthermore, is itself complicated. This is because the semilunar hinges of the leaflets supported by the two sinuses that give rise to the coronary arteries (Fig. 1.3a) extend beyond the anatomic junction of the arterial sinusal walls with the supporting ventricular structures. This means that, in these two sinuses, which are adjacent to the pulmonary trunk, there are small crescents of myocardium incorporated at their base, with the myocardial support being

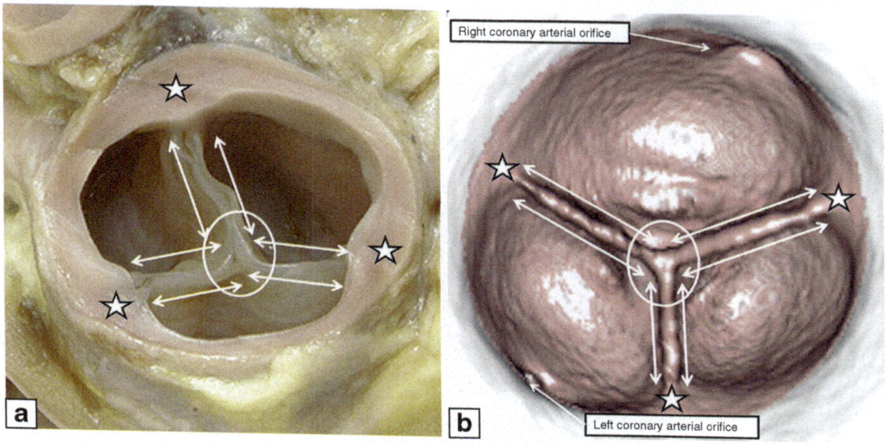

Fig. 1.2 The images show the arterial aspect of the closed aortic valve as seen in an anatomical specimen (Panel **a**) and a "fish-eye" view of a reconstructed computed tomographic dataset obtained from a patient undergoing analysis of coronary arterial disease. The *stars* show the peripheral attachments of the semilunar hinges of the moving components of the root at the sinu-tubular junction. These are known traditionally as the commissures. When defined anatomically, however, a "commissure" is the zone of apposition between two adjacent parts, as shown by the *white* arrows. Since it is unlikely that "commissure" will be used to describe anything other than the peripheral attachments of the hingelines, we will describe the junctional areas as the zones of apposition. As is seen from both panels, these fit snugly together when the valve is competent. The authors retain their intellectual copyright in the images from which these figures were prepared

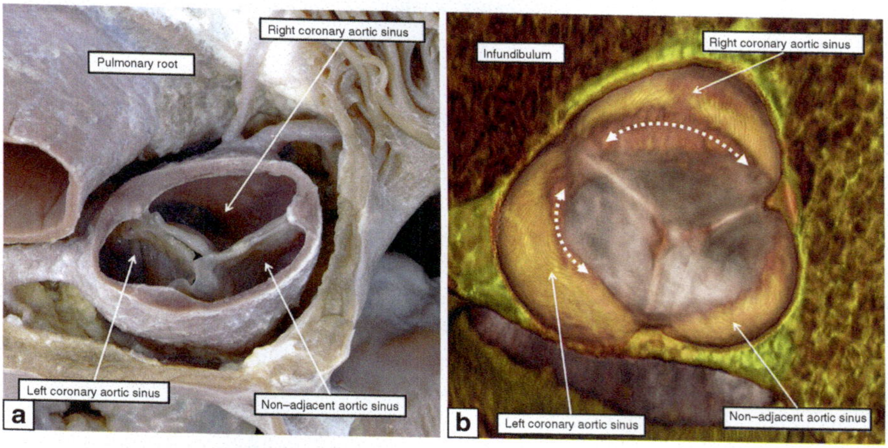

Fig. 1.3 The images show the optimal convention for naming the sinuses of the aortic root. The two sinuses adjacent to the pulmonary root give rise to the coronary arteries. The root is viewed from the arterial aspect in the specimen shown in panel **a**. The third sinus, which does not usually give rise to a coronary artery, is not adjacent to the pulmonary root. It can, however, on rare occasions give rise to a coronary artery. We prefer, therefore, to describe the sinus as being non-adjacent. The image obtained by virtual dissection of a computed tomographic dataset obtained from a patient undergoing analysis for coronary arterial disease (Panel **b**), orientated to match the image shown in panel **a**, reveals the presence of the small crescents of myocardium incorporated at the base of the two sinuses which give rise to the coronary arteries (*white double headed dotted arrows*). The authors retain their intellectual copyright in the images from which these figures were prepared

greater in the right coronary than the left coronary sinus (Fig. 1.3b). There is no myocardium, however, incorporated at the base of the third aortic sinus, which is opposite to the pulmonary trunk (Fig. 1.3a). The leaflet of the aortic valve supported by this sinus is in fibrous continuity with the aortic, or anterior, leaflet of the mitral valve. In most instances, this sinus is called the non-coronary sinus. This is usually an appropriate designation. Very rarely, however, a coronary artery can take its origin from this sinus [5]. In such circumstances, it makes no sense to name the sinus as being "non-coronary". We prefer, therefore, to identify the sinus as being non-adjacent (Fig. 1.3a).

When we assess the aortic root in opened fashion (Fig. 1.1b), we then recognise further components of the root which, until relatively recently, have received scant attention from clinicians. These are the interleaflet triangles [6]. Part of the subvalvar component of the root, and hence part of the left ventricular cavity, they are distal to the virtual basal plane created by joining together the proximal attachments of the semilunar leaflets. They separate, furthermore, the cavity of the left ventricle from either the pericardial space, or the tissue plane between the aortic root and the subpulmonary infundibulum. We will describe, in a subsequent section, the relationships of these triangles in detail, since in many ways an appreciation of their location is the key to understanding the overall valvar anatomy [6]. As can be seen from Fig. 1.1b, nonetheless, the triangles occupy the spaces within the root located on the ventricular aspects of the semilunar hinges of the leaflets. It is these semilunar hinges, therefore, which mark the haemodynamic ventriculo-arterial junction. They separate the parts of the root which, during catheterisation procedures, register aortic as opposed to left ventricular pressures. These haemodynamic ventriculo-arterial junctions, however, are markedly different from the anatomic junctions between the proximal extent of the arterial walls of the valvar sinuses and the supporting ventricular structures [7]. As already explained, it is because the semilunar hinges cross this anatomic ventriculo-aortic junction that the crescents of myocardium are incorporated at the bases of the two sinuses giving rise to the coronary arteries (Fig. 1.3b). And, as also explained, the virtual basal plane marking the entrance of the root is constructed by joining together the proximal attachments of the leaflets.

It is the virtual nature of this plane that creates the perhaps biggest persisting problem in reaching consensus on naming the components of the root, namely the nature of the so-called "annulus". In the sense that the boundaries of the virtual plane created by joining together the nadirs of the semilunar hingelines form a little ring, there is justification in taking the basal ring to represent the valvar annulus. This is the approach taken by clinicians when measuring the dimensions of the root. In contrast, many, but not all, surgeons consider the semilunar hinges of the leaflets to represent the valvar annulus [1]. When reconstructed, however, these hingelines take the form of a coronet rather than a little ring (Fig. 1.4). The semilunar hingelines also extend through the full length of the root, with the dimensions of their diameters varying according to whether measured at the level of the virtual basal plane, the mid-sinusal level, or at the sinutubular junction (Fig. 1.5). For better or worse, furthermore, it is the diameter of the virtual basal plane that is measured by echocardiographers and angiographers when accounting for the valvar "annulus". This, therefore, is the plane that should probably now

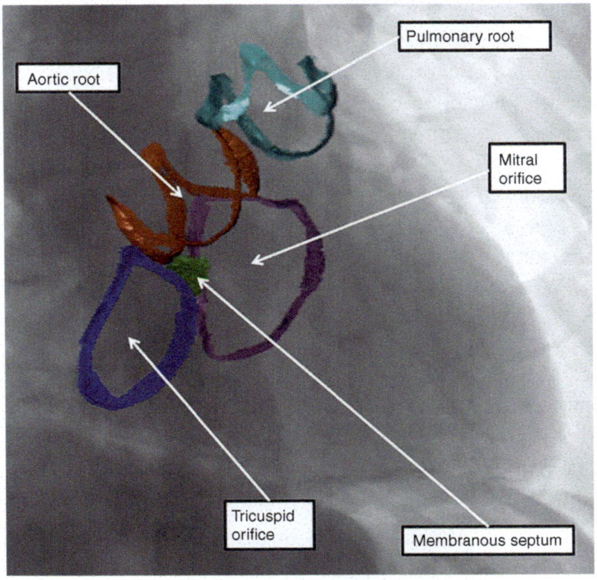

Fig. 1.4 The image is prepared by reconstructing the hingelines of the attachments of the valvar leaflets as seen in a computed tomographic dataset obtained from a patient undergoing investigation for coronary arterial disease. It shows that, although the hinges of the atrioventricular valves are attached in relatively annular fashion, the hinges of the arterial valves produce a coronet arrangement when viewed in three dimensions. The authors retain their intellectual copyright in the image from which this figure was prepared

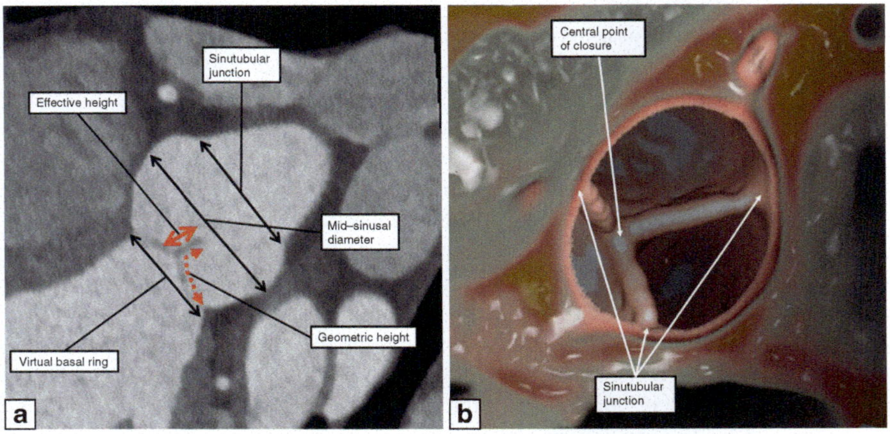

Fig. 1.5 The image in Panel **a** shows a section taken through a computed tomographic dataset obtained from an individual undergoing assessment for suspected coronary arterial disease. The section is cut through the nadirs of the right coronary and the non-adjacent aortic valvar sinuses. It shows how the dimensions of the root vary in terms of its distal, middle, and proximal boundaries, with the proximal border formed by joining together the attachments of the hinges of the valvar leaflets (See also Figs. 1.6 and 1.7). The solid and dotted double-headed *red arrows* show the so-called effective and geometric heights of the valvar leaflets. Note that the line of closure of the leaflets is no more than half way up the height of the arterial root. This is confirmed by the reconstructed images shown in Panel **b**. The central point of coaptation of the closed leaflets is appreciably proximal to their peripheral attachment at the sinutubular junction. The authors retain their intellectual copyright in the images from which these figures were prepared

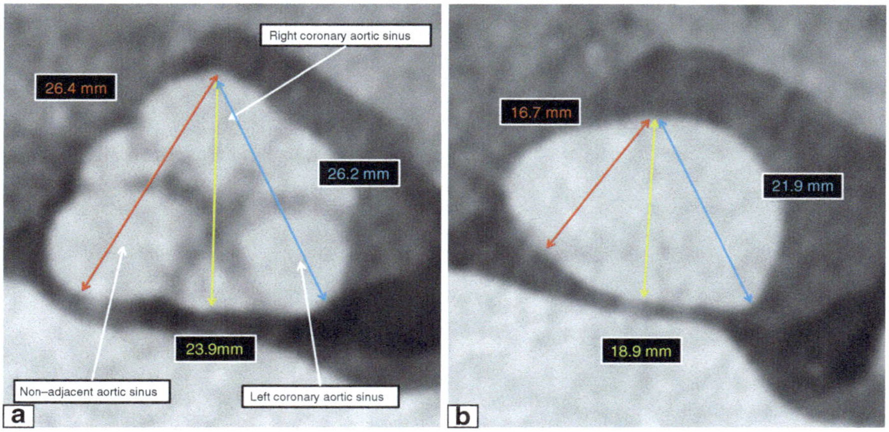

Fig. 1.6 The images show the potential problems in measuring the dimensions of the aortic root at the level of the basal ring (Panel **b**) as opposed to mid-sinusal level (Panel **a**). The cross-sections are taken from the computed tomographic dataset used to create Fig. 1.5. When measuring at mid-sinusal level, the bisected diameter is shorter than the distance measured from sinus to sinus. At the level of the virtual basal ring, because of the ovoid shape of the basal component of the root, the measurements taken from sinus to sinus (*red and blue double headed arrows*) themselves vary, and also vary relative to the section that bisects the root (*yellow double headed arrow*). The sections indicated by the *red and yellow arrows* are shown in Fig. 1.7. The authors retain their intellectual copyright in the images from which these figures were prepared

be taken as the clinical annulus [8], although it must be remembered that many surgeons will still describe the valvar coronet as the surgical annulus [9]. A case can be made, therefore, for distinguishing between the surgical and the echocardiographic annuluses [10].

Acceptance that the virtual basal plane represents the echocardiographic annulus, nonetheless, is not without its own problems. This is because, when measured at mid-sinusal level, or at the sinutubular junction, the aortic root is more-or-less circular, and there is little difference in the dimensions of its diameters (Compare Figs. 1.6 and 1.7). This is not the case when assessing the shape of the virtual basal plane. Rather than being circular, it is decidedly ovoid. Hence, there are potentially significant differences when assessing the root in terms of measurements taken from the nadirs of the valvar leaflets as opposed to planes that bisect the root (Fig. 1.8). Because of these potential problems, it is more sensible nowadays to measure the area of the entrance to the root using three-dimensional techniques (Fig. 1.5), rather than seeking to use a solitary measurement to represent the valvar "annulus" (Fig. 1.8). It is then also necessary to recognise that, when the valvar leaflets are in their closed position (Fig. 1.2), the central point of coaptation is no more than half-way up the length of the root (Fig. 1.5). This is the area recognised by surgeons as the effective height of the leaflets, to be distinguished from their geometric height, which is achieved when the leaflets are lying in their open position within the valvar sinuses [11].

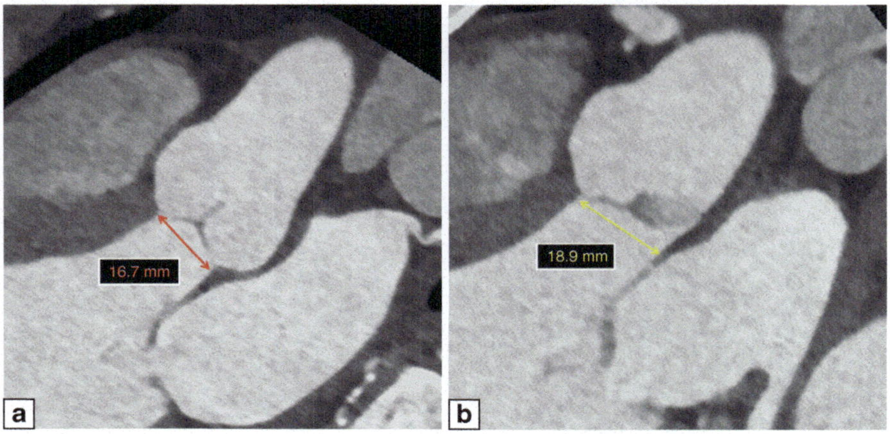

Fig. 1.7 The images show two sections taken through the computed tomographic dataset used to produce Figs. 1.5 and 1.6. Panel **a** shows a parasternal long axis cut taken through the nadirs of the right coronary and non-adjacent aortic valvar sinuses. It is contrasted, in panel **b**, with a cut taken from the nadir of the right coronary sinus to the zone of apposition between the left coronary and non-adjacent aortic valvar leaflets, this plane bisecting the aortic root. The cut from nadir-to-nadir underestimates the diameter of the root by one-eighth. The authors retain their intellectual copyright in the images from which these figures were prepared

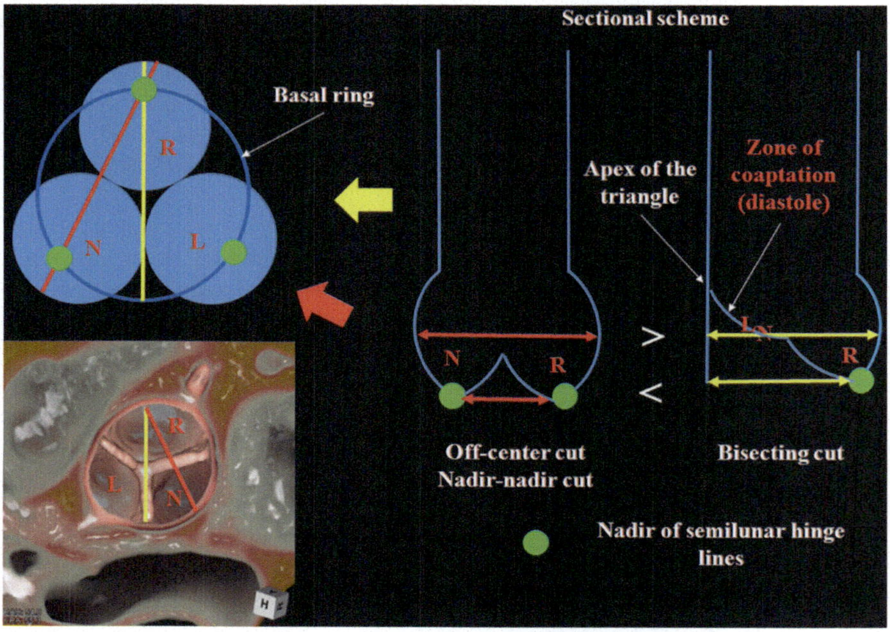

Fig. 1.8 The panels illustrate the potential problems in providing accurate measurements of the virtual basal plane, which is the "echocardiographic annulus", when assessing the dimensions from nadir to nadir of the valvar leaflets, rather than taking a measurement that bisects the aortic root. The upper *left* hand panel shows the arrangement as seen from the ventricular base, whereas the lower *left* panel shows a virtual dissection as viewed from the atrial aspect. The *red and yellow arrows* show dimensions comparable to those shown in Figs. 1.6 and 1.7. The authors retain their intellectual copyright in the images from which these figures were prepared

1.3 Attitudinal Anatomy of the Root

Another of the problems that continue to plague a full understanding of the anatomy of the aortic root is the ongoing penchant of anatomists and cardiologists to describe the heart in so-called "Valentine" location, as if removed from the body and positioned on its apex, rather than as it lies in the body. There is no excuse now for continuing to use this approach to naming components of the heart. Not only does it break the cardinal rule of human anatomy, namely that all structures within the body should be named using the so-called "anatomical position", with the subject standing upright and facing the observer, but the anatomy itself is now increasingly demonstrated in the clinical setting using three-dimensional techniques which show the heart in its bodily location. The most egregious example of the use of the Valentine approach is the naming of the coronary artery that is inferior and interventricular as being posterior and descending (Fig. 1.9) [12]. Less obvious is the naming of the aortic valvar sinuses. If designated as being right coronary, left coronary, and non-adjacent, the constraints of the Valentine approach are removed, since these terms themselves do not depend on the relationships between the sinuses and the bodily coordinates. The right coronary sinus, however, is located anteriorly relative to the two other sinuses when the heart is normally located, with the non-adjacent and left coronary sinuses being positioned side-by-side, with the non-adjacent sinus to the right (Fig. 1.9).

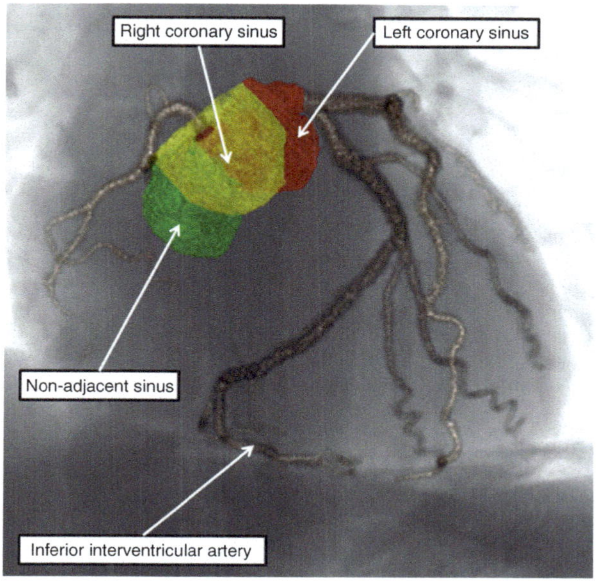

Fig. 1.9 The aortic valvar sinuses have been reconstructed from a computed tomographic dataset prepared from an individual undergoing assessment for suspected coronary arterial disease. They are shown as seen from the front. The right coronary aortic sinus, shown in *yellow*, is positioned in front of the non-adjacent, and left coronary sinuses, shown in *green and red*, respectively. Note that the so-called "posterior descending artery", which in this individual arises from the circumflex artery, is interventricular and located inferiorly. The authors retain their intellectual copyright in the image from which this figure was prepared

1.4 Location of the Aortic Root Within the Heart

Assessment of the cardiac base from the atrial aspect shows how the aortic root forms its centrepiece (Fig. 1.10). Viewing the cardiac silhouette from the front confirms the central location of the root, positioned as it is at the junction of the left ventricular outflow tract and the intrapericardial component of the ascending aorta (Fig. 1.11). The current ability to separate the components of the heart by interrogation of computed tomographic datasets confirms that the so-called "right" chambers of the heart are, in reality, located anteriorly relative to their presumed left-sided counterparts. The aortic root is wedged between the anteriorly positioned infundibulum of the right ventricle and the anterior attachment of the atrial septum (Fig. 1.10). Unlike the right ventricle, which possesses a completely muscular outflow tract, the infundibulum, which lifts the leaflets of the pulmonary valve away from the cardiac base, the outflow tract of the left ventricle is relatively short, and has no discrete anterior boundary. Its posterior boundary is formed by the extensive area of fibrous continuity between the leaflets of the aortic and mitral valves. It is the attachments of this so-called aortic-mitral curtain which anchor the aortic and mitral valves to the roof of the left ventricle (Figs. 1.12 and 1.13). When the left ventricle is opened, it is easier to recognise the thickenings of both ends of the aortic-mitral curtain. These areas are the so-called right and left fibrous trigones. As shown in Figs. 1.12 and 1.13, it is the attachment of the trigones to the summits of the

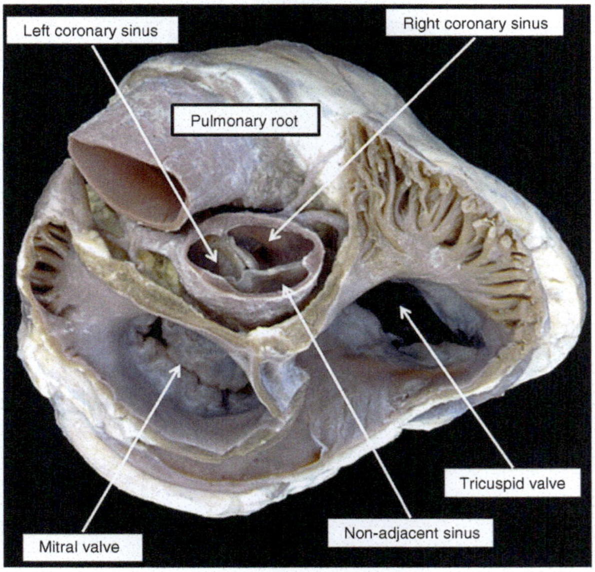

Fig. 1.10 The heart has been dissected by removing the larger part of the atrial myocardium, along with the arterial trunks. It is viewed from the atrial aspect, showing the central location of the aortic root within the cardiac base. The authors retain their intellectual copyright in the image from which this figure was prepared

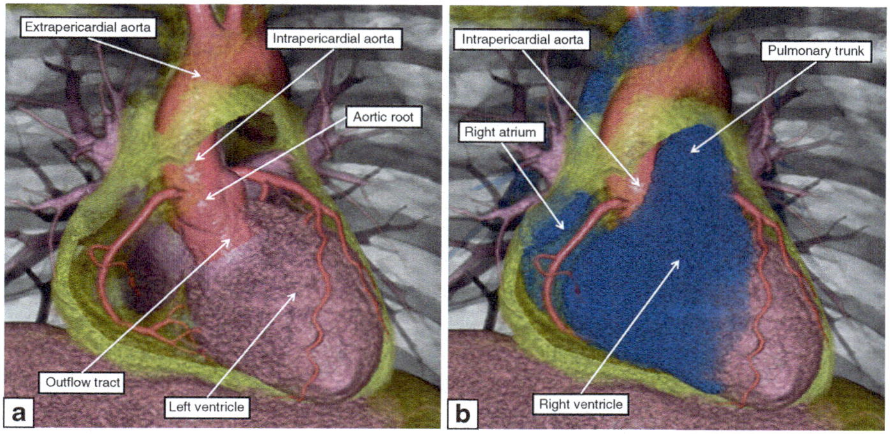

Fig. 1.11 The images are prepared using a computed tomographic dataset obtained from an individual undergoing assessment for suspected coronary arterial disease. The images in panel **a** shows the extent of the pericardial cavity, which is separating the intra-and extrapericardial components of the ascending aorta. The dataset has been coloured so as to show the subvalvar component of the left ventricle. In panel **b**, the components of the so-called right heart have been added. As can be seen, in reality the right heart chambers are anterior to their supposedly left counterparts, with the aortic root wedged between the infundibulum of the right ventricle and the posteriorly located left atrium. The authors retain their intellectual copyright in the images from which these figures were prepared

ventricular walls which anchors the combined valvar unit within the base of the left ventricle. The right fibrous trigone itself is then usually in fibrous continuity with the membranous part of the ventricular septum. The septal component then forms the right wall of the proximal part of the aortic root and the right-sided cardiac chambers (Fig. 1.12). The conjoined structure formed centrally within the cardiac base from the right trigone and the membranous septum is also the strongest part of the insulating plane between the atrial and ventricular chambers. It is the so-called central fibrous body (Fig. 1.14). The membranous septum itself is also continuous distally with the fibrous tissue that fills the gap found on the ventricular aspect of the right aortic and non-adjacent valvar sinuses as the hinge lines of the leaflets supported by these sinuses come together at the sinutubular junction. Such areas of fibrous tissue are also found on the ventricular aspect of the junctional zones between the other valvar sinuses. It is an appreciation of the locations and the relationships of these areas of fibrous tissue separating the distal attachments of the valvar sinuses, the so-called interleaflet fibrous triangles [6], that underscores the overall understanding of the anatomy of the aortic root.

It is the basal continuation of the membranous part of the ventricular septum that constitutes the largest of the triangles. As already shown and discussed, the

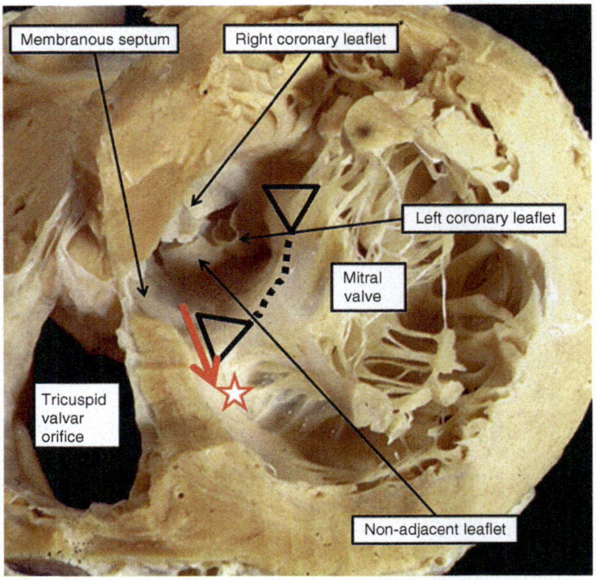

Fig. 1.12 The heart has been sectioned across the short axis of the ventricular mass, and is viewed from the ventricular apex. The image shows the attachments of the aortic mitral curtain (*dotted black line*) through the right and left fibrous trigones (*black open triangles*) to the roof of the left ventricle. Note that there is an inferior extension from the subvalvar outflow tract that interposes between the inferior part of the muscular ventricular septum and the leaflets of the mitral valve. In consequence, the leaflets of the mitral valve are hinged from the ventricular septum only towards the crux of the heart (*white star with red borders*). The space between the septum and the valvar leaflets (*red arrow*) is known as the postero-inferior diverticulum of the outflow tract (See Fig. 1.13). The authors retain their intellectual copyright in the image from which this figure was prepared

membranous septum itself separates the medial wall of the aortic root from the right-sided heart chambers (Fig. 1.12). It is the attachment of the hinge of the septal leaflet of the tricuspid valve to its right side that separates the septum into its atrioventricular and interventricular components. Viewing the area from the right side in a virtual dissection shows how the attachment of the inner heart curvature, known as the ventriculo-infundibular fold, separates the membranous septum from the apex of the interleaflet triangle. The two components of the membranous septum, separated from each other by the hinge of the septal leaflet of the tricuspid valve, are obviously inside the heart. The interleaflet triangle, in contrast, separates the most distal part of the left ventricular outflow tract, within the aortic root, from the right side of the transverse pericardial sinus. The right coronary artery runs through this space as it extends from its sinusal origin to reach the right atrioventricular groove

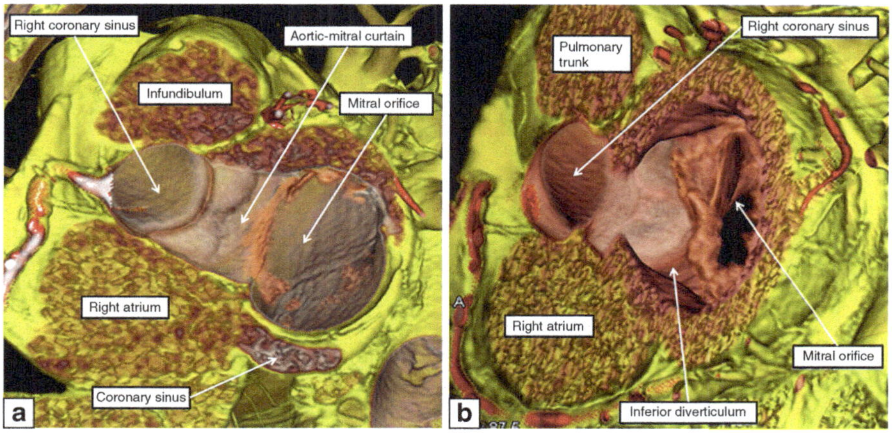

Fig. 1.13 The images are prepared by virtual dissection of a computed tomographic dataset obtained from an individual undergoing assessment for suspected coronary arterial disease. They are cuts through the cardiac base, viewed from the ventricular apex, and replicate the image prepared from a specimen as shown in Fig. 1.12. Panel **a** shows how the aortic root is positioned between the atrial chambers posteriorly and the infundibulum of the right ventricle anteriorly. The cut is taken apical to the roof of the left ventricle, which is formed by fibrous continuity between the leaflets of the aortic and mitral valves. Panel **b** is prepared by angling the section plane so as to show that the postero-inferior extension of the left ventricular outflow tract, which interposes between the mitral valvar orifice and the inferior part of the muscular ventricular septum. The authors retain their intellectual copyright in the images from which these figures were prepared

(Fig. 1.15). This relationship to the rightward margin of the transverse sinus is well demonstrated by removing the interleaftet triangle in the autopsied heart, and again viewing the specimen from the right side. The dissection in the autopsied heart (Fig. 1.16a) confirms the location of the triangle of Koch as shown by the virtual dissection, and again shows the landmarks that permit prediction of the course of the atrioventricular conduction axis, a feature of great surgical significance. Sectioning a virtual dataset then shows the relationships between the fibrous triangle and membranous septum to the extracardiac and intracardiac spaces, respectively (Fig. 1.16b).

The triangle that fills the space on the ventricular aspects of the two aortic valvar sinuses that support the coronary arteries is the smallest of the three triangles. It separates the distal extent of the aortic root from the tissue plane that, in turn, is located between the anterior aspect of the root and the free-standing muscular subpulmonary infundibulum (Fig. 1.17). The third triangle, filling the space between the ventricular aspects of the left coronary and non-adjacent aortic sinuses, is continuous apically with the extensive area of fibrous continuity which forms the aortic-mitral curtain (Fig. 1.13). This triangle again separates the distal extent of the aortic

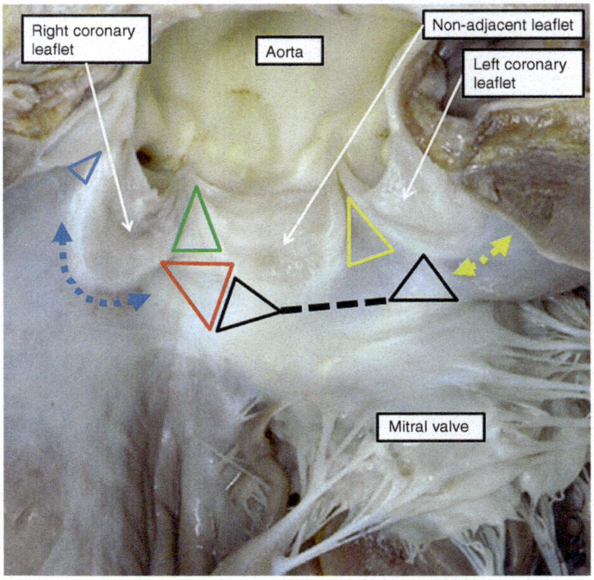

Fig. 1.14 The aortic root has been opened through a cut across the left coronary aortic sinus, and is viewed from the front. The aortic-mitral curtain, formed from fibrous continuity between the aortic leaflet of the mitral valve, the non-adjacent leaflet of the aortic valve, and part of the left coronary aortic valvar leaflet, forms the roof of the left ventricle. The ends of the area of fibrous countinuity (*dashed black line*) are thickened to form the right and left fibrous trigones (*black open triangles*). The right trigone is continuous in the medial wall of the aortic root with the membranous component of the ventricular septum (*red triangle*), which in turn is continuous with the fibrous interleaflet triangle interposed between the right coronary and the non-adjacent aortic valvar sinuses (*green triangle*). Note the continuity of the interleaflet triangle between the non-adjacent and the left coronary aortic sinuses (*yellow triangle*) with the aortic-mitral continuity. Note also the shorter interleaflet triangle (*blue triangle*) between the two coronary aortic sinuses. It is only the two leaflets supported by the sinuses giving rise to the coronary arteries that also have attachment to the left ventricular muscular walls (*blue and yellow dashed double headed arrows*). The authors retain their intellectual copyright in the image from which this figure was prepared

root from the transverse sinus of the pericardial cavity. Due to its more posterior location, however, this triangle is related to the middle component of the transverse pericardial sinus. It is the anterior interatrial groove that forms the posterior boundary of the pericardial sinus in this location, with the atrial septum and the oval fossa directly behind the atrial walls (Fig. 1.18). Bachmann's bundle, made up of the aggregated cardiomyocytes that preferentially conduct the cardiac impulse from the sinus node to the left atrium, extends through these atrial walls.

The location of the triangles can be appreciated by taking histological sections through the aortic root at mid-sinusal level (Fig. 1.19a) and at the level of the

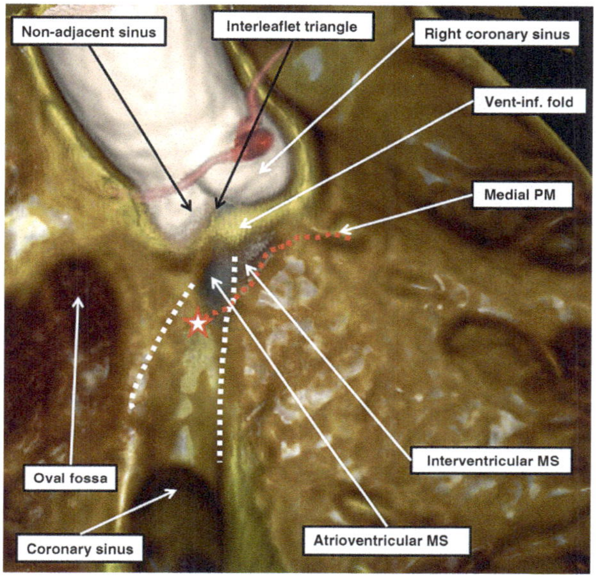

Fig. 1.15 The virtual dissection is prepared from a computed tomographic dataset obtained from an individual undergoing assessment for suspected coronary arterial disease. It shows the boundary between the right coronary and the non-adjacent aortic valvar sinuses as viewed from the *right* side. Note how the ventriculo-infundibular (Vent-inf.) fold separates the interleaflet triangle, which is outside the heart, from the membranous septum. It is the septal leaflet of the tricuspid valve that divides the membranous septum (MS) into its atrioventricular and interventricular components, with the hinge line continuing inferiorly to form the anterior boundary of the triangle of Koch, which is shown by the *white dotted lines*. The *white star with red borders* show the location of the atrioventricular node at the apex of Koch's triangle, with the *red dotted line* showing the site of the atrioventricular conduction axis, with the right bundle branch emerging in the right ventricle beneath the origin of the medial papillary muscle (PM). The authors retain their intellectual copyright in the image from which this figure was prepared

membranous septum virtual basal plane (Fig. 1.19b). The overall relationship of the root is then better demonstrated by interrogation of datasets prepared during life using multidetector computed tomography. A section from such a dataset taken through the cardiac base shows the root sandwiched between the atrial chambers and the infundibulum of the right ventricle (Fig. 1.20a). By combining the information obtained with sectioning the different levels of the root (Fig. 1.19), we can then construct a cartoon showing the location of the sinuses as seen attitudinally, emphasising the location of the support provided by the underlying venticular components, with only a small part of the basal circumference being muscular, the larger parts being fibrous (Fig. 1.20b—compare with Fig. 1.19).

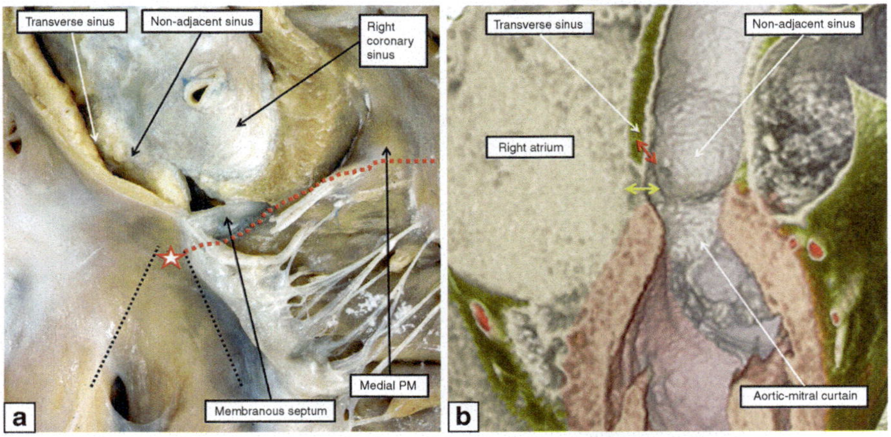

Fig. 1.16 The dissection shown in Panel **a** is made by removing the interleaflet triangle that separates the right coronary and non-adjacent aortic valvar sinuses, along with the portion of the ventriculo-infundibular fold adjacent to the atrioventricular junction so as to reveal the interventricular component of the membranous septum. The heart is then viewed from the *right* side. The *dotted black lines* show the location of the triangle of Koch, with site of the atrioventricular node marked by the *white star with red borders* (compare with Fig. 1.15). The *red dotted line* shows the course of the atrioventricular conduction axis, with the right bundle branch tracking towards the medial papillary muscle (PM). The section in panel **b** is a long axis section through the interleaflet triangle (*double headed red arrow*) and the membranous septum (*double headed yellow arrow*). Note that the fibrous interleaflet triangle separated the distal extent of the aortic root from the transverse pericardial sinus. The authors retain their intellectual copyright in the images from which these figures were prepared

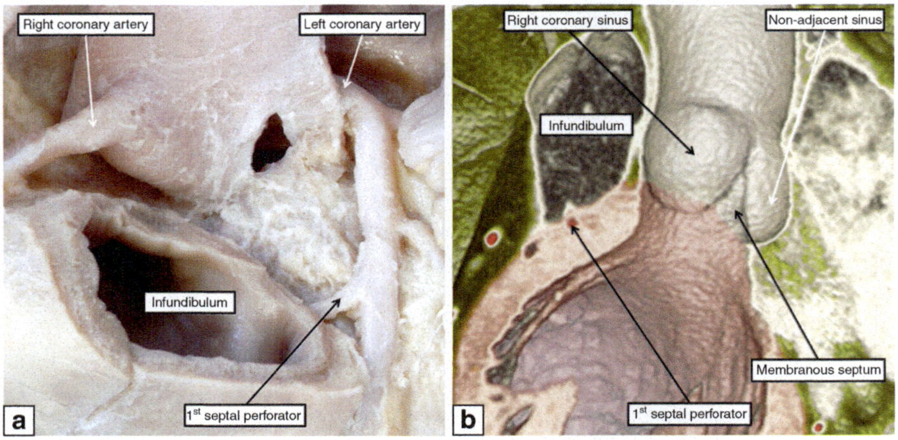

Fig. 1.17 The dissection shown in Panel **a** is made by first removing the pulmonary valve and its supporting free-standing infundibular sleeve from the base of the heart, and then removing the fibrous interleaflet triangle interposed between the right and left coronary aortic valvar sinuses. Note the location of the first septal perforating artery. The image in panel **b** comes from a computerised tomographic dataset, and shows the relationship between the anterior wall of the aortic root in the area of the interleaflet triangle and the subpulmonary infundibulum. The authors retain their intellectual copyright in the images from which these figures were prepared

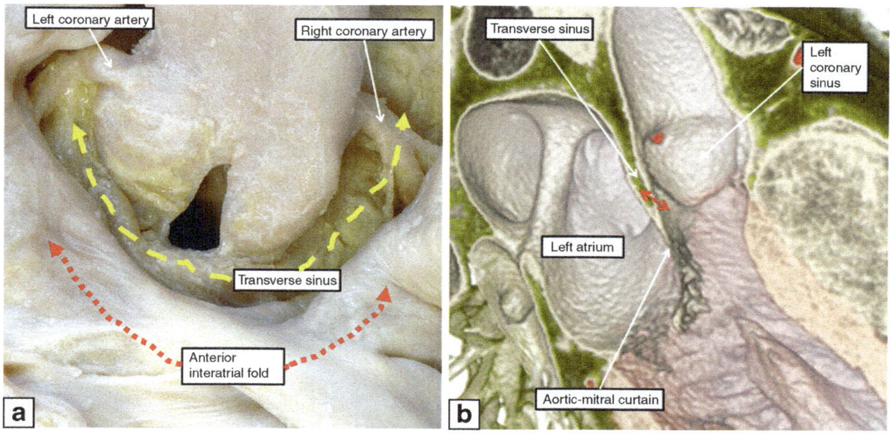

Fig. 1.18 The dissection in Panel **a** is made by removing the fibrous interleaflet triangle interposed between the non-adjacent and left coronary aortic valvar sinuses, and photographing the aortic root from behind. Bachmann's bundle runs through the anterior interatrial fold. Panel **b** shows how the interleaflet triangle (*double headed red arrow*) separates the distal extent of the aortic root from the transverse pericardial sinus. The section is viewed from the *right* side. The authors retain their intellectual copyright in the images from which these figures were prepared

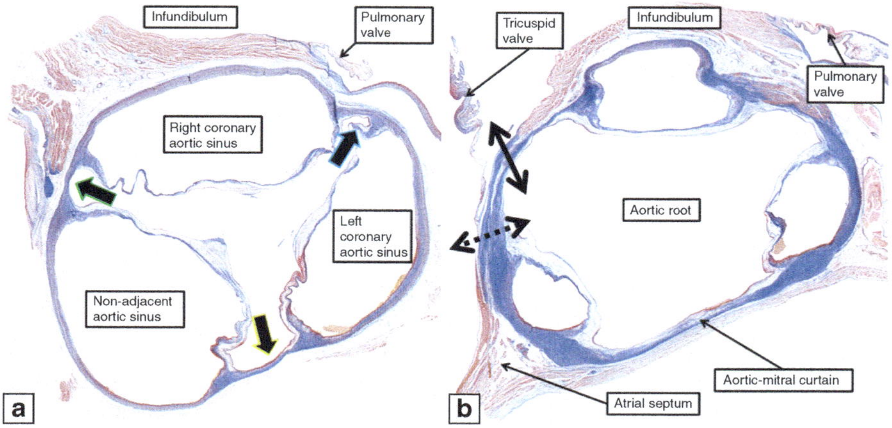

Fig. 1.19 The sections are taken through a human aortic root sectioned in its short axis. Panel **a** is at mid-sinusal level, and shows the interleaflet triangles separating the ventricular aspect of the root from extracardiac tissues. The *black arrow* with *green borders* shows the basal part of the triangle continuous with the membranous septum, as revealed by panel **b**, which is taken closer to the ventricular apex. This panel shows how the hinge of the septal leaflet of the tricuspid valve separates the membranous septum into its atrioventricular (*dotted double headed black arrow*) and interventricular (*solid double headed black arrow*) components. The *black arrow* with *blue borders* shows the triangle separating the root from the subpulmonary infunbibulum, while the *black arrow* with *yellow borders* shows how the triangle between the non-adjacent and left coronary aortic sinuses is continuous apically with the aortic-mitral curtain. The images are created using original material prepared by Professor Nigel Brown, St George's Medical University, and are reproduced with his kind permission. Professor Brown retains his intellectual copyright in the images from which the figures were prepared

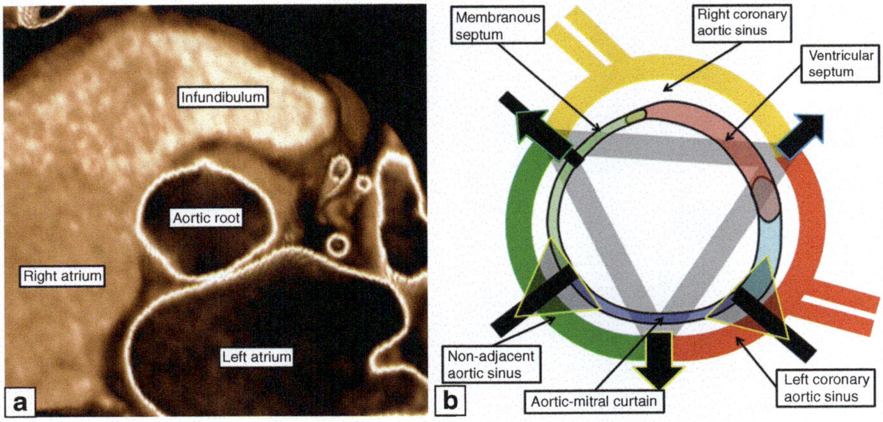

Fig. 1.20 The image obtained by sectioning the computed tomographic dataset (Panel **a**), viewed from the ventricular apex in attitudinally appropriate fashion, shows the central location of the root, with the atrial chambers posterior and the infundibulum of the right ventricle to the front. The cartoon shown in Panel **b** then combines the information regarding the relationships of the different parts of the root. The *black arrows* with coloured borders show the locations of the three interleaflet fibrous triangles (Compare with Fig. 1.19). The authors retain their intellectual copyright in the images from which these figures were prepared

1.5 Surgical Anatomy of the Aortic Root

As shown in Fig. 1.4, reconstruction of the semilunar hinges of the aortic valvar leaflets produces a coronet-like configuration. It is the remnants of these attachment of the leaflets within the root, when the leaflets themselves have been removed during replacement of the aortic valve, that surgeons use to anchor the sutures used to secure the placement of valvar prostheses (Fig. 1.21). It is, presumably, for this reason that many surgeons continue to describe these lines of attachment as the valvar "annulus". There is, however, no specific anatomic structure forming the alleged annulus over and above the attachment of the leaflets to the supporting structures. The semilunar lines of attachment mark the haemodynamic ventriculo-arterial junction, but they cross the anatomic ventriculo-arterial junction. It is the extent of the overall attachments of the leaflets, furthermore, which defines the extent of the root. As described in the previous section, the interleaflet triangles separate the tips of the valvar hinges as they come together at the sinutubular junction. The locations of these spaces between the sinuses can then be used as sites of incision to enlarge the congenitally narrowed root. Thus, it is incisions made through the interleaflet triangle that separates the non-coronary and the left coronary aortic sinuses, continuing proximally into the aortic-mitral curtain, which provides the substrate for the Nicks-Manougian approach to enlargement of the root [13]. Incisions through the interleaflet triangle separating the right and left coronary aortic sinuses, continuing anteriorly into the subpulmonary infundibulum, underscore

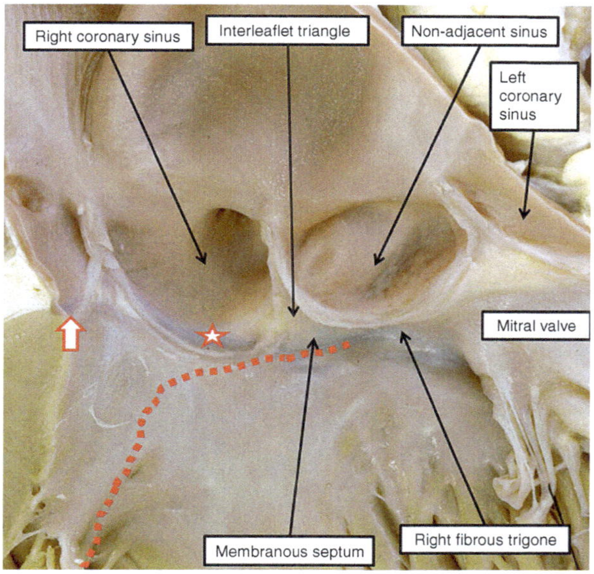

Fig. 1.21 The dissection is made by opening the aortic root through the left coronary aortic sinus, and removing the leaflets of the aortic valve. This reveals the semilunar valvar hinges, described by many cardiac surgeons as the valvar "annulus". Note that the nadirs of the hinges of the leaflets guarding the sinuses giving rise to the coronary arteries extend proximally beyond the anatomic ventriculo-arterial junction so that crescents of myocardium are incorporated within the bases of the sinuses (*white star and white arrow with red borders*). The *red dotted line* shows the proximal extent of the atrioventricular conduction axis and the left bundle branch (see also Fig. 1.22). The authors retain their intellectual copyright in the image from which this figure was prepared

the Rastan-Konno approach. It is not possible, however, to enlarge the root through the triangle between the right coronary and the non-adjacent aortic sinuses. This is because the membranous septum forms the base of this triangle, and the atrioventricular conduction axis penetrates through the atrioventricular component of the septum. This anatomy itself, of course, is of major surgical significance. It is now also of major concern to interventional cardiologists, since bundle branch block is a well-recognised complication of transcutaneous insertion of aortic valvar prostheses [14]. So as to appreciate the adjacency of the conduction axis to the valvar structure, we cannot do better than consult the original cartoon prepared by Tawara [15] when he first described the location of the conduction axis (Fig. 1.22). As can be seen from his reconstruction, the fan formed by the fascicles of the left bundle branch descends onto the smooth left ventricular septal surface just beneath the nadir of the hinge of the right coronary aortic leaflet. It is this relationship that provided the necessary information for the interventional cardiologist so as to avoid iatrogenic disturbances of rhythm [14]. For the cardiac surgeon, providing that sutures are placed within the remaining semilunar hinges of the valvar leaflet during valvar replacements, there should be no danger of damaging the components of the atrioventricular conduction axis.

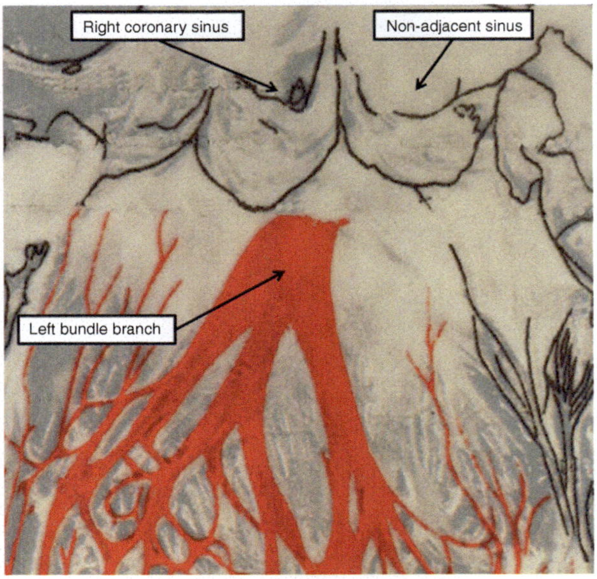

Fig. 1.22 The image is modified from the original reconstruction prepared by Tawara [15] to show the location of the left bundle branch

Conclusion

The aortic root is the central part of both the heart and the left ventricular outflow tract. It is delimited by the semilunar lines of attachment of the valvar leaflets. These leaflets are suspended predominantly from the aortic valvar sinuses of Valsalva. The most proximal attachments of the two leaflets supported by the sinuses which give rise to the coronary arteries, however, cross the anatomic ventriculo-arterial junction. This means that small crescents of myocardium are incorporated as the bases of both these sinuses. Three-dimensional reconstruction of the overall arrangement of the valvar hinges produces a coronet-like configuration. It is the hinges that are described by some cardiac surgeons as the valvar annulus. Clinical diagnosticians, in contrast, tend to describe the diameter of the virtual plane constructed by joining together the nadirs of attachment of the leaflets as the "annulus". There is no anatomic structure corresponding to this plane. The dimensions of the root, furthermore vary markedly not only according to the depth measurements are taken within the root, but also depending on whether they are taken from the nadirs of adjacent leaflets or by bisecting the root. These various discrepancies emphasise the importance of distinguishing between the surgical and clinical annuluses. They also indicate that appropriate measurement should take into account the full extent and configuration of the root.

References

1. Sievers HH, Hemmer G, Beyersdorf F, Moritz M, Moosdorf R, Lichtenberg A, et al. The everyday used nomenclature of the aortic root components: the Tower of Babel? Eur J Cardiothorac Surg. 2012;41:478–82.

2. Anderson RH, Loukas M. The importance of attitudinally appropriate description of cardiac anatomy. Clin Anat. 2009;22:47–51.
3. Mori S, Spicer DE, Anderson RH. Revisiting the anatomy of the living heart. Circ J. 2016;80(1):24–33.
4. Lin CY, Chung FP, Lin YL, Chong E, Chang SL, Lo LW, et al. Radiofrequency catheter ablation of ventricular arrhythmias originating from the continuum between the aortic sinus of Valsalva and the left ventricular summit: electrocardiographic characteristics and correlative anatomy. Heart Rhythm. 2016;13:111–21.
5. Garg A, Ogilvie BC, McLeod AA. Anomalous origin of the left coronary artery from the non-coronary sinus of Valsalva. Heart. 2000;84:136.
6. Sutton JP III, Ho SY, Anderson RH. The forgotten interleaflet triangles: a review of the surgical anatomy of the aortic valve. Ann Thorac Surg. 1995;59:419–27.
7. Anderson RH. Clinical anatomy of the aortic root. Heart. 2000;84:670–3.
8. Frater RWM, Anderson RH. How can we logically describe the components of the arterial valves? J Heart Valve Dis. 2010;19:438–40.
9. Anderson RH. Defining the enigmatic annulus of the aortic valve. Eur J Cardiothorac Surg. 2016;49:101–2.
10. Loukas M, Bilinsky E, Bilinsky S, Blaak C, Tubbs RS, Anderson RH. The anatomy of the aortic root. Clin Anat. 2014;27:748–56.
11. Bierbach BO, Aicher D, Issa OA, Bomberg H, Graber S, Glombitza P, Schafers HJ. Aortic root and cusp configuration determine aortic valve function. Eur J Cardiothorac Surg. 2010;38:400–6.
12. Loukas M, Aly I, Tubbs RS, Anderson RH. The naming game: a discrepancy amongst the medical community. Clin Anat. 2015;29(3):285–9. https://doi.org/10.1002/ca.22666.
13. Anderson RH, Lal M, Ho SY. Anatomy of the aortic root with particular emphasis on options for its surgical enlargement. J Heart Valve Dis. 1996;5(Suppl III):S 249–57.
14. Piazza N, Onuma Y, Jesserun E, Kint PP, Maugenest AM, Anderson RH, de Jaegere PPT, Serruys PW. Early and persistent intraventricular conduction abnormalities and requirements for pacemaking after percutaneous replacement of the aortic valve. J Am Coll Cardiovasc Interv. 2008;1:310–6.
15. Tawara S. Das Reizleitgssystem des Saugetierherzens. Jena: Gustav Fischer; 1906.

Aortic Root Anatomy and Physiology

2

Ruggero De Paulis and A. Salica

2.1 Introduction

The aortic root is a complex region of the heart anatomy. It is positioned immediately above the left ventricle as a bridge between the ventricle and the ascending aorta and has relationship to all cardiac chambers [1]. It could be considered the "centerpiece" of the heart (Fig. 2.1).

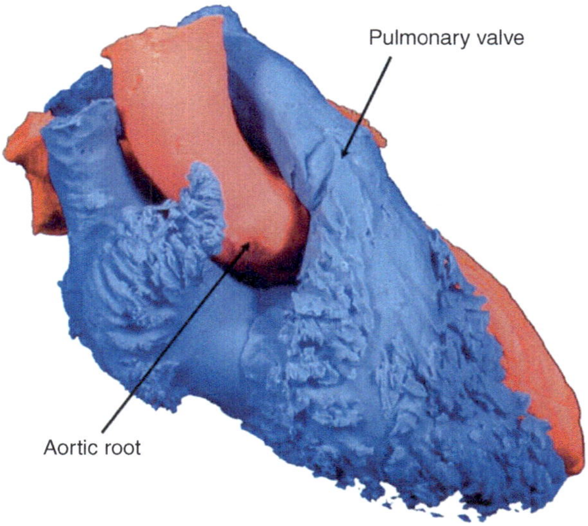

Fig. 2.1 Aortic root has relationship to all cardiac chambers

R. De Paulis • A. Salica (✉)
Cardiac Surgery Department, European Hospital, Via Portuense 700, Rome 00149, Italy
e-mail: salicandrea@gmail.com

K. Fattouch et al. (eds.), *Advances in Treatments for Aortic Valve and Root Diseases*, https://doi.org/10.1007/978-3-319-66483-5_2

Wide spread of valve sparing surgery and the introduction of transcatheter aortic valve replacement (TAVI) in the clinical practice, rise up the interest about its anatomy and allows the newer insights.

Schematically, the aortic root is characterized by a dilatation, the sinuses of Valsalva (SV) that starts immediately above the crown like attachment of the aortic leaflets and finishes with a narrowing, the sino-tubular junction (STJ), immediately before the tubular tract of the ascending aorta.

In addition to its anatomical function, housing the aortic valve, it plays a role in the physiology of the aortic leaflets interacting with the blood flow dynamics during the entire cardiac cycle [2, 3].

2.2 Anatomical Definition

Despite aortic root is a well-defined anatomic unit, there is still no concerns as how best to describe the aortic root in terms of single components [4]. From a surgical point of view and to simplify the argument the aortic root is divided in: the aortic annulus (AAn), the aortic leaflets (AL), the sinuses of Valsalva (SV), and the sino-tubular junction (STJ).

2.3 Aortic Annulus (Ventriculo-Aortic Junction, Interleaflets Triangles, Crown-like Leaflets Attachment and Sino-tubular Junction)

Despite the aortic annulus represents one of the most studied anatomical region of the heart, it remains an enigmatic entity. In the daily clinical practice, aortic annulus has more than one definition. In fact, in case of aortic valve replacement surgery, surgeons commonly considered as aortic annulus, the *locus* of the attachment of the valvar leaflets in between the left ventricle and the sinuses of Valsalva [5], while in case of valve sparing surgery, the aortic annulus is identified in a place immediately under the nadir of the leaflets very close to the virtual basal ring (VBR). On the other hand, the VBR constructed by joining together the *nadir* of each leaflets in a circular shape, is used and analysed by Cardiologists when providing measurements of the diameter of the aortic annulus.

Despite these simple and practical definitions have been widely accepted, aortic annulus is anatomically much more complex and characterized by a clear three-dimensional morphology.

As stated by El Khoury, aortic annulus could be identified in a functional unit, the functional aortic annulus (FAA), composed by (1) the STJ, (2) the semilunar attachments of the aortic leaflets and (3) the virtual line joining together the nadirs of each leaflet with the respective interleaflet triangles (VBR) [6].

The basal attachment of the aortic leaflets describes three semilunar lines with a characteristic crown-like fashion. These semilunar lines represent the hemodynamic boundary line between the LVOT and the arterial system. This hemodynamic annulus significantly differ from the anatomical boundary line between the LVOT and the arterial system. This locus is represented by the VAJ that is the anatomical connection where the LVOT join the aortic tissues, as we described in the dedicated section.

Every single semilunar line has a *nadir* that overlap the LVOT in its most distal portion, and a *zenith* that rise and join the sino-tubular junction that represent their upper attachment. The STJ, also known as the supra-aortic ridge, represents the upper portion of the aortic annulus.

2.4 The Sino-tubular Junction

The sino-tubular junction joins upwards the tubular portion of the aorta and downwards the sinuses of Valsalva and the aortic commissure with which is in direct continuity. On the aortic lumen the STJ usually presents a slightly raised ridge of thickened aortic wall, while on the outside it is smooth and. The sino-tubular junction takes on the contour of the three sinuses, thus it is not perfectly circular and evidences a mildly trefoil or scalloped outline.

STJ play a fundamental role in the structure of the aortic root and in the function of the aortic valve being a component of the functional aortic annulus [6]. It has specific geometrical relationship with the other components of the root. In fact, despite the area of the STJ increased with age and with hypertensive cardiomyopathy [7], in normal healthy hearts echocardiographic diameter of the STJ is about 75% of the maximal sinus diameter [8], while is larger than aortic annulus at the level of the VBR with a ratio of 1.3.

2.5 The Ventriculo Aortic Junction and the Virtual Basal Ring

While the VBR represents a virtual line, with a functional relevance, the VAJ represents a real anatomical site where ventricular structures (muscular septum, membranous septum, mitro-aortic curtain), join the arterial system. Schematically, it is represented by an almost circular line constructed joining the base of the interleaflet triangles with the lower third of the sinuses of Valsalva, slightly above the nadir of the aortic leaflets [9, 10] (Fig. 2.2).

Analyzing the anatomical features of the three sinuses of Valsalva, it has been observed that the VAJ is characterized by peculiar differences per each sinus. In fact, the three leaflets have different relationships with the ventricular muscle, the mitro-aortic junction and the membranous septum. Left ventricular fibers insert the aortic root wall with muscular inclusions at the level of the right coronary sinuses, left/right commissure and a part of the left coronary sinuses towards the right sinus. The right/non coronary commissure takes relationship with the membranous septum, while the non coronary sinus and the non/left coronary commissure have relationships with the mitro-aortic curtain. For these reasons the VAJ describes an

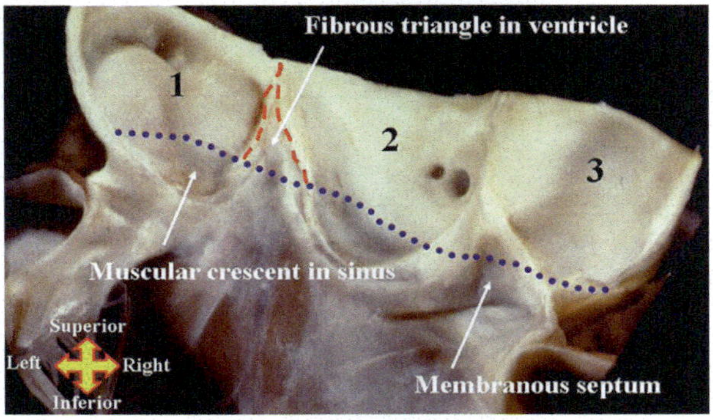

Fig. 2.2 The purple dotted line indicates the Ventriculo Aortic Junction

almost circular line, with a slight tridimensional morphology. In fact, the VAJ is farther at the level of the right coronary sinus and closer at the level of the non coronary sinus respect to the VBR.

While the VBR is positioned at the level of the nadir of the aortic leaflets and never crosses their basal attachment, the VAJ crosses in several point the semilunar line of the aortic leaflets that runs up and down the VAJ. For this reason, the crown-like line divides the aortic root in sub-valvar and supra-valvar regions. The supra-valvar region, despite contains ventricular cells (at the level of the VAJ), is an aortic portion, while the sub-valvar region, despite contains aortic fibro-elastic cells (the interleaflet triangles), is a ventricular portion [10].

These anatomical relationships between the basal attachment of the aortic leaflets, the VBR and the VAJ have to be considered when aortic valve sparing surgery or single aortic annuloplasty is performed.

2.6 Aortic Leaflets, Commissures and Interleaflets Triangles

The normal aortic valve is composed of three leaflets that represent the moving parts of the valve. They have a crimpled surface facing the aorta and a smoother surface facing the ventricle.

Each leaflet is composed of a free margin that is slightly thicker than the basal portion and is responsible of the closure of the valve during the diastole. The apposition zone, the “lunule”, is on the ventricular surface of the free margin and represents the place where each leaflet meets the adjacent leaflets during valvar closure. At the mid-portion of the “lunule”, there is a further thickening called the “nodule of Arantius”. Leaflets fenestrations above the closure line are common.

The basal margin of the leaflets is attached in a semilunar fashion to the aortic root. This basal attachment has the nadir below the VAJ and the zenith at the level of the STJ, where each leaflet, joining the adjacent leaflet, form the three commissures respectively. Beneath the apex of the commissures, a thin layer of fibrous tissue go downstairs, between the respective leaflets, towards the VAJ and forms the final part the LVOT. These thinner areas of fibrous wall, are described as the interleaflet triangles and separates the inside of the left ventricle from the extra-cardiac space.

The total area of the leaflets is about 40% greater than that of the aortic root, with the largest area measured in the non-coronary leaflet and the smallest to the left coronary leaflet in the majority of cases [4, 9].

2.7 The Sinuses of Valsalva

The three-dimensional space of the aortic root surrounding the aortic leaflets are known as the sinuses of Valsalva. The sinuses of Valsalva represent the most proximal portion of the arterial system above the aortic valve. In a cross-sectional view the three bulges have a clover shape, and due to its physiological morphology, characterized by a dilatation, the root is much wider at the midpoint of the sinuses than at either the STJ or at the basal attachment of the leaflets.

In theoretical terms, all three sinuses of the root are identical, however two of them give rise to the coronary arteries and are named the right and the left coronary sinuses. A crescent of ventricular musculature, relative to the VAJ, is incorporated all along the base of the right coronary sinus and in the part of the left coronary sinuses close to the right sinus. The third sinus, called the non-coronary aortic sinus, has exclusively arterial wall. In fact, the basal part of this sinus is made up of a portion of the mitro-aortic curtain thus at this level the VAJ and the VBR coincide.

2.8 The Aortic Root

In the previous paragraphs the principal components of the aortic root have been treated as single units to better analyze their characteristics. Now the aortic root will be described in its integrity.

Although, the aortic root could be schematize with an approximately cylindrical and symmetrical shape, its real morphology is more complex with several peculiarity and a slightly asymmetrical shape. It is well known that the internal height and volume of each sinus was found to be different. The LCS was systematically found to be the smallest sinus while the RCS was found to be similar to the NCS, that in many cases appears to be the higher and larger one [7, 11, 12]. In fact, the aortic root follows the natural curvature of the entire ascending aorta and the presence of a tilt angle of 5.5°–11° between the VBR and STJ planes have been widely observed [7, 11, 12].

In addition to this characteristic, aortic root has an internal or intravascular and an external or extravascular face with proper peculiarity in terms of dimensions and histology along the root circumference. As of fresh aortic roots studies from human cadavers, the internal root height is higher than the respective external height. In fact, the internal height is measured from the VBR to the STJ, while the external root height is measured from the VAJ to the STJ. In this setting, the nonplanar nature of the VAJ significantly affects these measurements. Briefly, the external root height

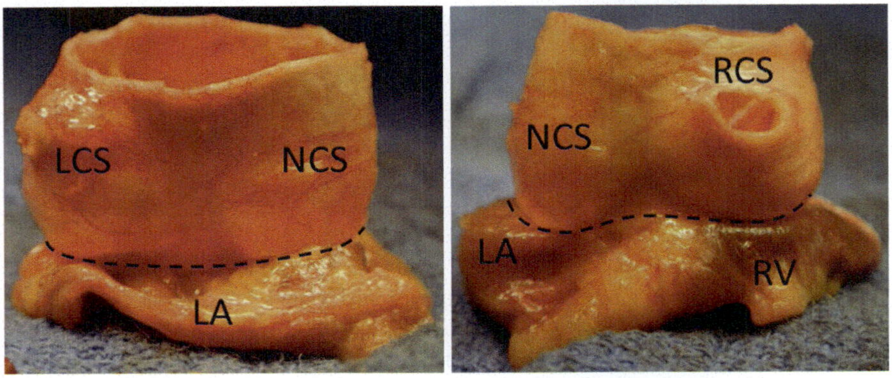

Fig. 2.3 The Virtual Basal Ring has a planar bidimensional shape, while the Ventriculo Aortic Junction has a nonplanar shape (*dotted lines*)

is significantly shorter on the side of the RCS compared with the NCS and LCS (Fig. 2.3) [13].

As we well known, the presence of muscular inclusions, place the VAJ farer from the VBR and nearer to the STJ, while the absence of crescents make the VAJ closer to the VBR minimizing the difference between the internal and external height.

In particular, the presence of muscular fibers of the LVOT into the right coronary sinus, left/right commissure, and half of the left coronary sinus, rise the VAJ significantly higher respect to the VBR and closer to the STJ (At the level of the right/non commissure the presence of the basal attachment of the septal leaflet of the tricuspid valve into the lower part of the membranous septum acts as a boundary that definitely place the VAJ over the VBR and closer to the STJ). On the contrary, in correspondence of the non coronary sinus, non/left coronary commissure and part of the left coronary sinus, the absence of muscular crescents nears the VAJ closer to the VBR [13].

From the histologic point of view, the thickness of the VAJ is variable along the aortic root circumference as the presence of muscular inclusions thicken the respective portion of the root. In fact, the left/right commissure and the right coronary sinus are significantly thicker (maximum thickness at the level of the right coronary sinus with 4.6 mm) than the right/non commissure, non coronary sinus, left/non coronary commissure and left coronary sinus where muscular inclusion of the left ventricle give way to the membranous septum and mitro-aortic curtain, with a mean thickness lower than 1 mm (Fig. 2.4). For these reasons the overall mean thickness of the root is about 3 mm [13].

Differently from the VAJ, the VBR, so-called the echocardiographic “annulus”, is no more than a virtual plane, created by connecting together the nadirs of the hingelines of the individual leaflets, without a real anatomic counterpart. Despite it has been considered a circular line, recently its elliptical shape has been well

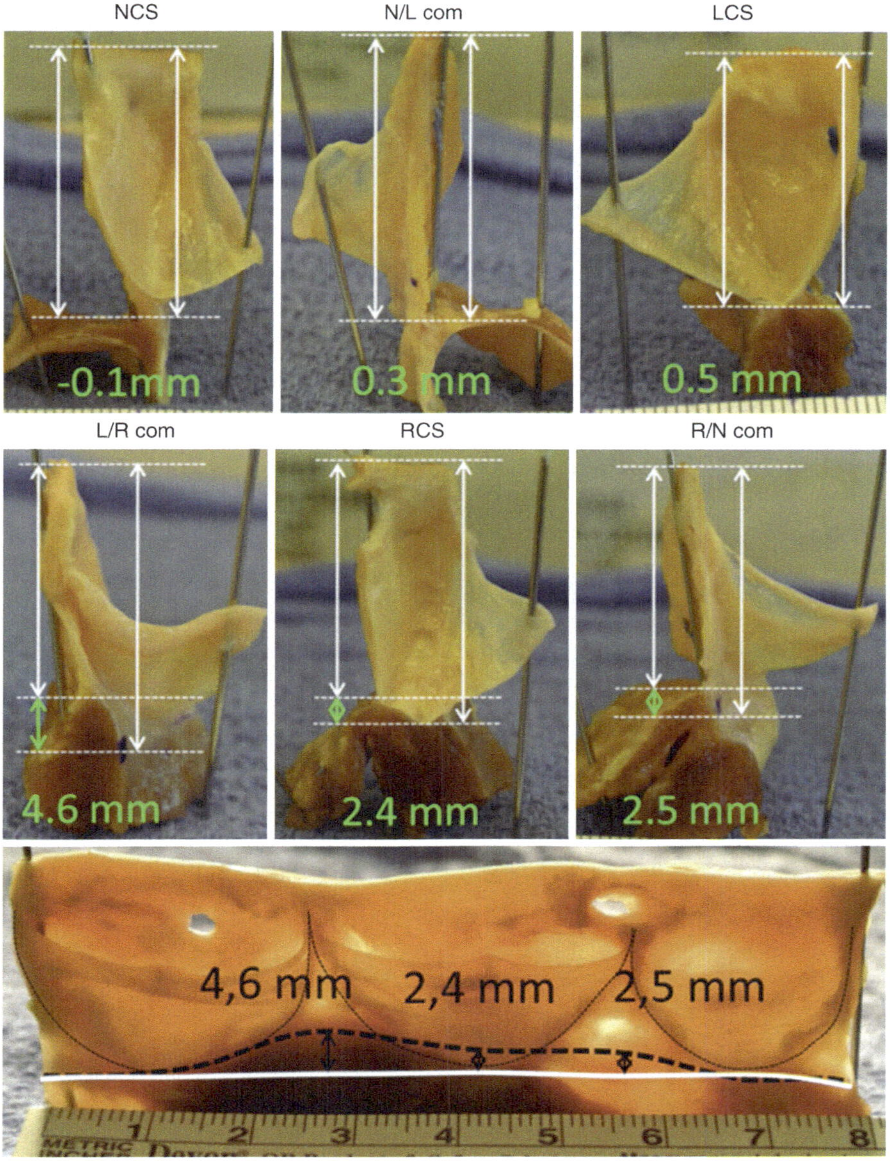

Fig. 2.4 The lines evidence the different thickness of the VAJ along the aortic root. The left/right commissure and the right coronary sinus are significantly thicker than the right/non commissure, non coronary sinus, left/non coronary commissure and left coronary sinus where muscular inclusion of the left ventricle give way to the membranous septum and mitro-aortic curtain, with a mean thickness lower than 1 mm

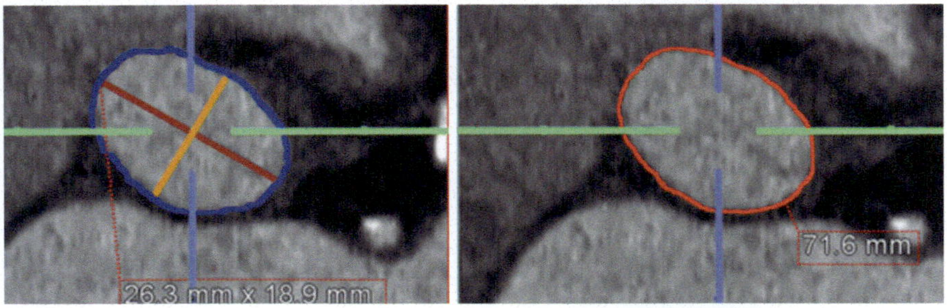

Fig. 2.5 *In vivo* CT scan studies evidenced the elliptical shape of the Virtual Basal Ring

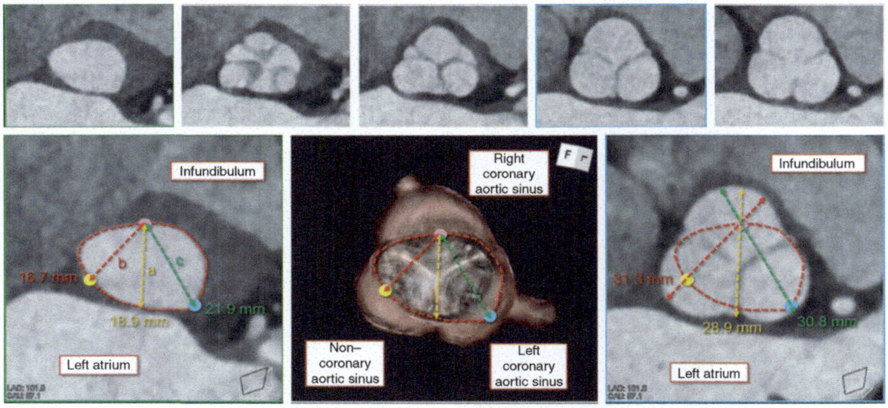

Fig. 2.6 Due to the elliptical shape of the Virtual Basal Ring, its diameters will vary if measured using bisecting as opposed to off-center nadir-to-nadir cuts. In fact, measuring the VBR diameters using the bisecting cuts (*yellow line*) and the right and left off-center cuts (*green line*), has been evidenced that bisecting cuts have been proved to provide diameters significantly larger than those measured with the off-center cuts

described with in vivo CT scan studies (Fig. 2.5) [14]. It follows, therefore, that the measured diameters of the ring will vary if measured using bisecting as opposed to off-center nadir-to-nadir cuts. In fact, measuring the VBR diameters using the bisecting cuts and the right and left off-center cuts, has been evidenced that bisecting cuts have been proved to provide diameters significantly larger than those measured with the off-center cuts [15] (Fig. 2.6).

Differently from the right ventricle, with its free-standing infundibulum, in which muscular crescents are found at the base of each pulmonary sinuses, the aortic VBR goes through the mitro-aortic curtain, under the non-coronary leaflet and through the muscular crescents, under the coronary leaflets. The hypothesis that these different types of tissues influence the elliptical shape of the VBR, as observed in CT scan studies, appears suggestive.

2.9 Physiology from a Surgical Point of View

The aortic root is a well-defined anatomical unit, which has been proved to play a major role in reducing stress on aortic valve cusps and in optimizing ejection to warrant hemodynamic efficiency without structural deterioration of the aortic leaflets throughout life [16, 17].

A normal aortic valve starts to open even before forward blood flow. A slight increase of the diameter at level of the VAJ takes place before the ejection. In fact, during the isovolumetric phase of the left ventricle the contraction of the muscular fibers present at the level of the VAJ acts enlarging the "aortic annulus", while at the same time, intraventricular pressure is transmitted through the inter-leaflet triangle up to the commissures. Both these mechanisms act to enlarge the terminal portion of the LVOT before isotonic contraction and forward blood flow. Thus aortic valve starts to open before forward flow, promoting the ejection phase of the systole. This interaction between aortic root and the contraction of the left ventricle promotes smooth leaflets opening movements during the systole contributing to the reduction of the energy loss across the aortic valve.

During the cardic cycle, pulsatility of the blood flow produces complex fluid structures that interacts with the aortic root.

Several studies have been attempt to clarify the synergistic role that blood flow and the surrounding structures, as the sinuses of Valsalva, have in the opening and closing movements of the aortic leaflets, and a complex interaction has been demonstrated [2, 18–20].

In normal subjects, three distinct phases of aortic leaflets movement were observed during the ejection phase of the systole: a rapid leaflets opening, a slow systolic closure, and a rapid leaflets closing movement [21]. As soon as the forward blood flow starts, the aortic leaflets open with a rapid movement. Contemporary, as the blood flow reaches the STJ, the peripheral portion of the bloodstream curls down into the sinuses of Valsalva forming vortex structures. Then, because of these fluid structures, the "eddy currents", inside the sinuses, leaflets starts to close before forward flow has ended. This phenomenon produces a slow systolic closure, that promotes a smooth valve closure with minimal stress once, at the end of the systole, blood flow reverse generating the rapid leaflets closing movement [16, 17, 21, 22].

The wide diffusion of aortic valve sparing procedures renewed the interest about the role and the physiology of the aortic root, with particular interest about the importance of the sinuses space reconstruction.

Leyh and colleagues in a foundamental study enhanced the importance and the role of the aortic root, as a dynamic structure, in the physiology of the aortic leaflets. Authors observed that after root replacement with recreation of a sinus-like space without aortic annulus stabilization (remodeling technique), the aortic leaflets opening velocity was similar to that evidenced in normal subjects. In contrast, in patients who received aortic annulus stabilization without sinuses reconstruction (reimplantation technique) the velocity of leaflets opening was significantly faster than in normal subjects with phenomena of impacts of the leaflets against the respective Dacron wall during the ejection phase of the cardiac cycle. During the end of the systole, the slow closing motion, was not evidenced in the absence of sinus space. The missing sinus vortices impair the ability of leaflets to start to close before the onset of flow deceleration and reverse.

These observations enhance the great importance of the dynamic role of the aortic root in terms of fluid structures formation and spatial modification of the root during the cariac cycle. In fact, enlargement of the "aortic annulus" at the level of the VAJ, during the isometric phase of the systole, before ejection phase, was similar between remodeling and normal population, while was significantly reduced in reimplantation subjects. This mechanism promotes and prepare the opening of the aortic leaflets before forward flow. Presence of the sinuses space promotes and houses the natural vortices of the blood flow. During the systolic forward flow allows the physiological spatial disposition of the aortic leaflets, preventing their contact with the Dacron wall, and after the peak systolic flow, vortices existing inside the sinuses, allows a smooth leaflets closure yet before reverse flow starts [3].

These aspects were recently confirmed by fluid dynamics *in vitro* experiments. It appears that the presence of sinus-like space reconstruction, independently from its distensibility, plays an important and probably additive role in allowing a progressive increase in valve leaflets opening during the ejection phase of the systole. Presence of sinus-like space, promotes an instrumental interaction between the aortic leaflets opening and the flow structures (vortices) present in the pulsatile flow field, that results in improving the pressure drop and the energy loss across the aortic valve [2, 23].

In fact, comparing hydrodynamic performance of the aortic valve in straight vs Valsalva root models by the use of *in vitro* dedicated test benches, resulted that presence of the sinus of Valsalva was determinant to improve the hemodynamic performance of the aortic valve both in pulsatile and continuous flow regimes. In fact, as reported by Yoganathan and co-workers [24], continuous flow studies can be helpful to characterize energy losses of prosthetic valves, especially at the flow phase corresponding to peak systole, where it has been demonstrated that quasi-stationary flow conditions might be assumed [25]. In these test the presence of the sinuses of Valsalva evidenced a better hydrodynamic performance of the aortic valve respect the straight root models with a significant reduction in terms of pressure drop during the peak systolic ejection phase. This observations suggest that flow separation regions generated by the flow, act as a functional obstruction in the absence of sinuses of Valsalva reducing (1) the complete opening of the aortic leaflets and (2) the lumen available to forward flow, resulting in a pressure drop across the aortic valve. On the contrary, in presence of appropriate space and architecture (represented by sinuses of Valsalva), aortic leaflets are free to complete valve opening with low pressure drops. This phenomenon could possibly be caused by the flow recirculation regions (vortices) forming above the aortic valve. These vortices find a natural housing in the sinuses expansion, which has an immediate effect in more space available for leaflet expansion [2].

Over these dynamic or systolic properties, the role of sinuses of Valsalva is also related to the reduction of stress distribution on the root components.

Finite-elements studies which compared cylindrical straight graft and pseudosinuses graft with normal root, observed that the pseudosinuses model evidenced the closest leaflets stress and strain pattern to the normal aortic root and concluded that natural sinus space as well as sinus-like space reconstruction appear to be instrumental in reduction of leaflet's stress and strain during the diastolic phase of the cardiac cycle [26]. These observations could rising the potential advantages of sinuses reconstructions in valve sparing operations in terms of aortic valve durability.

Sinuses of Valsalva play an instrumental role also in stress and strain distribution on the coronary ostia in root surgery. Bentall procedure, with straight and Valsalva Dacron graft, and aortic root of normal subjects have been investigated with a finite elements in terms of stress and strain on the coronary ostia. Stress distribution on the coronary ostia appear comparable between Valsalva and normal healthy root, while in Straight models, without a pseudosinus-space recreation, a significantly incremented stress on coronary ostia respect normal subjects was evidenced. In particular, a direct comparison among Valsalva and Straight configurations indicates that coronary ostia sutured to a straight Dacron graft had to sustain a 40% higher stress compared with coronary ostia sutured to a Valsalva graft [27].

In conclusion, the complex role of the aortic root is comprised in its anatomy.

Its peculiar geometry interacts with the dynamic fluid structures of the arterial blood flow during the entire cardiac cycle. During the diastole the sinuses of Valsalva minimize mechanical stress on the entire root components, in particular on aortic leaflets and on the coronary ostia. During the systole, promotes opening movements of the leaflets minimizing the energy loss across the aortic valve.

These features are physiologic for the durability of the aortic valve and for the optimal left ventricular function.

References

1. Cook AC, Anderson RH. Attitudinally correct nomenclature. Heart. 2002;87:503–6.
2. Salica A, Pisani G, Morbiducci U, Scaffa R, Massai D, Audenino A, Weltert L, Guerrieri Wolf L, De Paulis R. The combined role of sinuses of Valsalva and flow pulsatility improves energy loss of the aortic valve. Eur J Cardiothorac Surg. 2016;49(4):1222–7.
3. Leyh RG, Schmidtke C, Sievers HH, Yacoub MH. Opening and closing characteristics of the aortic valve after different types of valve preserving surgery. Circulation. 1999;100:2153–60.
4. Ho SY. Structure and anatomy of the aortic root. Eur J Echocardiogr. 2009;10:i3–i10.
5. Pretre R, Kadner A, Dave H, Bettex D, Genoni M. Tricuspidisation of the aortic valve with creation of a crown-like annulus is able to restore a normal valve function in bicuspid aortic valves. Eur J Cardiothorac Surg. 2006;29:1001–6.
6. El Khoury G, Glineur D, Rubay J, Verhelst R, d'Acoz Y, Poncelet A, Astarci P, Noirhomme P, van Dyck M. Functional classification of aortic root/valve abnormalities and their correlation with etiologies and surgical procedures. Curr Opin Cardiol. 2005;20:115–21.
7. Sliver MA, Roberts WC. Detailed anatomy of the normally functioning aortic valve in hearts of normal and increased weight. Am J Cardiol. 1985;55:454–61.

8. Tamàs E, Nylander E. Echocardiographic description of the anatomic relations within the normal aortic root. J Heart Valve Dis. 2007;16:240–6.
9. Anderson RH. The surgical anatomy of the aortic root. Multimed Man Cardiothorac Surg. 2007;2007(102):mmcts.2006.002527. https://doi.org/10.1510/mmcts.2006.002527.
10. Anderson RH, Devine W, Ho SY, Smith A, McKay R. The myth of the aortic annulus: the anatomy of the subaortic outflow tract. Ann Thorac Surg. 1991;52:640–6.
11. Berdajs D, Lajos P, Turina M. The anatomy of the aortic root. Cardiovasc Surg. 2002;10:320–7.
12. Choo SJ, McRae G, Olomon JP, St George G, Davis W, Burleson-Bowles CL, et al. Aortic root geometry: pattern of differences between leaflets and sinuses of Valsalva. J Heart Valve Dis. 1999;8:407–15.
13. De Kerchove L, El Koury G. Anatomy and pathophysiology of the ventriculo-aortic junction: implication in aortic valve repaire surgery. Ann Cardiothorac Surg. 2013;2(1):57–64.
14. Blanke P, Russe M, Leipsic J, et al. Conformational pulsatile changes of the aortic annulus: impact on prosthesis sizing by computed tomography for transcatheter aortic valve replacement. JACC Cardiovasc Interv. 2012;5:984–94.
15. Mori S, Anderson RH, Tahara N, et al. The differences between bisecting and off-center cuts of the aortic root: the three-dimensional anatomy of the aortic root reconstructed from the living heart. Echocardiography. 2017;34:1–9.
16. Thubrikar MJ, Bosher LP, Nolan SP. The mechanism of opening of the aortic valve. J Thorac Cardiovasc Surg. 1979;77:863–70.
17. Thubrikar MU, Nolan SP, Aoud J, Deck JD. Stress sharing between the sinuses and leaflets of canine aortic valve. Ann Thorac Surg. 1986;42:434–40.
18. De Hart J, Peters GWM, Shreurs PJG, Baaijens FTP. A three-dimensional computational analysis of fluid-structure interaction in the aortic valve. J Biomech. 2003;36:103–12.
19. Morbiducci U, Ponzini R, Rizzo G, Cadioli M, Esposito A, Montevecchi FM, et al. Mechanistic insight into the physiological relevance of helical blood flow in the human aorta. An in vivo study. Biomech Model Mechanobiol. 2011;10:339–55.
20. Kvitting JPE, Ebbers T, Wingström L, Engvall J, Olin CL, Bolger AF. Flow patterns in the aortic root and the aorta studied with time-resolved, 3-dimensional, phase contrast magnetic resonance imaging: implication for aortic valve-sparing surgery. J Thorac Cardiovasc Surg. 2004;127:1602–7.
21. Higashidate M, Tamiya K, Beppu T, Imai Y. Regulation of the aortic valve opening. J Thorac Cardiovasc Surg. 1995;110:496–503.
22. Bellhouse BJ, Bellhouse FH. Mechanism of closure of the aortic valve. Nature. 1968;217:86–7.
23. Pisani G, Scaffa R, Ieropoli O, Dell'Amico EM, Maselli D, Morbiducci U, et al. Role of the sinuses of Valsalva on the opening of the aortic valve. J Thorac Cardiovasc Surg. 2013;145:999–1003.
24. Yoganathan AP, Cape EG, Sung HW, Williams FP, Jimoh A. Review of hydrodynamic principles for the cardiologist: applications to the study of blood flow and jets by imaging techniques. J Am Coll Cardiol. 1988;12:1344–53.
25. Yellin EL, Peskin CS. Large amplitude pulsatile water flow across an orifice. J Dyn Sys Meas Control. 1975;97:92–5.
26. Grande-Allen KJ, Cochran RP, Reinhall PG, Kunzelmann KS. Re-creation of sinuses is important for sparing the aortic valve: a finite element study. J Thorac Cardiovasc Surg. 2000;119:753–63.
27. Weltert L, De Paulis R, Scaffa R, Maselli D, Bellisario A, D'Alessandro S. Re-creation of a sinuslike graft expansion in Bentall procedure reduces stress at the coronary button anastomoses: a finite element study. J Thorac Cardiovasc Surg. 2009;137(5):1082–7.

Functional Anatomy and Dynamics of the Aortic Root

3

Xiao Zhou, Mani A. Vannan, and Khalil Fattouch

The anatomy of the aortic root is a sophisticated structure uniquely designed to optimize its function. Each component of the aortic root (Fig. 3.1) is deliberately assembled to allow the stroke volume to be ejected as a laminar flow with minimal resistance and minimal tissue wear and tear [1]. This organized action of the components of the aortic root is critical to the efficiency of the left ventricular pump, normal coronary blood flow, and the distinctive flow pattern in the aorta [2–6]. Thus, an understanding of the functional anatomy of the aortic root is essential to understand the clinical consequences of the disruption of this complex structure. This understanding also is key to the surgical repair techniques aimed to restore

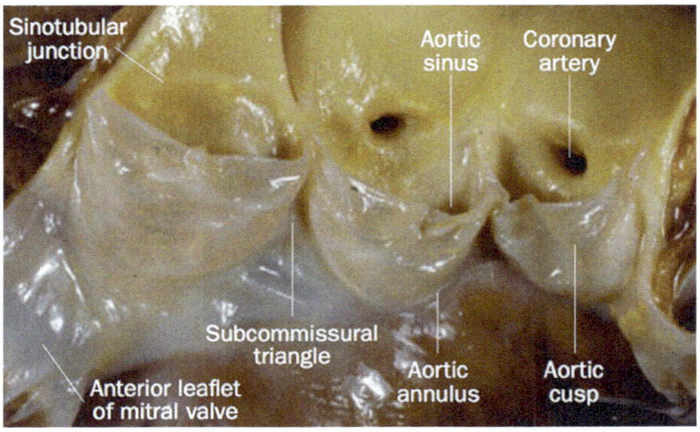

Fig. 3.1 Surgical anatomy of the components of the aortic root. The annulus, the inter-leaflet triangles (subcommissural triangle), aortic leaflets, sinuses of Valsalva and the sino-tubular junction comprise the aortic root. (Reproduced with permission from David TE. Surgical treatment of aortic valve disease. Nat Rev Cardiol. 2013;10:375–86)

X. Zhou, M.D., Ph.D. • M.A. Vannan, M.B.B.S. (✉) • K. Fattouch, M.D.
Echo Department, PLA Chinese Hospital, Beijing, China

Marcus Heart Valve Center, Piedmont Heart Institute, Atlanta, GA, USA
e-mail: mani.vannan@piedmont.org

K. Fattouch et al. (eds.), *Advances in Treatments for Aortic Valve and Root Diseases*, https://doi.org/10.1007/978-3-319-66483-5_3

this sophisticated anatomy in various diseases of the aortic root. The following section will first describe the structure of the aortic root and in the second part describe the coordinated functioning of this complex yet intuitively efficient structure.

3.1 Anatomy

3.1.1 Annulus

The *annulus* refers to a circular boundary which defines the nadir of the attachments of the leaflets to the aortic valve. This circular boundary is morphologically non-existent hence sometimes referred to as he virtual ring (or the basal ring, Fig. 3.2). The annulus is the boundary measured by echocardiography and other imaging modalities to size the prosthesis used in surgical aortic valve replacement (SAVR) or trans-catheter aortic valve implantation (TAVI). It is also used as the reference location to describe the position of aortic valve (AV) prosthesis as intra-, sub- or supra-valvular [7, 8]. The annulus is also the smallest orifice through which stroke volume is ejected. Next, the ring formed by junction of the aortic tissue with the ventricular myocardium forms the *anatomic ventriculo-arterial junction* (or ring, VAJ), which is distal to the basal ring [9]. Lastly, the semi-lunar attachment of the leaflets to the aortic wall forms a coronet like ring which identifies the separation of

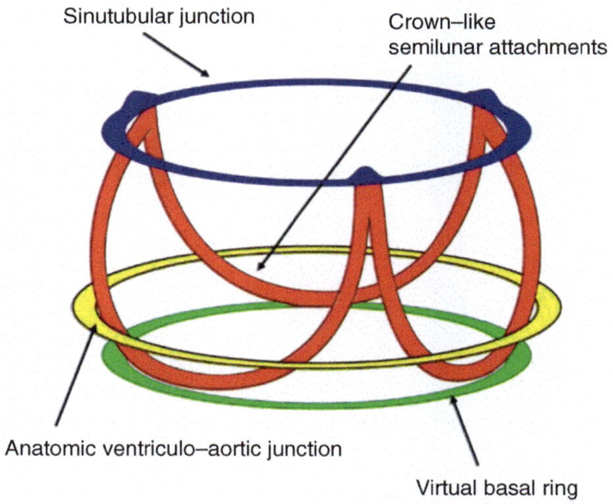

Fig. 3.2 Illustrates the three rings of the aortic root. The basal ring (hinge) is the lowest point of the insertion of the leaflets. The anatomic VAJ marks the junction of the aortic tissue with the ventricular myocardium, and the crown like attachment of the aortic leaflets to the aortic wall forms the hemodynamic VAJ. *VAJ* ventriculo-arterial junction. (Adapted from Tilea I, Suciu H, Tilea B, Tatar CM, Ispas M, Serban RC. In: Aikawa E, editor. Anatomy and function of normal aortic valvular complex. Calcific aortic valve disease. InTech; 2013. https://doi.org/10.5772/53403

the ventricular and aortic hemodynamics and is called the *hemodynamic VAJ* [6]. This separates the portions of the fibrous aortic root exposed to ventricular pressures which are the most superior portions of inter-leaflet triangles, and the basal portions of the sinus of Valsalva (left ventricular portions) which are exposed to the aortic pressures. The hemodynamic VAJ is distal to both the basal ring and the ring formed by the anatomic VAJ (Fig. 3.2).

3.1.2 Leaflets

The leaflets provide the main sealing mechanism of the central aortic orifice, and are the structural and hemodynamic boundary between the left ventricle (LV) and the aorta. The trileaflet morphology of the AV is best suited to allow the passage of systolic ejection flow with minimal resistance [10]. There is a constant mathematical relationship between the free edge length and the geometric height of the leaflets: the bases are ~1.5 times the free edge length, and the latter is 1.6–2.2 times the height of the leaflets [11]. The normal leaflet *free edge lengths* range from 26 to 35 mm (average ~31 mm), and *geometric height* from 12 to 19 mm (average ~14.5 mm). The *effective leaflet height* is the vertical distance between the annular plane and the tips which is usually 7–12 mm. The NCC tends be the largest (because most of the systolic flow occurs over this leaflet) followed by the RCC and LCC. About 50% of the leaflet height and 30% of the leaflet surface area are used for effective sealing of the valve orifice in diastole. The fibrous and thin co-apting ventricular surfaces of the adjacent leaflets are called the *lunulae*, and are about 2–4 mm in height. The nodular thickening at the center of the free edge of the leaflets on the ventricular surface are called the *nodule of Arantius* which aid in the competence of the closed AV. The length of the cusp apposition during closure is called the *coaptation length* which is 5–6 mm, thus the closure point is below the inferior portion of the lunulae. Furthermore, the the closure point does not necessarily correspond to the geometric center of the AV orifice. The *co-aptation height* measured by imaging as the vertical distance between the annular plane and the tip of the closed leaflets is essentially the effective leaflet height measured intraoperatively, and is 7–12 mm [12–14]. Lastly, the belly of the leaflets forms a sphere with their respective sinus of Valsalva (SOV). Figures show the morphological characteristics of the aortic leaflets described in this section.

3.1.3 Commissures and Inter-Leaflet Triangles

The distal parts of the crown like attachment of the leaflets into the aortic wall, where the insertion of the adjacent leaflets run parallel are called *commissures*. This is usually at are slightly below the sino-tubular junction (STJ). Sometimes the co-apting peripheral portions of the free edge of the leaflets are included in the term commissures. But, this is best avoided [15]. The internal distance between the commissures varies between 19 and 20 mm and the external distance between 24 and 25 mm. The spaces beneath the apices formed by the three commissures are referred to as *inter-leaflet triangles* (also called sub-commissural triangles) [16]. The interleaflet spaces beneath the NCC are fibrous and the one between the RCC and LCC is muscular. The inter-leaflet triangle between the NCC and LCC is continuous with the aorto-mitral curtain which leads to the anterior mitral valve leaflet. The inter-leaflet space between the NCC and RCC is continuous with the membranous inter-ventricular septum which contains the Bundle of His. The two inter-leaflet spaces of the NCC constitutes 55% of the circumference of the attachment of the annulus to the LVOT, whereas the space between LCC and RCC occupies the other 45% of the circumference. The apices of the inter-leaflet triangles of NCC represent potential communication sites with the pericardium, and the apex of the space between the LCC and RCC is a potential communication site with the tissue between the aorta and the sub-pulmonary infundibulum.

3.1.4 Sinuses of Valsalva and the Sino-Tubular Junction

The *sinuses* are bulges of the aortic root which extend from the insertion of the leaflets to the STJ. There are three sinuses which are named after the origin of the coronary arteries: left, right and non. The right SOV tend be the largest followed by the right and then left. The walls of sinuses are made of aortic tissue albeit thinner than the rest of the aorta, and at the bottom the wall of the sinuses consist of varying amount of ventricular tissue. The distal part of the SOV where the commissures are located form a tubular ridge called the *STJ* which is mostly made of elastic tissue. The STJ is most superior portion of the aortic root and marks the boundary between the aortic root and the ascending aorta [6, 8, 15]. The STJ is not a perfect circle but is scalloped consistent with the contours of the three sinuses. In the adults, the diameter of the STJ is about 10% (up to 15% in younger adults and 20% in children) smaller than the annular diameter, so that shape of the aortic root is a truncated cone. The coronary ostia are normally located in the two anterior sinuses, usually just below the STJ. But, the location of the ostia are variable and may arise from the center of the SOV or just above the STJ. The right coronary ostium shows the most variation.

3.2 Functional Anatomy

All the components of the aortic root function as a single unit during systole and diastole to maximize trans-valvular flow and LV filling, respectively. During LV ejection, the lower parts of the until are exposed to LV pressures and the upper parts of the root are exposed to aortic pressures. This means the upper part, specifically the STJ, expands during systole so that the shape of the root becomes a cylinder. This change is shape from a truncated cone to a cylinder is a specific adaptation to reduce resistance to flow [17]. Additionally, during systolic ejection blood flows back from the STJ along the walls of the SOV forming vortices in the latter behind the leaflets and then flowing back along central stream of the ejected blood. These vortices prevent apposition of the leaflets against the aortic wall which helps to prevent occlusion of coronary ostia. Furthermore, this mid SOV position of the leaflets helps in atraumatic closure during late systole and diastole. After ejection, in late-systole, the eddy currents in the SOV promote the movement of the belly of the leaflets towards each other so that the valve closure is almost complete. Then, in early diastole, complete sealing is accomplished by gentle apposition of the free-edge of the leaflets preventing damage to the thin lunulae. Although the SOV does not have direct role in the competency of the valve and the eddy currents are generated at the level of the STJ, the shape of the SOV aids in the persistence of the vortices. Furthermore, the spherical shape of the of the SOV in diastole is a significant adaptation to reduce the stress on the closed leaflets which is about four times higher than the SOV. The outward movement of the SOV walls (making them more spherical) helps to absorb some of the stress and reduce wear and tear of the leaflets. In fact, this leaflet-SOV assembly is a crucial mechanism by which the atraumatic sealing of the central orifice of the aortic root is accomplished [6, 10, 18, 19].

The inter-leaflet triangles are also crucial in the optimal function of the aortic root. They allow the leaflet-SOV assembly, described above, to function independently to ensure valve competency [18]. Dilatation of the VAJ causes the two subcommissural triangular spaces beneath the NCC to become more obtuse which reduces leaflet coaptation length and results in AR [14]. Also, even though the tissue of these triangles is thin and exposed to ventricular pressures, it is strong enough to withstand these pressures an contribute the dynamic changes of the base of the aortic root. The base of the root expands during ventricular filling and shrinks during ejection, thus following the behavior of the ventricle. The fact that 45% of the circumferential attachment of the inter-leaflet triangle to the annulus is muscular is a key contributor to this dynamic aorta-ventricle interaction [6, 18]. The inter-leaflet triangles also support prosthetic valves which are partially sewn to these structures during SAVR. The VAJ is also non-planar: it is above the basal ring 2.3–4.6 mm from the left/right commissure to right/non-commissure. This means that the external height of the non/left commissure is higher than the other two commissures. This has implications for optimal dissection of the aortic root during valve-sparing surgery and external annuloplasty procedures [20].

The free edge of the leaflets are much longer than the inter-commissural distance of the leaflets which is necessary for the optimal opening and closing during systole and diastole, respectively. The lunulae of the leaflets may often develop fenestrations as in the elderly, but rarely cause AR since these are above the closure line. Also, even though the leaflets are avascular, they are not inert structures, instead they actively remodel in response to stretch such as dilatation of the STJ which increase the inter-commissural distance. Through activation of nerve endings in the leaflets which respond to stretch, the free edge length and the height of the leaflets increase. This helps to maintain adequate co-aptation to prevent AR. However, the extent to which the height of the leaflets can increase is significantly less than the extent to which the free-edge length can increase [21]. This means that proportional increase in height and length (area) of the leaflets which match the increase in STJ diameter will be compensatory to prevent AR. However, relative lack of leaflet area (mainly due to lack of proportional remodeling of leaflet height) compared to the STJ diameter may result in central AR (Fig. 3.3). In fact, the height to STJ diameter ratio is as good as the leaflet area to STJ ratio in predicting central AR [22–24]. Eccentric AR may develop when the free-edge length is excessive compared to the height (Length/Height ratio > ~2.2) causing prolapse of the leaflet edge [24].

Thus, the aortic root is a sophisticated structure in which the complex anatomical arrangement of the individual component is intricately designed to function as a unit to enable to seamless conduct of stroke volume and provide sealing of the aortic orifice. It is also the hemodynamic connection between the LV and the systemic pressure and its macroscopic and microscopic anatomy is uniquely designed to minimize resistance to flow and trauma to the components while maximizing its functional efficiency.

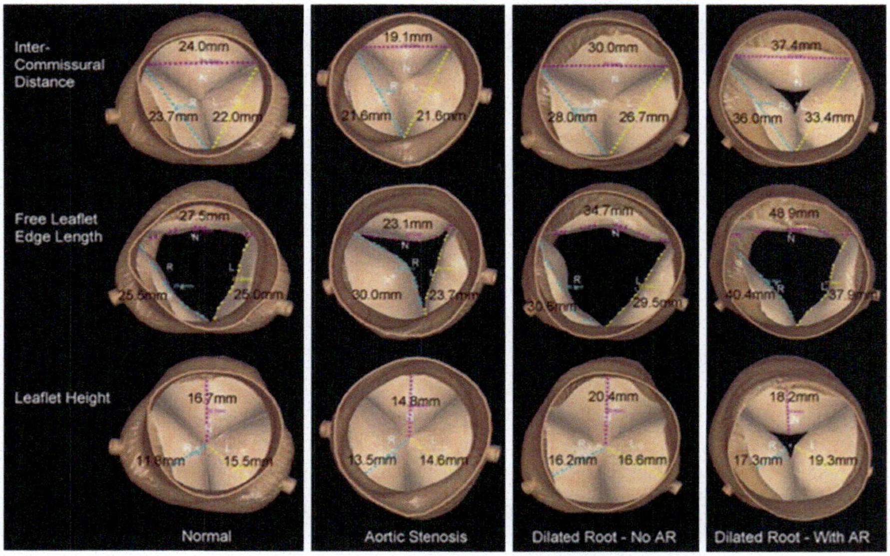

Fig. 3.3 Leaflet remodeling in dilatation of the STJ. With progressive increase in the inter-commissural distance due to dilatation of the STJ, leaflet length and height increase to maintain effective sealing of the central aortic orifice. This prevents AR or minimizes the degree of AR (*middle panel*). However, when the compensatory remodeling of the height of the leaflet is attenuated or reaches its maximum capacity, effective co-aptation is no longer possible and significant AR ensues (*right panel*). Whether the AR is central or eccentric is dependent on the relative excess of the free-edge length compared to the height of the leaflets. (Modified and reproduced with permission from Calleja A, Thavendiranathan P, Ionasec RI, Houle H, Liu S, Voigt I, Sai Sudhakar C, Crestanello J, Ryan T, Vannan MA. Automated quantitative 3-dimensional modeling of the aortic valve and root by 3-dimensional transesophageal echocardiography in normals, aortic regurgitation, and aortic stenosis: comparison to computed tomography in normals and clinical implications)

References

1. Thubrikar MJ. The aortic valve. 1st ed. Boca Raton, FL: CRC; 1981.
2. Bellhouse BJ, Bellhouse FH. Mechanism of closure of the aortic valve. Nature. 1968;217:86–7.
3. Bellhouse BJ, Bellhouse FH, Reid KG. Fluid mechanics of the aortic root with application to coronary flow. Nature. 1968;219:1059–61.
4. Thubrikar M, Piepgrass WC, Bosher LP, et al. The elastic modulus of canine aortic valve leaflets in vivo and in vitro. Circ Res. 1980;47:792–800.
5. Brewer RJ, Deck JD, Capati B, et al. The dynamic aortic root. Its role in aortic valve function. J Thorac Cardiovasc Surg. 1976;72:413–7.
6. Charitos EI, Sievers HH. Anatomy of the aortic root: implications for valve-sparing surgery. Ann Cardiothorac Surg. 2013;2:53–6.
7. Anderson RH. Clinical anatomy of the aortic root. Heart. 2000;84:670–3.
8. Anderson RH. The surgical anatomy of the aortic root. Multimed Man Cardiothorac Surg. https://doi.org/10.1510/mmcts.2006.002527.
9. de Kerchove L, Jashari R, Boodhwani M, Duy KT, Lengel B, Gianello P, Nezhad ZM, Astarci P, Noirhomme P, El Khoury G. Surgical anatomy of the aortic root: implication for valve-sparing reimplantation and aortic valve annuloplasty. J Thorac Cardiovasc Surg. 2015;149:425–33.
10. Robicsek F, Thubrikar MJ, Cook JW, Fowler B. The congenitally bicuspid aortic valve: how does it function? Why does it fail? Ann Thorac Surg. 2004;77:177–85.
11. Kunzelman KS, Grande KJ, David TE, Cochran RP, Verrier ED. Aortic root and valve relationships. Impact on surgical repair. J Thorac Cardiovasc Surg. 1994;107:162–70.
12. David TE, Feindel CM. An aortic valve-sparing operation for patients with aortic incompetence and aneurysm of the ascending aorta. J Thorac Cardiovasc Surg. 1992;103:617–22.
13. David TE, Feindel CM, Bos J. Repair of the aortic valve in patients with aortic insufficiency and aortic root aneurysm. J Thorac Cardiovasc Surg. 1995;109:345–52.
14. David TE. Surgical treatment of aortic valve disease. Nat Rev Cardiol. 2013;10:375–86.
15. Sievers HH, Hemmer W, Beyersdorf F, Moritz A, Moosdorf R, Lichtenberg A, Misfeld M, Charitos EI, on behalf of the Working Group for Aortic Valve Surgery of the German Society of Thoracic and Cardiovascular Surgery. The everyday used nomenclature of the aortic root components: the tower of Babel? Eur J Cardiothorac Surg. 2012;41:478–82.
16. Underwood MJ, El Khoury G, Deronck D, Glineur D, Dion R. The aortic root: structure, function, and surgical reconstruction. Heart. 2000;83:376–80.
17. Lansac E, Lim HS, Shomura Y, Lim KH, Rice NT, Goetz W, Acar C, Duran CMG. A four-dimensional study of the aortic root dynamics. Eur J Cardiothorac Surg. 2002;22:497–503.
18. Sutton JP III, Ho SY, Anderson RH. The forgotten interleaflet triangles. A review of the surgical anatomy of the aortic valve. Ann Thorac Surg. 1995;59:419–27.
19. Furukawa K, Ohteki H, Cao ZL, Doi K, Narita Y, Minato N, Itoh T. Does dilatation of the sinotubular junction cause aortic regurgitation? Ann Thorac Surg. 1999;68:949–54.
20. de Kerchove L, El Khoury G. Anatomy and pathophysiology of the ventriculo-aortic junction: implication in aortic valve repair surgery. Ann Cardiothorac Surg. 2013;2:57–64.
21. Schafers HJ, Schmied W, Marom G, Aicher D. Cusp height in aortic valves. J Thorac Cardiovasc Surg. 2013;146:269–74.
22. Calleja A, Thavendiranathan P, Ionasec RI, Houle H, Liu S, Voigt I, Sai Sudhakar C, Crestanello J, Ryan T, Vannan MA. Automated quantitative 3-dimensional modeling of the aortic valve and root by 3-dimensional transesophageal echocardiography in normals, aortic regurgitation, and aortic stenosis: comparison to computed tomography in normals and clinical implications. Circ Cardiovasc Imaging. 2013;6(1):99–108.
23. Kim DH, Handschumacher MD, Levine RA, Sun BJ, Jang JY, Yang DH, Kang JW, Song JM, Kang DH, Lim TH, Song JK. Aortic valve adaptation to aortic root dilatation: insights into the mechanism of functional aortic regurgitation from 3-dimensional cardiac computed tomography. Circ Cardiovasc Imaging. 2014;7:828–35.
24. Regeer MV, Kamperidis V, Versteegh MI, Schalij MJ, Marsan NA, Bax JJ, et al. Three-dimensional transoesophageal echocardiography of the aortic valve and root: changes in aortic root dilation and aortic regurgitation. Eur Heart J Cardiovasc Imaging. 2016.

Part II

Imaging

4 Multimodality Imaging Assessment of Aortic Stenosis

Raluca Dulgheru and Patrizio Lancellotti

4.1 Introduction

In AS patients, transthoracic echocardiography (TTE) remains the first choice modality to diagnose the disease, assess its severity and its consequences on cardiac geometry and function. It is widely available, non invasive and relatively cheap. However, several other imaging techniques, such as exercise stress echocardiography (ESE), cardiac computed tomography (CT), cardiac magnetic resonance (CMR) and positron emission CT (PET-CT) have been developed over the years and proved to be useful for severity assessment, risk stratification and treatment planning of patients with calcific AS.

4.2 Potential Problems Related to AS Severity Assessment by Echocardiography

The criteria proposed by the guidelines to identify severity in AS patients are a peak transvalvular velocity (Vmax) >4 m/s, a mean pressure gradient (MG) >40 mmHg and an effective orifice area (EOA) <1.0 cm^2 or an EOA indexed (EOAi) <0.6 cm^2/m^2 [1]. The guidelines emphasize the need for a multi-parametric approach

R. Dulgheru, M.D.
Department of Cardiology, University of Liège Hospital, GIGA Cardiovascular Sciences, Heart Valve Clinic, CHU Sart Tilman, Avenue de l'hôpital, n1, Liège 4000, Belgium
e-mail: eralucadulgheru@yahoo.com

P. Lancellotti, M.D., Ph.D. (✉)
Department of Cardiology, University of Liège Hospital, GIGA Cardiovascular Sciences, Heart Valve Clinic, CHU Sart Tilman, Liège, Belgium

GVM Care and Research, E.S. Health Science Foundation, Lugo, RA, Italy
e-mail: plancellotti@chu.ulg.ac.be

K. Fattouch et al. (eds.), *Advances in Treatments for Aortic Valve and Root Diseases*, https://doi.org/10.1007/978-3-319-66483-5_4

to confirm severity, but make no specific comments regarding the mutually inclusiveness/exclusiveness of these criteria [1].

In patients without low left ventricular ejection fraction (LVEF) an agreement between hemodynamic parameters defining severity, EOA and MG is expected. Awareness that a poor left ventricular (LV) systolic function may lead to a significant decrease in LV stroke volume (SV), and to consequently lower gradients due to the dependency of gradients on flow, makes the issue of discordance between EOA and MG less unexpected in AS patients with reduced LVEF. The role of dobutamine stress echocardiography (DSE) is well established in this setting aiming to distinguish between severe and pseudosevere AS by increasing flow rate across the valve [2]. However, in patients with preserved LVEF, although preserved LVEF does not necessarily imply preserved LV systolic function or normal transvalvular flow rate/SV, discordance between EOA and MG may lead to uncertainty regarding AS severity and to erroneous patient management.

Discordant values (EOA <1.0 cm^2 and MG <40 mmHg) are not uncommon and have been observed in up to 25–30% of patients with a LVEF >50% [3]. Identification of a separate group of patients with severe AS, as defined by an EOA <1.0 cm^2, preserved LVEF, but low flow conditions (i.e. SVi <35 mL/m^2) and lower than expected gradients (i.e. MG <40 mmHg), the so called "paradoxical low flow low gradient AS" helped in understanding the apparent discordance between MG and EOA in patients with preserved LVEF [4]. In these patients, pronounced LV remodeling with small volume cavity size, impaired diastolic filling, as well as a reduced LV longitudinal systolic function could explain the low SV index (SVi) and lower than expected MG in the presence of a truly severe AS [4]. However, this entity is rather infrequent (prevalence between 3 and 7% in recent studies on asymptomatic patients) [5, 6] and cannot account for all cases of discrepancy between EOA and gradients in patients with preserved LVEF, as Minners et al. pointed out [3]. There are patients with discordance between EOA and MG despite normal flow, as well as patients with low flow and unexpectedly high gradients (i.e. MG >40 mmHg). It has been suggested that the discordance may be partly explained by an inherent inconsistency between the criteria proposed by the guidelines, i.e. between the EOA and MG and EOA and Vmax, respectively [3]. The criteria are inconsistent from two standpoints [7]. First, cut-off values to define severity and decide surgery come from catheter based studies. Yet, nowadays evaluation of AS is made using Doppler techniques. EOA and MG obtained by echocardiography are thus not interchangeable with catheter-derived EOA and MG. Due to pressure recovery phenomenon, echo-based gradients are always higher than their catheter based counterpart. Consequently, EOA is always lower when assessed by Doppler echocardiography using the continuity equation. On the other hand, according to the Gorlin formula, the MG that theoretically corresponds to an EOA of 1.0 cm^2 in a patient with a normal cardiac output (i.e. a cardiac output of 6 L/min and heart rate of 80 bpm) would not be 40 mmHg, but 34 mmHg. Conversely, for a MG of 40 mmHg the theoretical EOA would be 0.8 cm^2 [8]. Lowering of the cut off value for EOA that defines severe AS to 0.8 cm^2 was suggested in order to reconcile some of these discrepancies [3]. However, several echocardiography based studies, that graded severe AS according to the cut-off value for EOA <1 cm^2, irrespective of the MG, have shown that this particular value holds a predictive power for detecting excess mortality and morbidity [9, 10]. Outcome studies of patients with an EOA between 0.8 and 1.0 cm^2 managed medically would be required to allow lowering the EOA threshold of severity below 0.8 cm^2 [7].

The integration of flow pattern (low flow or normal flow) and its relation to gradient into the classification of AS has been proposed recently. This would allow correct interpretation of the relationship between EOA and MG and help in the identification of a certain "pathophysiologic type of AS" [11]. This classification does not only help understanding the physiopatholgy behind each AS patient, but gives also important prognostic information [5, 12–15]. Presence of a low flow state seems to be associated with a higher mortality rate and worse outcomes in patients with AS [12, 15].

The new classification has as a central element an EOA <1.0 cm^2 and divides severe AS into four categories, according to the flow-gradient relationship: (1) normal flow/high gradient (NF/HG); (2) normal flow/low gradient (NF/LG); (3) low flow/high gradient (LF/HG) and (4) low flow/low gradient AS (LF/LG). To date, a low flow state is defined as a SVi <35 mL/m^2, and this cut-off value has been validated by several studies [4, 6]. Some authors prefer as definition a CI <3 L/min/m^2. However, it has to be emphasized that SVi seems more appropriate since gradients depend on flow per beat, not on flow per minute. More importantly, recent studies have confirmed that a SVi <35 mL/m^2 in severe AS with preserved LVEF is markedly associated with an increase risk of mortality [6]. Careful interpretation of a low SVi is necessary in obese patients, in which the prevalence of low-flow states may be overestimated by applying this cut-off value.

4.3 Grading AS—Step by Step Approach

4.3.1 Imaging Work-Up

In patients with discordant findings with 2D TTE, a multimodality approach is necessary (Figs. 4.1 and 4.2). This multi-modality approach may include 2D TOE, 3D TTE and/or 3D TOE, MDCT with the analysis of valve calcium score, DSE or ESE, CMR and even PET/CT.

4.3.2 2D Transthoracic Echocardiography, Step-by-Step Approach

A complete 2D echocardiographic report should contain information regarding valve morphology, give hints regarding etiology of AS, quantify AS severity and assess upstream consequences. Complete hemodynamic description of valve stenosis includes systematic reporting of EOA (by continuity equation), EOAi, Vmax, MG and SVi. Left ventricular outflow tract diameter (LVOTd) should always be

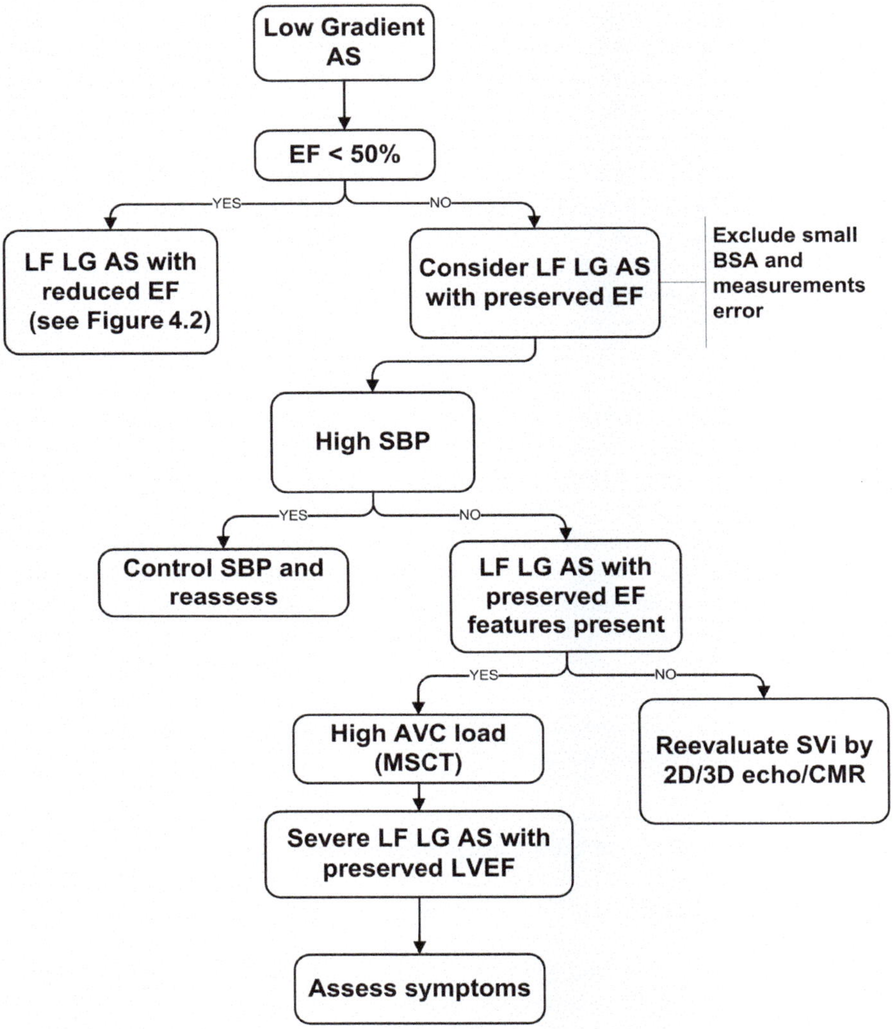

Fig. 4.1 Imaging work-up in patients with low gradient aortic stenosis regardless of the left ventricle ejection fraction

reported to allow accurate monitoring of stenosis progression during follow-up. Systematic blood pressure measurement before each echocardiographic study is strongly recommended in order to avoid underestimation of severity (in hypertensive patients) and to allow computation of valvuloarterial impedance (Zva), an important predictor of LV dysfunction and clinical outcome in severe AS patients

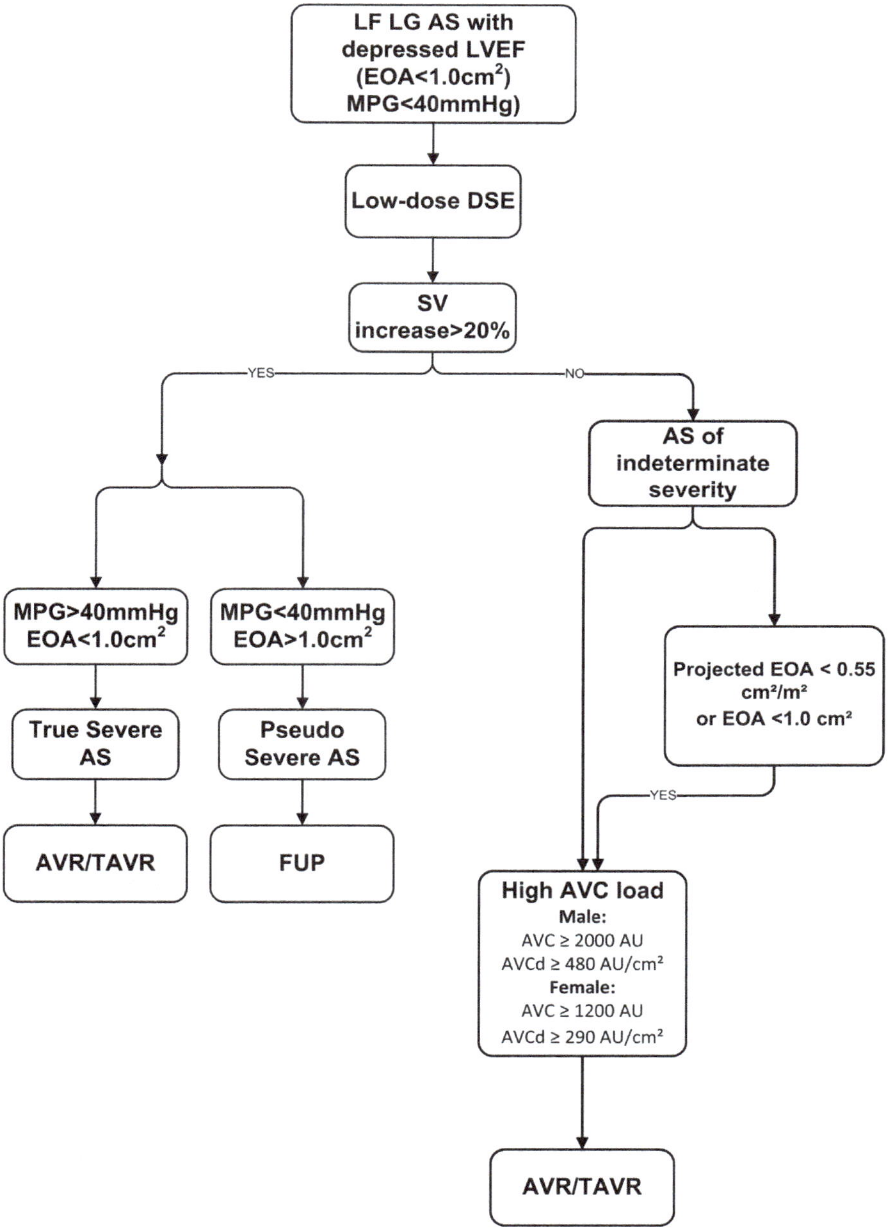

Fig. 4.2 Imaging work-up in patients with low flow low gradient aortic stenosis and depressed left ventricle ejection fraction

[16–18]. Systematic measurement of BP allows the estimation of systemic arterial compliance, which can be severely reduced in up to 40% of patients with AS [16] and contributes to the increased LV afterload and thus to progression of LV dysfunction. Systematic measurement of ascending aorta diameter 1 cm downstream of the sinotubular junction in systole is equally important to allow correction for pressure recovery and avoid overestimation of AS severity in patients with small ascending aortas (i.e. diameter of the sinotubular junction <3.0 cm) in which pressure recovery is significant [16, 19]. The pattern of LV response to chronic pressure overload is highly variable from one patient to another and it can involve concentric LV remodeling, concentric or eccentric LV hypertrophy. The high inter-individual variability of LV remodeling is little understood. Age, sex, obesity, metabolic syndrome and diabetes mellitus are some of the factors known to influence the pattern of LV remodeling [20–22]. Most will agree to the fact that hemodynamically significant AS can be ruled out in the presence of a normal LV (without concentric remodeling/hypertrophy). Thus, assessment of indexed LV mass, as well as assessment of relative wall thickness (RWT) is an important step through the understanding of AS. Moreover, severe LV hypertrophy or remodeling has been associated to worse myocardial function [23], increased risk of untoward cardiac events [24] and increased operative and late mortality after AVR [25]. LVEF, as assessed by the Simpson's biplane method using 2D echocardiography is the only parameter of LV systolic function included in the current guidelines on which decision regarding AVR is made and should be assessed and reported systematically.

Transvalvular gradients are known to be flow-dependent. EOA, as assessed by the continuity equation, is regarded as a less flow dependent parameter. It has the disadvantage of being more prone to error measurement because of its calculation based on different cardiac cycles and using several assumptions (i.e. CSA_{LVOT} assumed to be circular, flow pattern in the LVOT assumed to be laminar). Guidelines advise to use both MG and EOA to assess AS severity, and concordance between these measurements is expected. When those two parameters are concordant, AS is considered with a high degree of certitude as being severe and further decision making regarding the need for AVR is based on the presence of symptoms and/or LV dysfunction (i.e. LVEF <50%). When the two parameters are in disagreement (EOA <1.0 cm^2, but MG <40 mmHg), careful reviewing of the continuity equation is advised to exclude error measurements (LVOT diameter, elliptical geometry of $LVOT_{CSA}$, SV calculation by other modality than the Doppler method), as well as indexation of EOA to the BSA to avoid overestimation of severity (i.e. EOA <1.0 cm^2, but indexed EOA >0.6 cm^2/m^2) in patients with small BSA.

If discordances persist after careful exclusion of error measurements and the Svi is <35 mL/m^2, careful analysis of LV geometry and function and exclusion of other diseases that may lead to a low flow state should be performed. In patients with no other significant valvular disease (mitral stenosis, significant mitral or tricuspid regurgitation) or other cardiac dysfunction that may explain the low flow state, LFLG AS with preserved LVEF should be suspected. In these patients, severe LV concentric remodeling/hypertrophy, restrictive LV physiology and altered longitudinal LV function may lead to a low SVi despite a "preserved LVEF". If the echocardiographic features that characterize LF LG AS with preserved LVEF are absent, one has to make sure that SVi is not erroneously underestimated or that SBP values are not elevated and thus, responsible of the low-flow state [26].

If 2D measurements are considered adequate, but the discordance still persists, a multi-modality approach may be needed to ascertain AS severity.

Patients with normal flow (i.e. SVi $\geq$ 35 mL/m^2), an EOA <1.0 cm^2 and/or indexed EOA <0.6 cm^2/m^2, but a MG <40 mmHg, if no overestimation of SVi and no underestimation of MG has been done, are considered to have NF LG AS. Outcome studies have shown that they have the best prognosis during follow-up, closer to patients with moderate AS [5].

It is equally important to exclude by color flow and PW Doppler acceleration of flow in the LVOT related to basal septal hypertrophy because this may lead to an overestimation of SVi and of EOA and misclassification of AS.

Concordance between EOA and MG in both patients with preserved and reduced LVEF does not pose any problem to confidently classify AS as severe. In patients with low EF, analysis of SVi helds prognostic information [12].

4.3.3 2D Transoesophageal Echocardiography

2D TOE has the advantage of a higher spatial resolution and is very useful to grade AS severity in patients with poor transthoracic acoustic windows in which measurement of the LVOTd and aortic valve area (AVA) by planimetry is impossible. Measurement of EOA is also possible using the continuity equation provided that a good alignment with transaortic flow direction from the transgastric view is achieved. If available, 2D TOE should be completed by a 3D TOE study. Its advantages are discussed in the paragraph below. However, it has to be emphasized that AVA by planimetry is a measurement of the maximal geometrical AV orifice opening during systole and conceptually and numerically different from EOA calculated by the continuity equation. Planimetered AVA is usually larger than EOA, therefore the two values should not be interchanged.

4.3.4 3D Echocardiography

3D TTE has the disadvantage of being dependent on transthoracic acoustic window and having a lower spatial resolution that 3D TOE. In brief, 3D echocardiography (both TTE and TOE) can be used to allow a more accurate assessment of AS severity in the following ways: (1) guided planimetry of the anatomic aortic valve area (AVA) using the biplane method (usually with 3D TTE); (2) offline planimetry of the AVA using a 3D dataset that is cropped to allow direct planimetry at the leaflet tips (usually with 3D TOE); (3) optimized computation EOA using the continuity equation and the planimetry of the cross sectional area (CSA) of the LVOT without any geometrical assumption from a 3D dataset; this allows for a more accurate assessment of LV SV, since LVOTd measurement by 2D echocardiography is the greatest potential source of error in the continuity equation; this modality improves assessment of EOA in patients with an elliptical LVOT, in which EOA may be underestimated because the LVOTd measured by 2D echocardiograph, which is the sagittal diameter may be smaller than coronal diameters; (4) likewise, a 3D full volume acquisition focused on the LV allows estimation of the 3D SV (as the difference between 3D end-diastolic and 3D end-systolic volumes) that can be used to calculate more accurately EOA by the continuity equation. It is important to understand that 2D/3D anatomic AVA obtained by planimetry is not interchangeable with EOA, obtained by the continuity equation. The hemodynamic burden related to aortic valve stenosis seems to be more closely related to EOA, than to anatomic AVA [7]. Due to flow constraint distal to the anatomic stenosis, EOA is always smaller than AVA. An inverse relation (measured EOA > AVA) should prompt for careful reassessment of all measurements to check for possible sources of error.

3D TOE has yet another important role: it may help in patient selection for TAVI, since accurate aortic annulus sizing is critical for correct selection of prosthesis size (avoid paravalvular regurgitation which has been associated with worse survival after TAVI [27] and annular rupture during TAVI. Three-dimensional imaging techniques (3D TOE, MDCT and CMR) are superior to two dimensional imaging techniques for measurement of aortic annulus size and to assess its geometry [28]. Many centers that perform TAVI interventions prefer MDCT as the technique of choice for valve sizing due to its higher spatial resolution, but 3D TOE can be used as well to measure: the minimum and maximum aortic annulus diameter, the aortic annulus perimeter and area that otherwise would be impossible to measure by 2D techniques. It has been shown that aortic annulus sizing using 3D TOE lowers the risk of paravalvular regurgitation when compared to 2D TOE [28].

4.3.5 Stress Echocardiography

There are two main stress modalities that can be used to assess patients with AS: (1) DSE, usually appropriate for patients with LFLG AS with depressed LVEF to test the LV and the valve, and (2) ESE, suitable for asymptomatic patients with the aim of helping in risk stratification. ESE has little added value in AS severity assessment.

DSE is useful in patients with AS and depressed LVEF to test the LV and interpret AS severity in the light of flow-gradient interaction. It has both diagnostic and prognostic value. In the presence of LV systolic dysfunction in patients with an EOA <1.0 cm^2 and a SVi <35 mL/m, due to the flow dependency of gradients, the MG is often lower than 40 mmHg. In this setting, without performing a DSE, the severity of AS remains unknown. Two entities can fit into this echocardiographic pattern (LV systolic dysfunction, i.e. LVEF <50%, EOA <1.0 cm^2, MG <40 mmHg and SVi <35 mL/m^2): true severe AS (TS AS) and pseudo-severe AS (PS AS). Low-dose (up to 20 µg/min/kg) DSE is the key exam to distinguish between them [29]. The separation of TS from PS AS is very important because the outcome and management of these patients are different. Patients with PS AS have survival curves comparable with patients with non valvular LV systolic dysfunction when treated medically and AVR does not seem to bring any benefit to this subset of patients [30]. By opposition, patients with TS AS benefit from the relief of valve obstruction. According to ESC guidelines, TS AS is defined as an increase in MG to >40 mmHg, a small change in EOA (EOA <0.3 cm^2) and/or an EOA $\leq$ 1.0–1.2 cm^2 with DSE [31]. ACC/AHA guidelines, TS AS is defined by an increase in MG >40 mmHg (or increase in Vmax $\geq$ 4 m/s) with an EOA $\leq$ 1.0 cm^2 at any stage of DSE [2]. Patients with TS AS have a highly fibrotic and calcified aortic valve and LV systolic dysfunction is a result of valve stenosis. PS AS is characterized by a significant increase in EOA ($\geq$0.3 cm^2) and/or an EOA >1.2 cm^2 with a MG remaining lower than 40 mmHg. It is not the valve disease that triggers LV dysfunction in patients with pseudosevere AS, but an intrinsic myocardial disease. In these patients the valve is only mildly or moderately calcified, but the failing LV is not able to build up enough pressure to open the aortic leaflets to an EOA >1.0 cm^2.

The changes in MG and EOA during DSE depend on the magnitude of flow increase achieved with dobutamine. Thus, the major drawback of DSE is that the distinction between TS and PS AS is not possible if the transaortic flow rate/SV does not increase adequately. In most cases, an increase in SV >20% is sufficient to distinguish with high accuracy TS from PS AS. Whenever SV increase is <20% the discordance between EOA and MG may persist after DSE and AS severity remains unknown. To overcome this limitation, Blais et al. have proposed the computation of projected EOA (EOAproj) at a standard flow rate of 250 mL/s to distinguish PS from TS AS [32]. An EOAproj >1.0 cm^2 or an indexed EOAproj >0.55 cm^2/m^2 were used as cut-off values to distinguish TS from PS AS. Moreover, EOAproj proved to be an important predictor of outcome in LF LG AS with depressed LVEF [33]. In patients in whom computation of EOAproj does not clear up the disease severity, flow-independent methods, such as the aortic valve calcium score by MDCT may be useful to distinguish TS from PS AS [34].

4.3.6 MDCT

CT is a 3D technique that can be used, just like 3D echocardiography to improve assessment of AS severity by measurement of AVA or, combined with Doppler echocardiography, to allow EOA calculation. This technique is especially useful in patients with contraindication to TOE and poor transthoracic acoustic windows. In patients with a difficult parasternal window, the LVOTd is sometimes impossible to measure and any inaccuracy in its measurement can be translated into a poor estimation of EOA and a misclassification of the AS severity (1 mm of error in LVOTd measurement leads to an error of 0.01 cm^2 of EOA). If TOE is contraindicated, cardiac CT can be used to measure AVA and the CSA_{LVOT} by direct planimetry with a very high spatial resolution, thus helping in the assessment of AS severity. Measurement of the LVOT CSA can be then combined with Doppler echocardiography to allow calculation of SV and introduced into the continuity equation to estimate EOA. This overcomes the limitation of cardiac

CT which, when used alone, can provide the anatomic AVA, but not the EOA. Exposure to ionizing radiation precludes the use of cardiac CT as a follow up modality, especially in younger patients. Assessment of AVC by MDCT proved to be a flow-independent and robust parameter that helps in assessing severity of AS in patients with low-flow states [34]. AVC has been shown to correlate well with AS hemodynamic severity [34–36]. According to recent studies this relationship seems to be influenced by gender: aortic leaflets with hemodynamically significant valve stenosis are lighter in women than in men, even when accounting for BSA and aortic annulus CSA [34, 37]. It is thus important to remember that the cut-off values of AVC and AVCd (i.e. AVCd = AVC/CSA of the aortic annulus) that are indicative of hemodynamically significant AS are not interchangeable between males and females. This study on 646 patients with AS, proposed as cut-off values to diagnose severe AS an AVC ≥ 1200 AU for women and ≥2000 AU in men, and an AVCd ≥ 290 AU/cm^2 and ≥480 AU/cm^2, respectively [34]. In routine clinical practice assessment of AVC and AVCd by MDCT has little value to severity assessment in patients with concordant MG and EOA at echocardiography, but may help in risk-stratification [38]. In patients with discordant findings, AVC and AVCd are highly valuable, especially in patients in which DSE is not feasible or provides discordant/inconclusive results. Cardiac CT is particularly useful for assessment of patients in which TAVI is being contemplated. Although some experienced centers may use 3D TOE, the use of CT scan for measurement of aortic annulus diameter, leaflet length and annular to coronary ostia distance before TAVI has become routine in most centers.

4.3.7 CMR

CMR proved to be useful to assess both AVA and EOA using the continuity equation. It can be used to quantify AS severity in patients with difficult transthoracic acoustic windows and contraindication for TOE. However, its main role in patients with AS is to help in risk stratification by its ability to characterize the pattern and volume of myocardial fibrosis [39, 40].

4.3.8 PET/CT

Recent studies have advanced the concept that PET/CT, by targeting the degree of calcification and inflammation within the aortic valve leaflets, may be used to assess disease activity in AS [41]. PET uses dedicated tracers (a positron emitter such as 18F-fluoride bound to a vehicle, such as fluorodeoxyglucose-FDG) to target a specific biochemical processes in a tissue of interest, such as inflammation in the aortic valve leaflets, and uses PET detectors to build a 3D image of the positron emission events at the sites of tracer accumulation in that specific tissue. PET/CT is not used to assess AS severity but to derive information regarding disease activity [42]. It combines the anatomical information from CT with the functional information derived from PET.

4.4 Follow-Up and Risk Stratification

AS is a progressive disease and severity portends an adverse prognosis. Eighty-two percent, 67% and 33% of the asymptomatic patients with a baseline echocardiographic study indicating severe AS will develop symptoms at 1 year, 2-years and 5 years follow up, respectively, if not treated surgically [43]. Mortality in symptomatic patients approximates 2% per month. Moreover, to date, the exact rate of progression in an individual patient is impossible to predict. Therefore, follow-up of patients with AS is mandatory and the interval between each outpatient clinic visit has to be chosen wisely to allow timely decision regarding AVR, before sudden death, symptom or LV systolic dysfunction occur. For this purpose, the AHA/ACC guidelines recommend assessment by TTE every 3–5 years in patients with mild AS (Vmax between 2 and 2.9 m/s), every 1–2 years in moderate AS (Vmax <3.9 m/s) and every 6–12 months in patients with severe AS and normal flow (Vmax ≥ 4 m/s) [2]. The ESC guidelines recommend evaluation of asymptomatic severe AS every 6 months (spontaneous reported symptoms, change in exercise tolerance ideally with an exercise test, and change in echocardiographic parameters) and of moderate asymptomatic AS yearly. Mild AS is to be followed-up each 2–3 years [31]. ACC/AHA guidelines underline that follow-up of patients with asymptomatic severe AS may be better achieved in a heart valve clinic. The aim during a heart valve clinic consultation is to help in the selection of the timing and the type of valve procedure that will optimize the risk-benefit of the procedure and patients outcome. To date, the decision to refer patients to valve replacements/implantation procedures is based on AS severity, presence and severity of symptoms, degree of myocardial dysfunction, presence of predictors of rapid progression and short-term unfavorable outcome, and presence and types of comorbidities.

The natural history of calcific AS is characterized by a longstanding asymptomatic period. During this period, the risk of sudden death is relatively low, less than 1% per year [43]. This risk is lower than the risk of surgery (of about 2.5%) and prosthesis related complications thus, prophylactic surgery is not recommended. Current guidelines advocate delaying AVR until symptom develop or LV systolic dysfunction ensues because the benefit of AVR clearly outweighs the risks [2, 31]. However in highly experienced centers and in patients with low-surgical risk in which some predictors of adverse outcome have been identified, surgery may be proposed earlier. Thus, besides assessment of severity and symptoms, a heart valve clinic consultation should focus also on finding predictors of disease progression and adverse outcome in each individual patient so that asymptomatic patient whom may benefit from early elective surgery to be promptly identified and treated. Risk stratification usually starts with resting echocardiography derived parameters, but a multi-modality approach may be necessary (Fig. 4.3).

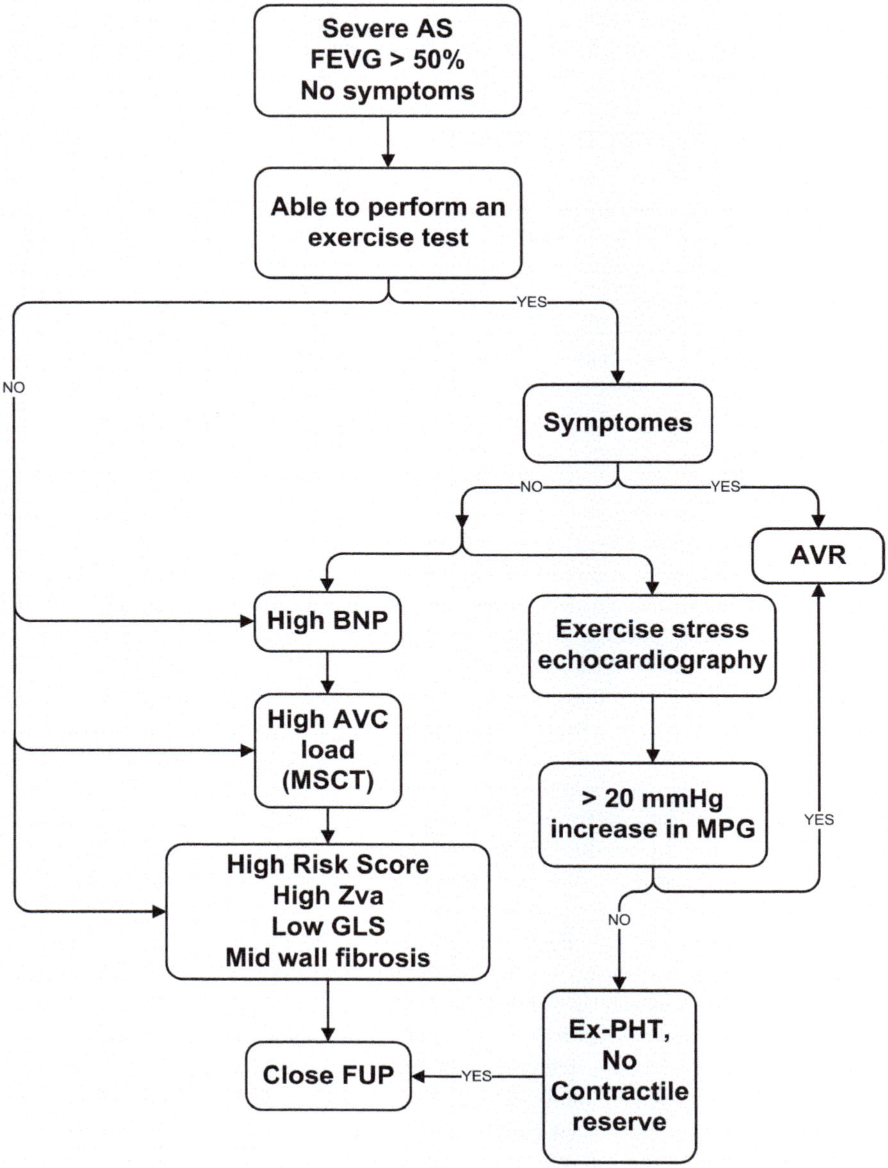

Fig. 4.3 Risk stratification using multi-modality imaging in asymptomatic severe aortic stenosis

4.4.1 Role of Resting Echocardiography in Risk Stratification

Valvular, arterial, and ventricular parameters derived from resting echocardiography can be used to help in risk stratification of patients with severe AS. Vmax is clearly a strong predictor of worse outcome in AS [44, 45]. Event-free survival gets significantly worse as Vmax increases [45]. The degree of aortic calcification (moderate-to-severe vs. mild) is also predictive of worse outcome and when associated to an increase of Vmax $\geq$ 0.3 m/year identifies a group of patients even at higher risk [46]. This criterion is currently a class IIa indication for AVR in the ESC guidelines [31]. Several parameters of LV longitudinal systolic function (such as a peak systolic mitral annular velocity s' assessed by tissue Doppler imaging $\leq$4.5 cm/s or a GLS $\leq -15.9\%$) have been used as prognostic markers in asymptomatic patients with AS and preserved LVEF [18]. Analysis of LV diastolic function seems to have an added value over symptom development and LVEF in patients with severe AS [47].

4.4.2 Role of Stress Echocardiography in Risk Stratification

ESE combines an exercise ECG test performed on a dedicated tilting table equipped with a cycloergometer at its end, with Doppler TTE that allows continuous monitoring during exercise of LV function, valve hemodynamics and pulmonary systolic artery pressure. ESE is suitable for all asymptomatic patients with severe AS and preserved LVEF able to perform an exercise test. Exercise induced typical angina and syncope are clearly evidence of symptomatic AS and ESE is contraindicated in these patients. However, self reported exercise induced dyspnea is difficult to link to AS, especially in elderly patients, because dyspnea may have a plurifactorial cause. Moreover, elderly patients may unconsciously and progressively reduced their level of activity to avoid symptoms, whenever AS is critical. Therefore, an exercise test can be useful to unmask symptoms in those patients who deny being symptomatic and to identify an abnormal response during exercise testing that can be linked to the presence of severe AS. ESC guidelines strongly advocate exercise testing in patients with severe AS [31]. AHA/ACC guidelines give it a class IIa indication [2]. The positive predictive value of exercise testing is higher in younger patients, 79% as opposed to 56% in patients >70 years old, with similar negative predictive values [48]. Thus, an abnormal response to exercise in a young patient is very likely related to AS, whilst in an elderly patient, a positive test may lack specificity. Conversely, a negative test in an elderly patient is reassuring and the patient is likely to remain asymptomatic until the 1 year follow up. An exercise test is considered normal if no angina, near-syncope/syncope, no limiting dyspnea at low workloads, no complex ventricular arrhythmias develop during exercise. An inadequate increase in BP with exercise (i.e. <20 mmHg) is also considered abnormal. At least 80% of the age-predicted heart rate should be reached in the absence of symptoms before stopping the test. A positive exercise test has been shown to predict the rapid onset of symptoms and cardiac death [49]. Dizziness has the highest positive predictive value for symptom development. Dyspnea at high workloads with rapid resolution during recovery phase should not be interpreted as a positive test.

ESE can be used in patients with AS to assess symptom development and adaptation to exercise, to which other important information can be added. However it is worth mentioning that there is no class indication in either of the guidelines for exercise testing in the form of ESE. Based on individual preference and experience patients with severe AS and preserved LVEF may be tested for symptom development on an upright bicycle/treadmill before undergoing an ESE on the tilting table. ESE has an additive prognostic value above and beyond clinical data, resting echocardiography, and exercise testing [50–53]. Parameters related to valve hemodynamics, LV function, and sPAP are targeted. Apart from changes in E/e'- an estimate of LV filling pressure- that is obtained at low level exercise (before e'- and a'- wave fusion), all other parameters should be obtained throughout each step of the test (baseline, low, medium, high levels) and at peak exercise. ESE is an excellent tool to help in risk stratification of asymptomatic patients with moderate or severe AS.

An increase in MG $\geq$ 18–20 mmHg with exercise proved to be associated with an increased risk of cardiac-related events [50, 51]. From a pathophysiological standpoint this significant increase in MG with exercise may reflect a more advanced valvular disease (a hemodynamically more severe AS at rest, hence higher increase in gradients for a given flow rate during exercise or a more rigid/non compliant aortic valve, hence no or minimal enlargement of EOA with increase in flow rate, or both). However, exercise-induced changes in MG should always be interpreted in the light of exercise induced changes in LV function and SV. Normally, transaortic gradients increase with exercise due to increase in flow rate. Decrease of MG at one point during exercise may reflect the inability of the LV to adapt to the acute increase in afterload imposed by exercise [54]. The outcome of patients with this biphasic response (initial increase followed by a subsequent decrease in MG) is yet unknown. Analysis of LV systolic function during exercise may provide additional prognostic information in asymptomatic patients with AS. Limited LV contractile reserve (i.e. decrease or limited increase in LVEF) is associated with future symptom development and cardiac death and to an abnormal response to exercise [50, 55]. LV longitudinal systolic function proved to be a more sensitive modality to detect early changes in LV function in patients with AS and a more powerful parameter in predicting exercise intolerance, symptom development and outcomes, above and beyond LVEF [56–58]. It was suggested that a post-exercise increase in mitral annular s'-wave velocity >5 cm/s or an exercise induced increase in GLS by >−1.4% may be used to define the presence of contractile reserve in patients with AS [53, 59]. LV contractile reserve, as assessed by GLS, is more frequently altered in patients with an abnormal exercise test [53]. Exercise induced PHT is yet another ESE derived parameter that can help in risk stratification in asymptomatic patients with severe AS. In one recent study, exercise PHT (i.e. defined as a sPAP during exercise >60 mmHg) was independently associated with a twofold increase in risk of cardiac events at 3-years follow-up. An alarming high rate of cardiac death (12%) was found in patients who developed exercise PHT [52]. Pulmonary hypertension already present at rest is a strong predictor of poor outcomes in severe AS. Yet, patients with resting PHT (i.e. sPAP >50 mmHg) are rarely asymptomatic. The role of resting PHT in risk stratification of asymptomatic patients is thus limited. However, ESE is able to unmask exercise-PHT in asymptomatic patients with severe AS and thus help in risk assessment.

4.4.3 MDCT in Risk Stratification

It has been recently shown that measuring AVC load provides incremental prognostic value for survival, beyond clinical and resting Doppler echocardiographic assessment. Severe AVC (i.e. AVC $\geq$ 1200 AU in women and $\geq$2000 AU in men; AVCd $\geq$ 290 AU/cm^2 in women and $\geq$480 AU/cm^2 in men) independently predicted excess mortality in this large multicentric prospective study [38]. Assessment of AVC may thus be considered not only for diagnostic purposes in LFLG AS but also for risk stratification in all AS patients irrespective of the concordance/discordance of the Doppler echocardiographic parameters. To avoid unnecessary and potentially harmful irradiation related to repeated exposure, MDCT should probably best be performed whenever other biological, CMR, resting or stress echocardiography derived markers indicate a high risk patient. It can be useful for risk stratification in asymptomatic severe AS patients with concordant findings at echocardiography and in patients unable to perform an ESE.

4.4.4 CMR in Risk Stratification

CMR using late gadolinium enhancement facilitates noninvasive assessment of replacement fibrosis within the myocardium. Up to 38% of patients with moderate or severe AS may exhibit a midwall pattern of myocardial fibrosis and this pattern has been associated to a eightfold increase in mortality in one study [39]. The presence of LGE predicted higher postoperative mortality and worse all-cause survival and cardiovascular diseases related survival at 5 year follow-up after surgical AVR in symptomatic patients with severe AS [40]. Diffuse myocardial fibrosis can be evaluated using equilibrium contrast CMR with T1-mapping. The technique has been validated in patients with severe AS and has been shown to correlate with symptomatic status, but outcome studies are needed [60, 61]. More recently, CMR proved to be useful for tissue valve characterization in patients with AS [62]. CMR accurately quantified lipid, fibrous and calcium components within the aortic valve cusps in 16 patients with severe AS. The hypothetical advantage of AV leaflet characterization by CMR would be the early detection and longitudinal follow-up of valvular lesions in AS, that may theoretically help in risk stratification [62]. However, data on this topic are still limited to allow implementation of tissue valve characterization by CMR in routine clinical practice.

4.4.5 PET/CT in Risk Stratification

18F-sodium fluoride (18F-NaF) and 18F-fluorodeoxyglucose (18F-FDG) was used to assess leaflets calcification and inflammation, respectively, in 101 patients with calcific AS [41]. The magnitude of increased 18F-NaF activity within the aortic leaflets correlated well with disease severity [41]. Increased 18F-NaF was found in all patients with severe AS and in 91% of patients with hemodynamically significant

AS. By opposition, the association of increased 18F-FDG uptake with increasing AS severity was weaker, suggesting that calcification is the predominant pathological process in AS, while inflammation is the leading process in the early stages of AS, i.e. aortic sclerosis stage. 18F-NaF PET/CT holds promise as a biomarker of disease activity and as a predictor of disease progression in AS. To this regard, a small monocentric study validated the use of 18F-NaF as a marker of calcification activity against histological markers of active calcification (osteocalcin and tissue nonspecific alkaline phosphatase) and showed that it is a good predictor of the progression in aortic valve calcium score by MDCT at 1 year [42]. According to this study, 18F-NaF binds more readily to regions of developing calcium in aortic valve leaflets and acts like a marker of calcification activity, providing distinct information to calcium scoring which can detect sites of valve calcification but may not make the distinction between a quiescent and an ongoing calcification process [42]. Larger multicentric studies with longer follow-up periods and outcome analysis are needed to confirm the role of 18F-NaF PET/CT as a tool to stratify risk in AS. Its use as a follow-up imaging modality is still limited by the radiation exposure.

Conclusion

Normal flow high gradient severe AS does not pose any diagnostic problems and transthoracic echocardiography is usually enough for an accurate diagnosis. In asymptomatic patients, ESE, CMR and aortic valve calcium score by MDCT may be helpful for risk stratification. Low gradient AS is more challenging and needs a multimodality approach for a final and accurate diagnosis. Low gradient AS with reduced LVEF needs DSE to ascertain between true-severe AS and pseudo-severe AS and to assess the presence of contractile reserve, an important predictor of high perioperative mortality. Fibrosis assessment with CMR may be particularly informative in these patients with low gradient severe AS and reduced LV systolic function and a powerful predictor of mortality. MDCT with the assessment of aortic valve calcium score is the only available flow-independent parameter available to help severity grading of low flow AS patients and proved to be an independent predictor of excess mortality in calcific AS patients. All these multi-modality imaging techniques are available and ready for use in clinical practice in patients with AS. Care has to be taken to make the optimal choice between these techniques depending on the clinical question to be answered.

QCM

1. Regarding AS severity grading, which of the following affirmations is false:
   (a) MDCT with evaluation of aortic valve calcium score can be used when echocardiographic findings are discordant
   (b) Dobutamine stress echocardiography can be used in patients with low flow low gradient AS and reduced LVEF
   (c) PET-CT is useful
   (d) Effective orifice area as measured by the continuity equation is usually lower than the anatomic valve area by planimetry

2. During the echocardiographic evaluation of a patient with AS, systemic hypertension will:
   (a) Lead to the recording of a higher transvalvular gradient
   (b) Overestimate the stenosis severity (through the influence on transaortic pressure gradient)
   (c) Does not influence the transvalvular pressure gradients
   (d) May lead to the underestimation of AS severity because gradients may be lower
3. In asymptomatic severe AS with preserved ejection fraction and no echocardiographic discordances, the following modalities can be used for risk stratification:
   (a) Dobutamine stress echocardiography
   (b) Exercise stress echocardiography
   (c) MDCT
   (d) CMR

References

1. Baumgartner H, Hung J, Bermejo J, et al. Echocardiographic assessment of valve stenosis: EAE/ASE recommendations for clinical practice. Eur J Echocardiogr. 2009;10:1–25.
2. Nishimura RA, Otto CM, Bonow RO, et al. 2014 AHA/ACC guideline for the management of patients with valvular heart disease: executive summary: a report of the American College of Cardiology/American Heart Association task force on practice guidelines. J Am Coll Cardiol. 2014;63:2438–88.
3. Minners J, Allgeier M, Gohlke-Baerwolf C, et al. Inconsistencies of echocardiographic criteria for the grading of aortic valve stenosis. Eur Heart J. 2008;29:1043–8.
4. Hachicha Z, Dumesnil JG, Bogaty P, Pibarot P. Paradoxical low flow, low gradient severe aortic stenosis despite preserved ejection fraction is associated with higher afterload and reduced survival. Circulation. 2007;115:2856–64.
5. Lancellotti P, Magne J, Donal E, et al. Clinical outcome in asymptomatic severe aortic stenosis: insights from the new proposed aortic stenosis grading classification. J Am Coll Cardiol. 2012;59:235–43.
6. Eleid MF, Sorajja P, Michelena HI, et al. Survival by stroke volume index in patients with low-gradient normal EF severe aortic stenosis. Heart. 2014.
7. Pibarot P, Dumesnil JG. Improving assessment of aortic stenosis. J Am Coll Cardiol. 2012;60:169–80.
8. Carabello BA. Aortic stenosis. N Engl J Med. 2002;346:677–82.
9. Pai RG, Varadarajan P, Razzouk A. Survival benefit of aortic valve replacement in patients with severe aortic stenosis with low ejection fraction and low gradient with normal ejection fraction. Ann Thorac Surg. 2008;86:1781–9.
10. Barasch E, Fan D, Chukwu EO, et al. Severe isolated aortic stenosis with normal left ventricular systolic function and low transvalvular gradients: pathophysiologic and prognostic insights. J Heart Valve Dis. 2008;17:81–8.
11. Dumesnil JG, Pibarot P, Carabello B. Paradoxical low flow and/or low gradient severe aortic stenosis despite preserved left ventricular ejection fraction: implications for diagnosis and treatment. Eur Heart J. 2010;31:281–9.
12. Herrmann HC, Pibarot P, Hueter I, et al. Predictors of mortality and outcomes of therapy in low-flow severe aortic stenosis: a Placement of Aortic Transcatheter Valves (PARTNER) trial analysis. Circulation. 2013;127:2316–26.

13. Clavel MA, Dumesnil JG, Capoulade R, et al. Outcome of patients with aortic stenosis, small valve area, and low-flow, low-gradient despite preserved left ventricular ejection fraction. J Am Coll Cardiol. 2012;60:1259–67.
14. Mohty D, Magne J, Deltreuil M, et al. Outcome and impact of surgery in paradoxical low-flow, low-gradient severe aortic stenosis and preserved left ventricular ejection fraction: a cardiac catheterization study. Circulation. 2013;128:S235–42.
15. Eleid MF, Sorajja P, Michelena HI, et al. Flow-gradient patterns in severe aortic stenosis with preserved ejection fraction: clinical characteristics and predictors of survival. Circulation. 2013;128:1781–9.
16. Briand M, Dumesnil JG, Kadem L, et al. Reduced systemic arterial compliance impacts significantly on left ventricular afterload and function in aortic stenosis: implications for diagnosis and treatment. J Am Coll Cardiol. 2005;46:291–8.
17. Hachicha Z, Dumesnil JG, Pibarot P. Usefulness of the valvuloarterial impedance to predict adverse outcome in asymptomatic aortic stenosis. J Am Coll Cardiol. 2009;54:1003–11.
18. Lancellotti P, Donal E, Magne J, et al. Risk stratification in asymptomatic moderate to severe aortic stenosis: the importance of the valvular, arterial and ventricular interplay. Heart. 2010;96:1364–71.
19. Baumgartner H, Steffenelli T, Niederberger J, Schima H, Maurer G. "Overestimation" of catheter gradients by Doppler ultrasound in patients with aortic stenosis: a predictable manifestation of pressure recovery. J Am Coll Cardiol. 1999;33:1655–61.
20. Carroll JD, Carroll EP, Feldman T, et al. Sex-associated differences in left ventricular function in aortic stenosis of the elderly. Circulation. 1992;86:1099–107.
21. Page A, Dumesnil JG, Clavel MA, et al. Metabolic syndrome is associated with more pronounced impairment of left ventricle geometry and function in patients with calcific aortic stenosis: a substudy of the ASTRONOMER (Aortic Stenosis Progression Observation Measuring Effects of Rosuvastatin). J Am Coll Cardiol. 2010;55:1867–74.
22. Lund BP, Gohlke-Barwolf C, Cramariuc D, et al. Effect of obesity on left ventricular mass and systolic function in patients with asymptomatic aortic stenosis (a Simvastatin Ezetimibe in Aortic Stenosis [SEAS] substudy). Am J Cardiol. 2010;105:1456–60.
23. Cramariuc D, Cioffi G, Rieck AE, et al. Low-flow aortic stenosis in asymptomatic patients: valvular-arterial impedance and systolic function from the SEAS Substudy. JACC Cardiovasc Imaging. 2009;2:390–9.
24. Cioffi G, Faggiano P, Vizzardi E, et al. Prognostic effect of inappropriately high left ventricular mass in asymptomatic severe aortic stenosis. Heart. 2011;97:301–7.
25. Orsinelli DA, Aurigemma GP, Battista S, Krendel S, Gaasch WH. Left ventricular hypertrophy and mortality after aortic valve replacement for aortic stenosis. A high risk subgroup identified by preoperative relative wall thickness. J Am Coll Cardiol. 1993;22:1679–83.
26. Eleid MF, Nishimura RA, Sorajja P, Borlaug BA. Systemic hypertension in low-gradient severe aortic stenosis with preserved ejection fraction. Circulation. 2013;128:1349–53.
27. Kodali SK, Williams MR, Smith CR, et al. Two-year outcomes after transcatheter or surgical aortic-valve replacement. N Engl J Med. 2012;366:1686–95.
28. Altiok E, Koos R, Schroder J, et al. Comparison of two-dimensional and three-dimensional imaging techniques for measurement of aortic annulus diameters before transcatheter aortic valve implantation. Heart. 2011;97:1578–84.
29. de Filippi CR, Willett DL, Brickner E, et al. Usefulness of dobutamine echocardiography in distinguishing severe from nonsevere valvular aortic stenosis in patients with depressed left ventricular function and low transvalvular gradients. Am J Cardiol. 1995;75:191–4.
30. Fougeres E, Tribouilloy C, Monchi M, et al. Outcomes of pseudo-severe aortic stenosis under conservative treatment. Eur Heart J. 2012;33:2426–33.
31. Vahanian A, Alfieri O, Andreotti F, et al. Guidelines on the management of valvular heart disease (version 2012): the Joint Task Force on the Management of Valvular Heart Disease of the European Society of Cardiology (ESC) and the European Association for Cardio-Thoracic Surgery (EACTS). Eur J Cardiothorac Surg. 2012;42:S1–44.
32. Blais C, Burwash IG, Mundigler G, et al. The projected valve area at normal flow rate improves the assessment of stenosis severity in patients with low flow aortic stenosis: the multicenter TOPAS (Truly or Pseudo Severe Aortic Stenosis) study. Circulation. 2006;113:711–21.

33. Clavel MA, Burwash IG, Mundigler G, et al. Validation of conventional and simplified methods to calculate projected valve area at normal flow rate in patients with low flow, low gradient aortic stenosis: the multicenter TOPAS (True or Pseudo Severe Aortic Stenosis) study. J Am Soc Echocardiogr. 2010;23:380–6.
34. Clavel MA, Messika-Zeitoun D, Pibarot P, et al. The complex nature of discordant severe calcified aortic valve disease grading: new insights from combined Doppler echocardiographic and computed tomographic study. J Am Coll Cardiol. 2013;62:2329–38.
35. Messika-Zeitoun D, Aubry MC, Detaint D, et al. Evaluation and clinical implications of aortic valve calcification measured by electron-beam computed tomography. Circulation. 2004;110:356–62.
36. Cueff C, Serfaty JM, Cimadevilla C, et al. Measurement of aortic valve calcification using multislice computed tomography: correlation with haemodynamic severity of aortic stenosis and clinical implication for patients with low ejection fraction. Heart. 2011;97:721–6.
37. Aggarwal SR, Clavel MA, Messika-Zeitoun D, et al. Sex differences in aortic valve calcification measured by multidetector computed tomography in aortic stenosis. Circ Cardiovasc Imaging. 2013;6:40–7.
38. Clavel MA, Pibarot P, Messika-Zeitoun D, et al. Impact of aortic valve calcification, as measured by MDCT, on survival in patients with aortic stenosis: results of an international registry study. J Am Coll Cardiol. 2014;64:1202–13.
39. Dweck MR, Joshi S, Murigu T, et al. Midwall fibrosis is an independent predictor of mortality in patients with aortic stenosis. J Am Coll Cardiol. 2011;58:1271–9.
40. Barone-Rochette G, Pierard S, De Meester dR, et al. Prognostic significance of LGE by CMR in aortic stenosis patients undergoing valve replacement. J Am Coll Cardiol. 2014;64:144–54.
41. Dweck MR, Jones C, Joshi NV, et al. Assessment of valvular calcification and inflammation by positron emission tomography in patients with aortic stenosis. Circulation. 2012;125:76–86.
42. Dweck MR, Jenkins WS, Vesey AT, et al. 18F-sodium fluoride uptake is a marker of active calcification and disease progression in patients with aortic stenosis. Circ Cardiovasc Imaging. 2014;7:371–8.
43. Pellikka PA, Sarano ME, Nishimura RA, et al. Outcome of 622 adults with asymptomatic, hemodynamically significant aortic stenosis during prolonged follow-up. Circulation. 2005;111:3290–5.
44. Otto CM, Burwash IG, Legget ME, et al. Prospective study of asymptomatic valvular aortic stenosis. Clinical, echocardiographic, and exercise predictors of outcome. Circulation. 1997;95:2262–70.
45. Rosenhek R, Zilberszac R, Schemper M, et al. Natural history of very severe aortic stenosis. Circulation. 2010;121:151–6.
46. Rosenhek R, Binder T, Porenta G, et al. Predictors of outcome in severe, asymptomatic aortic stenosis. N Engl J Med. 2000;343:611–7.
47. Bruch C, Stypmann J, Grude M, et al. Tissue Doppler imaging in patients with moderate to severe aortic valve stenosis: clinical usefulness and diagnostic accuracy. Am Heart J. 2004;148:696–702.
48. Das P, Rimington H, Chambers J. Exercise testing to stratify risk in aortic stenosis. Eur Heart J. 2005;26:1309–13.
49. Alborino D, Hoffmann JL, Fournet PC, Bloch A. Value of exercise testing to evaluate the indication for surgery in asymptomatic patients with valvular aortic stenosis. J Heart Valve Dis. 2002;11:204–9.
50. Lancellotti P, Lebois F, Simon M, et al. Prognostic importance of quantitative exercise Doppler echocardiography in asymptomatic valvular aortic stenosis. Circulation. 2005;112:I377–82.
51. Marechaux S, Hachicha Z, Bellouin A, et al. Usefulness of exercise-stress echocardiography for risk stratification of true asymptomatic patients with aortic valve stenosis. Eur Heart J. 2010;31:1390–7.
52. Lancellotti P, Magne J, Donal E, et al. Determinants and prognostic significance of exercise pulmonary hypertension in asymptomatic severe aortic stenosis. Circulation. 2012;126:851–9.
53. Donal E, Thebault C, O'Connor K, et al. Impact of aortic stenosis on longitudinal myocardial deformation during exercise. Eur J Echocardiogr. 2011;12:235–41.

54. Lancellotti P, Moonen M, Garweg C, Pierard LA. Image. Afterload mismatch revealed by an exercise biphasic response in aortic stenosis. Arch Cardiovasc Dis. 2009;102:593–4.
55. Marechaux S, Ennezat PV, LeJemtel TH, et al. Left ventricular response to exercise in aortic stenosis: an exercise echocardiographic study. Echocardiography. 2007;24:955–9.
56. Lancellotti P, Donal E, Magne J, et al. Impact of global left ventricular afterload on left ventricular function in asymptomatic severe aortic stenosis: a two-dimensional speckle-tracking study. Eur J Echocardiogr. 2010;11:537–43.
57. Lancellotti P, Moonen M, Magne J, et al. Prognostic effect of long-axis left ventricular dysfunction and B-type natriuretic peptide levels in asymptomatic aortic stenosis. Am J Cardiol. 2010;105:383–8.
58. Lafitte S, Perlant M, Reant P, et al. Impact of impaired myocardial deformations on exercise tolerance and prognosis in patients with asymptomatic aortic stenosis. Eur J Echocardiogr. 2009;10:414–9.
59. Van Pelt NC, Stewart RA, Legget ME, et al. Longitudinal left ventricular contractile dysfunction after exercise in aortic stenosis. Heart. 2007;93:732–8.
60. Flett AS, Hayward MP, Ashworth MT, et al. Equilibrium contrast cardiovascular magnetic resonance for the measurement of diffuse myocardial fibrosis: preliminary validation in humans. Circulation. 2010;122:138–44.
61. Flett AS, Sado DM, Quarta G, et al. Diffuse myocardial fibrosis in severe aortic stenosis: an equilibrium contrast cardiovascular magnetic resonance study. Eur Heart J Cardiovasc Imaging. 2012;13:819–26.
62. Le Ven F, Tizon-Marcos H, Fuchs C, et al. Valve tissue characterization by magnetic resonance imaging in calcific aortic valve disease. Can J Cardiol. 2014;30:1676–83.

5 Multimodality Imaging Assessment of Aortic Regurgitation

Denisa Muraru, Luigi P. Badano, and Shizhen Liu

5.1 Introduction

Aortic regurgitation (AR) is a common valvular heart disease secondary to either congenital or acquired conditions. AR causes both pressure and volume overload of the left ventricle (LV), resulting in LV cavity dilation, eccentric hypertrophy and, ultimately, systolic dysfunction. Echocardiography is the primary imaging modality to assess and follow patients with AR, and the recent three-dimensional (3D) capabilities enable to appreciate the functional complexity of the aortic valve (AV) complex in the beating heart [1]. The only effective treatment of patients with severe AR is surgery. Multi-modality imaging plays a pivotal role in establishing the optimal timing of intervention, before irreversible LV dysfunction develops, and also in planning the surgical procedure (repair versus replacement; ascending aorta replacement etc).

In this chapter, we review the comprehensive echocardiographic workup of patients with AR and the role of more advanced imaging modalities to ascertain the diagnosis and assess the ascending aorta.

5.2 Normal Anatomy of Aortic Valve Complex

Usually clinicians refer to AV by describing its three semilunar cusps, named right, left and non-coronary based on the location of the coronary Ostia. However, the AV is a more complex structure formed by different components and including the three

D. Muraru (✉) • L.P. Badano
Department of Cardiac, Thoracic and Vascular Sciences, University of Padua, Via Giustiniani 2, Padua 35128, Italy
e-mail: denisa.muraru@gmail.com

S. Liu, M.D., Ph.D.
Marcus Heart Valve Center, Piedmont Heart Institute, Atlanta, GA, USA

K. Fattouch et al. (eds.), *Advances in Treatments for Aortic Valve and Root Diseases*, https://doi.org/10.1007/978-3-319-66483-5_5

cusps, the annulus and the aortic root, creating the so-called "aortic valve complex".

The spatial configuration of the AV cusps is three-dimensional and resembles a crown (Fig. 5.1) [1]. In the normal AV, the insertion of the cusps at the level of the aortic root wall forms three prominent semilunar ridges (or hingelines), separated by three interleaflet triangles. Thus, the true anatomic aortic annulus is not the ring projected at the most basal insertion of AV cusps—as usually defined and measured with various imaging techniques—but actually it is a crown-like 3D structure. The aortic root, comprising the Valsalva sinuses and the fibrous interleaflet triangles, provides support for AV cusps. The AV cusps are also attached peripherally at the sino-tubular junction, which represents the distal boundary of the aortic root. Both Valsalva sinuses and sino-tubular junction are integral parts of the AV closure mechanism, so any significant dilatation of these structures will result in AR.

Due to its central location in the heart, the aortic root has a complex relationship to the cardiac chambers and valves. The aortic root and proximal ascending aorta have spatial relationships with both atria. The aortic root lies to the right and posterior to the subpulmonary infundibulum. The posterior margins of the aortic root are wedged between the orifices of the two atrio-ventricular valves. Approximately 1/3 of the aortic root at the level of ventriculo-anatomic junction (in correspondence to the non-coronary and left AV cusps) is connected to the anterior mitral leaflet via the fibrous continuity (aortic-mitral curtain), while the remaining 2/3 of its circumference are muscular and correspond to the interventricular septum. The interleaflet triangle between the non-coronary and right coronary cusp is crossed on its right side by the hinge of the septal tricuspid leaflet, which divides the septum into atrio-ventricular and interventricular components. These spatial relationships are crucial for understanding the functional interplay

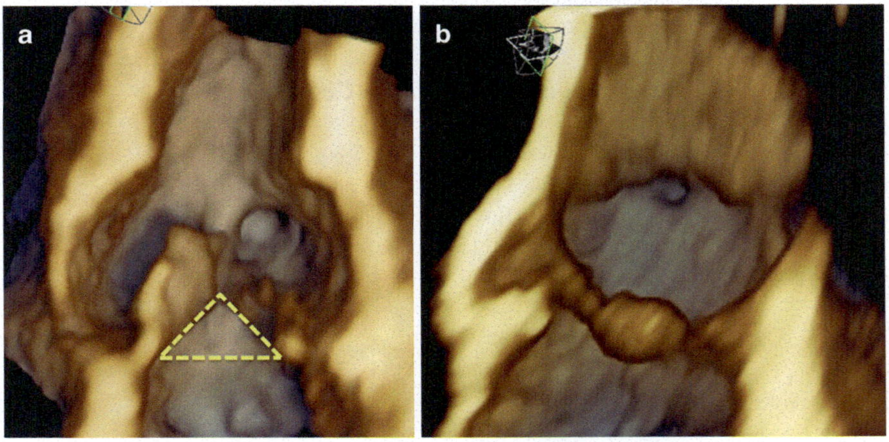

Fig. 5.1 Anatomy of the aortic root complex by 3D transesophageal imaging, showing its crown-like configuration, Valsalva sinuses, interleaflet triangles (**a**) and the left main coronary ostium (**b**)

of the aortic valve and root with the atrio-ventricular valves and are best appreciated using 3D imaging modalities.

5.3 Aetiology of Aortic Regurgitation

The aetiologies of AR fall into two broad categories: (1) primary structural abnormalities of AV cusps and (2) secondary geometric changes of AV cusps, caused by abnormalities of the aortic root.

Primary structural abnormalities of the AV include both congenital and acquired diseases.

Congenital causes include various anatomic variants of AV morphology, such as bicuspid (most often), quadricuspid and unicuspid AV, leading to isolated AR or combined valvular stenosis and regurgitation (Fig. 5.2). Among the acquired

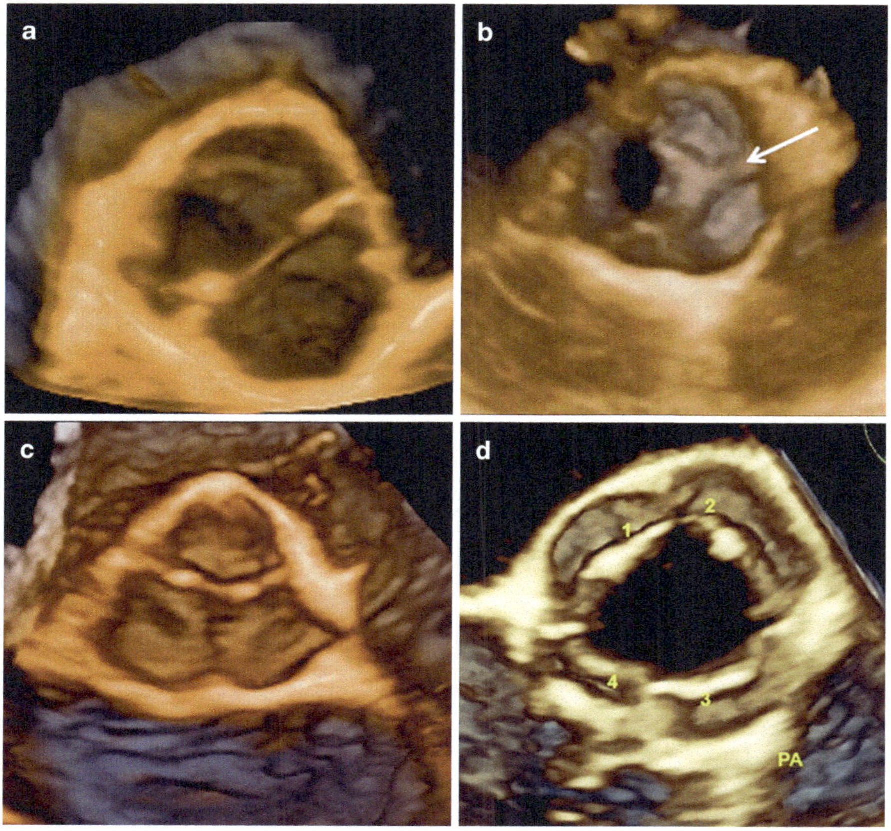

Fig. 5.2 Congenital morphologic variants of aortic valve: true bicuspid (**a**), bicuspid with rafe (**b**), tricuspid (**c**), and quadricuspid (**d**, courtesy of Dr. Alex Felix, Brazil)

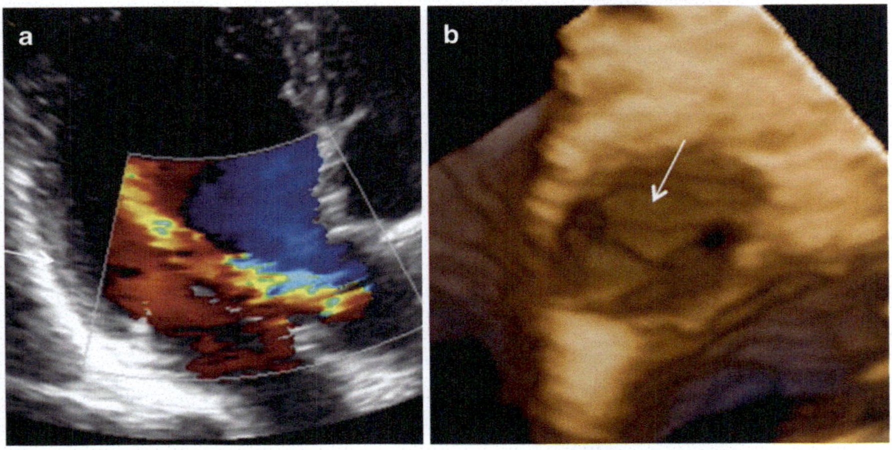

Fig. 5.3 Eccentric degenerative aortic regurgitation (**a**). The exact mechanism was identified by 3D transthoracic echocardiography as due to right coronary cusp prolapse (**b**, *en face* view from ventricular perspective)

valvular lesions, the most frequent aetiologies of AR are: degenerative calcific valve disease, endocarditis, rheumatic valve disease, cusp prolapse due to degenerative disease (Fig. 5.3), radiation therapy, connective tissue diseases etc.

Acute AR is a rare condition that may result from endocarditis, aortic dissection, blunt chest trauma or iatrogenic complications of procedures (TAVI, aortic balloon valvuloplasty etc).

Bicuspid aortic valves are frequently associated with aortic dilation either at the level of the sinuses of Valsalva or, more frequently, in the ascending aorta. The morphologic variant of bicuspid valve is correlated with the risk of ascending aortic dilation, i.e. greater risk if non-coronary cusp is fused either with the right or left coronary cusp [2].

The accurate determination of AR aetiology is crucial for patient management, and is commonly based on the integration of patient history, clinical data and characteristic echocardiographic aspects [3].

5.4 Functional Classification of Aortic Regurgitation

A systematic assessment and reporting of the AR mechanism is important, particularly when surgical procedures for AV repair are contemplated.

The most common functional classification is the adapted Carpentier classification for AR [4]:

- Type 1: Enlargement of the aortic root with normal cusp motion
- Type 2: Excessive cusp motion, with cusp prolapse due to excessive cusp tissue or commissural disruption.

- Type 3: Poor cusp tissue quality or quantity, including cusp retraction, extensive degenerative calcifications (≥grade 3), congenitally abnormal valves, endocarditis or other etiology leading to cusp thickening, fibrosis and calcifications.

Type 1 can be subcategorized in four groups: 1a with enlargement of both sino-tubular junction and ascending aorta; 1b with dilation of sino-tubular junction and sinuses of Valsalva; 1c with dilation of aortic annulus (ventriculo-arterial junction); and 1d with cusp perforation [5].

Cusp prolapses can be further categorized in three groups: cusp flail (eversion of the cusp into the LV outflow tract), partial or distal cusp prolapse, and whole cusp prolapse.

This classification provides the surgeon with a functional description of the AV lesions, that helps him in choosing the most appropriate surgical technique. In general, most type 1 and 2 AR lesions are considered as "repairable" in the absence of significant calcifications, while type 3 are deemed as nonrepairable. Also the extent and localization of calcifications are important for planning surgery. Moderately calcified AV cusps with calcifications limited to their free margins could be amenable to repair, while heavily calcified valves with calcifications involving the cusp bodies are generally replaced with valve prostheses [4].

5.5 Quantification of Aortic Regurgitation Severity

Echocardiographic assessment of AR includes integration of data from Doppler indices of AR severity with 2D/3D imaging of the AV, aortic root dimensions, and LV size and function [6]. Transthoracic echocardiography (TTE) is recommended as the first-line imaging modality in assessing AR severity, and should include a series of qualitative, semi-quantitative and quantitative parameters (Figs. 5.4, 5.5, and 5.6, Table 5.1). Frequently, TTE is sufficient to evaluate the presence and the severity of chronic AR.

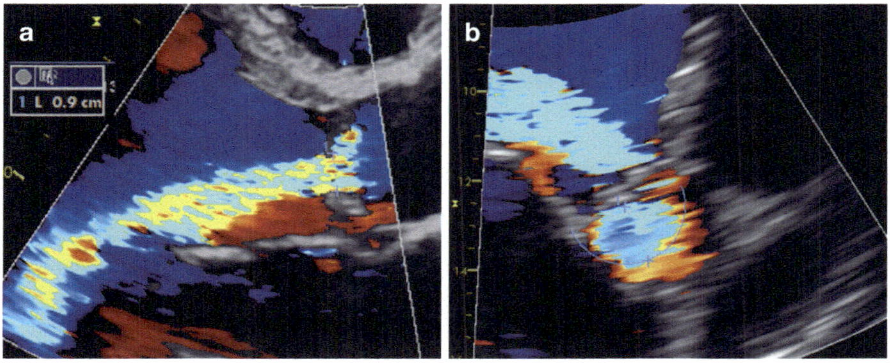

Fig. 5.4 Quantification of regurgitation severity by color Doppler indices reflecting a severe aortic insufficiency: vena contracta (**a**) and PISA radius (**b**)

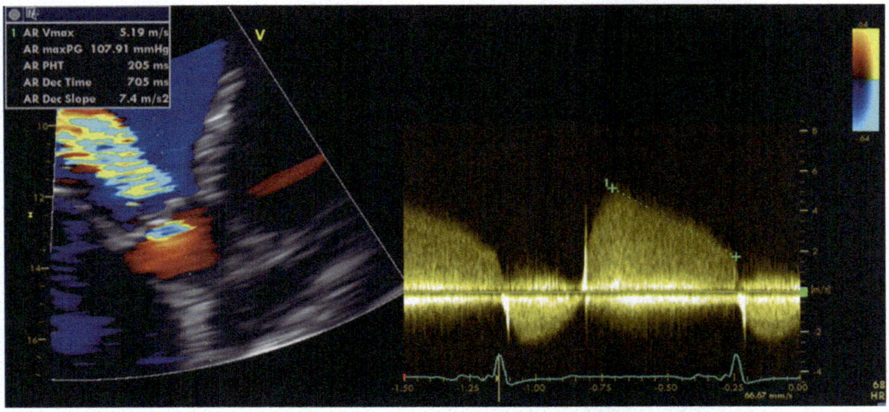

Fig. 5.5 Quantification of aortic regurgitation severity using pressure-half time (PHT)

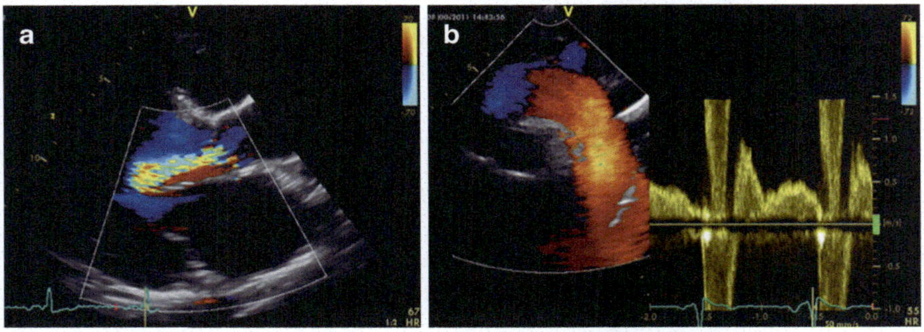

Fig. 5.6 Doppler features of severe aortic regurgitation: wide origine jet (**a**) with significant holodiastolic reverse flow in descending aorta (**b**)

Acute severe AR is more challenging to diagnose than chronic AR based on color Doppler. Commonly, the diagnosis of acute AR is based on a high index of suspicion (i.e. patient with endocarditis or aortic dissection with acute heart failure signs or cardiogenic shock etc) and on several Doppler signs, including brief AR jet with low velocity, often eccentric, with short deceleration time, normal LV and left atrial volumes. If acute AR is suspected, a low threshold for performing a TEE examination is advisable.

Transesophageal echocardiography (TEE) (Fig. 5.7) is reserved for a more detailed assessment and can be useful to further clarify the mechanism of AR, as well as for a better appreciation of AV complex anatomy. TEE improves the diagnostic accuracy of TTE in several scenarios associated with AR, such as endocarditis and aortic valve masses, acute aortic dissection or congenital aortic valve abnormalities. The detailed understanding and characterization of the AR mechanism by TEE is particularly important when valve-sparing aortic surgery, valve repair surgery or transcatheter procedures are contemplated.

Table 5.1 Echocardiographic assessment of aortic regurgitation (AR) severity (adapted after [6])

Parameters	Severe if	Comments
Aortic valve morphology	Coaptation defect, cusp flail, visible regurgitation orifice	Data from both long- and short-axis views of the valve using 2D/3D echocardiography is recommended
Color Doppler flow	Central jet with large width at its origin and significant proximal convergence zone without baseline shift	Jet width is less reliable in eccentric jets
Continuous-wave Doppler signal	High density profile with steep deceleration	Signal density and slope cannot reliably discriminate moderate from severe AR
Diastolic flow reversal in descending thoracic aorta	Holodiastolic flow reversal with end-diastolic velocities >20 cm/s and larger velocity-time integral (VTI) than the VTI of the systolic forward flow	Affected by aorta compliance
Diastolic flow reversal in abdominal aorta	Present	Specific sign; may be absent despite severe AR
Vena contracta width	≥6 mm	
Pressure half-time	<200 ms	Specific sign; may be absent in chronic severe AR Affected by LV diastolic pressure, aorta compliance, vasodilator therapy
Effective regurgitant orifice area	≥30 mm^2	Not feasible in eccentric jets or heavily calcified valves
Regurgitant volume	≥60 mL	
Left ventricular volumes	Significantly increased	May be normal in acute severe AR 2D echo diameters and volumes may underestimate the true LV size (3D echo is recommended whenever feasible)

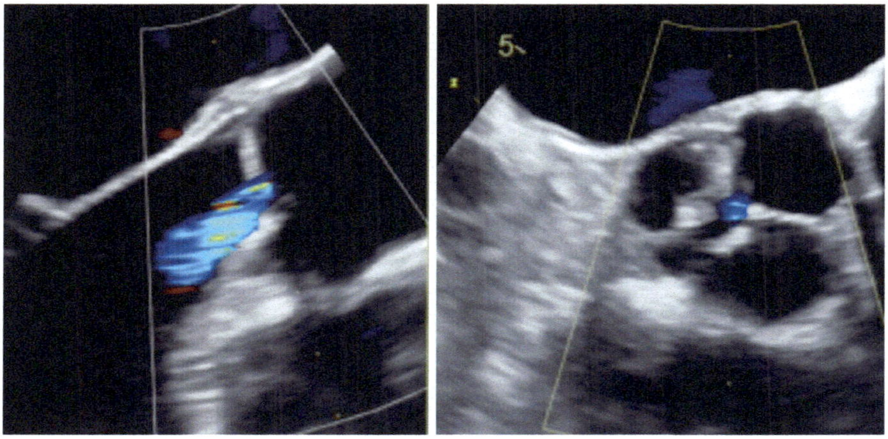

Fig. 5.7 Biplane 2D imaging by transesophageal echocardiography, showing a thickened aortic valve with three cusp morphology and a central jet of aortic regurgitation

5.6 Multi-Modality Imaging

5.6.1 3D Echocardiography

In patients with AR, the stereoscopic geometry of AV complex and its real-time dynamics can be more easily appreciated and interpreted using 3D echocardiography (3DE) (Fig. 5.8). Dynamic *en face* 3D views of AV can be obtained from both aortic and ventricular perspectives (Fig. 5.9). In general, the aortic perspective of the AV is best suited for assessing valve morphology (i.e. bicuspid versus tricuspid), while the ventricular perspective is useful for assessing cusp prolapse, visualizing vegetations or subvalvular obstructions. 3D TEE provides superior spatial resolution of AV cusps and it is the method of choice when a definite diagnosis cannot be made by transthoracic 3DE.

Imaging the AV by transthoracic 3DE can be achieved from either parasternal or apical approach. The 3D data set acquisitions are usually done as multi-beat ECG-gated ("stitched" volumes) or real-time 3D zoom images. For assessing AR jet, a 3D color Doppler data set is obtained using a multi-beat acquisition in order to optimize the temporal resolution.

Precise description of AV morphology (mono- versus bi-, tri- or quadri-cuspid valve, Fig. 5.2) is important to guide patient management (e.g. indication for TAVI or for surgical replacement of ascending aorta, screening of family members etc), to schedule the frequency of follow-up exams or to plan surgical AV repair techniques. By two-dimensional (2D) echocardiography, false-positive and false-negative diagnoses of bicuspid AV may arise from incomplete demonstration of all three leaflet closure lines due to inadequate AV cross-section and continuous through-plane motion of the valve, making difficult to perfectly align the transversal plane exactly

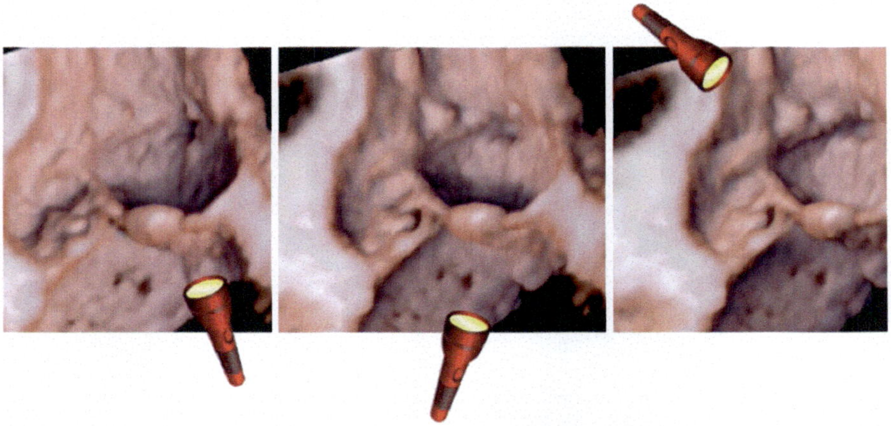

Fig. 5.8 Use of anatomic maps and virtual light source to enhance the visualization of anatomic details on 3D data sets, such as coronary ostia and extension and distribution of aortic root calcific plaques

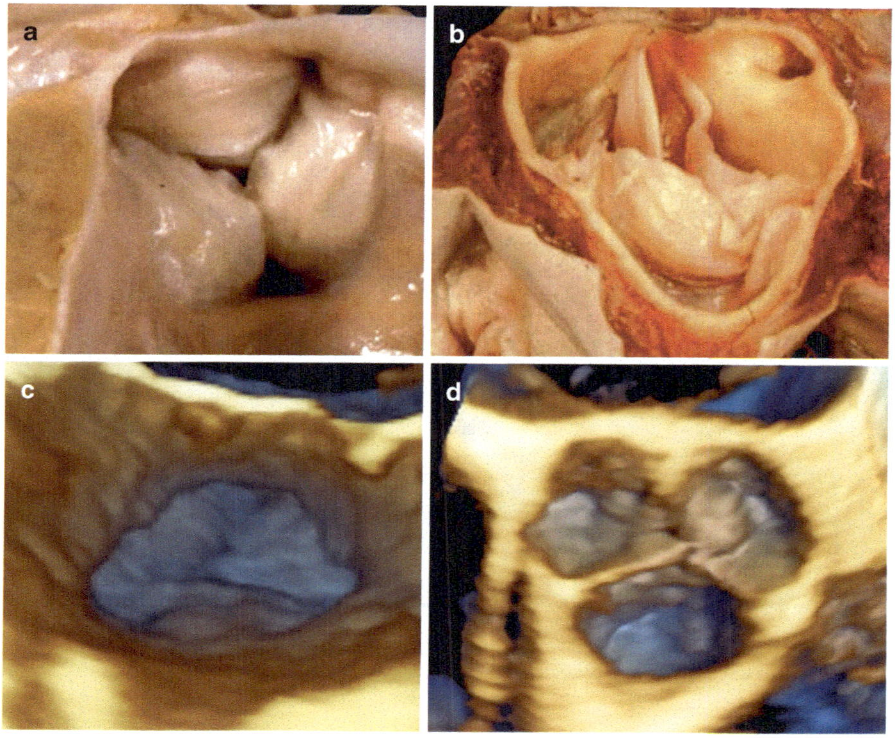

Fig. 5.9 Anatomic specimens (**a**, **b**, courtesy of Prof Cristina Basso, Cardiovascular Pathology, University of Padua) versus 3D echocardiography imaging (**c**, **d**) of the aortic valve seen from the ventricular and from the aortic root perspectives. On the ventricular perspective, the elliptical shape of the left ventricular outflow tract can be appreciated. On the aortic root perspective, the three-cusp morphology with degenerative structural alterations and a small regurgitant orifice between noncoronary and left cusps can be appreciated

at the leaflet tips at end-systole. Dynamic 3D rendering of AV from aortic perspective allows the discrimination between a tricuspid valve and a bicuspid valve with a raphe in doubtful cases by conventional echocardiography [1].

In a comparative study of 2D TEE and epicardial 3DE against surgical findings, epicardial 3DE was more sensitive than 2D TEE in detecting morphologic abnormalities of AV documented intra-operatively (leaflet deficiency, prolapse/perforation, commissural fusion) [7].

Recent insights from 3D TEE showed that, in patients with aortic root dilation, aortic cusps might undergo a process of adaptation by increasing their size and that central AR results from an insufficient remodelling of AV cusps in relation to the aortic root cross sectional area [8]. Conversely, in patients with eccentric AR, there is a relative abundance of cusp tissue resulting in relative cusp prolapse. In type 1 central AR, valve-sparing root replacement techniques (remodelling or reimplantation technique) may be sufficient to reduce the aortic root diameter to match the

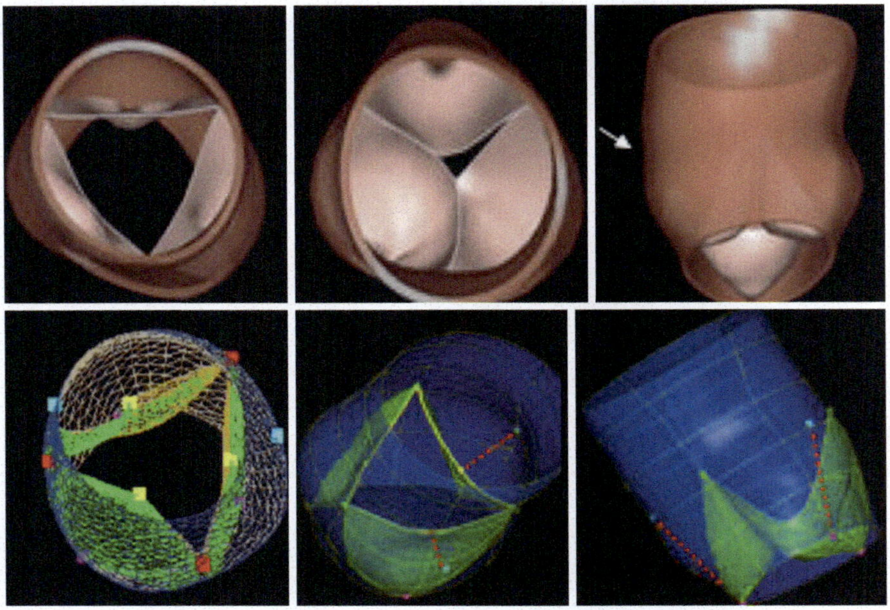

Fig. 5.10 Automated quantitative, patient-specific modelling of the aortic root and the aortic valve from 3D transesophageal echocardiographic data sets

aortic valve cusp size. However, in eccentric AR, cusp reconstruction with plication, triangular resection, or resuspension may be needed [9]. In addition to the AR mechanism, the ratio between closed cusp area and aortic root area at the sino-tubular junction level might help in determining which AV reconstructive technique is most appropriate [8]. Advanced tools to quantify the geometry of AV leaflets and aortic root from 3DE data sets are currently being evaluated. Using highly performant software algorithms applied on 3D TEE data sets, an automated quantitative, patient-specific modelling of the aortic root and the AV can be achieved within minutes (Fig. 5.10). Figure 5.11 shows an example of quantitative 3D TEE of the aortic root in a patient with AR where the relative lack of cusp tissue (inadequate height despite significant increase in length) result in development of a central regurgitant orifice. These pre-operative data from 3DE are also valuable to predict optimal graft size and are highly promising for determining the need for cusp remodelling in patients with AR selected for valve-sparing root surgery [1].

The assessment of AR severity by 2D color Doppler is limited by numerous geometric assumptions regarding the shape of the regurgitant orifice and the position of the tomographic plane exactly in the middle of the regurgitant orifice. 3D color Doppler data sets can be cropped in multiple transversal planes exactly perpendicular to the AR jet direction, in the proximity of the jet origin at the AV level, in order to identify and planimeter the smallest color jet area— the vena contracta area. This approach had a good accuracy to discriminate between different AR grades at angiography [10] and was found to be more accurate than conventional Doppler parameters when compared with cardiac magnetic resonance (CMR) [11]. A cut-off value of 32 mm^2 for 3D vena contracta area to identify severe AR has been recently

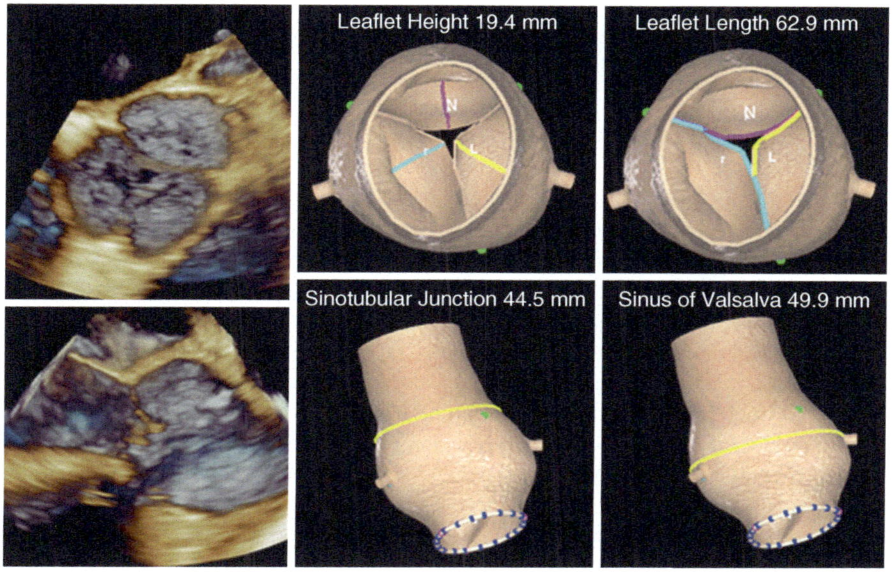

Fig. 5.11 Automated quantitative 3-D TEE modelling of the aortic root in aortic regurgitation. The panel on the left shows 3-D short-axis (above) and long-axis orientations of the aortic root in a patient with AR. The short-axis orientation shows a central regurgitant orifice. The middle panel shows 3-D leaflet height (average) of 19.4 mm and STJ diameter of 44.4 mm. The right panel shows the leaflet length of 62.9 mm and SoV diameter of 49.9 mm. Thus, the ratio of the height to the STJ is 0.44 which is less than the cut-off of 0.49 which results is significant AR. Similarly, the ratio of the length to the height is 3.44 (≥2.2 causes significant AR). Also, the ratio of the height to SoV diameter is 0.39 and <0.49 is causative of significant AR

proposed by a small single-center study [12], requiring validation from larger studies. However, color gain, wall filter settings, and variability of aliasing velocities, limited temporal and spatial resolution may affect the accuracy and reproducibility of 3D vena contracta area. Although 3D color Doppler is promising and conceptually superior to 2D color, this method still requires further validation for its application for clinical purposes.

5.6.2 Stress Echocardiography

Exercise echocardiography leads to increase in systemic pressure, but also in heart rate, shortening the diastolic duration and therefore being less useful for grading the severity of AR [13].

In the asymptomatic patient with severe AR, exercise echocardiography can be used to elicit patient symptoms, to assess his/her functional capacity and contractile reserve. The assessment of LV contractile reserve and longitudinal function during exercise allows to identify an early LV dysfunction in asymptomatic patients with severe AR [14, 15].

In the symptomatic patient with moderate AR, stress echocardiography can be useful to detect other coexisting reasons for patient symptoms, such as inducible ischemia, significant rise in pulmonary pressure during exercise (>60 mmHg), or LV ejection fraction that fails to increase during stress [13].

5.6.3 Cardiac Magnetic Resonance

Cardiac magnetic resonance can be used in selected patients with moderate and severe AR and suboptimal echocardiographic images for the quantification of AR and/or LV volumes and function. Moreover, patients with discrepancy between symptoms and AR severity by echocardiography (i.e. symptomatic patient with moderate AR by Doppler echocardiography measures), or with discrepancy between 2D echocardiographic features and Doppler data (i.e. significant enlargement of the left ventricle and moderate AR by Doppler measures) can be also considered for a CMR study [2]. Other scenario when CMR may be indicated is represented by the patient with multiple valvular lesions, when he quantification of AR by Doppler echocardiography is challenging. CMR can also be used for assessing and following patients with both AR and dilation of the thoracic aorta, especially if young, as it avoids the radiation exposure in comparison with computed tomography (CT) and because CMR measurements are generally less variable at longitudinal follow-up than conventional echocardiographic quantifications of AR severity and LV remodelling.

Steady-state free precession (SSFP) acquisitions with ECG gating can be used to evaluate the AV morphology and orifice area.

AR with/without stenosis results in turbulent flow, generating signal voids, which appear as dark "jets" emanating from the AV (Fig. 5.12). The identification of a

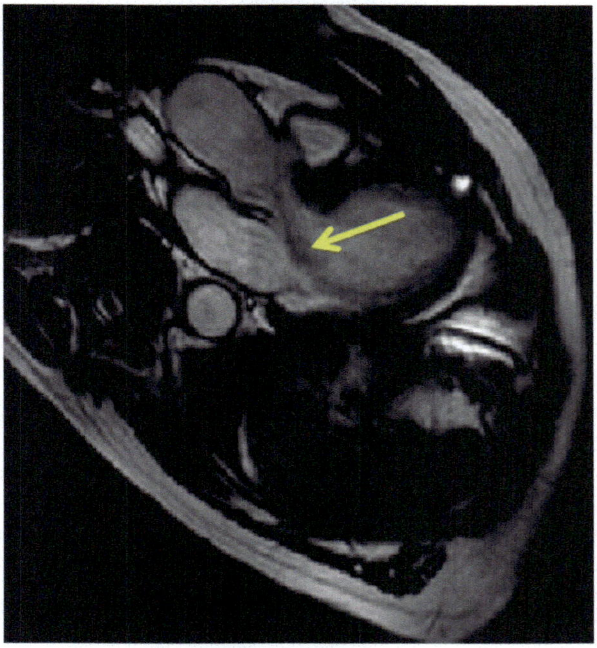

Fig. 5.12 Example of severe eccentric jet of aortic regurgitation visualized in 3-chamber phase-contrast cine CMR image in a patient with dilated ascending aorta. Courtesy of Dr. Gianluca Pontone, Centro Cardiologico Monzino, Milan (Italy)

signal void is helpful in diagnosing AR, however its magnitude depends on a number of factors (the echo time, flip angle, imaging plane).

Therefore, the qualitative assessment of regurgitant jet signal void of AR has significant limitations and should be interpreted with caution.

Quantification of AR at CMR can be done either by through-plane phase-contrast velocity mapping, or by stroke volume method. However, these methods are not as widely used or standardized as Doppler flow measurements.

CMR flow mapping allows the measurement of forward flow (FF) and regurgitant flow (RF) across the AV, and the calculation of the regurgitant fraction as 100 × RF/FF (%). A cut-off value of regurgitant fraction of 33% by CMR, associated with LV end-diastolic volume > 246 mL, predicts the development of indication for surgery within 3 years [16]. The stroke-volume method is applicable only in AR patients without other valve insufficiency or shunt lesions, and is based on the calculation of the regurgitant volume as the difference between LV stroke-volume and right ventricular stroke volume.

The costs, limited availability, long examination time, as well as presence of CMR-incompatible pacemakers or other metallic devices, renal insufficiency and claustrophobia limit the application of CMR for routinely assessing patients with AR. Moreover, the partial volume effects and the difficulty to visualize highly mobile structures (i.e. small masses and vegetations) may affect the accuracy of interpretation by CMR.

5.6.4 Computed Tomography (CT)

There is no current clinically validated method for measuring flow velocity or flow volume using CT. Yet, CT is a highly valuable imaging modality for assessing patients with dilated aorta and type 1 secondary AR.

Common indications for CT include: (1) dilated aorta in patients with unsatisfactory acoustic window; (2) comprehensive assessment of entire aorta for quantifying aortic dilation or coarctation in patients with bicuspid AV (Fig. 5.13); (3) rapid rule out of aortic dissection; (4) assess valve morphology, aortic calcifications and atheromatous plaques; (5) rule out significant coronary artery disease in patients with indication for surgery for severe AR and low probability of coronary atherosclerosis.

Cardiac CT allows a reliable quantification of AV calcifications (in the same manner as coronary calcium scores are obtained and expressed as Agatston score) and its excellent spatial resolution enables the characterization of large vegetations or tumors attached to AV cusps (>1 cm) or the measurement of regurgitant valve orifice area by planimetry. The sensitivity of CT for evaluating AR severity can be limited in case of coexisting mild AV stenosis or in the presence of significant calcifications.

In endocarditis-relate complications, CT is a valuable diagnostic tool for assessing perivalvular abscess or pseudoaneurysms, as well as other infections embolic complications, such as septic pulmonary or renal emboli.

Despite CT images are fast and easy to acquire in many patients, the need for radiation exposure and contrast injection material are significant limitations against its more widespread use.

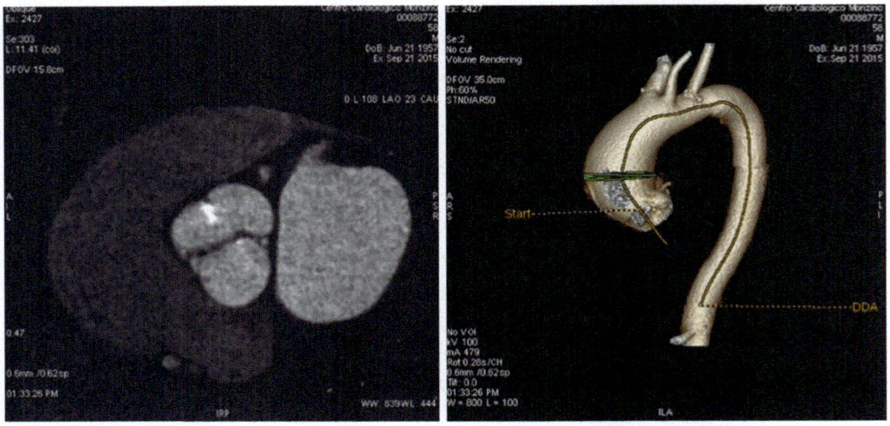

Fig. 5.13 Dilation of ascending aorta (56 mm) in a patient with bicuspid aortic valve (fusion of right and noncoronary cusps, *left panel*), visualized by cardiac CT with 3D reconstruction (*right panel*). Courtesy of Dr. Gianluca Pontone, Centro Cardiologico Monzino, Milan (Italy)

5.6.5 Cardiac Catheterization

Cardiac catheterization is rarely needed to assess the severity of AR. Cardiac catheterization should be performed with aortic root angiography and measurements of LV pressure to assess the severity of AR, aortic root dimensions and LV function.

In AR, the LV stroke volume measured angiographically is greater than the forward stroke volume determined by the Fick cardiac output, and the difference corresponds to the AR regurgitant fraction.

The aortic pressure tracing in AR typically reveals a rapid upstroke and an increased systolic pressure, due to increased stroke volume, with a rapid fall and near equalization of aortic and LV pressures at the end of diastole. The pulse pressure is therefore widened in severe AR. In chronic severe AR, the LV end-diastolic pressure is normal or slightly elevated, since the compliance of the LV is also increased. Conversely, in acute AR, the LV pressure tracing shows a steep rise in diastolic pressure and a markedly elevated end-diastolic pressure, while the aortic systolic pressure is reduced and the pulse pressure is smaller.

Current guidelines recommend cardiac catheterization only in patients in whom the findings of non-invasive imaging techniques have provided results that are inconsistent or discordant with clinical assessment [17].

References

1. Muraru D, Badano LP, Vannan M, Iliceto S. Assessment of aortic valve complex by three-dimensional echocardiography: a framework for its effective application in clinical practice. Eur Heart J Cardiovasc Imaging. 2012;13:541–55.
2. Nishimura RA, Otto CM, Bonow RO, Carabello BA, Erwin JP III, Guyton RA, et al. 2014 AHA/ACC guideline for the management of patients with valvular heart disease: a report

of the American College of Cardiology/American Heart Association Task Force on Practice Guidelines. J Am Coll Cardiol. 2014;63:e57–185.
3. Lancellotti P, Tribouilloy C, Hagendorff A, Moura L, Popescu BA, Agricola E, et al. European Association of Echocardiography recommendations for the assessment of valvular regurgitation. Part 1: aortic and pulmonary regurgitation (native valve disease). Eur J Echocardiogr. 2010;11:223–44.
4. Le Polain de Waroux JB, Pouleur AC, Goffinet C, Vancraeynest D, Van Dyck M, Robert A, et al. Functional anatomy of aortic regurgitation: accuracy, prediction of surgical repairability, and outcome implications of transesophageal echocardiography. Circulation. 2007;116:I264–9.
5. Zoghbi WA, Adams D, Bonow RO, Enriquez-Sarano M, Foster E, Grayburn PA, et al. Recommendations for noninvasive evaluation of native valvular regurgitation: a report from the American Society of Echocardiography Developed in Collaboration with the Society for cardiovascular magnetic resonance. J Am Soc Echocardiogr. 2017.
6. Lancellotti P, Tribouilloy C, Hagendorff A, Popescu BA, Edvardsen T, Pierard LA, et al. Recommendations for the echocardiographic assessment of native valvular regurgitation: an executive summary from the European Association of Cardiovascular Imaging. Eur Heart J Cardiovasc Imaging. 2013;14:611–44.
7. De Castro S, Salandin V, Cavarretta E, Salvador L, Valfre C, Caselli S, et al. Epicardial real-time three-dimensional echocardiography in cardiac surgery: a preliminary experience. Ann Thorac Surg. 2006;82:2254–9.
8. Regeer MV, Kamperidis V, Versteegh MI, Schalij MJ, Marsan NA, Bax JJ, et al. Three-dimensional transoesophageal echocardiography of the aortic valve and root: changes in aortic root dilation and aortic regurgitation. Eur Heart J Cardiovasc Imaging. 2016.
9. Boodhwani M, de Kerchove L, Glineur D, Poncelet A, Rubay J, Astarci P, et al. Repair-oriented classification of aortic insufficiency: impact on surgical techniques and clinical outcomes. J Thorac Cardiovasc Surg. 2009;137:286–94.
10. Fang L, Hsiung MC, Miller AP, Nanda NC, Yin WH, Young MS, et al. Assessment of aortic regurgitation by live three-dimensional transthoracic echocardiographic measurements of vena contracta area: usefulness and validation. Echocardiography. 2005;22:775–81.
11. Perez de Isla L, Zamorano J, Fernandez-Golfin C, Ciocarelli S, Corros C, Sanchez T, et al. 3D color-Doppler echocardiography and chronic aortic regurgitation: a novel approach for severity assessment. Int J Cardiol. 2013;166:640–5.
12. Sato H, Ohta T, Hiroe K, Okada S, Shimizu K, Murakami R, et al. Severity of aortic regurgitation assessed by area of vena contracta: a clinical two-dimensional and three-dimensional color Doppler imaging study. Cardiovasc Ultrasound. 2015;13:24.
13. Garbi M, Chambers J, Vannan MA, Lancellotti P. Valve stress echocardiography: a practical guide for referral, procedure, reporting, and clinical implementation of results from the HAVEC Group. JACC Cardiovasc Imaging. 2015;8:724–36.
14. Wahi S, Haluska B, Pasquet A, Case C, Rimmerman CM, Marwick TH. Exercise echocardiography predicts development of left ventricular dysfunction in medically and surgically treated patients with asymptomatic severe aortic regurgitation. Heart. 2000;84:606–14.
15. Vinereanu D, Ionescu AA, Fraser AG. Assessment of left ventricular long axis contraction can detect early myocardial dysfunction in asymptomatic patients with severe aortic regurgitation. Heart. 2001;85:30–6.
16. Myerson SG, d'Arcy J, Mohiaddin R, Greenwood JP, Karamitsos TD, Francis JM, et al. Aortic regurgitation quantification using cardiovascular magnetic resonance: association with clinical outcome. Circulation. 2012;126:1452–60.
17. Vahanian A, Alfieri O, Andreotti F, Antunes M, Barón-Esquivias G, Baumgartner H, et al. Guidelines on the management of valvular heart disease (Version 2012). Eur Heart J. 2012;33:2451–96.

Stress Echocardiography in Aortic Valve Disease

6

Julien Magne, Erwan Donal, Dania Mohty, and Luc A. Pierard

Aortic disease, including aortic stenosis (AS) and aortic regurgitation (AR) is the most common valvular disease and the third most prevalent form of cardiovascular disease in the Western world. The prevalence of aortic disease is around 2–7% in patients >65 years old with 1–2% of AR and 1–5% of AS [1]. This prevalence is increasing with population aging. Aortic disease is now regarded as a growing health problem with sizeable economic impact, especially with ageing population and increased exposure to risk factors related to AS development paralleling obesity and metabolic disorders epidemic. Together, these considerations suggest that the burden of AS and AR will markedly increase over the next 25 years.

The diagnosis of AS and AR is classically based on transthoracic echocardiography (TTE) and may be complemented by other imaging modalities. After a long asymptomatic phase, patients with aortic disease may have an increased risk of harmful cardiovascular events such as symptom occurrence and/or deterioration, ventricular dysfunction, heart failure and even death.

There is general agreement that when severe AS or AR is accompanied by one or more symptoms (e.g. fatigue, exercise intolerance, breathlessness, chest pain, syncope or resuscitated sudden death) aortic valve replacement (AVR) (i.e. surgical- [SAVR] or trans-catheter- [TAVR]) is recommended because of well-established dismal outcome of non-operated symptomatic cases, with relatively low

J. Magne, Ph.D. (✉) • D. Mohty, M.D., Ph.D.
Department of Cardiology, Dupuytren University Hospital, Inserm U1094, Limoges University, Limoges, France
e-mail: jumagne8@gmail.com

E. Donal, M.D., Ph.D.
Cardiology Department and CIC-IT 804, CHU Rennes, Rennes, France

L.A. Pierard, M.D., Ph.D.
Department of Cardiology, Heart Valve Clinic, University Hospital Sart Tilman, University of Liège, Liège, Belgium

K. Fattouch et al. (eds.), *Advances in Treatments for Aortic Valve and Root Diseases*, https://doi.org/10.1007/978-3-319-66483-5_6

peri-operative mortality and morbidity after AVR. Thus, symptomatic severe AS or AR are class I indication for surgery in most recent guidelines [2, 3]. The measurement of LV ejection fraction (LVEF) is mandatory for the management of these patients and in case of impaired LV function (i.e. LVEF < 50%) aortic valve intervention is also recommended (class I).

In asymptomatic patients with preserved LV function, the timing of surgery remains controversial and in this regard, the role of exercise stress echocardiography is crucial. It is important to emphasize that exercise test is contraindicated in patients with symptoms and AS. Low dose dobutamine stress echo is more appropriate in patients with AS and depressed LVEF.

In patients with AS, stress echocardiography has been extensively studied. By contrast, there is very few data illustrating the role of stress echocardiography in AR.

6.1 Exercise Stress Echocardiography: Definition and Practical Use

Exercise stress echocardiography refers to TTE performed during exercise. Good training and large experience are required and the use of an adequate exercise stress table and room settings are mandatory (Fig. 6.1). Frequent blood pressure measurements (i.e. at each stage of the test) and continuous 12-lead ECG should to be recorded. The measurement of hemodynamic parameters is preferably performed at peak exercise. Nevertheless, the recording of loops or Doppler signals may be performed throughout the test. The targeted parameters are valve hemodynamics, LV function and systolic pulmonary arterial pressure (SPAP). Exercise-induced change in the LV filling pressure estimation (i.e. E/e′ ratio) should be obtained at low level of exercise (usually around 100–110 bpm) in order to avoid E- and A-waves fusion and to ensure good tissue Doppler imaging quality.

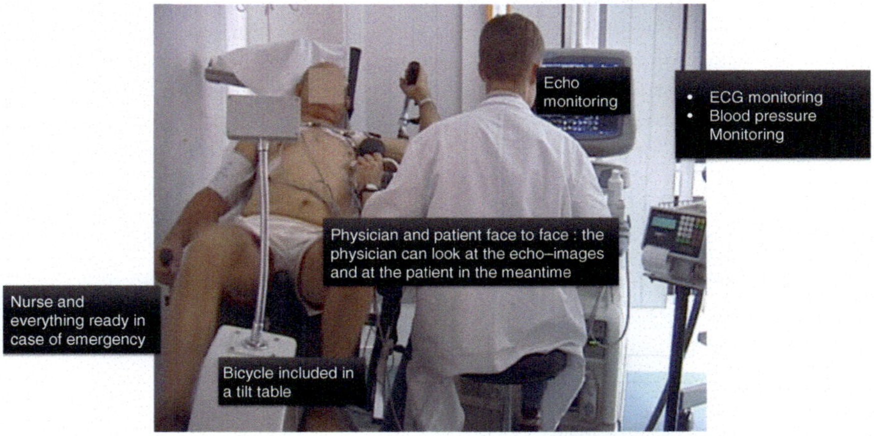

Fig. 6.1 Stress echocardiography lab settings

The dynamic changes in trans-aortic mean pressure gradient and in systolic pulmonary arterial pressure (SPAP) need to be assessed throughout the test, from rest to peak exercise with also measurement at low and intermediate levels of exercise. The biphasic hemodynamic and mechanical responses of both the LV and the aortic valve may be frequent. Hence, it is of high importance to obtain images recording throughout the test in order to reveal this singularity [4].

Early marked increase in trans-aortic mean pressure gradient (e.g. at 70% of the targeted maximal heart rate) may indicate more severe and advanced stage of the disease with significant clinical and outcome implications. Similarly, fast increase in SPAP may indicate poor adaptation of pulmonary vascular function, reduced pulmonary compliance and increased pulmonary resistance.

The assessment of exercise-induced changes in LV systolic function may also very useful. Worsening in LV wall contractility typically indicates an ischemic damage due to coronary artery disease, excessive afterload or both. The use of wall motion score, or more recently the use of 2D speckle tracking imaging, may help to quantify such abnormalities which do not necessarily indicate the presence of significant coronary artery disease. The absence of LV contractile reserve may be a powerful marker of prognosis. The LV contractile reserve is defined as an exercise-induced increase in LV ejection fraction (>5%). The longitudinal myocardial function (derived from tissue Doppler imaging or 2D speckle tracking) may be assessed during exercise and be used as surrogate marker of LV contractile reserve (Fig. 6.2). However, prognostic cut-off value still remains to be defined and validated.

Of note, to the best of our knowledge, exercise-induced increase in AR has never been reported.

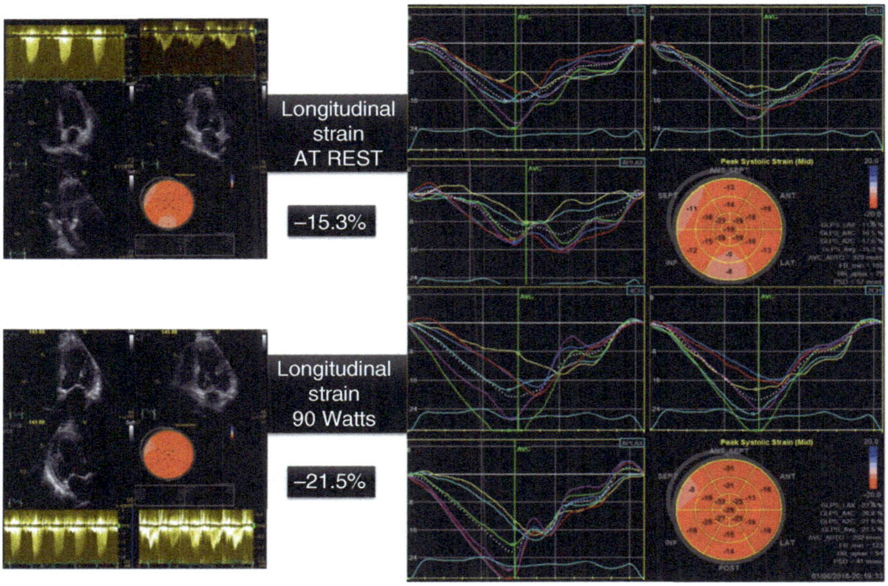

Fig. 6.2 LV contractile reserve using 2D strain

6.2 Clinical and Prognostic Value of Exercise Stress Echocardiography

6.2.1 In Patients with AR

Only few studies, including a small number of patients, have evaluated significant AR using exercise echocardiography [5, 6]. When performed, attention should be focused on LV ejection fraction at exercise. The absence of contractile reserve, i.e. decrease in LVEF ≥5% at exercise—seems to be predictive of LV impairment after surgery. In addition, exercise stress testing can be used to assess symptomatic status and functional capacity in patients with AR. In this regard, exercise stress echocardiography may help to confirm that patients are really asymptomatic or, in opposition, may reveal exertional symptoms.

Asymptomatic patients with a moderately enlarged LV secondary to severe AR and evidence of latent LV dysfunction as assessed using exercise stress echocardiography (i.e. failure to increase LVEF during test) may be strictly followed with short intervals (3–6 months). Surgery may be envisaged but there is no recommendation in the current guidelines. Further data are mandatory in this population.

6.2.2 In Patients with AS

6.2.2.1 Exercise-Induced Changes in Mean Pressure Gradient

The increase in trans-valvular pressure gradient may reflect the presence of either a more severe AS (the more severe the stenosis at rest, the higher the increase in gradient for a given flow rate during exercise) and/or a non-compliant and rigid aortic valve (no or minimal improvement of aortic valve orifice area during test). The latter phenomenon could be related to the presence of highly calcified aortic valve, which is, in turn, considered as an important marker of outcome [7]. The exercise-induced changes in aortic mean pressure gradient should, however, be analyzed in the light of the exercise-induced changes in LV stroke volume. Indeed, markedly increase in LV stroke volume in response to exercise may directly affect the aortic mean pressure gradient, even in the presence of aortic valve opening reserve. In contrast, in highly calcified aortic stenosis, without improvement in aortic valve area during exercise, mild increase in LV stroke volume may produce significant increases in mean aortic pressure gradient.

In asymptomatic moderate to severe AS (valve area <1.2 cm^2), exercise-induced changes in LV function or AS indices are predictive of outcome. An increase in mean trans-aortic pressure gradient by ≥18–20 mmHg during exercise (Fig. 6.3), which may occur in 21–35% of patients, is associated with an increased risk of cardiac events. This has been underlined in two studies, whose one multi-centric.

An exercise-induced increase in mean pressure gradient >18 mmHg has suggested incremental prognostic value over resting echocardiographic data and

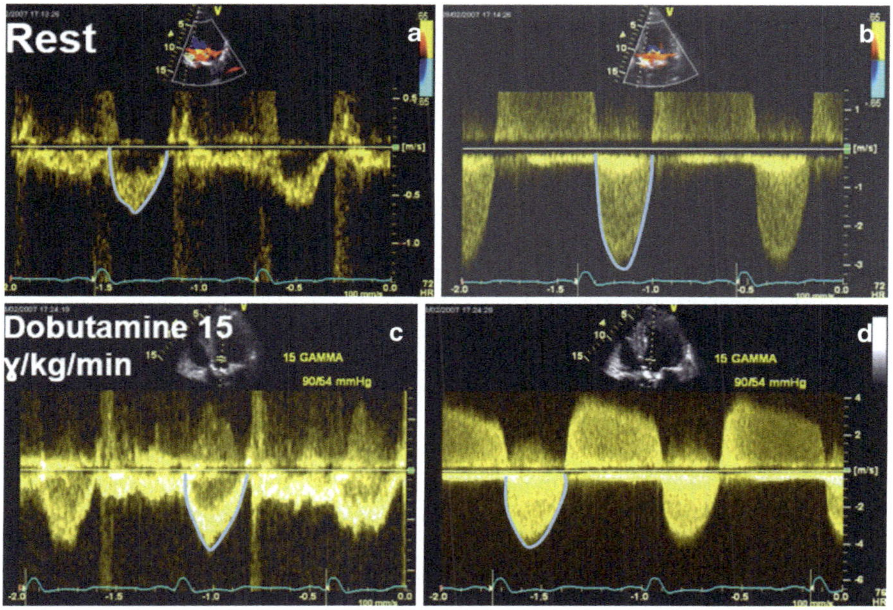

Fig. 6.3 Exercise-induced changes in trans-aortic mean pressure gradient >20 mmHg

exercise ECG [8]. This was confirmed later in a multicenter study reporting the resting and exercise echocardiographic data of 186 "truly" asymptomatic patients (i.e. without abnormality during an exercise test) with at least moderate AS [9]. An exercise-induced increase in mean trans-aortic pressure gradient >20 mmHg was identified as a powerful independent predictor of poor outcome with a 3.8-fold increase in risk of cardiac event (including indication for aortic valve replacement).

6.2.2.2 LV Contractile Reserve

The assessment of the adaptation of LV function during exercise is of clinical interest. Patients with a decrease or limited increase (<5%) in LVEF during exercise are more likely to exhibit an abnormal response to exercise and cardiac-related events during follow-up [10–12]. Abnormal response to exercise (defined as excessive symptoms, fall or <20 mmHg increase in systolic blood pressure and ≥2 mm ST segment depression) was associated with a maladaptation of the LVEF during exercise (decrease or only mild increase).

Others parameters of LV function were used to define the presence or absence of LV contractile reserve. Although derived from small sample sizes study and without external validation, exercise-induced increase in S′-wave velocity >5 cm/s [13] or changes in global longitudinal strain >−1.4% [10] may also be used to assess the presence of LV contractile reserve.

6.2.2.3 Exercise-Induced Changes in Systolic Pulmonary Arterial Pressure

Resting high SPAP and the presence of pulmonary hypertension (PH) (i.e. SPAP >50 mmHg) in patients with severe AS seem to be associated with a poor prognosis [14, 15], a higher mortality rate after valve replacement [16] and represent an independent predictor of hospital mortality and postoperative major adverse cardiovascular and cerebrovascular events [17]. Furthermore, PH is a strong determinant of outcome following TAVI [18].

Exercise PH is generally considered as a predictor of occurrence of resting PHT during the follow-up, development of symptoms and/or outcome in various cardiac diseases [19, 20], including valvular heart disease [18, 21–23].

In a prospective series of 105 "truly" asymptomatic patients with severe AS in whom exercise stress echocardiography was performed, 55% of patients developed exercise PH. Exercise PH development was essentially driven by exercise parameters of diastolic dysfunction burden (i.e. indexed LV end-diastolic volume, exercise e′-wave velocity and exercise-induced changes in indexed left atrial area). More interestingly, the presence of exercise PH doubles the risk of 3-year cardiac event, including higher rate of cardiovascular deaths.

Practically, the measurement of SPAP throughout the exercise could provide useful additive information. However, the dynamic changes in SPAP and the occurrence of exercise PH should be cautiously interpreted and analyzed in light of age, exercise load (especially when symptoms and PH occur at early stage of exercise), and changes in systemic blood pressure and in cardiac output.

6.3 Clinical Implications

In the 2012 ESC guidelines [2], AVR is indicated in asymptomatic severe AS, if the exercise test is abnormal, particularly in case of symptom development (class I, evidence C) or asymptomatic hypotension (class IIa, evidence C). In 2014 ACC/AHA guidelines [3], the indication of AVR is a class IIa in asymptomatic patients with severe AS and equivocal symptoms. Consequently, regarding the most recent expert consensus, it seems reasonable to perform AVR in asymptomatic severe AS patients with preserved LV function but in the presence of exercise abnormalities, i.e. "false" asymptomatic patients.

In patients without exercise abnormalities, i.e. "true" asymptomatic, exercise stress echocardiography may be very useful. Indeed, patients with inconclusive or negative exercise test but with comorbidities and intermediate age (65–75 years old) might have some hemodynamic or LV function alterations that comprehensive exercise echocardiographic test could reveal.

Although the place of exercise stress echocardiography remains weak in current guidelines from both ESC and ACC/AHA, exercise-induced changes in mean transaortic pressure gradient, in LVEF, in LV longitudinal myocardial function and in SPAP may identify a subset of patients with hidden and early consequences of the increased LV afterload produced by the AS. The current ESC guidelines indicate that AVR may be considered in asymptomatic patients with severe AS, normal LV ejection fraction and increase of mean pressure gradient during exercise by

>20 mmHg (class IIb, evidence C). In addition, and despite no clear recommendations, the ESC guidelines state that exercise stress echocardiography may provide prognostic information in asymptomatic severe AS by assessing the changes in LV function. Furthermore, the dramatic increase in cardiovascular event and death observed in patients with occurrence of PH could promote early surgery in these patients. At least, referral to dedicated valvular heart disease clinic [24] and close follow-up (3- to 6-month follow-up) could be indicated. However, this management strategy needs to be confirmed by further prospective data from various centres.

6.4 Low-Dose Dobutamine Stress Echocardiography

In patients with AS and depressed LVEF, more particularly in those with low flow—low gradient (LFLG) AS, low dose dobutamine stress echocardiography may be useful. Indeed, these patients may have a reduced aortic valve area because of inadequate forward LV stroke volume due to underlying cardiomyopathy relative, i.e. "pseudo-severe" AS, or may have fixed severe AS with afterload mismatch, i.e. "true" severe AS (Fig. 6.4). Low dose dobutamine stress TTE is helpful to differentiate patients with pseudo to those with true severe AS.

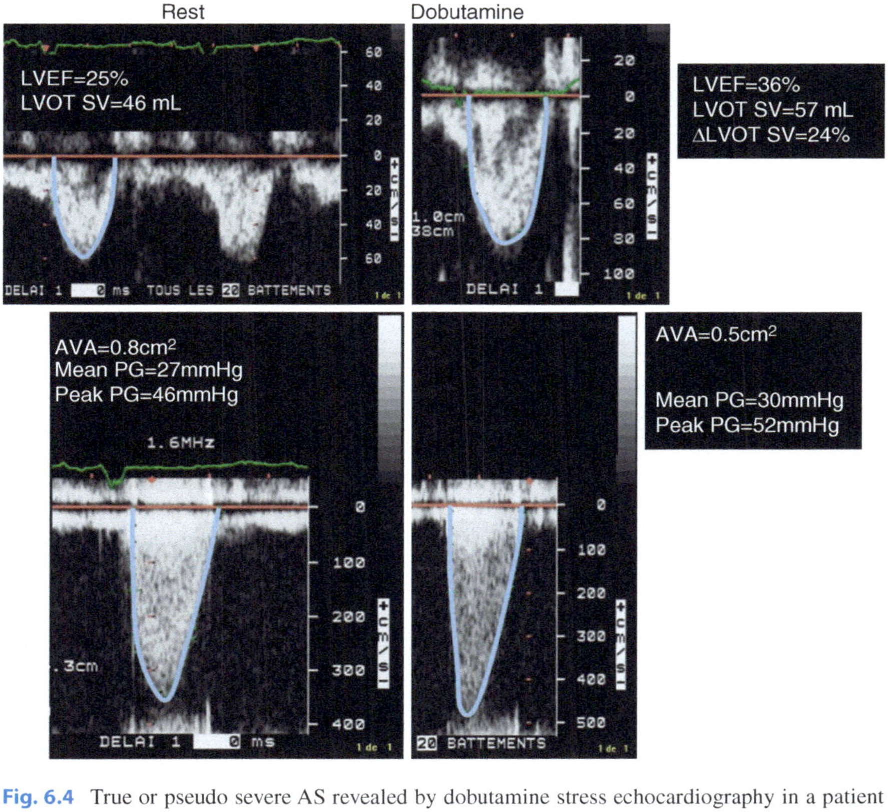

Fig. 6.4 True or pseudo severe AS revealed by dobutamine stress echocardiography in a patient with LFLG AS

In this setting, a dobutamine challenge is recommended to determine the absence or the presence and extent of flow reserve. A low to moderate dose of dobutamine protocol should be used in order to obtain the maximal inotropic effect without chronotropic response. Dobutamine is usually started at 5 μg/kg/min (even 2.5 μg/kg/min may be preferable in very sick patients with poor LV function) and may be increased to 20 μg/kg/min. The duration of each stage and the mode of dose increment at each step are not standardized, with variation from 3 to 5 min and from 2.5 to 5 μg/kg/min. Blood pressure and 12 lead ECG need to be carefully monitored. The test should be stopped when one of the following criteria appears:

- the maximal dose reached
- increase in heart rate >10–20 beats/min
- obvious inotropic response.

With TTE, Doppler measurement of trans-aortic mean pressure gradient and forward LV stroke volume should be performed at each dose of dobutamine. Increase in mean pressure gradient and limited changes in aortic valve area (remaining <1 cm^2), paralleling the improvement of LV contractility is a suggestive sign of "true" severe AS.

The assessment of LV flow reserve, as defined as increase in forward LV stroke volume ≥20% from baseline, need to be performed [25].

In the absence of LV flow reserve, the assessment of AS severity remains challenging and the discrimination between "true" and "pseudo"-severe AS remains unreliable. In this context, the estimation of the projected aortic valve area at normal flow rate may be helpful [7, 26]. Furthermore, the use of CT scan and aortic valve calcium score measurement if of high interest.

6.5 Decision-Making Following Dobutamine Stress Echocardiography in LFLG Severe AS

In patients with LFLG AS, the operative risk is well stratified by dobutamine stress echocardiography. Patients with LV flow reserve and "true" severe AS have an acceptable operative risk. Valve replacement is recommended in most of these patients and usually leads to improved functional status and survival. By opposition, in the absence of LV flow reserve, the operative mortality is prohibitive and the opportunity to perform TAVI should be discussed.

Conclusion

Stress echocardiography in patients with aortic valve disease may be useful to guide decision making and stratify the risk of these patients. In asymptomatic patients with severe AS, exercise stress echocardiography may provide incremental clinical and prognostic value, beyond physical examination and resting echocardiography. Low-dose dobutamine stress echocardiography is particularly helpful in patients with LFLG AS and depressed LV ejection fraction. In patients with AR, the role of stress echocardiography is weaker and there is a profound need for new data from large sample size studies.

MCQ 1: a Dobutamine stress echocardiography is recommended for patients:

1. with a low flow low gradient, depressed LV ejection fraction
2. who are asymptomatic
3. who did a pulmonary oedema independently of the LV ejection fraction
4. with a significant mitral regurgitation associated with the AS
5. with a pulmonary hypertension

Response: 1

MCQ 2: in asymptomatic patients with a severe AS

1. a conventional exercise stress test is contra-indicated
2. an exercise stress echocardiography could be proposed for monitoring the pulmonary pressures
3. an exercise stress echocardiography could be proposed for monitoring the trans-aortic pressure gradient
4. an exercise stress echocardiography could be proposed for looking for a significant coronary artery disease
5. for making sur that the AS is really severe

Responses: 2, 3, 5

MCQ 3: an exercise stress echocardiography in AS is

1. mandatory for every single patient
2. is possible in asymptomatic patients and might help for guiding the strategy
3. has been demonstrated useless as compare to the calcium scoring
4. is recommended with a class I and level of evidence A in the most recent guidelines for asymptomatic patients
5. is proposed by guidelines at the ESC level

Responses: 2, 5

References

1. Nkomo VT, Gardin JM, Skelton TN, Gottdiener JS, Scott CG, Enriquez-Sarano M. Burden of valvular heart diseases: a population-based study. Lancet. 2006;368(9540):1005–11.
2. Vahanian A, Alfieri O, Andreotti F, Antunes MJ, Baron-Esquivias G, Baumgartner H, et al. Guidelines on the management of valvular heart disease (version 2012): The Joint Task Force on the Management of Valvular Heart Disease of the European Society of Cardiology (ESC) and the European Association for Cardio-Thoracic Surgery (EACTS). Eur Heart J. 2012;33(19):2451–96.
3. Nishimura RA, Otto CM, Bonow RO, Carabello BA, Erwin JP III, Guyton RA, et al. 2014 AHA/ACC guideline for the management of patients with valvular heart disease: executive

summary: a report of the American College of Cardiology/American Heart Association Task Force on practice guidelines. J Am Coll Cardiol. 2014;129(23):2440–92.
4. Lancellotti P, Moonen M, Garweg C, Pierard LA. Afterload mismatch revealed by an exercise biphasic response in aortic stenosis. Arch Cardiovasc Dis. 2009;102(6–7):593–4.
5. Wahi S, Haluska B, Pasquet A, Case C, Rimmerman CM, Marwick TH. Exercise echocardiography predicts development of left ventricular dysfunction in medically and surgically treated patients with asymptomatic severe aortic regurgitation. Heart. 2000;84(6):606–14.
6. Forsberg LM, Nylander E, Tamás É. Exercise echocardiography predicts postoperative left ventricular remodeling in aortic regurgitation. Scand Cardiovasc J. 2014;48(1):4–12.
7. Clavel MA, Burwash IG, Mundigler G, Dumesnil JG, Baumgartner H, Bergler-Klein J, et al. Validation of conventional and simplified methods to calculate projected valve area at normal flow rate in patients with low flow, low gradient aortic stenosis: the multicenter TOPAS (True or Pseudo Severe Aortic Stenosis) study. J Am Soc Echocardiogr. 2010;23(4):380–6.
8. Lancellotti P, Lebois F, Tombeux C, Simon M, Chauvel C, Pierard LA. Quantitative exercise echocardiographic assessment of asymptomatic aortic valve stenosis: prognostic implications. Circulation. 2004;110(17):III-709.
9. Marechaux S, Hachicha Z, Bellouin A, Dumesnil JG, Meimoun P, Pasquet A, et al. Usefulness of exercise-stress echocardiography for risk stratification of true asymptomatic patients with aortic valve stenosis. Eur Heart J. 2010;31(11):1390–7.
10. Donal E, Thebault C, O'Connor K, Veillard D, Rosca M, Pierard L, et al. Impact of aortic stenosis on longitudinal myocardial deformation during exercise. Eur J Echocardiogr. 2011;12(3):235–41.
11. Marechaux S, Ennezat PV, LeJemtel TH, Polge AS, de Groote P, Asseman P, et al. Left ventricular response to exercise in aortic stenosis: an exercise echocardiographic study. Echocardiography. 2007;24(9):955–9.
12. Lancellotti P, Karsera D, Tumminello G, Lebois F, Pierard LA. Determinants of an abnormal response to exercise in patients with asymptomatic valvular aortic stenosis. Eur J Echocardiogr. 2007;9(3):338–43.
13. Van Pelt NC, Stewart RA, Legget ME, Whalley GA, Wong SP, Zeng I, et al. Longitudinal left ventricular contractile dysfunction after exercise in aortic stenosis. Heart. 2007;93(6):732–8.
14. Cooper R, Ghali J, Simmons BE, Castaner A. Elevated pulmonary artery pressure. An independent predictor of mortality. Chest. 1991;99(1):112–20.
15. McHenry MM, Rice J, Matlof HJ, Flamm MD Jr. Pulmonary hypertension and sudden death in aortic stenosis. Br Heart J. 1979;41(4):463–7.
16. Copeland JG, Griepp RB, Stinson EB, Shumway NE. Long-term follow-up after isolated aortic valve replacement. J Thorac Cardiovasc Surg. 1977;74(6):875–89.
17. Carnero-Alcazar M, Reguillo-Lacruz F, Alswies A, Villagran-Medinilla E, Maroto-Castellanos LC, Rodriguez-Hernandez J. Short- and mid-term results for aortic valve replacement in octogenarians. Interact Cardiovasc Thorac Surg. 2010;10(4):549–54.
18. Magne J, Pibarot P, Sengupta PP, Donal E, Rosenhek R, Lancellotti P. Pulmonary hypertension in valvular disease: a comprehensive review on pathophysiology to therapy from the HAVEC Group. JACC Cardiovasc Imaging. 2015;8(1):83–99.
19. Van De Bruaene A, La GA, Prior DL, Voigt JU, Delcroix M, Budts W. Pulmonary vascular resistance as assessed by bicycle stress echocardiography in patients with atrial septal defect type secundum. Circ Cardiovasc Imaging. 2011;4(3):237–45.
20. Shim CY, Kim SA, Choi D, Yang WI, Kim JM, Moon SH, et al. Clinical outcomes of exercise-induced pulmonary hypertension in subjects with preserved left ventricular ejection fraction: implication of an increase in left ventricular filling pressure during exercise. Heart. 2011;97(17):1417–24.
21. Magne J, Lancellotti P, Pierard LA. Exercise pulmonary hypertension in asymptomatic degenerative mitral regurgitation. Circulation. 2010;122(1):33–41.
22. Magne J, Lancellotti P, O'Connor K, Van de Heyning CM, Szymanski C, Pierard LA. Prediction of exercise pulmonary hypertension in asymptomatic degenerative mitral regurgitation. J Am Soc Echocardiogr. 2011;24(9):1004–12.

23. Lancellotti P, Magne J, Donal E, O'Connor K, Dulgheru R, Rosca M, et al. Determinants and prognostic significance of exercise pulmonary hypertension in asymptomatic severe aortic stenosis. Circulation. 2012;126(7):851–9.
24. Lancellotti P, Rosenhek R, Pibarot P, Iung B, Otto CM, Tornos P, et al. ESC Working Group on Valvular Heart Disease position paper—heart valve clinics: organization, structure, and experiences. Eur Heart J. 2013;34(21):1597–606.
25. Monin JL, Monchi M, Gest V, Duval-Moulin AM, Dubois-Range JL, Gueret P. Aortic stenosis with severe left ventricular dysfunction and low transvalvular pressure gradients. J Am Coll Cardiol. 2001;37(8):2101–7.
26. Blais C, Burwash IG, Mundigler G, Dumesnil JG, Loho N, Rader F, et al. The projected valve area at normal flow rate improves the assessment of stenosis severity in patients with low flow aortic stenosis: the multicenter TOPAS study. Circulation. 2004;110(17):III-745.

7 Multimodality Imaging Assessment of Prosthetic Aortic Valve

Mohamed-Salah Annabi, Erwan Salaun, Bernard Cosyns, Patrizio Lancellotti, and Philippe Pibarot

7.1 Introduction

Valvular heart disease afflicts more than 100 million persons worldwide and this number is continuously increasing due to the increased incidence of degenerative valvular heart disease with population ageing. Aortic valve disease, and particularly aortic stenosis, is the most common valvular disease [1, 2]. Implantation of a prosthetic heart valve (PHV) currently remains the only available option for the treatment of severe aortic valve disease. Aortic valve replacement (AVR) account for two thirds of all surgical valve procedures [1–3]. Since its introduction in the 1960, AVR has dramatically improved the longevity and quality of life of patients with aortic valve disease. However, this procedure is not a definitive cure, and the native valve disease is often traded for a "prosthetic valve disease". PHVs indeed suffer from several limitations including suboptimal hemodynamics, increased thrombogenicity, and limited durability [4]. There are two main types of PHVs that can be used for surgical AVR: bioprostheses or mechanical valves. The main drawback of the mechanical valves is the thromboembolic risk and thus the life-time requirement for anticoagulation. The main

M.-S. Annabi • E. Salaun • P. Pibarot (✉)
Department of Medicine, Québec Heart and Lung Institute/Institut Universitaire de Cardiologie et de Pneumologie de Québec, Laval University, Québec, QC, Canada
e-mail: Philippe.Pibarot@med.ulaval.ca

B. Cosyns
Cardiology Department (CHVZ), In Vivo Molecular and Cellular Imaging Center, Universitair Ziekenhuis Brussel, Brussel, Belgium

P. Lancellotti, M.D., Ph.D.
Department of Cardiology, University of Liège Hospital, GIGA Cardiovascular Sciences, Heart Valve Clinic, CHU Sart Tilman, Liège, Belgium

GVM Care and Research, E.S. Health Science Foundation, Lugo, RA, Italy

K. Fattouch et al. (eds.), *Advances in Treatments for Aortic Valve and Root Diseases*, https://doi.org/10.1007/978-3-319-66483-5_7

limitation of bioprosthetic valves is the limited durability and the need of re-operation in case of structural valve failure. In the past decades, there has been a shift away from mechanical valves toward greater use of bioprosthetic valves, particularly in patients >65 years of age [1]. Increasingly, younger patients or those with an active lifestyle opt for a bioprosthetic valve to avoid anticoagulation despite its shorter durability compared to a mechanical valve. Transcatheter AVR (TAVR) has emerged as a valuable alternative to surgical AVR for patients at extreme, high or intermediate surgical risk. The number of patients receiving transcatheter PHVs is increasing exponentially.

Although PHV dysfunctions and complications are rare, they are potentially life threatening [1, 4]. While routine assessment and follow-up almost exclusively rely on Doppler-echocardiography, other imaging modalities may be useful when valve dysfunction is suspected or when there is discordance between the echocardiographic assessment and the patient's clinical status [5].

In this chapter, we present a state-of-the-art overview of the use of Doppler-echocardiographic and the complementary role of multi-modality imaging for the assessment of PHV integrity and function following AVR.

7.2 Different Types of Prosthetic Valves

7.2.1 Mechanical Valves

There are three basic types of mechanical prosthetic valves: bi-leaflet, tilting disk, and ball-cage (Fig. 7.1). The St. Jude bi-leaflet valve is the most frequently implanted mechanical prosthesis worldwide. It consists of two pyrolytic semi-circular disks with a slit-like central orifice between the two leaflets and two larger semi-circular

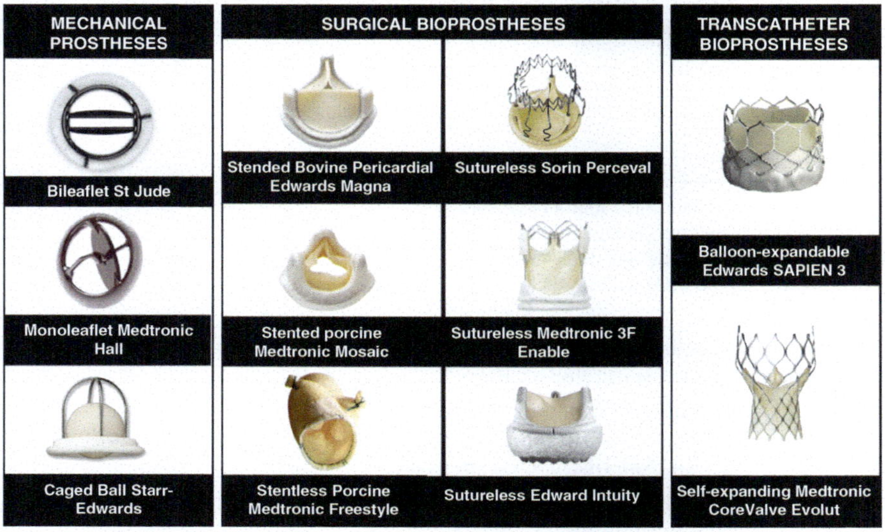

Fig. 7.1 Different types of prosthetic valve models

orifices laterally. The opening angle of the leaflets relative to the annulus plane ranges from 75 to 90°. The Carbomedics valve is a variation of the St. Jude prosthesis that can be rotated to prevent limitation of leaflet excursion by subvalvular tissue.

Tilting-disk or mono-leaflet valves use a single circular disk that rotates within a rigid annulus to occlude or open the valve orifice. The disk is secured by lateral or central metal struts. The opening angle of the disk relative to the valve annulus ranges from 60 to 80° resulting in two orifices of different size.

The bulky Starr-Edwards ball-cage valve, the oldest commercially available prosthetic heart valve first used in 1965, is now very rarely implanted. The ball-cage valve is more thrombogenic, and has less favorable hemodynamic performance characteristics, than either bi-leaflet or tilting disk valves.

Currently available mechanical valves have excellent long-term durability, with up to 45 years for the Starr-Edwards valve and more than 30 years for the St. Jude valve. Structural valve failure (strut fracture with disk embolization, ball variance, etc.) of these prostheses is nowadays extremely rare. Ten-year freedom from valve-related death exceeds 90% for both St. Jude and Carbomedics bi-leaflet valves. All patients with mechanical valves require life-long anticoagulation with a vitamin K antagonist (VKA). Long-term issues associated with mechanical valves include infective endocarditis, paravalvular leaks, hemolytic anemia, thromboembolism/valve thrombosis, pannus in-growth, and hemorrhagic complications related to anticoagulation.

7.2.2 Biological Valves

Tissue or biological valves include stented and stentless bioprostheses (porcine, bovine), homografts (or allografts) from human cadaveric sources, and autografts of pericardial or pulmonic valve origin (Fig. 7.1). They provide an alternative, less thrombogenic heart valve substitute for which long-term anticoagulation in the absence of additional risk factors for thromboembolism is not required.

7.2.2.1 Stented Bioprosthetic Valves

The traditional design of a bioprosthetic valve consists of three biologic leaflets made from the porcine aortic valve or bovine pericardium treated with glutaraldehyde to reduce its antigenicity. The leaflets are mounted on a metal or polymeric stented ring; they open to a circular orifice in systole, resembling the anatomy of the native aortic valve (Fig. 7.1). The vast majority of bioprosthetic valves are treated with anti-calcifying agents or processes. One limitation of earlier generations of bioprosthetic valves was their limited durability due to structural valve deterioration (SVD), typically beginning after 5–7 years following AVR and becoming more frequent after 10–15 years. The process of SVD is accelerated in younger patients, in those with systemic arterial hypertension or phospho-calcic disorders (e.g. end-stage renal disease), and, possibly, in pregnant women. With newer generations of bioprosthetic pericardial valves, the durability is excellent with SVD rates of 2–10% at 10 years, 10–20% at 15 years, and 40% at 20 years [6, 7].

7.2.2.2 Stentless and Sutureless Bioprosthetic Valves

Stentless bioprosthetic valves were developed to improve hemodynamics and potentially reduce mechanical stress on valve leaflets and therefore the risk of SVD (Fig. 7.1). The stentless bioprostheses can be implanted with the subcoronary technique or the root replacement technique. The widespread utilization of this type of valve has, however, been limited by the implantation technique that is more challenging than for other substitutes. More recently, Sutureless stented bioprosthetic valves have been developed to decrease the complexity and duration of valve implantation (Fig. 7.1).

7.2.2.3 Transcatheter Bioprosthetic Valves

TAVR is a valuable alternative to surgical AVR in patients with symptomatic severe aortic stenosis considered to be at extreme, high or intermediate surgical risk. Several hundreds of thousands of patients have undergone TAVR in the past decade. Two main types of transcatheter heart valves (THVs) are currently used: balloon-expandable valves and self-expanding valves (Fig. 7.1).

The first two generations of the Edwards balloon-expandable THVs comprised three leaflets fabricated with equine pericardium (Cribier-Edwards) or bovine pericardium (Edwards SAPIEN) mounted in a stainless steel frame, available in two sizes 23 and 26 mm. The Edwards SAPIEN XT and SAPIEN 3 balloon expandable valves consist of a three-leaflet pericardial bovine valve mounted in a cobalt chromium frame, available in 20, 23, 26 and 29 mm sizes. The main limitation of this new type of PHV is the relatively high rate of paravalvular regurgitation (PVR). Mild to moderate PVR occurs in 30–80% of cases with 5–20% being moderate to severe (VideoClip#11) [8–10]. Moderate-severe PVR is associated with a 2-fold increase in mortality [11]. The third generation SAPIEN 3 valve includes a skirt to reduce PVR. Recent data suggested a reduction of moderate-severe PVR incidence to less than 5% [9].

The first generation of the CoreValve system consisted of a self-expanding nitinol frame with a bovine pericardial valve. The second generation of the CoreValve consisted of three leaflets of porcine pericardium seated higher in the nitinol frame to provide true supra-annular placement. The third generation (EVOLUT R) differs slightly from the previous one in the sealing skirt to reduce paravalvular PVR, and it is available in 26, 29 and 31 mm sizes.

Approximately 75–85% of TAVR procedures are now performed via a transfemoral approach [1, 9]. With the reduction in the sheath sizes (now 14F or 16F for most THVs), the balance is anticipated to shift even more toward the transfemoral approach. The transfemoral approach is associated with lower risk of morbidity and mortality and faster recovery of LV function compared to alternative access approaches (trans-apical, trans-aortic, trans-subclavian etc.).

7.2.2.4 Homografts and Autografts

Aortic valve homografts are harvested from human cadavers within 24 h of death and are treated with antibiotics and cryopreserved at −196°C. They are preferred for management of aortic valve and root endocarditis in the active phase. Neither immune-suppression nor routine anticoagulation is required. However, long-term durability beyond 10 years is not superior to that for current generation pericardial valves [12] and re-operation may be technically more challenging.

In the Ross procedure, the patient's own pulmonary valve or autograft is harvested as a small tissue block and inserted in the aortic position as a complete root replacement with re-implantation of the coronary arteries [12]. The pulmonic valve and right ventricular outflow tract are then replaced with either an aortic or pulmonary homograft. With appropriate patient selection and performance of the procedure by expert surgeons, operative mortality rates are <1% and 20-year survival rates are similar to the general population [13]. Advantages of the autograft include the ability to increase in size during childhood growth, excellent hemodynamic performance characteristics, lack of thrombogenicity, and resistance to infection. However, there is a substantial valve failure rate of the pulmonary homograft [14].

7.3 Doppler Echocardiographic Assessment of Prosthetic Aortic Valves

Doppler echocardiography is the primary imaging modality to assess the structural integrity and function of PHVs as well as the impact on cardiac chambers dimensions and function at baseline (i.e. at the time of AVR) and during follow-up [5].

7.3.1 Baseline Assessment and Timing of Follow-up

An initial transthoracic echocardiographic (TTE) examination performed 6 weeks to 3 months after PHV implantation is recommended to assess the results of surgery and serve as a baseline for comparison should complications or deterioration occur later during follow-up. Repeat TTE as well as transesophageal echocardiography (TEE) is recommended if there is a change in clinical symptoms or signs suggesting valve dysfunction. In patients with a bioprosthetic valve, routine annual TTE follow-up is recommended after year 5 by the European Association of Cardiovascular Imaging (EACVI) and American Society of Echocardiography (ASE) guidelines [5, 15] but not until year 10 by the 2014 AHA/ACC guidelines. Recent studies estimate that 25–30% of patients with a bioprosthesis implanted for less than 10 years in the aortic position have some degree of valve degeneration/dysfunction at TTE exam [7, 16]. In patients with mechanical valves, routine annual TTE is not indicated in the absence of a change in clinical status [1].

A complete echocardiogram includes two-dimensional imaging of the prosthetic valve, evaluation of the valve leaflet/occluder morphology and mobility, measurement of the transprosthetic velocity and gradients, valve EOA, Doppler velocity index, estimation of the degree of regurgitation, evaluation of left ventricular size and systolic function and calculation of systolic pulmonary arterial pressure [5, 15]. PVR is more common following TAVR vs. surgical AVR and the measurement of valve EOA is more challenging in THVs than in surgical valves due to the presence of the valve stent in the LV outflow tract. The evaluation of THV follows the same principles used for the evaluation of surgical prosthetic valves with some specifics and caveats. Transesophageal echocardiography (TEE) is more likely to be needed for mechanical valves and for THVs to evaluate valve morphology, paravalvular region, and associated complications.

7.3.2 Morphologic Characteristics

A ball-caged mechanical PHV displays a cage and the moving echo of the ball on the aortic side. In 2D echo, the metallic struts create highly reflective echoes and the poppet moves forward and backward in the cage. On M-mode, the cage, the sewing ring, and the ball provide four distinct echoes. ***With tilting-disc (monoleaflet) PHVs***, a single echo moving up and down can be seen on the LV side. The opening angle of the disc relative to the valve stent ranges from 60 to 80° resulting in two orifices of different size. On M-mode, the opening of the valve forms an intense echo with multiple reverberations. ***In bileaflet PHVs***, two separate hemi-discs can be visualized. The opening angle of the leaflets relative to the annulus plane ranges from 75 to 90°, with the open valve consisting of three orifices: a smaller, slit-like central orifice between the leaflets, and two larger semi-circular orifices laterally.

In biological valves the leaflets appear thin (<1 mm) with unrestricted motion and no evidence of prolapse [5, 15]. Their 2D and M-mode appearances reveal a box-like opening in systole, similar to that of native aortic valves. The sewing ring and the struts of surgical PHVs (the 3 struts are visualized in the short-axis view) are however more echogenic and may cause acoustic shadowing, which can limit the visualization of the leaflets. In THVs the visualization of the leaflets may also be limited by the shadowing and artefacts caused by the stent. The implantation depth of THVs can be measured in the parasternal long-axis view by measuring the portion of the stent that is below the aortic annulus. An implantation depth superior to 6 mm is associated with a greater risk of PVR and atrioventricular conduction disorders requiring a pacemaker implantation [17]. Stentless aortic bioprostheses, aortic homografts, or pulmonary autografts have a similar appearance to that of native aortic valves, except for an increased thickness in the LV outflow tract and the ascending aorta. Early after implantation, a stentless valve inserted with the subcoronary technique may be surrounded by haematoma and oedema, which generally regress within the first weeks or months after AVR and is associated with improvement in hemodynamics. TEE is superior to TTE to assess valve leaflet morphology and mobility and detect the presence of valve leaflet thickening/calcification and restricted opening.

7.3.2.1 Artefacts

Prosthetic materials, particularly in mechanical models, cause acoustic shadowing, reverberations, refraction, and mirror artefacts, which often affect imaging quality [5, 15]. To overcome these problems multiple including off-axis views may be used, preferably at lower gain settings. The posterior aspect of aortic PHVs may be shadowed on TTE while the anterior aspect may be shadowed on TEE [15, 18].

Microbubbles (or cavitations), exclusively seen in mechanical prostheses, are characterized by a discontinuous stream of rounded, strongly echogenic, fast moving transient echoes. They are localized at the inflow zone. They are probably due to carbon dioxide degassing and linked to hypercoagulability of blood near the valve.

Strands are thin, mildly echogenic, filamentous structures that are often <1 mm thick and >2 mm (up to 30 mm) length, and move independently from the PHV [19].

They can be observed on both mechanical and biological PHVs and are found in 6–45% of patients. They may have a fibrinous or a collagenous composition. The clinical relevance of strands remains unclear.

7.3.3 Hemodynamic Characteristics

The hemodynamic performance of most aortic PHVs is inferior to that of the normal native aortic valve [5]. All normally functioning aortic prostheses cause some degree of obstruction to blood flow which may vary depending on the model and size of prosthesis as well as the patient's body size [20]. Quantitative parameters of PHV function include peak transprosthetic flow velocity, peak and mean transprosthetic pressure gradients, effective regurgitant orifice (EOA) and Doppler velocity index (DVI).

7.3.3.1 Antegrade Flow Patterns and Clicks

The pattern of anterograde flow is unique to each valve and depends on the shape and number of orifices through which forward flows occur. The opening and closing of the leaflet/occluder, often referred to as clicks, manifest as brief, intense and high velocity signals at the beginning and at the end of the Doppler spectrum envelope, and is consistent in each cardiac cycle. In mono-leaflet PHVs, a dense and typically lower velocity jet arises from the major orifice, and a faint higher velocity jet from the minor orifice. Bileaflet PHVs generate three separate jets: dense, lower velocity jet arising from the two lateral orifices and a faint higher velocity jet arising from the central orifice. In Caged-ball PHVs, blood flow goes around the entire circumference of the ball and gives two curved side jets and a large wake in the central part. With bioprostheses, a single central anterograde flow pattern is observed. The flow pattern of THVs differs from that of surgical bioprostheses in the sense that there are two levels of flow acceleration at the inflow aspect of the valve: a first level when the flow enters into the apical portion of the valve stent and a second level when the flow passes through the prosthetic valve leaflets.

7.3.3.2 Transprosthetic Flow Velocity and Gradients

Transprosthetic gradients (ΔP) are measured by Doppler echocardiography using the simplified Bernoulli formula:

$$\Delta P = 4\left(V_2^{\,2}\right)$$

where V_2 is the transprosthetic velocity obtained by continuous-wave Doppler.

The peak velocity across the prosthesis is to some extent related to valve size with the smaller PHVs having higher velocities. However, in case of normally functioning bioprosthesis (where V2 is low) and/or high cardiac output or narrow LV outflow tract (LVOT) (where V1, i.e. velocity in LVOT obtained by pulsed wave Doppler, may be not negligible), estimation of the pressure gradient is more accurately determined by integrating the velocity proximal to the prosthesis into the Bernoulli equation.

Underestimation of the velocities and gradients may occur in case of failure to align the Doppler beam parallel with the highest velocity jet (ideal angle <20°). This can be addressed with multiple window interrogation including apical, right parasternal, suprasternal, and subcostal windows. Gradients may also underestimate the presence and severity of PHV stenosis in presence of any low flow state and/or elevated systemic blood pressure.

Overestimation of the gradients may occur in the following situation: (1) High flow states; (2) Mistaking mitral regurgitation flow signal for transaortic flow signal (MR starts earlier, lasts longer than aortic flow and has a less sharp spectral signal); (3) Presence of significant pressure recovery in any PHV or localized gradients in mechanical PHVs.

7.3.3.3 Effective Orifice Area (EOA)

The EOA is smaller than the anatomic orifice area (AOA) and it corresponds to the smallest area of the jet passing through the prosthesis as it exits the valve (i.e. vena contracta). Clinically, the flow contraction coefficient (EOA/AOA) varies from 0.90 to 0.71. From a pathophysiologic standpoint, the transvalvular pressure gradients are more closely related to the EOA than the AOA.

The prosthetic valve EOA is less flow dependent than the transprosthetic velocity or gradient, and is thus often a better index of intrinsic valve hemodynamic performance. However, this parameter is more prone to technical pitfalls and measurement errors. For both aortic and mitral prosthetic valves, the EOA should be calculated by the continuity equation method using the stroke volume measured using pulsed wave (PW) Doppler in the LVOT (Fig. 7.2) or rarely the right ventricular outflow tract (RVOT):

$$\text{EOA} = \text{CSA} * \text{VTI}_{\text{LVOT}} / \text{VTI}_{\text{PrV}}$$

where the VTI_{LVOT} is the velocity time integral of blood flow in the LVOT measured with PW Doppler in the LVOT just proximal to apical border of the PHV stent/sewing ring, and the VTI_{PrV} is the velocity time integral through the prosthetic valve obtained by continuous wave (CW) Doppler.

VTI_{PrV} tracing should include the total spectral envelope paying attention not to include the feathery part and the clicks. Because the sample volume should be apical to the PHV, the appropriate signal to measure the VTI_{LVOT} should have no opening or closing "clicks". In addition, because the modal velocity (i.e. the most frequently sampled velocity) should be measured, reducing the gain on the spectral Doppler is acceptable to eliminate the faint (less frequently sampled) higher velocity signals.

The measurement of the LVOT diameter is performed in the parasternal long-axis zoomed view with TTE or 120° mid-oesophageal view with TEE. This measurement is often challenging in the presence of an aortic PHV because of the reverberations and shadowing caused by the prosthesis components. LVOT diameter should be measured just proximal to the apical border of the stent from outer border to outer border of the stent (Fig. 7.2). Particular attention should be paid not to mistake the inner border of the prosthesis stent/ring for the inner edge of the

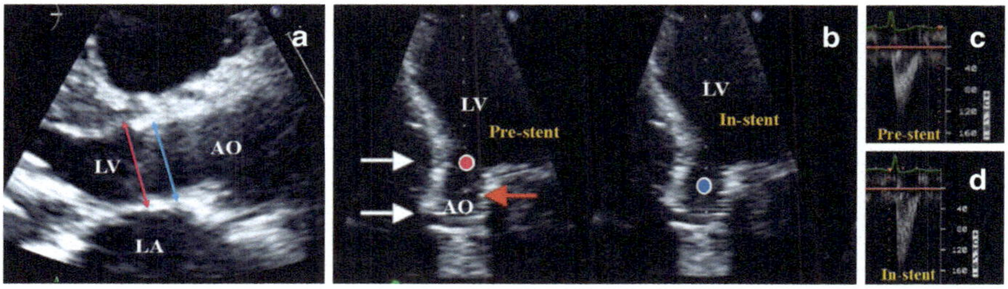

Fig. 7.2 Doppler-echocardiographic measure of stroke volume in presence of a balloon-expandable transcatheter heart valve. Panel (**a**) is a TTE parasternal long-axis zoomed view of the LVOT showing a SAPIEN 23 mm THV. With balloon-expandable THVs, there is a flow acceleration (see LVOT flow velocity at **d** versus **c**) within the apical portion of the stent (pulsed wave Doppler sample at the blue disc in **b**) and it is recommended to use the LVOT diameter (*pink double arrow* in **a**) and velocity (**c**) measured just proximal to the THV stent (pink disc in **b**) to calculate the stroke volume and then the effective orifice area. *White arrows*: aortic and apical borders of the THV stent. *Red arrow*: base of THV leaflets

LVOT. It is important to emphasize that the substitution of the LVOT diameter by the label prosthesis size in the continuity equation is not a valid method to determine the EOA of aortic prostheses. In normally functioning PHVs, the EOA should fall into the normal reference for that prosthetic valve type and size (Table 7.1).

In balloon-expandable THVs, the leaflets are attached close to the apical border of the stent and the flow is often accelerate in the inflow portion of the THV stent. It is thus recommended to measure the LVOT diameter and velocity immediately proximal to the apical end of the stent (Fig. 7.2) [21]. In self-expanding THVs, the leaflets are attached higher in the stent compared to balloon-expandable valves. There is thus no or minimal flow acceleration within the apical portion of the stent. Hence, in self-expanding valves with low implant depth, it may be preferable to measure the LV outflow tract diameter and velocity within the apical (first 5 mm) portion of the stent. As opposed to surgical PHVs, the EOA of a given prosthesis size varies significantly depending on the patient's aortic annulus size [22, 23]. Self-expanding THVs generally have somewhat larger EOAs and lower gradients compared to the balloon expandable THVs but higher incidence of PVR [24, 25].

7.3.3.4 Doppler Velocity Index (DVI)

The DVI is calculated as the ratio of the proximal peak flow velocity (or VTI) in the LVOT to the transprosthetic peak flow velocity (or VTI). For a normally functioning aortic prosthesis, the DVI is >0.30–0.35. Since the DVI is less dependent on valve size, it is helpful to screen for prosthetic valve stenosis, particularly when reliable measure of the LVOT diameter cannot be obtained to calculate the EOA.

7.3.3.5 Parameters of Flow Ejection Dynamics

In a normal aortic PHV, the contour of the CW flow velocity through the prosthesis generally has a triangular shape, with early peaking of the velocity and a short (<100 ms) acceleration time (i.e. the time from the onset of flow to maximal

Table 7.1 Normal reference values in cm² of effective orifice areas for the prosthetic aortic valves

Prosthetic valve size (mm)	**19**	**21**	**23**	**25**	**27**	**29**
Mechanical valves						
Medtronic-Hall	1.2 ± 0.2	1.3 ± 0.2	–	–	–	–
St. Jude Medical Standard	1.0 ± 0.2	1.4 ± 0.2	1.5 ± 0.5	2.1 ± 0.4	2.7 ± 0.6	3.2 ± 0.3
St. Jude Medical Regent	1.6 ± 0.4	2.0 ± 0.7	2.2 ± 0.9	2.5 ± 0.9	3.6 ± 1.3	4.4 ± 0.6
MCRI On-X	1.5 ± 0.2	1.7 ± 0.4	2.0 ± 0.6	2.4 ± 0.8	3.2 ± 0.6	3.2 ± 0.6
Carbomedics Standard and Top Hat	1.0 ± 0.4	1.5 ± 0.3	1.7 ± 0.3	2.0 ± 0.4	2.5 ± 0.4	2.6 ± 0.4
ATS Medical[a]	1.1 ± 0.3	1.6 ± 0.4	1.8 ± 0.5	1.9 ± 0.3	2.3 ± 0.8	–
Stented bioprosthetic valves						
Mosaic	1.1 ± 0.2	1.2 ± 0.3	1.4 ± 0.3	1.7 ± 0.4	1.8 ± 0.4	2.0 ± 0.4
Hancock II	–	1.2 ± 0.2	1.3 ± 0.2	1.5 ± 0.2	1.6 ± 0.2	1.6 ± 0.2
Carpentier-Edwards Perimount	1.1 ± 0.3	1.3 ± 0.4	1.50 ± 0.4	1.80 ± 0.4	2.1 ± 0.4	2.2 ± 0.4
Carpentier-Edwards Magna	1.3 ± 0.3	1.5 ± 0.3	1.8 ± 0.4	2.1 ± 0.5	–	–
Biocor (Epic)	1.0 ± 0.3	1.3 ± 0.5	1.4 ± 0.5	1.9 ± 0.7	–	–
Mitroflow	1.1 ± 0.2	1.2 ± 0.3	1.4 ± 0.3	1.6 ± 0.3	1.8 ± 0.3	–
Trifecta	1.4	1.6	1.8	2.0	2.2	2.4
Stentless bioprosthetic valves						
Medtronic Freestyle	1.2 ± 0.2	1.4 ± 0.2	1.5 ± 0.3	2.0 ± 0.4	2.3 ± 0.5	–
St. Jude Medical Toronto SPV	–	1.3 ± 0.3	1.5 ± 0.5	1.7 ± 0.8	2.1 ± 0.7	2.7 ± 1.0
Prima Edwards	–	1.3 ± 0.3	1.6 ± 0.3	1.9 ± 0.4	–	–
Transcatheter bioprosthetic valves						
Prosthetic valve size (mm)		**20**	**23**	**26**	**29**	**31**
Edwards SAPIEN		NA	1.57 ± 0.43	1.86 ± 0.51	NA	NA
Edwards SAPIEN XT		NA	1.39 ± 0.3	1.73 ± 0.42	2.08 ± 0.52	NA
Edwards SAPIEN 3		1.21 ± 0.23	1.46 ± 0.27	1.74 ± 0.36	1.91 ± 0.39	NA
Medtronic CoreValve [52]			1.47 ± 0.14	1.82 ± 0.48	1.94 ± 0.43	

[a]Adapted from [5]

velocity). However, the acceleration time is highly dependent on heart rate. To overcome this limitation, it is recommended to index the acceleration time to the LV ejection time. A ratio > 0.37 is suggestive of PHV stenosis.

7.3.3.6 Pressure Recovery and Localized High Gradient

In patients with a small aorta relative to the aortic valve EOA, a substantial proportion of the pressure initially lost between the LVOT and the vena contracta may be recovered downstream to the vena contracta. In these patients, transaortic gradients measured invasively by catheter is lower than that obtained by Doppler echocardiography. Not taking into account the pressure recovery may overestimate the severity of PHV stenosis. It is possible to correct the EOA for the extent of pressure recovery by calculating the energy loss coefficient: ELC = (EOA × AA/AA−EOA), where AA is the cross-sectional area of the aorta measured at about 1 cm downstream of the sino-tubular junction [26].

In bileaflet mechanical valves, a localized high velocity may be recorded by continuous wave Doppler through the central orifice of the valve. This may yield to an overestimation of gradient (by an average of 5–15%) and underestimation of EOA compared to cardiac catheterization.

7.3.3.7 Physiologic PHV Regurgitation

All mechanical PHVs have a regurgitant volume (2–10 mL) that may include a closing volume (necessary for closing the occluders), a washing volume (through the components) or both. This is theoretically to prevent blood stasis and thrombus formation. Normal leakage backflow jets are characterized by being narrow at their origin and symmetrical and usually have a homogeneous colour without significant aliasing. Of note, trace (<1 mL) central leakage may be seen in normally functioning bioprosthetic valves.

7.4 Additional Imaging Modalities

Additional imaging modalities, including TEE, cinefluoroscopy, cardiac MDCT, or CMR are generally not performed for routine evaluation of PHVs. However, these modalities may provide important additional information on the morphology and mobility of the valve leaflet/occluder and may help to corroborate the severity of PHV dysfunction.

7.4.1 Cinefluoroscopy

Cinefluoroscopy is the most accurate, economical, and least invasive technique to assess the valve occluder mobility in mechanical aortic prostheses [27, 28]. The opening/closing angles can be calculated in the fully open and closed positions for bileaflet or monoleaflet PHVs. This modality is useful to differentiate acquired PHV stenosis (abnormal occluder mobility) versus prosthesis-patient mismatch (normal mobility) in patients with high transprosthetic gradients. However cinefluoroscopy does not provide clues about the aetiology of reduced occluder mobility (thrombus vs. pannus vs. other).

7.4.2 Cardiac Computed Tomography

Cardiac multidetector computed tomography (MDCT) is a promising complementary technique for evaluation of PHVs. The image quality obtained is adequate for most PHVs except those containing cobalt-chrome alloy rings (e.g. Björk-Shiley and All-carbon tilting-disk prostheses), which cause severe prosthesis-related artefacts [29, 30].

Cardiac MDCT is useful: (1) to assess the morphology and mobility of the PHV leaflet/occluder, (2) to detect the underlying cause of valve obstruction (thrombus, pannus, calcific degeneration of bioprosthetic valve leaflets); and (3) to differentiate thrombus versus pannus [5, 31–34]. Moreover MDCT can be used to quantify the severity of bioprosthetic valve stenosis by measuring the valve anatomic orifice area by planimetry. The paravalvular complications of infective endocarditis may also be identified by MDCT. However, this modality is limited by its inability to assess flow and hemodynamics.

7.4.3 Cardiovascular Magnetic Resonance Imaging

Cardiac magnetic resonance imaging (CMR) with magnetic fields of 1.5 or 3.0 Tesla has been shown to be safe in patients with bioprosthetic or mechanical prosthetic valves. CMR can be used to measure: (1) the anatomic orifice area of bioprosthetic valves by cine CMR and planimetry; (2) the EOA of all types of prosthetic valves by phase-contrast CMR using the continuity equation principle or direct measurement of the vena contracta; (3) the aortic regurgitant volume and fraction using phase-contrast imaging [35–39]. This latter approach may be helpful to corroborate the severity of PVR following TAVR in patients for whom the grading of PVR at Doppler echocardiography is uncertain or discordant with the patient's symptomatic status. The repercussion of prosthesis dysfunction on LV volumes and function can also be assessed using standard cine CMR sequences.

7.4.4 Nuclear Imaging

Nuclear imaging may be useful to detect prosthetic valve endocarditis and associated septic embolism. Because the prosthetic valves are relatively small structures, fusion of the molecular imaging technique (positron emission tomography (PET)) or Single photon emission computed tomography (SPECT) with a robust anatomical imaging technique (MDCT) is necessary [40]. Otherwise, some recent studies suggest that ^{18}F–sodium fluoride PET/CT is also able to identify active tissue calcification and predict disease progression in patients with native aortic stenosis [41]. Future studies should to consider its applicability in the detection of active mineralization in the context of bioprosthetic structural degeneration.

7.5 Prosthetic Valve Dysfunction

Aortic PHV dysfunction, stenosis and/or regurgitation, is generally associated with abnormal valve leaflet/occluder morphology and/or mobility. Imaging may demonstrate the aetiology of dysfunction by showing evidence of leaflet degeneration (thickening, calcification, abnormal mobility) in bioprostheses, abnormal occluder/disc motion in mechanical PHVs, or excessive motion of the sewing ring (Table 7.2).

PHV dysfunction may be categorized into: (1) Structural valve dysfunction, (2) Non-structural valve dysfunction, and (3) Prosthesis-patient mismatch (PPM). Structural valve dysfunction is caused by an intrinsic deterioration of the structure of the PHV, which results in PHV stenosis or transvalvular regurgitation (Table 7.2). Non-structural dysfunction is any abnormality not intrinsic to the valve itself and includes dehiscence of sewing ring or mal-apposition of the stent (paravalvular regurgitation) or entrapment of the occluder by pannus, tissue, thrombus or suture. PPM is not a dysfunction of the prosthesis per se but rather an imbalance between the EOA of the prosthesis and the patient's body size (too small EOA in a too large patient).

7.5.1 Prosthesis-Patient Mismatch

PPM occurs when the valve EOA of a normally functioning prosthesis is too small in relation to the patient's body size (and thus cardiac output requirements), resulting in abnormally high postoperative velocities and gradients. The most widely accepted and validated parameter for identifying PPM is the indexed EOA, i.e., the EOA of the prosthesis divided by the patient's body surface area. Aortic PPM is defined as an EOA that is within the normal range of EOAs for the model and size of prosthesis implanted in the patient (Table 7.1) but that is too small when indexed for patient's body surface area. Aortic PPM is considered present when indexed EOA $<0.85\ cm^2/m^2$ and severe when $<0.65\ cm^2/m^2$). In obese patients (body mass index $\geq 30\ kg/m^2$), it is recommended to use lower cut-points of indexed EOA: $<0.70\ cm^2/m^2$ for overall PPM and $<0.55\ cm^2/m^2$ for severe PPM [5]. Moderate PPM may be quite frequent (20–70%), whereas the prevalence of severe PPM ranges from 2 to 10%. Patients with aortic PPM have worse functional class and exercise capacity, reduced regression of left ventricular hypertrophy, more adverse cardiac events, and increased risk of both perioperative and late mortality after aortic valve replacement when compared with patients who do not have PPM [42]. A greater clinical impact of aortic PPM is also observed in specific groups of patients such as those with pre-existing left ventricular dysfunction or severe left ventricular hypertrophy, and/or concomitant mitral regurgitation, as well as in those

Table 7.2 Role of the different imaging modalities for the assessment of aortic prosthetic valve dysfunction

	Prosthesis-patient mismatch	Thrombosis	Pannus	Structural valve deterioration	Paravalvular regurgitation	Endocarditis
Typical clinical features	Less improvement in symptoms after AVR. Recurrent heart failure.	Sudden onset of symptoms if significant PHV obstruction. May be associated with stroke or TIA. In mechanical PHVs, occurs at any time of FU, often associated with suboptimal anticoagulation. In bioprosthetic PHVs, occurs more frequently within the first months after AVR and is often subclinical (patient is asymptomatic).	Subclinical or progressive onset of symptoms at distance (>5 years) of AVR.	Progressive onset of symptoms and heart failure in case of bioprosthetic valve stenosis. Sudden onset of symptoms in case of bioprosthetic valve leaflet tear and acute regurgitation. Rare in mechanical PHVs.	THV: post procedural regurgitation associated with less improvement in symptoms and recurrent heart failure. Surgical bioprostheses: dehiscence at distance of surgery, new symptoms.	Subacute or acute sepsis with heart failure and/or embolic symptoms.
TTE	Normal valve leaflet morphology and mobility. Increased gradients. Normal EOA but small indexed EOA. Moderate: ≤ 0.85 cm^2/m^2 Severe: ≤ 0.65 cm^2/m^2	Presence of thrombus (i). Valve leaflets thickening/ reduced mobility. Increased gradients Small EOA and DVI. Transvalvular regurgitation.	Presence of pannus. Normal leaflet morphology but mobility may be reduced. Increased gradients. Small EOA and DVI.	Hyper-echogenic, thickened leaflets with reduced mobility and/or teared/avulsed leaflets. Increased gradients. Small EOA and DVI. Transvalvular regurgitation.	Paravalvular regurgitant jet(s) already present at the time of AVR (THV) or developing during FU (often associated with endocarditis). Localization of regurgitant jets and semi-quantitative assessment.	Presence of vegetation(s). New PHV regurgitation (transvalvular or paravalvular) or obstruction. Paravalvular complications: abscess, pseudoaneurysm, fistulae, dehiscence.

TEE	Normal valve leaflet morphology and mobility.	Mechanical valve: Mobile, globular hypo-echogenic mass attached to leaflet occluder or sewing ring/ stent or both. Bioprosthetic valve: diffuse or focal hypo-echogenic leaflet thickening (>2 mm) of at least one leaflet.	Small dense fixed hyper-echogenic structure.	Bioprosthetic valve: diffuse or focal hyper-echogenic leaflet thickening (>2 mm) of at least one leaflet.	Localization of regurgitant jets and semi-quantitative assessment. 3D Color Doppler: Measurement of the vena contracta.	Assessment of valvular and paravalvular lesions.
Cinefluoroscopy	Mechanical valve: Normal occluder mobility.	Mechanical valves: restriction of occluder motion.	Mechanical valves: possible restriction of occluder motion.	May identify severely calcified bioprosthetic valve leaflets.	THV: per-procedural angiography with semi-quantitative assessment with the Seller's classification.	Mechanical valve: possible restriction of occluder motion by a vegetation.
Cardiac CT	No pannus or thrombosis. Normal leaflet/ occluder morphology and mobility.	Mechanical valves: Presence of thrombus with lower attenuation (<200 HU) than fibrotic pannus (>200 HU) or Bioprosthetic valves: Hypo-attenuated leaflet thickening. Restricted mobility of leaflets on 4D CT.	Hypodense mass with a semi-circular anatomical configuration curved along and subvalvular to the valve ring.	Bioprosthetic valves: Presence of leaflet thickening/calcification and reduced mobility.		Assessment of paravalvular lesions.

(continued)

Table 7.2 (continued)

	Prosthesis-patient mismatch	Thrombosis	Pannus	Structural valve deterioration	Paravalvular regurgitation	Endocarditis
CMR				Measurement of GOA by planimetry. Phase contrast CMR: direct measurement of vena contracta or EOA by the continuity equation.	Phase-contrast imaging with measurement of backward flow volume and regurgitant fraction.	
Nuclear Imaging				^{18}F–Sodium fluoride PET/CT to identify active tissue calcification.		Abnormal activity around the site of all valve substitutes implantation detected by ^{18}F–FDG PET/CT (only if the prosthesis was implanted or >3 months) or radiolabelled leukocytes SPECT/CT.

DVI Doppler-velocity index, *EOA* effective orifice area, *GOA* geometric orifice area, *HU* Hounsfield Unit

<65–70 years. PPM is less frequent with TAVR compared to surgical AVR, particularly in the subset of patients with a small aortic annulus [43].

Besides the small indexed EOA, the other findings supportive of the presence of PPM are (Fig. 7.3): (1) the measured (unindexed) EOA is within 0.3 cm^2 of the normal reference value of EOA (Table 7.1); (2) the valve leaflet morphology and mobility are normal; (3) The high gradient is already present early after AVR and, as opposed to acquired PHV stenosis, there is no significant change in gradient or EOA during follow-up (Table 7.2).

One of the key imaging points to distinguish PPM from acquired PHV stenosis is to assess valve leaflet morphology and mobility (Fig. 7.3). TTE, TEE, cinefluoroscopy (mechanical valves) and/or MDCT can be used for this purpose (Table 7.2, Fig. 7.3).

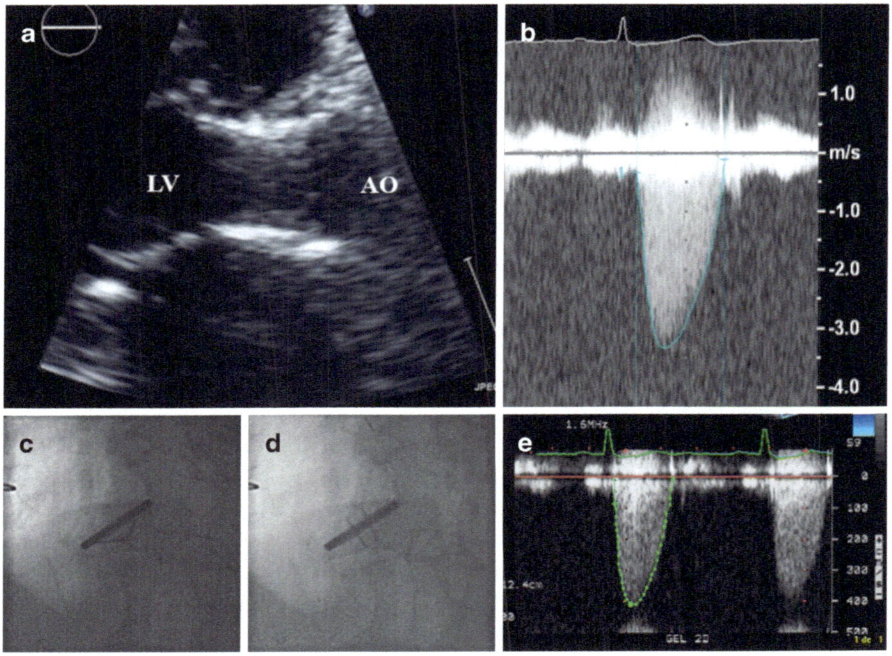

Fig. 7.3 Imaging features of prosthesis-patient mismatch. A transcatheter aortic valve prosthesis (SAPIEN XT 20 mm) with normal morphology and mobility of valve leaflets in parasternal long axis view in systole (Panel **a**) and a mechanical prosthesis (Carbomedics 19 mm) with normal leaflet motion as shown by cinefluoroscopy in diastole (Panel **c**) and systole (Panel **d**). Both valves had elevated transprosthetic gradients (Panel **b**: mean gradient 26 mmHg and Panel E: 39 mmHg, respectively) with a triangular shaped continuous wave Doppler velocity envelope and early peaking velocity. The acceleration time to LV ejection time ratio was <0.37 in both cases. The valve EOA calculated by continuity equation was 1.2 cm^2 (Doppler velocity index 0.35) for the SAPIEN XT valve and 1.06 cm^2 (Doppler velocity index: 0.32) for the mechanical Carbomedics 19 mm valve. These EOAs are within normal range. However, the indexed EOAs were <0.65 cm^2/m^2 (0.63 cm^2/m^2 and 0.53 cm^2/m^2, respectively). All these imaging findings are consistent with the presence of severe prosthesis-patient mismatch

7.5.2 Prosthetic Valve Stenosis

Echocardiographic detection and grading of PHV stenosis include assessment of valve leaflet morphology and mobility by TTE or TEE as well as evaluation of the hemodynamic severity of the stenosis using qualitative and semi-quantitative Doppler parameters (Table 7.3). Other imaging modalities can also be used to assess valve motion, structure, and function. Data should be interpreted according to the date of AVR, the model and size of prosthesis and the patient's hemodynamic conditions.

7.5.2.1 Thrombosis

Thrombus formation is the most common causes of obstruction of mechanical prostheses (≈0.3 to 8% per patient-year). Although less frequent and more insidious, it can also be observed in bioprostheses.

In mechanical PHVs, thrombosis can occur at any time after the surgery and it is often triggered by suboptimal anticoagulation [44]. In patients with (surgical or transcatheter) bioprosthetic valves, the risk of thrombosis is higher within the first 3 months and then to a lesser extent within the first 1–2 years after AVR [44, 45]. The incidence of clinical obstructive bioprosthetic valve thrombosis is around 0.5–1% per patient-year [45]. However, the incidence of subclinical thrombosis may higher (7–13%) particularly in THV [33, 46]. In subclinical thrombosis, valve leaflet thickening is often but not always associated with valve hemodynamic deterioration and the patient is asymptomatic [33, 47].

With significant obstructive PHV thrombosis, patients may present with acute or progressive onset of dyspnea and signs of heart failure, or systemic embolism. The diagnosis of PHV thrombosis should also be suspected in patients with an increase in transprosthetic gradient and a decrease in EOA compared with the previous echocardiographic exam, even if in the absence of any symptom (Table 7.2). With PHV thrombosis, TTE shows valve leaflet thickening with reduced mobility and an increase in mean transvalvular gradient >10 mmHg with concomitant decrease in EOA and DVI (Table 7.3, Fig. 7.4). The valve thrombosis may also be associated with a new transvalvular prosthetic valve regurgitation. However, TTE is often limited by the acoustic shadowing related to the prosthesis components and by the influence of others factors (pericardial effusion, emphysema, obesity, prior sternotomy). Thereby, TEE should be considered when there is suspicion of thrombosis at TTE.

In mechanical valves, the thrombus generally appears as a mobile, globular or linear, hypo-echogenic mass with density similar to that of the myocardium, which is attached to the valve occluder or sewing ring or both. The differential diagnosis between thrombus vs. pannus vs. endocarditis vegetation may be challenging and should take into account the clinical context. Cinefluoroscopy is helpful to assess the consequences of the thrombus, pannus, or vegetation on the mobility of the mechanical valve occluder but does not inform on the aetiology [28]. By measuring the leaflet opening and closing angles, cinefluoroscopy can detect even very subtle degree of restriction of the valve occluder before any hemodynamic or clinical deterioration occurs [5]. In patients with mechanical and bioprosthetic PHVs and inconclusive

Table 7.3 Imaging parameters and criteria for the identification and quantitation of prosthetic valve stenosis

	Normal	Possible stenosis	Significant stenosis
TTE/TEE/Cinefluoroscopy/CT			
Valve structure/leaflet morphology/mobility[a]	Normal	Often abnormal	Abnormal
Doppler quantitative parameters			
Peak velocity (m/s)	<3	3–4	≥4
Mean gradient (mmHg)	<20	20–35	≥35
Doppler velocity index	≥0.35	0.25–0.35	<0.25
Effective orifice area (cm^2)	>1.1	0.8–1.1	<0.8
Difference (Normal EOA[b]—Measured EOA)	<0.30	0.30–0.60	>0.60
Doppler semi-quantitative parameters			
Acceleration time (ms)	<80	80–100	>100
Acceleration time/LV ejection time	<0.32	0.32–0.37	>0.37
Changes in echo parameters during FU			
Increase in mean gradient (mmHg)	<10	10–19	≥20
Changes in echo parameters during stress echo			
Increase in mean gradient (mmHg)	<10	10–19	≥20

EOA effective orifice area, *FU* follow-up. Adapted from [5]

[a]Abnormal mechanical valves: occluder that is immobile or with restricted mobility, thrombus, or pannus; abnormal biologic valves: leaflet thickening/calcification, thrombus, or pannus

[b]For normal EOAs, see Table 7.1

assessment at TTE/TEE, MDCT could provide useful information on PHV structure and function. ECG-gated acquisitions enable dynamic evaluation of PHV leaflets of both mechanical and bioprosthetic valves, anatomic assessment in systole and diastole, and can differentiate between thrombosis and fibrotic pannus ingrowth on the basis of the Hounsfield units (Table 7.2). Thrombosis has lower attenuation than fibrotic pannus ingrowth (similar attenuation as the ventricular septum).

In bioprosthetic valves, thrombosis appears as diffuse hypo-echogenic thickening of valve leaflets that is generally associated with restriction of leaflet mobility (Fig. 7.4). With the more severe forms of THV thrombosis, there is a significant valve stenosis associated with significant hemodynamic deterioration (increase in mean gradient >20 mmHg during follow-up) and development of heart failure symptoms (Tables 7.2 and 7.3). However, in the majority of the cases THV thrombosis is subclinical, i.e. not associated with any symptom, and in many cases, there is no evidence of valve hemodynamic deterioration at TTE and the only detectable sign of THV thrombosis is the visualization of valve leaflet thickening. Because visualization of valve leaflets is often suboptimal at TTE, this modality may lack sensitivity for the identification of valve leaflet thickening and thus subclinical thrombosis. TEE or MDCT are superior to TTE to identify the presence of valve leaflet thickening and reduced mobility associated with subclinical thrombosis (Tables 7.2 and 7.3; Fig. 7.4).

7.5.2.2 Pannus

The incidence of pannus formation causing prosthesis obstruction is similar in biological and mechanical prostheses. Pannus generally occurs several years after AVR. Pannus are less commonly associated with suboptimal anticoagulation than thrombus, and is often subclinical or associated with a progressive onset of symptoms. At TTE or TEE pannus appears as a fixed echo-dense (density similar to pericardium) structure that is generally located at the inflow (more common) aspect of the PHV. With MDCT, pannus is visualised as a hypodense often semi-circular structure at the inflow of the PHV and, as opposed to thrombus, it is not attached to the valve leaflets of hinge mechanism. Pannus may cause some restriction in opening or closing of the valve leaflets, and therefore some degree of PHV stenosis or regurgitation, respectively. However, a pannus may also cause a subvalvular obstruction in the absence of any restriction in leaflet mobility.

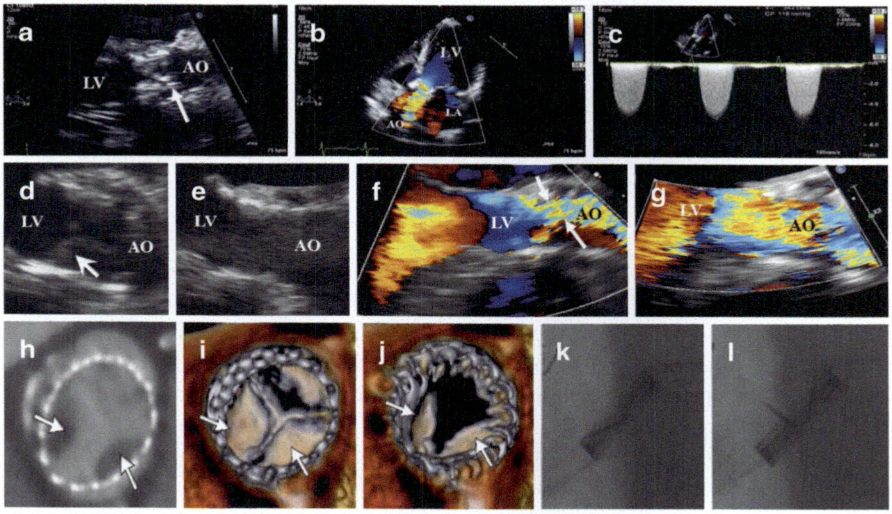

Fig. 7.4 Imaging features of prosthetic valve thrombosis. Panel **a**: TTE parasternal long-axis view of a patient with a transcatheter heart valve (SAPIEN 23 mm) implanted 3 months ago. This view shows thickened leaflets (*white arrow*) with echogenicity similar to myocardium. Panel **b**: TTE 5-chamber view showing turbulent "mosaic" flow (*white arrows*) across the THV. Panel **c**: very high transvalvular gradient with rounded-shaped and late peaking spectral continuous wave Doppler envelope of the aortic valve flow. The peak/mean gradients in this patient are 117/76 mmHg (versus 10/7 mmHg at discharge TTE); the EOA is 0.6 cm^2 and DVI is 0.18 (versus 1.8 cm^2 and 0.39 at discharge); the acceleration time/LV ejection time ratio is 0.55. Panels (**d** and **e**): TEE 120°mid-esophageal view of the valve leaflets (*arrows*) during systole in the same patient before (**d**) and after (**e**) coumadin treatment. There is evidence of valve leaflet thickening and markedly reduced mobility (**d**). After coumadin treatment, leaflet mobility is restored (**e**). Panels (**f** and **g**) show the color Doppler views before and after successful treatment with coumadin. There is a marked narrowing of the transvalvular flow (**f**) that is no longer present after anticoagulation therapy (**g**). Panel H is a MDCT image showing areas of hypo-attenuation at the base of 2 leaflets (*white arrows*) of an asymptomatic patient with a THV; this image is suggestive of subclinical valve thrombosis. Panels (**i**) (diastole) and (**j**) (systole) are 4D MDCT images of the same patient as in H showing restriction in the opening of the leaflets with thrombosis. Panels (**k**) (diastole) and (**l**) (systole) are cinefluoroscopy images showing a bileaflet mechanical valve restricted mobility of one leaflet. Panels (**h** to **j**) are adapted from [48] with permission from Massachusetts Medical Society

7.5.3 Structural Valve Deterioration

Mechanical prostheses have an excellent durability, and structural valve deterioration is extremely rare with contemporary valves, although mechanical failure (e.g., strut fracture, leaflet escape, occluder dysfunction caused by lipid adsorption) occurred with some models in the past. On the other hand, structural valve deterioration due to leaflet calcification and/or collagen fiber disruption is the major cause of bioprosthetic valve failure [4]. There is few data on the long-term follow-up of patients with THV and therefore the exact incidence of THV structural degeneration is not yet well established.

Structural valve deterioration may lead to leaflet stiffening and progressive stenosis or leaflet tear with ensuing often acute transvalvular regurgitation. Although structural valve deterioration of bioprostheses has long been considered a purely passive degenerative process, more recent studies suggest that active and potentially modifiable processes may be involved including lipid infiltration, inflammation, immune rejection, and active mineralization [4].

Structural valve degeneration is typically associated with valve leaflet thickening and calcification at TTE and/or TEE; the leaflets are hyper-echogenic with density similar to that of the prosthesis stent (Table 7.2 and Fig. 7.5). This process may lead to PHV stenosis and/or transvalvular regurgitation. In case of PHV stenosis, the mobility of the leaflets is reduced, the transvalvular flow jet visualized with color Doppler is narrowed and turbulent (Fig. 7.5), and there is a significant increase in gradient (absolute increase in mean gradient >10 mmHg) with concomitant decrease in EOA and DVI compared to the early post AVR TTE (Table 7.3). The measured EOA is substantially lower than the normal reference value of EOA for the model and size of implanted bioprosthesis (Tables 7.1 and 7.3). Structural deterioration may also lead to valve leaflet tear and PHV regurgitation (Fig. 7.5). Mineralization of the valve leaflets is the main culprit lesion for structural valve failure in bioprosthetic valves. Thus in the future, ^{18}F–sodium fluoride PET/CT may be provide a valuable tool for early detection of the mineralization process leading to structural deterioration of bioprosthetic valves [49].

7.5.4 Prosthetic Valve Regurgitation

Doppler echocardiography is the method of choice to localize and quantitate PHV regurgitation (Table 7.4). CMR may also be used when the grading of PHV regurgitation remains uncertain at TTE and/or when there is a discordance between the TTE grading of regurgitation and the patient's clinical status.

7.5.4.1 Transvalvular Regurgitation

The approach to detecting and grading PHV regurgitation is similar to that of native valves and involves color Doppler in multiple views and planes as well as the measurement of several Doppler-echocardiographic parameters (Table 7.4) [5, 15]. It is important to separate physiologic from pathologic prosthesis regurgitation. In the case of pathologic regurgitation, the origin of the regurgitant jet(s) should be localized to distinguish paravalvular from transvalvular regurgitation. In the late postoperative follow-up, the most frequent etiology of pathological transvalvular regurgitation is calcific degeneration and tear of valve leaflets in bioprosthetic valves (Fig. 7.5) and thrombus or pannus in mechanical valves. In addition, the stentless substitutes (stentless bioprostheses, homografts, autografts) are more likely than stented bioprostheses or mechanical valves to develop "functional" central aortic insufficiency due to continued dilation of the aortic root.

There is very limited data on the application and validation of semi-quantitative and quantitative parameters such as the width of the regurgitant jet or of the vena contracta, the effective regurgitant orifice area, and the regurgitant volume and fraction in the context of prosthetic valves [5, 15]. Given that all parameters of aortic regurgitation have important limitations and may be subject to measurement errors, a comprehensive multiparametric integrative approach is recommended (Table 7.4). The guidelines generally suggest to grade prosthetic valve regurgitation according to a 3-class scheme: i.e. mild, moderate and severe [5, 15]. However, some investigators recently suggested to use a more granular grading Scheme (5-class instead of 3-class), where the mild class is subdivided into two sub-classes: i.e. mild and mild-to-moderate and the moderate class into two sub-classes: i.e. moderate and moderate-to-severe [18].

7.5.4.2 Paravalvular Regurgitation

The incidence of PVR is similar in mechanical and biological surgical valves. However, PVR is more frequent following transcatheter AVR than after surgical AVR [18]. After surgical AVR, PVR depends on numerous factors including surgical technique, the size and type of the sewing ring, the position of the valve (annular vs. supra-annular), as well as the quality of the patient's tissues. New onset of PVR late after surgical AVR is often associated with endocarditis. PVR after TAVR is related to the presence and distribution of native aortic valve/annulus calcification, and THV undersizing and/or mal-positioning, which result in circumferential apposition of the THV stent on the native aortic annulus.

Localization of PVR may be difficult and requires TTE imaging in multiple on-axis and off-axis views, as well as TEE is some cases. At TTE, some PVR jets (especially those located laterally or medially) may only be visible on the parasternal short-axis view but, vice versa, other jets may be detected only in the apical views [18]. Indeed, PVR jets located posteriorly are often totally or partially masked in the parasternal short-axis or long-axis views because of the shadowing caused by the prosthetic valve stent. Apical views should thus be carefully examined to properly detect and quantitate these posterior jets. Hence, multi-window and multi-parametric approach is mandatory to properly identify and quantitate PVR by TTE following TAVR. TEE may be useful to improve visualization and quantitation of PVR jets, and especially those located posteriorly [18]. On the other hand, anterior jets may be underestimated with TEE.

Semi quantitative evaluation of the severity of PVR can be achieved by the estimation of the circumferential extent of the PVR jet(s) in the parasternal short-axis

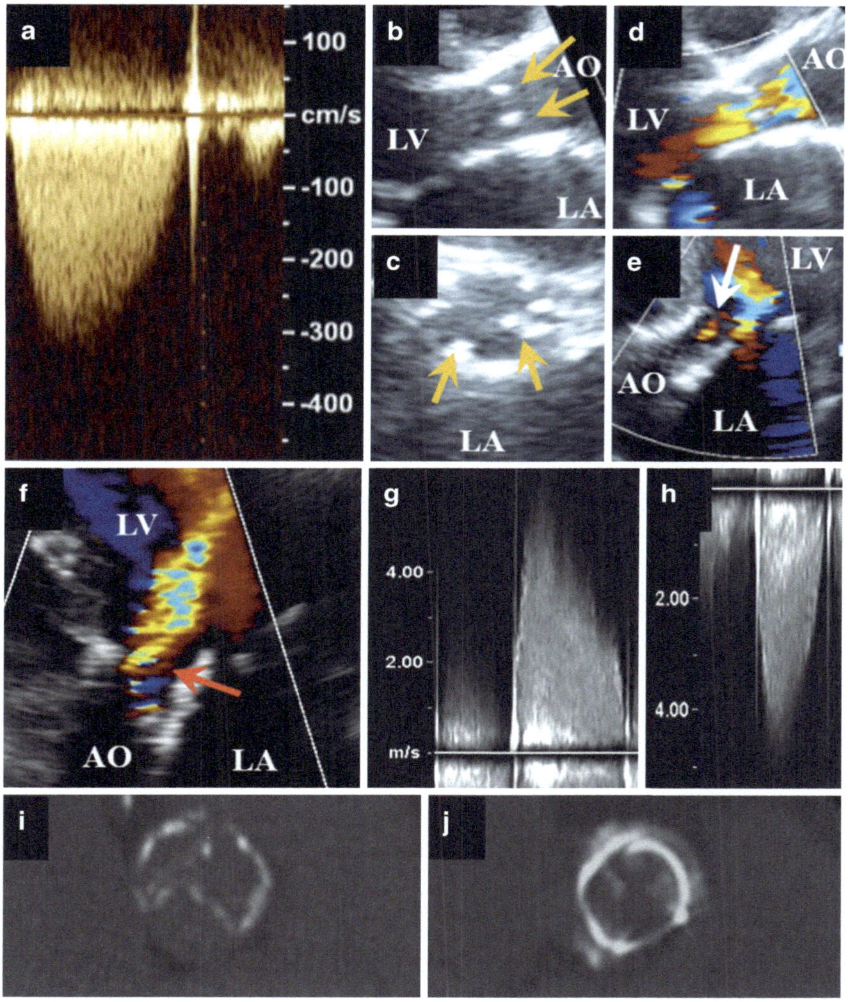

Fig. 7.5 Imaging features of prosthetic valve structural deterioration. Patient with a SAPIEN 3 transcatheter heart valve implanted 3 years ago, with a significant increase of peak/mean gradients (from 15/8 at discharge to 41/24 mmHg) (Panel **a**) and concomitant decrease in EOA (from 1.6 to 0.8 cm^2). Panels (**b** and **c**) are TTE parasternal images showing hyper-echogenic thickening of valve leaflets. The echo density of leaflets is similar to that of the THV stent. Panels (**d** and **e**) show narrowing of color Doppler transvalvular flow during systole (**d**) and a mild transvalvular aortic regurgitation during diastole (**e**). These findings (Panels **a** to **e**) are consistent with calcific structural degeneration of THV leaflets associated with moderate valve stenosis and mild regurgitation. Panels (**f** to **h**) show the TTE images of a surgical bioprosthetic valve implanted 15 years ago. There is a valve leaflet tear with severe transvalvular prosthetic valve regurgitation (*red arrow* in **f**). The continuous wave Doppler image (**g**) shows the aortic regurgitant signal with short pressure half time (200 ms). There is also markedly increased transprosthetic mean gradient (60 mmHg, **h**), which is, in part, due to the presence of moderate-to-severe PHV stenosis (i.e. aortic valve area: 1.0 cm^2) but also to the increased transprosthetic flow related to the prosthetic regurgitation. Panels (**i** and **j**) are MDCT images showing presence of leaflet calcification in a stentless porcine bioprosthesis (**i**) (volumetric leaflet calcification score = 1.35 mm^3) and in a stented pericardial bioprosthesis (**j**) (volumetric leaflet calcification score = 1.04 mm^3. Panels **i** and **j** are adapted from [31] with permission from BMJ Publishing Group Ltd

Table 7.4 Imaging parameters and criteria for the identification and quantitation of prosthetic valve regurgitation

	Mild	Moderate	Severe
TTE/TEE/Cinefluoroscopy/CT			
Valve structure/leaflet morphology/mobility[a]	Normal	Often abnormal	Abnormal
Doppler qualitative or semi-quantitative parameters			
Vena contracta width	<3	3–6	>6
Jet width in transvalvular jets (% LVOT diameter)	≤25	26–64	≥65
Pressure half time (ms)	Slow >500	200–500	Steep <200
Diastolic flow reversal in descending aorta	Absent- brief	Intermediate	Holodiastolic (end-diastolic velocity > 20 cm/s)
Circumferential extent (paravalvular) (%)	<10	10–29	≥30
Doppler quantitative parameters			
EROA (mm^2)	<10	10–29	≥30
Regurgitant volume (mL)[b]	<30	30–59	≥60
Regurgitant fraction (%)	<30	30–49	≥50
CMR			
Regurgitation fraction (%)	<30	30–49	≥50

EROA effective regurgitant orifice area, *LVOT* LV outflow tract. Adapted from [5]

[a]Abnormal mechanical valves: immobile occluder, dehiscence, or rocking (paravalvular regurgitation); abnormal biologic valves: cusps thickening/calcification or prolapse, dehiscence, or rocking (paravalvular regurgitation)

[b]Can be estimated as the difference of stroke volume in LVOT minus stroke volume in RV outflow tract (if no > mild pulmonary regurgitation) or at the mitral annulus (if no > mild mitral regurgitation)

view (Table 7.4 and Fig. 7.6). However, this parameter has not been well validated and is subject to many pitfalls [18]. It is thus important to also assess the other views (parasternal long-axis, apical 5- and 3-chamber); and the other parameters including the width of the jet(s) at its origin, the pressure half-time of the continuous wave Doppler signal of the regurgitant flow, and the estimation of the regurgitant volume by calculating the difference between the LV and RV stroke volumes (Table 7.4) [18]. The role of 3D Color Doppler echocardiography in quantitating PVR is promising but needs further investigation.

Phase-contrast velocity mapping during CMR is a reproducible, accurate and reliable method to quantify the regurgitant fraction in case of PHV regurgitation following transcatheter or surgical AVR, and has been shown to predict future clinical events (Table 7.4 and Fig. 7.6) [37, 39, 50].

7.5.5 Endocarditis

Patients with PHVs are at increased risk for infective endocarditis because of the foreign valve surface and sewing ring. Infective endocarditis occurs in 1–6% of

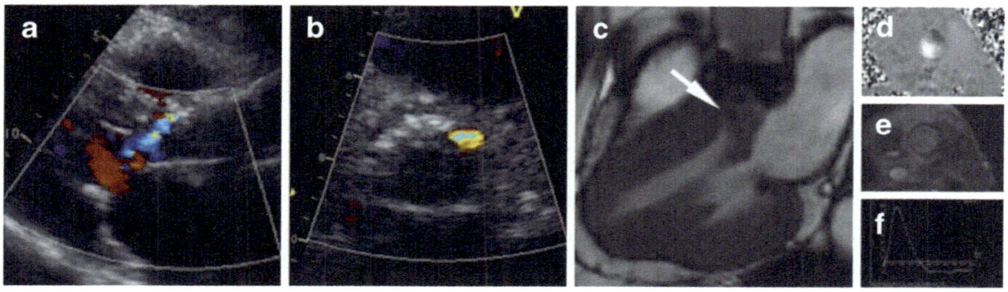

Fig. 7.6 Paravalvular regurgitation in a transcatheter heart valve. Panel **a**: TTE parasternal long-axis view with an eccentric paravalvular regurgitation (PVR) jet. Panel **b**: On the parasternal short axis view, the circumferential extent is about 10%. Panels (**c** to **f**) show CMR images showing in the long-axis view (**c**) an area with a loss of signal (*white arrow*) in diastole that extends from the anterior aspect of the THV stent to the left ventricular outflow tract. Panels (**d** and **e**) show phase imaging acquisitions obtained at the plane just distal to the THV stent and used to determine forward and retrograde flow (**f**) at the upper side of the THV. The regurgitation fraction was 13%, which confirms the presence of a mild aortic regurgitation

patients with PHVs accounting for 10–30% of all cases of infective endocarditis, and this is the most severe form [51]. The diagnosis is based on the Modified Duke Criteria and relies predominantly on the combination of positive blood cultures and echocardiographic evidence of prosthetic valve infection, including vegetations, paravalvular abscess, or a new paravalvular regurgitation. TEE is essential in patients with suspicion of PHV endocarditis and is superior to TTE to detect valvular and paravalvular lesions. MDCT allows to evaluate the presence and severity of paravalvular lesions. Finally recent studies suggested that increased uptake of ^{18}Fluorodeoxyglucose measured by positron emission tomography combined with computed tomography (PET-CT) may improve the early diagnosis of PHV endocarditis [40].

Conclusion

Doppler-echocardiography is the primary imaging modality to assess the structural and functional integrity of PHVs. The particular context of PHVs poses major challenges in terms of imaging and flow dynamics that push this modality to its limits. A comprehensive approach that integrates several parameters of PHV structure and function measured by TTE, TEE is key to appropriately detect and quantitate PHV dysfunction and complications. Other imaging modalities such as cinefluoroscopy, MDCT, CMR, and nuclear imaging are valuable additional tools in the diagnosis and management of PHV dysfunction and complications, particularly when Doppler-echocardiography is inconclusive or discordant with clinical status. TEE, cinefluoroscopy, and MDCT are particularly helpful to identify and quantify the abnormalities of the PHV leaflet/occluder morphology and mobility as well as the paravalvular lesions. CMR may be useful to corroborate the severity of PHV regurgitation.

7.6 Multiple Choice Questions

*: Right answer

7.6.1 Multiple Choice Question #1

At TTE exam performed 8 years after AVR, a male patient (65 y.o, body surface area: 1.95 m^2) with a 21 mm Mosaic bioprosthetic valve has a mean gradient of 32 mmHg, a valve EOA of 1.15 cm^2, and a DVI of 0.32. What is the most likely cause of the elevated transprosthetic gradient? (select only one answer):

1- PHV thrombosis
2- PHV endocarditis
*3- Prosthesis-patient mismatch
4- PHV structural valve degeneration
5- Measurement error.

7.6.2 Multiple Choice Question #2

In patients with aortic PHV, MDCT is useful for (you can select one or several answers):

*1- Identification of subclinical thrombosis in bioprosthetic valves
2- Quantitation of paravalvular regurgitation
3- Assessment of the hemodynamic severity of PHV obstruction
*4- Differentiation between PHV thrombus versus pannus
*5- Assessment of leaflet mobility in bioprosthetic and mechanical PHVs

7.6.3 Multiple Choice Question #3

Which are the TTE findings that can be used to differentiate a PHV stenosis from a prosthesis-patient mismatch (you can select one or several answers):

1- Mean transprosthetic gradient >20 mmHg
*2- Increase in mean gradient during follow-up > +10 mmHg
3- EOA <1.1 cm^2
*4- Difference between normal reference EOA and measured EOA > 0.3 cm^2
5- Indexed EOA < 0.85 cm^2/m^2
*6- Abnormal leaflet morphology/mobility

References

1. Lindman BR, Clavel MA, Mathieu P, Iung B, Lancellotti P, Otto CM, et al. Calcific aortic stenosis. Nat Rev Dis Primers. 2016;2:16006.
2. Iung B, Baron G, Butchart EG, Delahaye F, Gohlke-Barwolf C, Levang OW, et al. A prospective survey of patients with valvular heart disease in Europe: the Euro Heart Survey on valvular heart disease. Eur Heart J. 2003;24(13):1231–43.
3. Benjamin EJ, Blaha MJ, Chiuve SE, Cushman M, Das SR, Deo R, et al. Heart disease and stroke statistics-2017 update: a report from the American Heart Association. Circulation. 2017;135(10):e146–603.
4. Pibarot P, Dumesnil JG. Prosthetic heart valves: selection of the optimal prosthesis and long-term management. Circulation. 2009;119(7):1034–48.
5. Lancellotti P, Pibarot P, Chambers J, Edvardsen T, Delgado V, Dulgheru R, et al. Recommendations for the imaging assessment of prosthetic heart valves: a report from the European Association of Cardiovascular Imaging endorsed by the Chinese Society of Echocardiography, the Interamerican Society of Echocardiography and the Brazilian Department of Cardiovascular Imaging. Eur Heart J Cardiovasc Imaging. 2016;17(6):589–90.
6. Johnston DR, Soltesz EG, Vakil N, Rajeswaran J, Roselli EE, Sabik JF III, et al. Long-term durability of bioprosthetic aortic valves: implications from 12,569 implants. Ann Thorac Surg. 2015;99(4):1239–47.
7. Bourguignon T, Bouquiaux-Stablo AL, Candolfi P, Mirza A, Loardi C, May MA, et al. Very long-term outcomes of the Carpentier-Edwards Perimount valve in aortic position. Ann Thorac Surg. 2015;99(3):831–7.
8. Kodali SK, Williams MR, Smith CR, Svensson LG, Webb JG, Makkar RR, et al. Two-Year outcomes after transcatheter or surgical aortic-valve replacement. N Engl J Med. 2012;366(18):1686–95.
9. Thourani VH, Kodali S, Makkar RR, Herrmann HC, Williams M, Babaliaros V, et al. Transcatheter aortic valve replacement versus surgical valve replacement in intermediate-risk patients: a propensity score analysis. Lancet. 2016;387(10034):2218–25.
10. Leon MB, Smith CR, Mack MJ, Makkar RR, Svensson LG, Kodali SK, et al. Transcatheter or surgical aortic-valve replacement in intermediate-risk patients. N Engl J Med. 2016;374(17):1609–20.
11. Athappan G, Patvardhan E, Tuzcu EM, Svensson LG, Lemos PA, Fraccaro C, et al. Incidence, predictors, and outcomes of aortic regurgitation after transcatheter aortic valve replacement: meta-analysis and systematic review of literature. J Am Coll Cardiol. 2013;61(15):1585–95.
12. El-Hamamsy I, Eryigit Z, Stevens LM, Sarang Z, George R, Clark L, et al. Long-term outcomes after autograft versus homograft aortic root replacement in adults with aortic valve disease: a randomised controlled trial. Lancet. 2010;376(9740):524–31.
13. David TE, David C, Woo A, Manlhiot C. The Ross procedure: outcomes at 20 years. J Thorac Cardiovasc Surg. 2014;147(1):85–93.
14. Briand M, Pibarot P, Dumesnil JG, Cartier P. Mid-term echocardiographic follow-up after Ross operation. Circulation. 2000;102(19 Suppl 3):III-10–I-4.
15. Zoghbi WA, Chambers JB, Dumesnil JG, Foster E, Gottdiener JS, Grayburn PA, et al. Recommendations for evaluation of prosthetic valves with echocardiography and Doppler ultrasound: a report from the American Society of Echocardiography's Guidelines and Standards Committee and the Task Force on Prosthetic Valves, developed in conjunction with the American College of Cardiology Cardiovascular Imaging Committee, Cardiac Imaging Committee of the American Heart Association, the European Association of Echocardiography, a registered branch of the European Society of Cardiology, the Japanese Society of Echocardiography and the Canadian Society of Echocardiography, endorsed by the American College of Cardiology Foundation, American Heart Association, European

Association of Echocardiography, a registered branch of the European Society of Cardiology, the Japanese Society of Echocardiography, and Canadian Society of Echocardiography. J Am Soc Echocardiogr. 2009;22(9):975–1014.
16. Mahjoub H, Mathieu P, Sénéchal M, Larose É, Dumesnil JG, Després JP, et al. ApoB/ApoA-I ratio is associated with increased risk of bioprosthetic valve degeneration. J Am Coll Cardiol. 2013;61(7):752–61.
17. Mauri V, Reimanna A, Stern D, Scherner M, Kuhn E, Rudolph V, et al. Predictors of permanent pacemaker implantation after transcatheter aortic valve replacement with the SAPIEN 3. J Am Coll Cardiol Intv. 2016;9(21):2200–9.
18. Pibarot P, Hahn RT, Weissman NJ, Monaghan MJ. Assessment of paravalvular regurgitation following TAVR: a proposal of unifying grading scheme. JACC Cardiovasc Imaging. 2015;8(3):340–60.
19. Orsinelli DA. Prosthetic valve strands: clinically significant or irrelevant to management? J Am Soc Echocardiogr. 2009;22(8):895–8.
20. Pibarot P, Dumesnil JG. Valve prosthesis-patient mismatch, 1978 to 2011: from original concept to compelling evidence. J Am Coll Cardiol. 2012;60(13):1136–9.
21. Kappetein AP, Head SJ, Généreux P, Piazza N, Van Mieghem NM, Blackstone EH, et al. Updated standardized endpoint definitions for transcatheter aortic valve implantation: the Valve Academic Research Consortium-2 consensus document. Eur J Cardiothorac Surg. 2012;42(5):S45–60.
22. Clavel MA, Webb JG, Pibarot P, Altwegg L, Dumont É, Thompson C, et al. Comparison of the hemodynamic performance of percutaneous and surgical bioprostheses for the treatment of severe aortic stenosis. J Am Coll Cardiol. 2009;53(20):1883–91.
23. Shames S, Koczo A, Hahn R, Jin Z, Picard MH, Gillam LD. Flow characteristics of the SAPIEN aortic valve: the importance of recognizing in-stent flow acceleration for the echocardiographic assessment of valve function. J Am Soc Echocardiogr. 2012;25(6):603–9.
24. Nombela-Franco L, Ruel M, Radhakrishnan S, Webb JG, Hansen M, Labinaz M, et al. Comparison of hemodynamic performance of self-expandable corevalve versus balloon-expandable Edwards SAPIEN aortic valves inserted by catheter for aortic stenosis. Am J Cardiol. 2013;111(7):1026–33.
25. O'Sullivan KE, Gough A, Segurado R, Barry M, Sugrue D, Hurley J. Is valve choice a significant determinant of paravalular leak post-transcatheter aortic valve implantation? A systematic review and meta-analysis. Eur J Cardiothorac Surg. 2014;45(5):826–33.
26. Pibarot P, Garcia D, Dumesnil JG. Energy loss index in aortic stenosis: from fluid mechanics concept to clinical application. Circulation. 2013;127(10):1101–4.
27. Montorsi P, De Bernardi F, Muratori M, Cavoretto D, Pepi M. Role of cine-fluoroscopy, transthoracic, and transesophageal echocardiography in patients with suspected prosthetic heart valve thrombosis. Am J Cardiol. 2000;85(1):58–64.
28. Muratori M, Montorsi P, Maffessanti F, Teruzzi G, Zoghbi WA, Gripari P, et al. Dysfunction of bileaflet aortic prosthesis: accuracy of echocardiography versus fluoroscopy. J Am Coll Cardiol Img. 2013;6(2):196–205.
29. Habets J, Symersky P, van Herwerden LA, de Mol BA, Spijkerboer AM, Mali WP, et al. Prosthetic heart valve assessment with multidetector-row CT: imaging characteristics of 91 valves in 83 patients. Eur Radiol. 2011;21(7):1390–6.
30. Konen E, Goitein O, Feinberg MS, Eshet Y, Raanani E, Rimon U, et al. The role of ECG-gated MDCT in the evaluation of aortic and mitral mechanical valves: initial experience. AJR Am J Roentgenol. 2008;191(1):26–31.
31. Mahjoub H, Mathieu P, Larose É, Dahou A, Sénéchal M, Dumesnil JG, et al. Determinants of aortic bioprosthetic valve calcification assessed by multidetector CT. Heart. 2015;101(6):472–7.
32. Jilaihawi H, Asch FM, Manasse E, Ruiz CE, Jelnin V, Kashif M, et al. Systematic CT methodology for the evaluation of subclinical leaflet thrombosis. JACC Cardiovasc Imaging. 2017;10(4):461–70.
33. Makkar RR, Chakravarty T. Transcatheter aortic valve thrombosis; new problems, new insights. JACC Cardiovasc Interv. 2017;10(7):698–700.
34. Tanis W, Habets J, van den Brink RB, Symersky P, Budde RP, Chamuleau SA. Differentiation of thrombus from pannus as the cause of acquired mechanical prosthetic heart valve obstruction by non-invasive imaging: a review of the literature. Eur Heart J Cardiovasc Imaging. 2014;15(2):119–29.

35. Caruthers SD, Lin SJ, Brown P, Watkins MP, Williams TA, Lehr KA, et al. Practical value of cardiac magnetic resonance imaging for clinical quantification of aortic valve stenosis: comparison with echocardiography. Circulation. 2003;108(18):2236–43.
36. Garcia J, Markl M, Schnell S, Allen B, Entezari P, Mahadevia R, et al. Evaluation of aortic stenosis severity using 4D flow jet shear layer detection for the measurement of valve effective orifice area. Magn Reson Imaging. 2014;32(7):891–8.
37. Ribeiro HB, Le Ven F, Larose É, Dahou A, Nombela-Franco L, Urena M, et al. Cardiac magnetic resonance versus transthoracic echocardiography for the assessment and quantification of aortic regurgitation in patients undergoing transcatheter aortic valve implantation. Heart. 2014;100(24):1924–32.
38. Ribeiro HB, Orwat S, Hayek SS, Larose É, Babaliaros V, Dahou A, et al. Cardiovascular magnetic resonance to evaluate aortic regurgitation after transcatheter aortic valve replacement. J Am Coll Cardiol. 2016;68(6):577–85.
39. Salaun E, Jacquier A, Theron A, Giorgi R, Lambert M, Jaussaud N, et al. Value of CMR in quantification of paravalvular aortic regurgitation after TAVI. Eur Heart J Cardiovasc Imaging. 2016;17(1):41–50.
40. Saby L, Laas O, Habib G, Cammilleri S, Mancini J, Tessonnier L, et al. Positron emission tomography/computed tomography for diagnosis of prosthetic valve endocarditis: increased valvular 18F-fluorodeoxyglucose uptake as a novel major criterion. J Am Coll Cardiol. 2013;61(23):2374–82.
41. Dweck MR, Jenkins WS, Vesey AT, Pringle MA, Chin CW, Malley TS, et al. 18F-NaF uptake is a marker of active calcification and disease progression in patients with aortic stenosis. Circ Cardiovasc Imaging. 2014;7(2):371–8.
42. Dayan V, Vignolo G, Soca G, Paganini JJ, Brusich D, Pibarot P. Predictors and outcomes of prosthesis patient mismatch after aortic valve replacement. JACC Cardiovasc Imaging. 2016;9(8):924–33.
43. Pibarot P, Weissman NJ, Stewart WJ, Hahn RT, Lindman BR, McAndrew T, et al. Incidence and sequelae of prosthesis-patient mismatch in transcatheter versus surgical valve replacement in high-risk patients with severe aortic stenosis: a PARTNER trial cohort—a analysis. J Am Coll Cardiol. 2014;64(13):1323–34.
44. Roudaut R, Serri K, Lafitte S. Thrombosis of prosthetic heart valves: diagnosis and therapeutic considerations. Heart. 2007;93(1):137–42.
45. Latib A, Naganuma T, Abdel-Wahab M, Danenberg H, Cota L, Barbanti M, et al. Treatment and clinical outcomes of transcatheter heart valve thrombosis. Circ Cardiovasc Interv. 2015;8(4):1–8.
46. Hansson NC, Grove EL, Andersen HR, Leipsic J, Mathiassen ON, Jensen JM, et al. Transcatheter aortic heart valve thrombosis: incidence, predisposing factors, and clinical implications. J Am Coll Cardiol. 2016;68(19):2059–69.
47. del Trigo M, Munoz-Garcia AJ, Wijeysundera HC, Nombela-Franco L, Cheema A, Gutierrez E, et al. Incidence, timing and predictors of valve hemodynamic deterioration after transcatheter aortic valve replacement: Multicenter registry. J Am Coll Cardiol. 2016;67(6):644–55.
48. Makkar RR, Fontana G, Jilaihawi H, Chakravarty T, Kofoed KF, De Backer O, et al. Possible subclinical leaflet thrombosis in bioprosthetic aortic valves. N Engl J Med. 2015;373(21):2015–24.
49. Jenkins WS, Vesey AT, Shah AS, Pawade TA, Chin CW, White AC, et al. Valvular (18) F-fluoride and (18)F-fluorodeoxyglucose uptake predict disease progression and clinical outcome in patients with aortic stenosis. J Am Coll Cardiol. 2015;66(10):1200–1.
50. Nombela-Franco L, Eltchaninoff H, Zahn R, Testa L, Leon MB, Trillo-Nouche R, et al. Clinical impact and evolution of mitral regurgitation following transcatheter aortic valve replacement: a meta-analysis. Heart. 2015;101(17):1395–405.
51. Habib G, Lancellotti P, Antunes MJ, Bongiorni MG, Casalta JP, Del Zotti F, et al. 2015 ESC guidelines for the management of infective endocarditis: the task force for the management of infective endocarditis of the European Society of Cardiology (ESC) endorsed by: European Association for Cardio-Thoracic Surgery (EACTS), the European Association of Nuclear Medicine (EANM). Eur Heart J. 2015;36(44):3075–128.
52. Spethmann S, Dreger H, Schattke S, Baldenhofer G, Saghabalyan D, Stangl V, et al. Doppler haemodynamics and effective orifice areas of Edwards SAPIEN and CoreValve transcatheter aortic valves. Eur Heart J Cardiovasc Imaging. 2012;13(8):690–6.

Aortic-Mitral Coupling

8

Wendy Tsang, Karima Addetia, and Roberto M. Lang

Aortic-mitral coupling is the concept that aortic and mitral valve function are linked due to their anatomic connection. In this chapter, we will discuss not only the anatomy underlying this coupling but also the studies examining the effects of pathology on this coupling behavior.

8.1 Anatomy

The aortic and mitral valves are connected via a fibrous continuity known as the aortic-mitral curtain (Fig. 8.1). To appreciate the importance of this connection, it is necessary to understand the anatomy of the aortic and mitral valves as these valves themselves are part of a larger complex. The aortic valve is part of the aortic root complex, which is composed of the sinuses of Valsalva, the fibrous inter-cusp triangles and the valve cusps [1–3]. The transition from the left ventricle to the aortic root is defined by the basal attachment of the aortic valve cusps. While approximately two-thirds of the circumference of the lower portion of the aortic root is connected to the ventricular septum, the remaining one-third is connected to the mitral valve via the aortic-mitral curtain.

The mitral valve is part of a complex that includes the annulus, commissures, leaflets, chordae tendinae, papillary muscles, and left ventricle. The mitral annulus

W. Tsang, M.D., M.Sc.
Division of Cardiology, Department of Medicine, University of Toronto, Toronto General Hospital, University Health Network, Toronto, ON, Canada
e-mail: wendy.tsang@uhn.ca

K. Addetia, M.D. (✉) • R.M. Lang, M.D.
Section of Cardiology, Department of Medicine, Heart and Vascular Center, University of Chicago Medicine, Chicago, IL, USA
e-mail: kaddetia@medicine.bsd.uchicago.edu; rlang@medicine.bsd.uchicago.edu

K. Fattouch et al. (eds.), *Advances in Treatments for Aortic Valve and Root Diseases*, https://doi.org/10.1007/978-3-319-66483-5_8

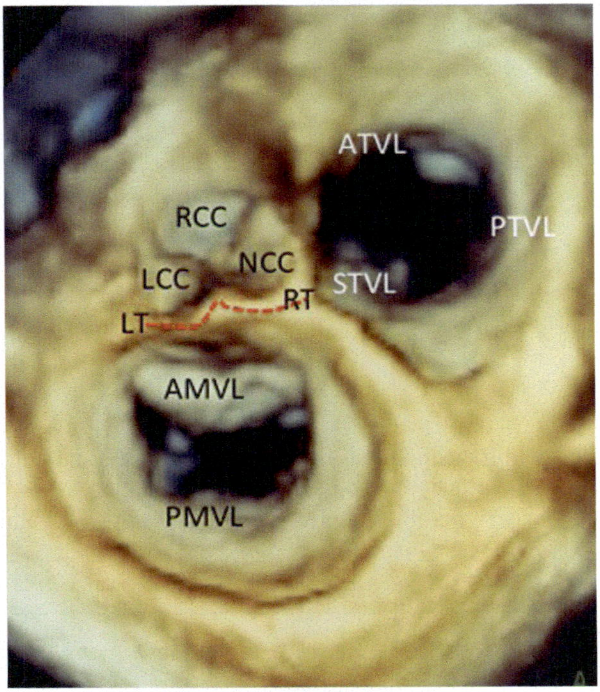

Fig. 8.1 Three-dimensional echocardiographic image demonstrating the location of the aortic-mitral curtain (*dashed red line*) in relation to the aortic and tricuspid valves. *AMVL* anterior mitral valve leaflet, *ATVL* anterior tricuspid valve leaflet, *LCC* left coronary cusp, *LT* left trigone, *NCC* non-coronary cusp, *PMVL* posterior mitral valve leaflet, *PTVL* posterior tricuspid valve leaflet, *RCC* right coronary cusp, *RT* right trigone, *STVL* septal tricuspid valve leaflet

is a fibromuscular ring to which the anterior and posterior mitral valve leaflets attach. It can be divided into the anterior and posterior annulus based on the insertion of the corresponding leaflets. The anterior portion of the annulus attaches to the right and left fibrous trigone. The right trigone is a fibrous area situated between the mitral, tricuspid, and non-coronary cusp of the aortic valve and membranous septum. The left trigone, is the fibrous area located between the left cusp of the aortic annuli and the most anterior portion of the mitral annulus [4]. The fibrous region between the left and right trigones forms part of the aortic-mitral curtain.

8.2 Normal Physiology

Given the anatomical link between the aortic and mitral valves, normal physiologic function of the aortic and mitral valves should be coupled [5]. However, prior to the development of three-dimensional echocardiography (3DE), this interdependence was not appreciated, as two-dimensional imaging techniques could not fully evaluate the complex three-dimensional interaction between these two valves. Thus, the aortic and mitral valves in humans were studied in isolation. However, with advances in 3DE this valvular coupling has now been studied in normal human hearts [6].

These studies have demonstrated that when mitral annular area is maximal during early diastole, aortic annular area is at its minimum (Fig. 8.2). Conversely, when

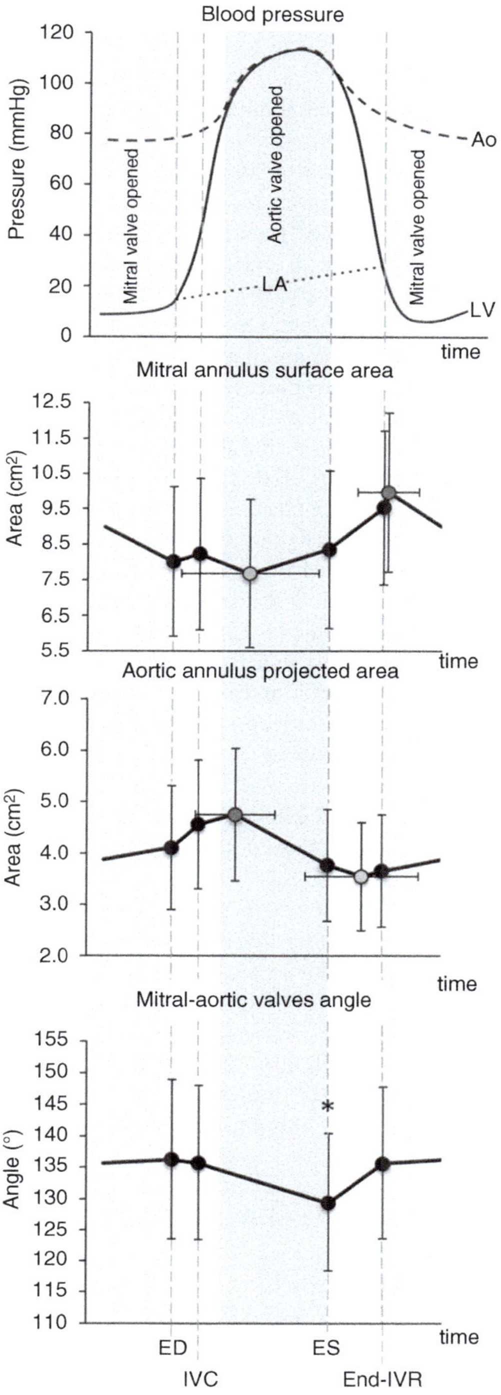

Fig. 8.2 Blood pressure diagram (*top*), in correspondence with measured MA surface area, AoA projected area and mitral-aortic valves angle computed at end-diastole, IVC, end-systole, and end of end-IVR (*vertical dashed lines*). Reprinted with permission from Veronesi F, et al. Circ Cardiovasc Imaging. 2009;2:24–31

mitral annular area is at its minimum during systole, aortic annular area is at its peak value. Thus, there is a synchronized reciprocal behavior between the mitral and aortic valves.

When regional annular areas are examined, important differences related to the aortic-mitral fibrous continuity are identified. The left and right semilunar portions of the aortic annulus showed the same behavior as the overall aortic annular area, while the non-coronary semi-lunar portion, which is connected to the aortic-mitral fibrous continuity showed no significant changes throughout the cardiac cycle. Also, the height of the commissure point between the non-coronary and the left cusps was significantly smaller than the other two commissural heights at all phases of the cardiac cycle. Dimensions of non-coronary inter-commissural distance and semi-lunar aortic annular segment were also significantly larger than left and right ones at end-isovolumic relaxation.

For the mitral valve, the anterior portion of the mitral annulus, which is connected to the aortic-mitral curtain, demonstrated less motion throughout the cardiac cycle than the posterior portion of the annulus. Additionally, maximum anterior mitral annular displacement was significantly smaller than the posterior one.

This relative 'fixedness' of the connected portions of the aortic and mitral annuli was also reflected by changes between the center and the angle between the valve annuli. Throughout the cardiac cycle, the aortic annular center remained in the same plane that contained the mitral annular center. However, during isovolumic contraction the aortic annular center moved outwards increasing the angle and distance between the aortic and mitral annular centers. Subsequently, during systole, both annular centers moved synchronously towards the apex. Then during isovolumic relaxation, the aortic annular center moved inward, reaching minimal distance between the aortic and mitral annuli. However, the narrowest angle between the aortic and mitral valves was found at end-systole. Finally, during diastole the aortic annular center moves towards the left ventricular base, attaining its original position.

Overall, these results suggest that the fibrous continuity acts as an anchor simultaneously affecting the dynamics of both valves and explains why the aortic and mitral valve behavior are coupled with reciprocal behavior during the cardiac cycle. This reciprocity may contribute to the efficiency of the heart as a pump because mitral annular contraction may facilitate aortic annular expansion leading to improved blood flow through the aortic valve during left ventricular ejection. Conversely, aortic annular contraction may facilitate mitral annular expansion, which improves blood flow through the mitral valve during left ventricular filling.

8.3 Impact of Aortic Valve Pathology

Given the knowledge of normal aortic-mitral valvular interaction, it suggests that diseases or surgical processes affecting one valve may have unanticipated effects on the dynamics of the other 'uninvolved' valve. Sclerocalcific aortic

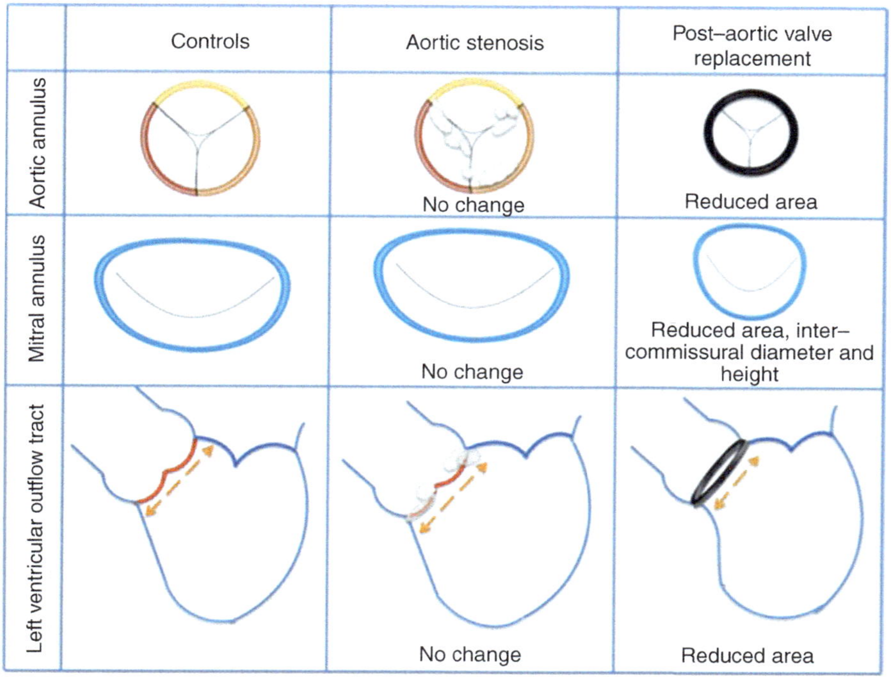

Fig. 8.3 Changes to the aortic and mitral valve in patients with severe aortic stenosis treated with surgical aortic valve replacement. Reprinted with permission from Tsang W, et al. J Am Soc Echocardiogr. 2013;26:606–14

stenosis (AS) is the most common valve disease in North America and treatment involves surgical valve replacement or the recently introduced aortic transcatheter valve implantation [7]. Aortic-mitral coupling has been studied in patients with isolated aortic stenosis undergoing surgical and transcather aortic valve replacement [8, 9].

First, in patients with severe aortic stenosis, there is a reduction in mitral annular motion although there are no changes in mitral annular area or height (Fig. 8.3). After surgical aortic valve replacement, there is a reduction in mitral annular area, height and displacement [8, 10, 11]. When the mitral annulus is examined more closely, it is observed that the inter-commissural but not the antero-posterior mitral annular distances were reduced. Additionally, the presence of the prosthetic valve not only resulted in a reduction in aortic annular area throughout the cardiac cycle but also prevented left ventricular outflow tract expansion.

These findings can be explained by the fact that during surgery, the prosthetic aortic valve ring is attached to the aortic-mitral curtain creating a fixed segment in the fibrous portion of the mitral annulus. Restriction of this segment of the mitral annulus results in a reduction in mitral annular area throughout the cardiac cycle, which is also the likely mechanism responsible for reduced mitral regurgitation post-aortic valve replacement noted in clinical studies [12]. In normal hearts, a reduction in mitral annular area during left ventricular ejection is required for mitral valve leaflet competency [13]. Thus, in patients with aortic stenosis and mitral regurgitation, after aortic valve replacement the smaller mitral annular area during left ventricular systole contributes to improved mitral valve leaflet competency reducing regurgitation severity.

The presence of mitral annular calcium may also increase the restriction in the mitral annulus post-surgery, amplifying the effect of the prosthetic aortic valve. Alternatively, it must be noted that following aortic valve replacement, left ventricular volume and pressure reduction secondary to a reduction in afterload may be an additional mechanism for the reduction in mitral annular area.

After surgical aortic valve replacement, the aortic annular area was significantly reduced throughout the cardiac cycle and was accompanied by a reduction in left ventricular outflow tract area, which affects left ventricular emptying dynamics. The reduction in left ventricular outflow tract area after aortic valve replacement is likely related to the reduction in aortic annular area resulting from the prosthetic ring, which prevents expansion of the anterior portion of left ventricular outflow tract. By suturing the aortic valve ring into the aortic annulus, there is fixation of the aortic-mitral annular continuity with resultant loss of mobility of the posterior portion of the left ventricular outflow tract, which is also the fibrous segment of the anterior mitral annulus. Thus, tethering from the prosthetic valve ring reduces the ability of the left ventricular outflow tract to increase in size during the cardiac cycle. Overall, surgical aortic valve replacement changes the geometry and dynamic three-dimensional motion of the aortic and mitral valves thus affecting left ventricular inflow and outflow patterns.

In another study where patients were treated with transcatheter aortic valve implantation, pre-implantation mitral annular height, area in addition to motion were significantly reduced (Fig. 8.4) [9]. This is in contrast to the surgical study where only mitral annular motion was reduced prior to valve replacement and is likely due to the more severe nature of the aortic stenosis in this population. Following transcatheter aortic valve implantation, mitral annular height and area remained reduced due to a predominant reduction in the mitral annular antero-posterior diameter. Mitral annular motion also remained reduced with a significantly wider end-systolic aortic-mitral annular angle.

Thus, in severe aortic stenosis and its treatment with transcatheter aortic valve implantation, there are two mechanisms by which mitral annular structure is affected. First, in severe aortic stenosis, mitral annular height, area and motion are reduced due to the calcification of the aortic-mitral fibrous continuity. Secondly, post-transcatheter aortic valve implantation patients with moderate-to-severe

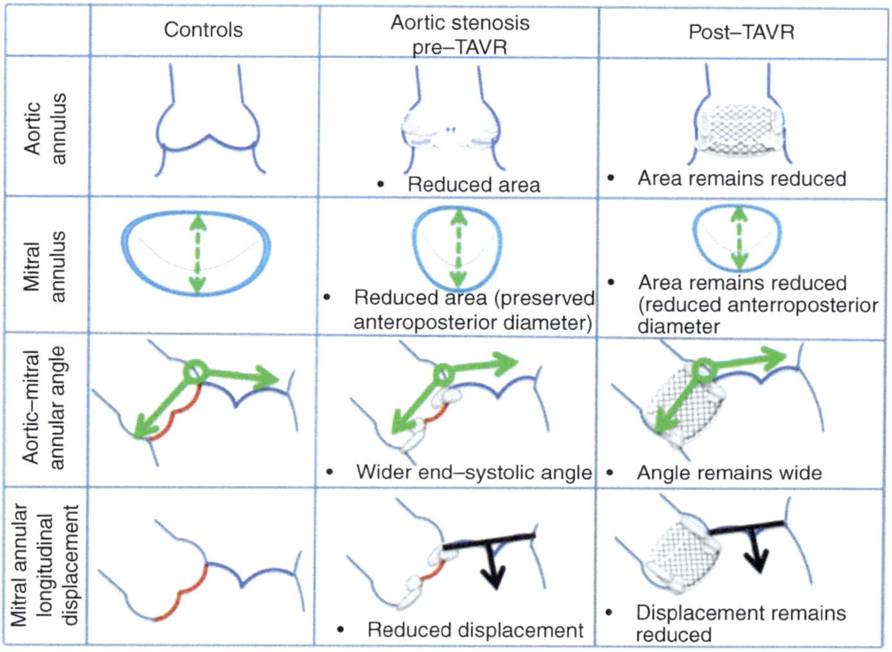

Fig. 8.4 Changes to the aortic and mitral valve in patients with severe aortic stenosis treated with transcatheter aortic valve implantation. Reprinted with permission from Tsang W, et al. Eur Heart J Cardiovasc Imaging. 2013;14:950–6

mitral annular calcification had significantly smaller mitral annular measurements compared to those with mild or no mitral annular calcification due to compression of the calcified aortic annulus against the aortic-mitral curtain by the transcatheter valve. The transcatheter valve strengthens aortic calcium along the aortic mitral curtain and reinforces anterior mitral annular calcium, which results in a reduction in mitral annular height, area and motion. This reinforcement also appears to restrict the normal hinge motion between the aortic and mitral annuli leading to a wider systolic angle.

The previous changes to the mitral annulus in patients with transcatheter aortic valve replacement are in contrast to the results of two other studies [11, 14]. The first paper compared surgical to transcatheter aortic valve replacement [11]. They found that mitral annular parameters measured before and after transcatheter aortic valve implantation were not significantly changed compared to changes seen with surgical aortic valve replacement. The authors concluded that transcatheter aortic valve implantation better preserved mitral annular geometry than surgical aortic valve replacement. Thus, transcatheter aortic valve replacement probably is a more physiologic approach. However, this study was limited in that it only studied ten patients in each group and had no control group.

In the second paper, 90 patients undergoing transcatheter aortic valve replacement were divided into two groups based on the presence or absence of mitral leaflet tethering [14]. While mitral annular parameters were smaller in the non-tethered group, there were no significant changes in mitral annular parameters when comparing these before and after transcatheter aortic valve implantation in both groups. While both groups experienced a reduction of mitral regurgitation post-valve implantation, leaflet tethering parameters and valvular-arterial impedance only decreased after aortic valve implantation in the leaflet-tethering group. Overall, the authors concluded that short-term improvement in mitral regurgitation was because of a decrease in valvular-arterial impedance and an improvement of mitral leaflet tethering rather than a change in mitral annular function.

8.4 Impact of Mitral Valve Pathology

Aortic-mitral coupling has also been studied in patients with mitral regurgitation undergoing mitral valve repair [15, 16]. These studies have demonstrated that there are no significant changes to aortic-mitral coupling or aortic annular dynamics when mitral valve disease with severe mitral regurgitation is present. However, post-mitral valve repair, it has been shown that the aortic valve annulus has reduced pulsatility and motion throughout the cardiac cycle due to the rigid structure of the mitral annuloplasty ring (Fig. 8.5). Thus, constriction imposed by mitral valve repair predominantly affects aortic annular dynamics and consequently the aortic-mitral coupling mechanism, and less so aortic valve morphology.

When patients who received complete versus partial mitral annuloplasty rings were studied, a significant impairment in left ventricular hemodynamics was observed in patients who received circumferential rings. These patients had a significant reduction in aortic annular compliance and flexibility [16]. Also, patients with complete rings had smaller effective mitral areas, which resulted from obstruction of the mitral valve orifice by the anterior mitral leaflet because opening movement was impaired through a posterior shift of the anterior mitral valve leaflet pivot point (Fig. 8.6). This impairment did not exist in patients who had flexible partial circumference rings because the anterior mitral valve leaflet is not fixed by the annuloplasty band and thereby allows 'natural' motion of the aortic-mitral fibrous continuity during the cardiac cycle.

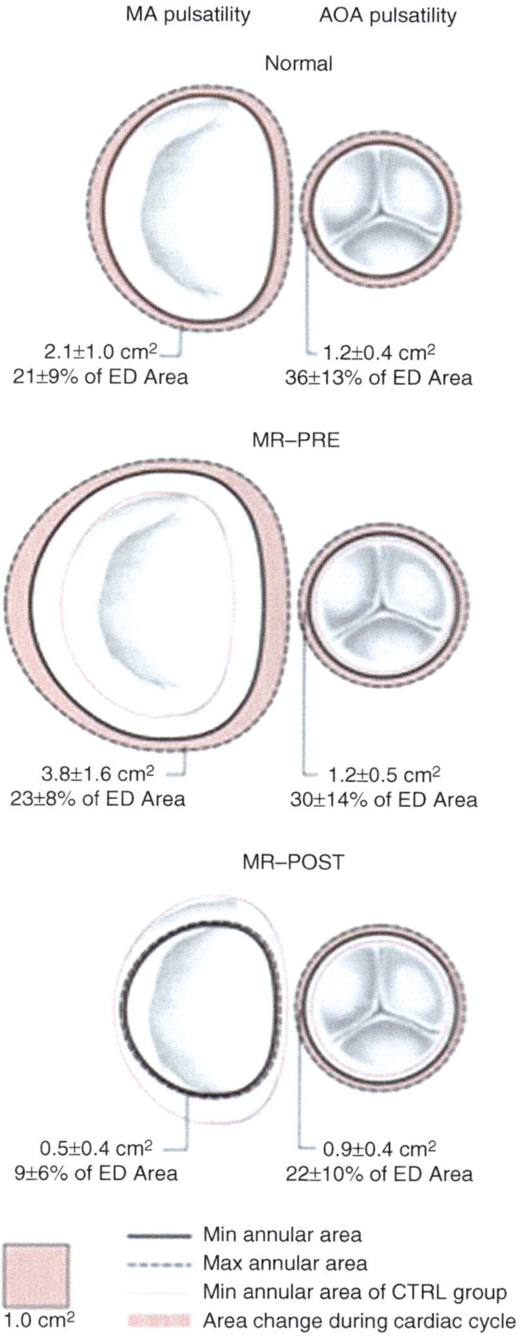

Fig. 8.5 Scale drawing of MA and AoA area and percentage area change (pulsatility) with respect to the end-diastolic (ED) frame in the control (CTRL) and MR patient groups before (MR-PRE) and after (MR-POST) repair with annuloplasty. For each patient group, maximal and minimal area for both the MA and the AoA are plotted, respectively, as *dashed* and *solid lines*. The *red*-shaded area represents the amount of annular size change. In MR-POST patients, this MA area change was almost invisible because of the constrictive effect of annuloplasty. The sizes of drawn annuli are to scale, and the proportion between annular diameters is respected in the graph. Reprinted with permission from Veronesi et al. J Am Soc Echocardiogr. 2012;25:524–31

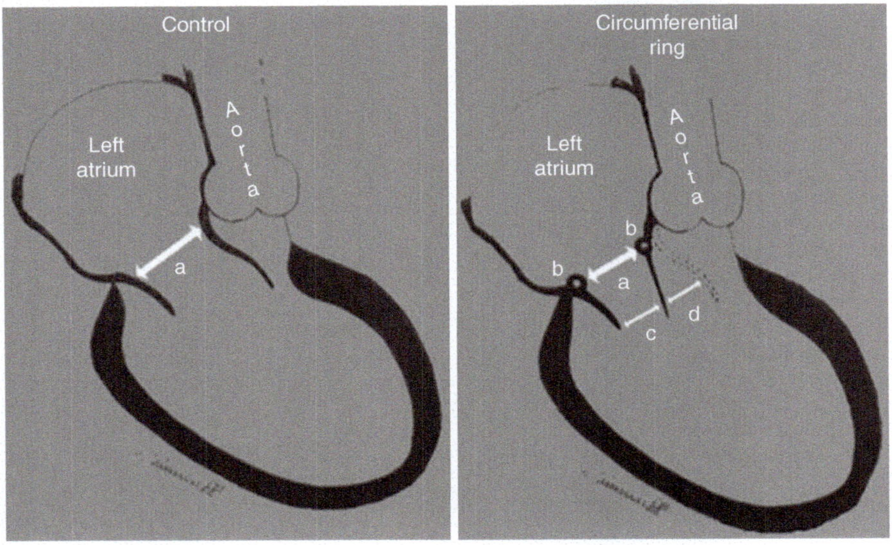

Fig. 8.6 Cartoon demonstrating changes to the mitral valve annulus with implantation of a circumferential annuloplasty ring. (**a**) mitral annular diameter; (**b**) circumferential ring; (**c**) the effective orifice diameter; (**d**) anterior mitral leaflet opening movement. Reprinted with permission from Caimmi PP. et al. Ann Thorac Surg. 2009;88:740–5

8.5 Summary

Due to their anatomic linkage, aortic and mitral valve function are coupled with reciprocal behavior during the cardiac cycle. Due to this relationship, disease processes and interventions affecting one valve have unintended effects on the other. The development of prosthetic valves or annulolasty rings for the aortic and mitral valves should assess the impact on aortic and mitral annular dynamics as these changes have an impact not only on their function but also ventricular function.

MCQ Questions

1. The aortic-mitral curtain does not include the following anatomic structures:
    a. One-third of the lower portion of the aortic root
    b. The region between the left and right trigone
    c. Portion of the left coronary cusp
    d. Portion of the right coronary cusp
2. During normal aortic-mitral coupling, the following is incorrect:
    a. Aortic annular area is at its minimum when mitral annular area is at its maximum.
    b. Aortic annular area is at its maximum when mitral annular area is at its maximum.

   c. Mitral annular area is at its minimum when aortic annular area is at its maximum.
   d. The anterior portion of the mitral annulus demonstrates less motion than the posterior portion of the mitral annulus throughout the cardiac cycle.
3. Which of the following are not affected by mitral valve repair by an annuloplasty ring?
   a. Aortic valve morphology
   b. Aortic annular dynamics
   c. Effective mitral area
   d. Anterior mitral valve leaflet motion

MCQ Answers:

1. **D**. The aortic-mitral curtain consists of the fibrous region between the aortic and mitral valves. This includes one-third of the lower portion of the aortic root and the fibrous region between the left and right trigone, which lies along the left and non-coronary cusp. The right coronary cusp is not part of the aortic-mitral continuity.
2. **B**. Due to aortic-mitral coupling, there is a synchronized reciprocal behavior between these two valves. When mitral annular area is maximal during early diastole, aortic annular area is at its minimum. Conversely, when mitral annular area is at its minimum during systole, aortic annular area is at its peak value. Also, due to its connection to the aortic-mitral curtain, the anterior portion of the mitral annulus is more 'fixed' compared to the posterior portion.
3. **A**. Aortic valve morphology is not affect by implantation of a mitral annuloplasty ring but aortic root dynamics, effective mitral area and motion of the anterior mitral valve leaflet are.

References

1. Piazza N, de Jaegere P, Schultz C, Becker AE, Serruys PW, Anderson RH. Anatomy of the aortic valvar complex and its implications for transcatheter implantation of the aortic valve. Circ Cardiovasc Interv. 2008;1(1):74–81.
2. Anderson RH. Clinical anatomy of the aortic root. Heart. 2000;84(6):670–3.
3. Underwood MJ, El Khoury G, Deronck D, Glineur D, Dion R. The aortic root: structure, function, and surgical reconstruction. Heart. 2000;83(4):376–80.
4. Berdajs D, Zund G, Camenisch C, Schurr U, Turina MI, Genoni M. Annulus fibrosus of the mitral valve: reality or myth. J Card Surg. 2007;22(5):406–9.
5. Lansac E, Lim KH, Shomura Y, Goetz WA, Lim HS, Rice NT, et al. Dynamic balance of the aortomitral junction. J Thorac Cardiovasc Surg. 2002;123(5):911–8.
6. Veronesi F, Corsi C, Sugeng L, Mor-Avi V, Caiani EG, Weinert L, et al. A study of functional anatomy of aortic-mitral valve coupling using 3D matrix transesophageal echocardiography. Circ Cardiovasc Imaging. 2009;2(1):24–31.
7. Bonow RO, Carabello BA, Chatterjee K, de Leon AC Jr, Faxon DP, Freed MD, et al. 2008 focused update incorporated into the ACC/AHA 2006 guidelines for the management of patients with valvular heart disease: a report of the American College of Cardiology/American

Heart Association Task Force on Practice Guidelines (Writing Committee to revise the 1998 guidelines for the management of patients with valvular heart disease). Endorsed by the Society of Cardiovascular Anesthesiologists, Society for Cardiovascular Angiography and Interventions, and Society of Thoracic Surgeons. J Am Coll Cardiol. 2008;52(13):e1–142.
8. Tsang W, Veronesi F, Sugeng L, Weinert L, Takeuchi M, Jeevanandam V, et al. Mitral valve dynamics in severe aortic stenosis before and after aortic valve replacement. J Am Soc Echocardiogr. 2013;26(6):606–14.
9. Tsang W, Meineri M, Hahn RT, Veronesi F, Shah AP, Osten M, et al. A three-dimensional echocardiographic study on aortic-mitral coupling in transcatheter aortic valve replacement. Eur Heart J Cardiovasc Imaging. 2013;14(10):950–6.
10. Mahmood F, Warraich HJ, Gorman JH 3rd, Gorman RC, Chen TH, Panzica P, et al. Changes in mitral annular geometry after aortic valve replacement: a three-dimensional transesophageal echocardiographic study. J Heart Valve Dis. 2012;21(6):696–701.
11. Vergnat M, Levack MM, Jackson BM, Bavaria JE, Herrmann HC, Cheung AT, et al. The effect of surgical and transcatheter aortic valve replacement on mitral annular anatomy. Ann Thorac Surg. 2013;95(2):614–9.
12. Ruel M, Kapila V, Price J, Kulik A, Burwash IG, Mesana TG. Natural history and predictors of outcome in patients with concomitant functional mitral regurgitation at the time of aortic valve replacement. Circulation. 2006;114(1 Suppl):I541–6.
13. Timek T, Dagum P, Lai DT, Green GR, Glasson JR, Daughters GT, et al. The role of atrial contraction in mitral valve closure. J Heart Valve Dis. 2001;10(3):312–9.
14. Shibayama K, Harada K, Berdejo J, Mihara H, Tanaka J, Gurudevan SV, et al. Effect of transcatheter aortic valve replacement on the mitral valve apparatus and mitral regurgitation: real-time three-dimensional transesophageal echocardiography study. Circ Cardiovasc Imaging. 2014;7(2):344–51.
15. Veronesi F, Corsi C, Sugeng L, Caiani EG, Weinert L, Mor-Avi V, et al. Quantification of mitral apparatus dynamics in functional and ischemic mitral regurgitation using real-time 3-dimensional echocardiography. J Am Soc Echocardiogr. 2008;21(4):347–54.
16. Caimmi PP, Diterlizzi M, Grossini E, Kapetanakis EI, Gavinelli M, Carriero A, et al. Impact of prosthetic mitral rings on aortomitral apparatus function: a cardiac magnetic resonance imaging study. Ann Thorac Surg. 2009;88(3):740–4.

9 4D Flow Imaging in Aortic Disease

Zhen Qian, Xiao Zhou, and Mani Vannan

9.1 Introduction

The hemodynamics in the cardiovascular system is believed to play a critical role in regulating the functions of the heart and the blood vessels [1]. Alterations in the blood flow pattern are closely related to the progression of cardiovascular diseases, and may contribute to the development of certain pathophysiologies [2]. Aortic hemodynamics is of particular importance, because of the extreme and abrupt variations of flow velocity and pressure presented in the aorta. Blood flow imaging in the aorta is conventionally done using the time-resolved (CINE) 2-dimensional phase-contrast magnetic resonance imaging (2D PC-MRI), which evaluates the flow velocity in a single direction through or within a user selected 2D imaging plane. Compared to echocardiography, PC-MRI flow imaging has a higher signal-to-noise ratio (SNR), and is not limited by the echo acoustic window in selecting the imaging plane, and therefore, achieves a better evaluation of the flow in the aorta.

In recent years, four-dimensional (4D) PC-MRI has been developed and performed in both research and clinical care to study the blood flow in the heart and the great vessels. The 4D PC-MRI data consist of the time-resolved flow velocity data in three orthogonal Cartesian directions (3D + time) in a 3D volumetric region of interest. Data acquisition is typically performed under a free-breathing condition using respiratory control techniques, such as the navigator gating and the self-gating methods. Compared to 2D flow imaging, 4D PC-MRI provides a full volumetric coverage of the region of interest, which makes it possible to retrospectively select

Z. Qian, Ph.D. (✉) • M. Vannan, M.B.B.S.
Department of Cardiovascular Imaging, Piedmont Heart Institute, Atlanta, GA, USA
e-mail: zhen.qian@piedmont.org; mani.vannan@piedmont.org

X. Zhou, M.D. Ph.D.
Department of Cardiology, Chinese PLA General Hospital, Beijing, China
e-mail: zhouxiaosmile@hotmail.com

K. Fattouch et al. (eds.), *Advances in Treatments for Aortic Valve and Root Diseases*, https://doi.org/10.1007/978-3-319-66483-5_9

the 2D slices or 3D sub-regions for the 3D flow quantification and analysis [3]. More importantly, a 4D PC-MRI scan allows more comprehensive visualization and quantification of the time-varying 3D blood flow pattern in a volume of interest, and potentially provides an avenue for the study of the complex relationship between cardiovascular hemodynamics and pathophysiology [4] in the development of cardiovascular disease.

9.2 Image Acquisition

Currently, 4D PC-MRI sequences are not widely available on the major commercial MR systems. Some vendors provide non-commercial 4D PC-MRI pulse sequences as part of a research package, and some institutions opt to develop their own in-house solutions. A major limitation of the current 4D flow imaging technique of the aorta is the lengthy acquisition time (10–15 min typically), which is too long for routine clinical scans. Alternative imaging techniques, such as radial sampling, under-sampling, and compressed sensing, have been developed in an attempt to accelerate 4D flow imaging. With these new technologies, the acquisition time of the 4D flow MRI in the near future may be significantly reduced, which will make the 4D PC-MRI study more applicable in clinical scenarios.

The free-breathing acquisition of 4D flow MRI in the aorta requires respiratory gating to eliminate motion artifacts. Different respiratory gating techniques, such as the navigator gating and self-gating techniques, have been proposed. In navigator gating, a commonly used navigator is the superior-inferior position of the diaphragm. Based on the position of the diaphragm, the navigator triggers MRI acquisition in a specified gating window of the respiratory cycle. The acceptance rate of the gating window is typically set to 50% [5]. When necessary, it needs to be adjusted to achieve a balance between the total scan time and the level of the respiratory motion artifacts.

4D PC-MRI encodes the blood flow velocity in all three space directions. An important imaging parameter of PC-MRI is the upper velocity encoding limit, which is conventionally termed as the Venc. Ideally, the Venc should equal to the maximum flow velocity. A higher flow velocity than the Venc leads to velocity aliasing, which appears as abrupt phase transitions in the flow image. A higher Venc, on the other hand, leads to a lower precision of the flow velocity measurement, and hence, a lower velocity-to-noise ratio. Therefore, before starting a 4D PC-MRI acquisition, the user should first estimate the maximum flow velocity in the region of interest based on the patient's specific pathophysiology, and set the Venc accordingly. For aortic flow imaging, the typical Venc is set to 150–200 cm/s. In patients with aortic diseases, such as aortic stenosis or coarctation, the Venc can be increased to 250–400 cm/s depending on the disease severity [3].

The scan parameters of 4D PC-MRI are determined based on considerations of both image quality and total scan time. The field of view in 4D flow imaging of the aorta is normally set to a sagittal oblique 3D volume that covers the entire thoracic aorta. Spatial and temporal resolutions are typically set to $<2.5 \times 2.5 \times 2.5$ mm^3 and

<40 ms, respectively [5]. In addition, clinical 4D PC-MRI acquisition is commonly performed as a part of a comprehensive cardiovascular MRI study, which often involves the use of MRI contrast agent. Performing 4D flow imaging after the contrast-enhanced studies, such as the myocardial perfusion exam and the delayed enhancement study, can improve the blood-to-tissue contrast and the velocity-to-noise ratio in the 4D PC-MRI images [6].

9.3 Image Pre-Processing

A number of sources may contribute to flow quantification errors in 4D PC-MRI. While some sources can be compensated and corrected automatically on the MRI scanner, there are two major phase errors that need to be addressed in the pre-processing step of the 4D flow data. First, the background phase offset induced by eddy currents has to be compensated. A common strategy is to identify the regions of static tissues in the 4D flow image using thresholding methods. Based on that, the user can estimate the eddy currents-induced background phase offset errors using polynomial fitting, and subsequently remove the phase offset from the 4D flow data [7]. Second, phase correction needs to be performed when phase aliasing occurs, for which, several phase-unwrapping algorithms have been proposed. Many research or preclinical software tools for 4D PC-MRI analysis provide semi-automated pre-processing functions for corrections of these two types of phase errors.

Segmentation and tracking of the aorta is a prerequisite of the flow visualization and quantification in 4D aortic flow imaging. For instance, flow pathline tracing should be performed only within the boundary of the aortic lumen. A common approach is to segment and track the aorta in the time-resolved 3D phase-contrast MR angiography, which can be derived from the 4D PC-MRI. Semi-automated segmentation algorithms have been developed to segment the aorta in PC-MR angiography by tracing the centerline.

9.4 Flow Visualization

Various 4D flow visualization tools have been developed for 4D PC-MRI in the aorta. The most commonly used methods include the flow velocity vector maps, the 3D streamlines, and the time-resolved 3D pathlines. The 3D streamline or pathline visualization technique traces the voxels or a set of down-sampled voxels in the aortic blood pool, and draw color-encoded lines along the traced trajectories to illustrate the blood flow [8]. 3D streamlines represent the flow velocity field at a single cardiac phase. In contrast, 3D pathlines trace the blood flow for a pre-defined period of time, and therefore, is best displayed dynamically. As shown in Fig. 9.1, visualization of the 3D flow pattern using the 3D streamlines and 3D pathlines techniques provides rich information of the aortic flow pattern, such as the locations and the velocities of the highspeed jet and the helical flow. For patients with aortic diseases,

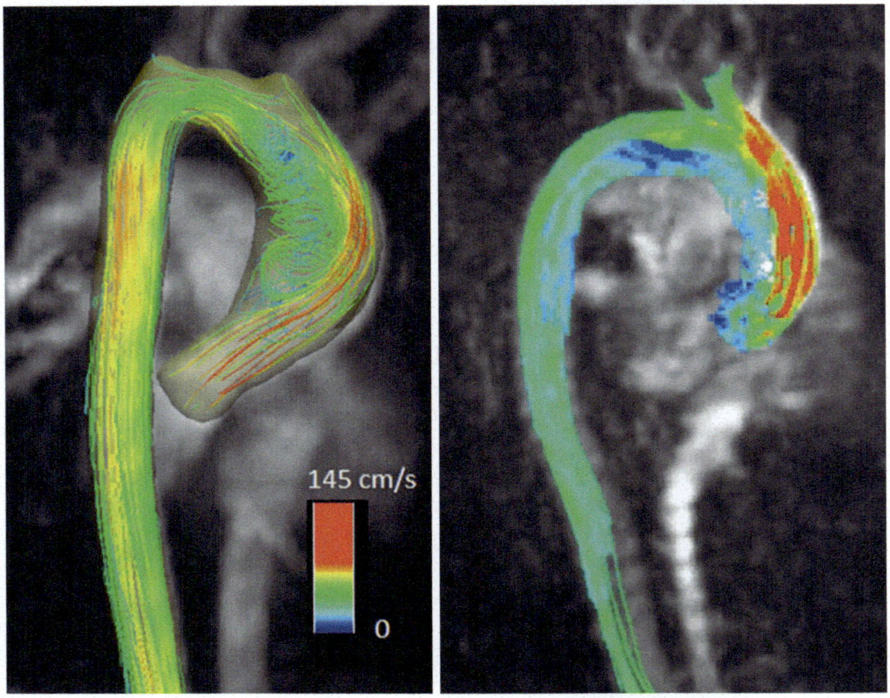

Fig. 9.1 Examples of 3D streamlines (*left hand side*) and 3D pathlines (*right hand side*) visualization of the 4D aortic flow in two patients with BAV. The line color represents the flow velocity and the orientation of the line represents the flow direction

such as aortic stenosis, aortic coarctation, and aortic dissection, visualization of the aortic flow is of particular interest. For example, in patients with bicuspid aortic valve (BAV), the skewed highspeed jet impinging on the convex wall of the ascending aorta can be visualized, which is believed to contribute to the development of aortic aneurysm. Furthermore, in patients with aortic dissection, 4D flow imaging can be used to visualize the position of the entry tears and the helical flow in the false lumen [9].

9.5 Flow Quantification

Because of the full volumetric coverage of the aorta, 4D PC-MRI provides a unique option of retrospective selection of the 2D slices or 3D sub-regions in the 3D field of view for 3D flow quantification and analysis. Besides the conventional 2D flow parameters, such as the transvalvular gradient and peak flow velocity, a number of advanced 4D blood hemodynamic markers have been proposed, and extensively tested in research.

Wall shear stress (WSS) is the shear force the blood flow exerted on the vessel wall. It can be estimated by taking the derivative of 4D flow velocity near the vessel wall boundary [10]. It is believed to play an important role in the regulations of the functions of the endothelial cell and the extracellular matrix in the vessel wall. Low WSS in the aorta has been associated with the development of atherosclerosis [2], and high WSS may lead to the dilation of the aorta and the formation of aortic aneurysm [11]. For example, in patients with aortic stenosis, the high velocity flow jet, depending on the flow direction and flow eccentricity, may result in high WSS in the ascending aortic wall. 4D flow imaging provides a promising and unique avenue to differentiate these patients with different prognoses.

Pulse wave velocity (PWV) is the propagation speed of the systolic wave front through the aorta. It is a direct indicator of the aortic wall stiffness and an important predictor of aortic disease progression in patients with hypertension and Marfan disease [12]. In order to measure PWV in 4D flow image, velocity waveforms are measured at selected sites along the centerline of the aorta. Then, PWV can be calculated as the ratio of the distance between measurement sites and the transit-time.

4D flow MRI has also been used to study the flow pattern in patients with aortic coarctation. Aortic flow eccentricity downstream of the coarctation has been observed by 4D flow MRI, which leads to the jet impingement on the descending aorta, and is believed to be associated with aortic dilation and aneurysm [13]. Alterations in the flow hemodynamic markers, such as the flow velocity, vorticity, WSS, and oscillatory shear index, have been reported after coarctation repair [14].

Other advanced hemodynamic markers derived from 4D flow imaging could include turbulent kinetic energy [15], energy dissipation [16], relative pressure fields [17], and flow displacement [18].

Conclusion

Over the past few years, 4D PC-MRI has become a promising diagnostic imaging tool for aortic diseases. Faster MRI acquisition techniques that have been recently developed will make 4D PC-MRI more clinically available in the near future. 4D flow MRI has unique advantages over the 2D PC-MRI technique, allowing more comprehensive visualization and quantification of the time-varying 3D blood flow pattern in a 3D volume. The novel 4D flow visualization and 3D hemodynamic markers derived from 4D flow image potentially provide a new avenue for the study of the complex interactions between hemodynamics and pathophysiology in the development of aortic diseases, and may help to improve patient outcome.

QCA

1. A major limitation of 4D PC-MRI that impedes its wide clinical acceptance is the lengthy imaging procedure. Which of the following methods have been used to shorten the imaging time of 4D PC-MRI? (Answers: A, C, D)
   A. Use parallel imaging technique.
   B. Use full k-space coverage.

   C. Use radial undersampling.
   D. Use compressed sensing.

2. Venc is an important imaging parameter for 4D PC-MRI. What do we need to know when setting up the Venc? (Answers: B, C, D)
   A. Venc should be set high enough to achieve adequate velocity-to-noise ratio.
   B. Ideally, Venc should be set to equal the highest flow velocity in the 3D field of view.
   C. Venc should be high enough to best avoid phase aliasing.
   D. Phase aliasing can be corrected using phase unwrapping software.

3. Patients with bicuspid aortic valve are at risk of aortic aneurysm formation. Which of the following hemodynamic markers can be used to stratify the risk? (Answers: A, B, D)
   A. Wall shear stress.
   B. Flow angle.
   C. Pulse wave velocity.
   D. Flow vorticity.

References

1. Richter Y, Edelman ER. Cardiology is flow. Circulation. 2006;113(23):2679–82.
2. Cheng C, Tempel D, van Haperen R, et al. Atherosclerotic lesion size and vulnerability are determined by patterns of fluid shear stress. Circulation. 2006;113(23):2744–53.
3. Stankovic Z, Allen BD, Garcia J, Jarvis KB, Markl M. 4D flow imaging with MRI. Cardiovasc Diagn Ther. 2014;4(2):173–92.
4. Eriksson J, Bolger AF, Ebbers T, Carlhäll C-J. Four-dimensional blood flow-specific markers of LV dysfunction in dilated cardiomyopathy. Eur Heart J Cardiovasc Imaging. 2012;14(5):417–24.
5. Dyverfeldt P, Bissell M, Barker AJ, et al. 4D flow cardiovascular magnetic resonance consensus statement. J Cardiovasc Magn Reson. 2015;17:72.
6. Hess AT, Bissell MM, Ntusi NAB, et al. Aortic 4D flow: quantification of signal-to-noise ratio as a function of field strength and contrast enhancement for 1.5T, 3T, and 7T. Magn Reson Med. 2015;73(5):1864–71.
7. Walker PG, Cranney GB, Scheidegger MB, Waseleski G, Pohost GM, Yoganathan AP. Semiautomated method for noise reduction and background phase error correction in MR phase velocity data. J Magn Reson Imaging. 1993;3(3):521–30.
8. Sengupta PP, Pedrizzetti G, Kilner PJ, et al. Emerging trends in CV flow visualization. JACC Cardiovasc Imaging. 2012;5(3):305–16.
9. Clough RE, Waltham M, Giese D, Taylor PR, Schaeffter T. A new imaging method for assessment of aortic dissection using four-dimensional phase contrast magnetic resonance imaging. J Vasc Surg. 2012;55(4):914–23.
10. Markl M, Wallis W, Harloff A. Reproducibility of flow and wall shear stress analysis using flow-sensitive four-dimensional MRI. J Magn Reson Imaging. 2011;33(4):988–94.
11. Bissell MM, Hess AT, Biasiolli L, et al. Aortic dilation in bicuspid aortic valve disease: flow pattern is a major contributor and differs with valve fusion type. Circ Cardiovasc Imaging. 2013;6(4):499–507.
12. Westenberg JJM, Scholte AJHA, Vaskova Z, et al. Age-related and regional changes of aortic stiffness in the Marfan syndrome: assessment with velocity-encoded MRI. J Magn Reson Imaging. 2011;34(3):526–31.

13. Allen BD, Barker AJ, Carr JC, Silverberg RA, Markl M. Time-resolved three-dimensional phase contrast MRI evaluation of bicuspid aortic valve and coarctation of the aorta. Eur Heart J Cardiovasc Imaging. 2013;14(4):399.
14. Frydrychowicz A, Markl M, Hirtler D, et al. Aortic hemodynamics in patients with and without repair of aortic coarctation: in vivo analysis by 4D flow-sensitive magnetic resonance imaging. Investig Radiol. 2011;46(5):317–25.
15. Dyverfeldt P, Hope MD, Tseng EE, Saloner D. Magnetic resonance measurement of turbulent kinetic energy for the estimation of irreversible pressure loss in aortic stenosis. JACC Cardiovasc Imaging. 2013;6(1):64–71.
16. Barker AJ, van Ooij P, Bandi K, et al. Viscous energy loss in the presence of abnormal aortic flow. Magn Reson Med. 2014;72(3):620–8.
17. Yang GZ, Kilner PJ, Wood NB, Underwood SR, Firmin DN. Computation of flow pressure fields from magnetic resonance velocity mapping. Magn Reson Med. 1996;36(4):520–6.
18. Sigovan M, Hope MD, Dyverfeldt P, Saloner D. Comparison of four-dimensional flow parameters for quantification of flow eccentricity in the ascending aorta. J Magn Reson Imaging. 2011;34(5):1226–30.

Part III

Aortic Valve Annuloplasty Techniques

External Aortic Ring Annuloplasty to Standardize Aortic Valve Repair

10

Emmanuel Lansac and Isabelle Di Centa

Degenerative tricuspid and bicuspid aortic insufficiency are the most common etiologies in Western countries, accounting for approximately 2/3 of the cases of aortic insufficiency in the Euro Heart Survey on valvular heart disease [1–3]. It is characterized by dilation the aortic annulus, sinuses and/or sinotubular junction (STJ) diameters preventing coaptation of pliable leaflets which may also be subjected to prolapse [3–6]. Dilation of the annulus is almost constantly present in annulo-aortic ectasia and dystrophic aortic insufficiency, especially in the setting of a bicuspid valve, where an untreated diameter greater than 25–28 mm has been identified as a risk factor for immediate and long term failure of valve repair, but also in isolated aortic insufficiency (AI) [4–13].

10.1 Surgical Anatomy for Aortic Annuloplasty

Two diameters ensure proper aortic valve function. The sinotubular junction is defined as the plane joining the three commissures. The circumferencial plane joining the lowest insertion points (nadirs) of the semilunar cusps has been defined either as the annulus, the virtual ring, the basal ring or the ventriculo-aortic junction [14–19]. As clearly stated in the literature [14–16], the term "annulus" is preferred, as it also corresponds to the echographic measurement of the aortic annulus diameter. As for mitral valve repair, annulus is the term used for anatomical description (mitral annulus), and ring for the prosthetic ring.

Electronic Supplementary Material The online version of this chapter (https://doi.org/10.1007/978-3-319-66483-5_10) contains supplementary material, which is available to authorized users.

E. Lansac (✉)
Département de Pathologie Cardiaque, Institut Mutualiste Montsouris, Paris, France
e-mail: emmanuel.lansac@imm.fr

I. Di Centa
Service de Chirurgie Vasculaire, Hôpital Foch, Suresnes, France

K. Fattouch et al. (eds.), *Advances in Treatments for Aortic Valve and Root Diseases*, https://doi.org/10.1007/978-3-319-66483-5_10

Indeed when the root is dissected externally down to the sub-valvular plane as is the case when performing an external ring annuloplasty (Fig. 10.1) or a Reimplantation procedure, the annulus is not divided into a "virtual ring" at the nadirs of the cusps and a "true anatomical ventriculo-aortic junction" located above the nadirs at mid-sinuses as described in non dissected hearts. On tricuspid aortic valves with non-dilated aortic roots, external dissection of the annulus may be achieved unequivocally down to the sub-valvular level below the nadir of the L and the NC cusps, and in 80% of the cases below or within 3 mm of the nadir of the R cusp. Interestingly, the location where the least amount of dissection towards the sub-valvular plane (i.e. highest dissected level above the annulus) that could be achieved is not the nadir of the R cusp, nor the region below the R-L commissure, but the region below the R-NC commissure where the base of that interleaflet triangle corresponds externally to the cross insertion of the membranous septum, right atrium wall, infundibulum and septal cusp of the tricuspid valve (Fig. 10.2). Moreover, the thickest tissue is located in the muscular part of the annulus with a mean thickness of 2.5 mm. as a result, external aortic annuloplasty using either a ring or a proximal suture of a Reimplantation tube graft would induce at least a 5 mm reduction of the annulus [14, 20].

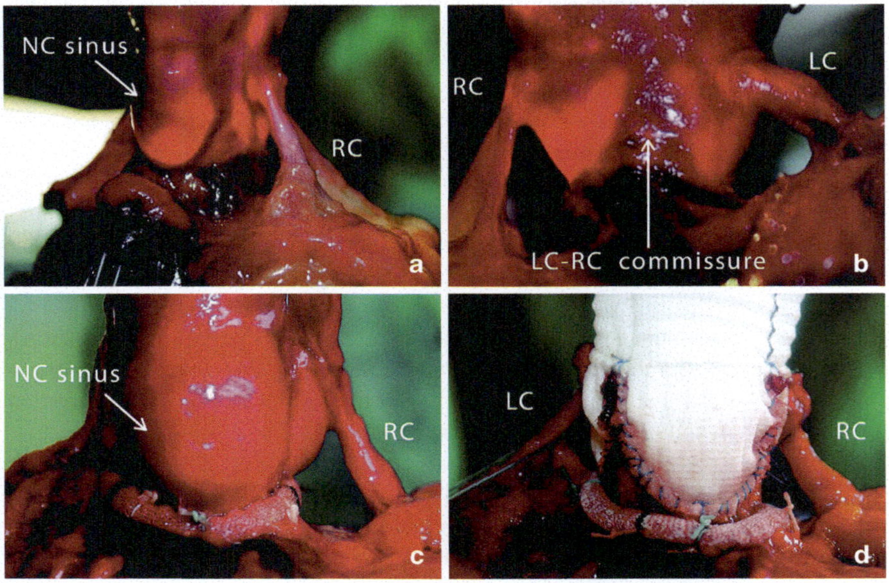

Fig. 10.1 Transillumination of the aortic root after dissection of the sub-valvular plane with view from the NC sinus (**a**) and from the RC-LC commissure (**b**). (**c**) Open ring (Extra-Aortic Open Ring, CORONEO, Inc.) for isolated aortic valve repair with sub-valvular annuloplasty without coronary detachment. (**d**) Remodeling root reconstruction associated to expansible aortic annuloplasty ring (Extra-Aortic Low Profile—25 mm diameter × 3 mm cross-section, CORONEO, Inc.) for root aneurysm repair with Dacron tube (Gelweave Valsalva, Vascutek, Inc.)

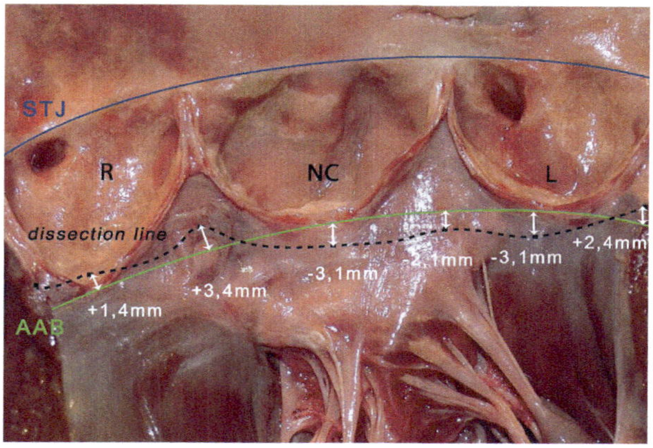

Fig. 10.2 (**a**) aortic root has been opened at commissural level in between the right and left coronary sinuses and spread apart, cusps removed. STJ (*blue line*) Sinotubular Junction, AAB (*green line*) aortic annulus; Scale drawing of the sub-valvular dissection plane line as well as schematic 3D aortic annular view from the R (**b**), NC (**c**) and L (**d**) cusps. *AAB* aortic annulus, *STJ* sinotubular junction

10.2 Rationale for Aortic Annuloplasty to Standardize Aortic Valve Repair

Aims of aortic valve repair technique are to restore proper valve coaptation, preserve or reconstruct the root and treat the annulus dilation [4–7, 10]. Depending on whether the sinuses of Valsalva and/or the tubular ascending aorta are dilated three phenotypes can be individualized: (1) aortic root aneurysms (sinuses of Valsalva >45 mm), (2) tubular ascending aortic aneurysm (sinuses of Valsalva <40–45 mm); (3) isolated AI (all diameters <40 mm) (Fig. 10.3) [5]. Prolapse may be due to an elongated free edge of myxoid leaflets or a ruptured congenital fenestration at commissural level or both.

Out of original valve sparing procedures, the Remodeling technique provides physiological movement of the cusp within the three reconstructed neo-sinuses, thus preserving root expansibility through the unhindered interleaflet triangles, but it does not address annulus dilation [21–24]. The Reimplantation procedure as an inclusion technique performs a sub-valvular annuloplasty through the proximal suture of the graft but withdraws the sinuses of Valsalva and includes the interleaflet triangles within the prosthesis, thus impairing root dynamics [9, 10, 22–24]. Furthermore, most failures of valve sparing procedures are due to cusp prolapse, either residual or induced by root reconstruction. Absence or incomplete cusp effective height resuspension has been identified as a risk factor for prolapse [8, 25–30].

Therefore, we developed a standardized approach to valve repair, towards a more systematic and physiological repair approach based on reduction of dilated root diameters (aortic annulus and sinotubular junction); respect of root dynamics (expansibility through the interleaflet triangles and reconstruction of sinuses of Valsalva) and resuspension of cusp effective height (Fig. 10.3) [4, 27, 28]. Depending on the phenotype of the ascending aorta, reduction of the sinotubular junction diameter will be achieved through a physiological reconstruction of the root according to the Remodeling technique (root aneurysm, sinuses of Valsalva ≥45 mm), a supracoronary graft (supracoronary aneurysm, sinuses of Valsalva <40–45 mm) or an STJ

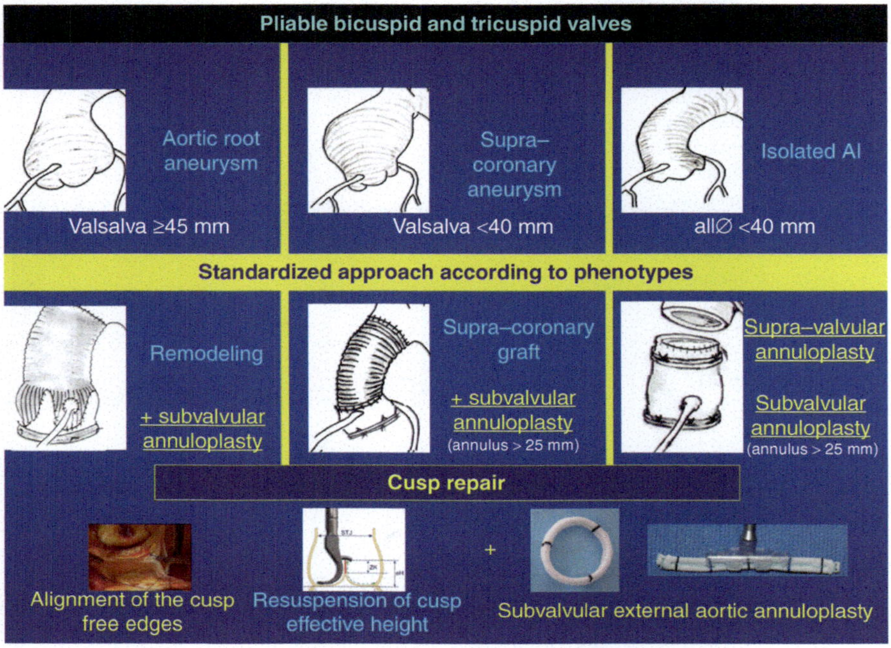

Fig. 10.3 Standardized and physiological approach to aortic valve repair according to each phenotype of ascending aorta

ring (isolated AI, sinus of Valsalva and tubular aorta <40 mm). External ring annuloplasty is systematically added when aortic annulus is ≥25 mm [4, 27, 28, 31, 32]. In case of tubular aorta aneurysm (sinuses of Valsalva < 40–45 mm), or isolated AI (all ascending aorta diameter <40 mm), an open external aortic ring is used in order to be placed under the coronary arteries without detaching them from the aortic wall (Fig. 10.3).

10.3 External Ring Device

These techniques were standardized by the development of a dedicated and calibrated manufactured expansible aortic ring (ExtraAortic ring, Coroneo Inc., Montreal) (Fig. 10.4) [32]. Goals of the ring are to reduce dilated diameters in diastole in order to increase valvular coaptation height, while maintaining root systolic expansibility to reduce stress on the leaflets. The properties of the device were tested *in vitro* and *in vivo* in an ovine model. The expansible ring produced significant reduction of aortic annular base and STJ diameters. Coaptation height was increased by 130% from 2.5 ± 0.7 mm to 6.2 ± 1.1 mm ($p < 0.001$). Mechanical testing on 6 month explanted samples revealed no significant differences in elastic modulus. Dynamics of the root were well preserved. Histomorphological studies showed incorporation of the material without degradation.

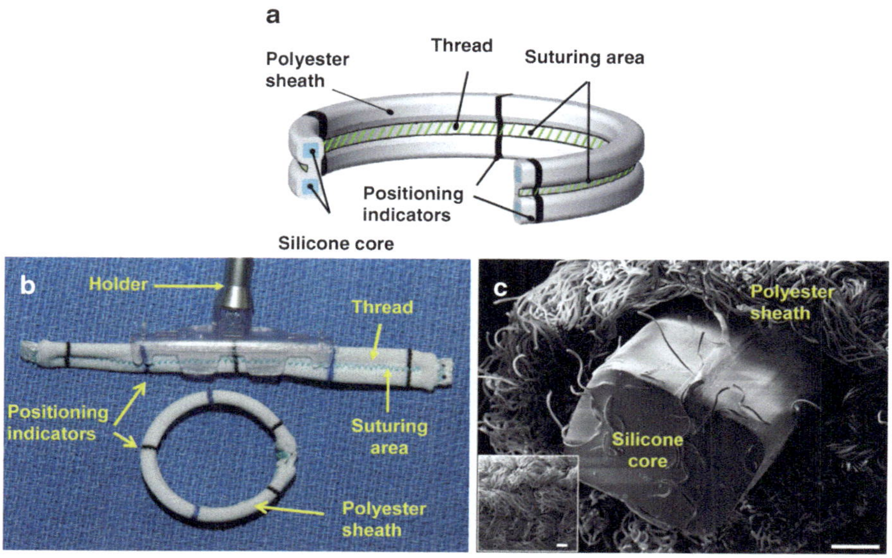

Fig. 10.4 Expansible aortic ring prior to implantation. (**a**) Cut-away schematic diagram of the device showing its key components. (**b**) Top: Prior to implantation, the ring is opened, mounted on a holder that is attached to handle. The *black* indicator marks on the ring facilitate optimal suture placement. Bottom: After implantation, the ends of the ring are fastened. (**c**) Scanning electronic microscope image showing a cross-section of the ring with its rectangular silicone core covered by polyester sheath (insert). Scale bars: 200 μm

10.4 Root Aneurysm: Surgical Steps of Remodeling Root Repair with an External Aortic Ring Annuloplasty [33, 34] (Figs. 10.5 and 10.6, Videos 10.1 and 10.2)

- *Dissection of the subvalvular plane*:

After resecting the sinuses of Valsalva, an external dissection of the aortic root is performed down to the aortic annulus. Cusp geometric height was assessed to detect valve retraction, defined as less than 16 mm for tricuspid cusps and less than 20 mm for the non fused cusp in bicuspid valves, which values are considered as cut off for valve replacement [29].

Native aortic annulus diameter is measured with Hegar dilators as it is the sole criterion for selecting the sizes of the aortic ring and of the graft used to remodel the aortic root (Gelweave Valsalva, Vascutek Ltd., Glasgow, United Kingdom) (Table 10.1). All patients underwent Remodeling root repair with cusp resuspension and subvalvular external aortic ring annuloplasty when the aortic annulus was ≥25 mm as measured intraoperatively with Hegar dilator. The expansible aortic ring diameter (ExAo) is undersized by one size relative to the measured native annulus diameter (Table 10.1).

Table 10.1 Criteria for choice of the aortic ring and tube graft diameters in case of aortic root aneurysm

	Aortic annular base Ø (Hegar dilators, mm)				
	25–27	28–30	31–33	34–39	>40
Tube graft Ø (mm)	26	28	30	32	34
Subvalvular aortic ring Ø (mm)	25	27	29	31	33

- *Placement of sub-valvular U-anchoring stitches for ring annuloplasty*:

Six "U" stitches (2-0 pledgeted polyester needle 25 or 26 mm) are placed circumferentially from inside-out in the subvalvular plane, below the nadir of each cusp and at the base of each interleaflet triangle, except between the right and non-coronary sinuses where the sixth stitch is placed externally on the atrium wall at the lowest level of dissection, in order to avoid potential lesion to the bundle of His or membranous septum.

- *First step of aortic cusp repair*

The first step of valve repair, done prior to root reconstruction, consists of aligning the cusp free edges and correcting any excess free margin length through central plicating stitches or cusp resection. A polypropylene 5 or 6/0 stay suture is passed through each noduli of Arantius. A grasper pulls outwards on the corresponding commissure while the two stitches at the level of the noduli of Arantia are retracted in the opposite direction. The excess length of free edge is then determined. Same step is performed for each hemi-cusp. Distance between the two stitches determines the area for the central plicating stitches to equalize each hemi-cusp free edge length (polypropylene 5 or 6/0-13).

- *Remodeling of the aortic root*

Remodeling of the aortic root is standardized by scalloping the Valsalva graft into three symmetrical neosinuses (placing the commissures at 120° in tricuspid valves) (Fig. 10.5) or into two symmetrical neosinuses (placing the commissures at 180° in bicuspid valves) (Fig. 10.7). The heights of the scallops are cut equally up to the transition point between circumferential and axial folds of the graft (corresponding to the diameter of the tube), thus ensuring that the commissures are placed at the same level.

The prosthesis is sutured following the sigmoid shape of the aortic annulus. Suture starts at the nadir of the left coronary sinus towards the commissure up to half of the sinus. The first stitch is knotted at the nadir of the sinus, in order to facilitate suture tension. Stitches are passed very close to the annulus following leaflet insertion. Another running suture is begun at the tip of the commissure towards corresponding hemi-sinus. Right and non coronary sinuses are then sutured.

This technique allows a bulging aspect of the neosinuses of Valsalva and the preservation of the interleaflet triangles.

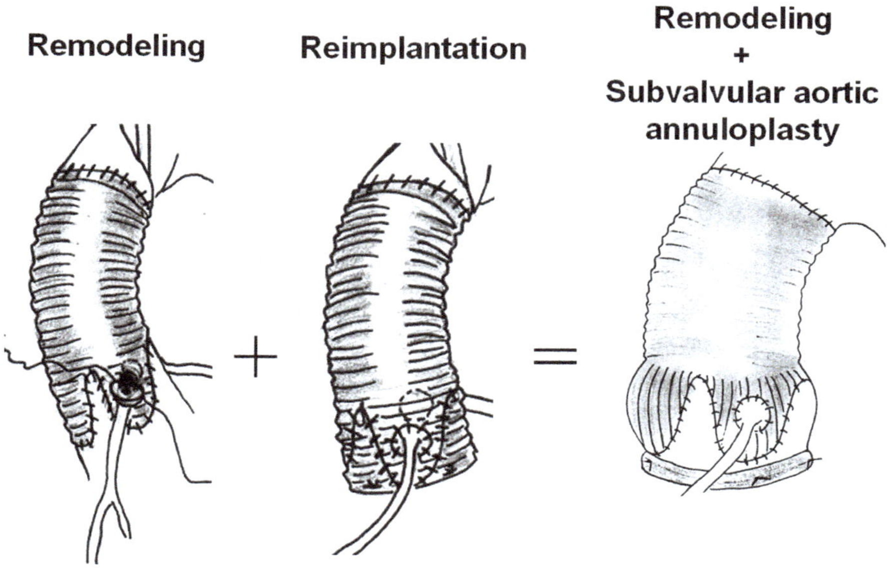

Fig. 10.5 Remodeling of the aortic root associated to an external subvalvular aortic annuloplasty (CAVIAAR technique), combining advantages of the original remodeling and reimplantation techniques

- *Second step of aortic cusp repair*

After remodeling of the aortic root is performed, commissural traction sutures are placed to mimic a pressurized aortic root in order to measure the effective height of each cusp. A dedicated cusp caliper is used to evaluate any residual or induced cusp prolapse according to the principle of Schäfers et al. (Fehling Instruments, Karlstein, Germany) [30]. Plicating stitches are added on the free edge of the culprit leaflet until an effective height of 9 mm is obtained.

- *Ring placement*

The six anchoring "U" stitches are passed around the expansible aortic ring (Extra-Aortic™, CORONEO, Inc., Montreal, QC, Canada) which is seated externally around the remodeled aortic root and tied in the subvalvular position.

- *Coronary reimplantation and final inspection*

The coronary ostia are then reimplanted according to the usual technique. The thicker part of the Gelweave graft can be cut to suture the coronaries ostia if they are ascensionned which is often the case for the right coronary button.

Distal anastomosis is performed using a 4–5/0 Prolene running suture in a standard fashion.

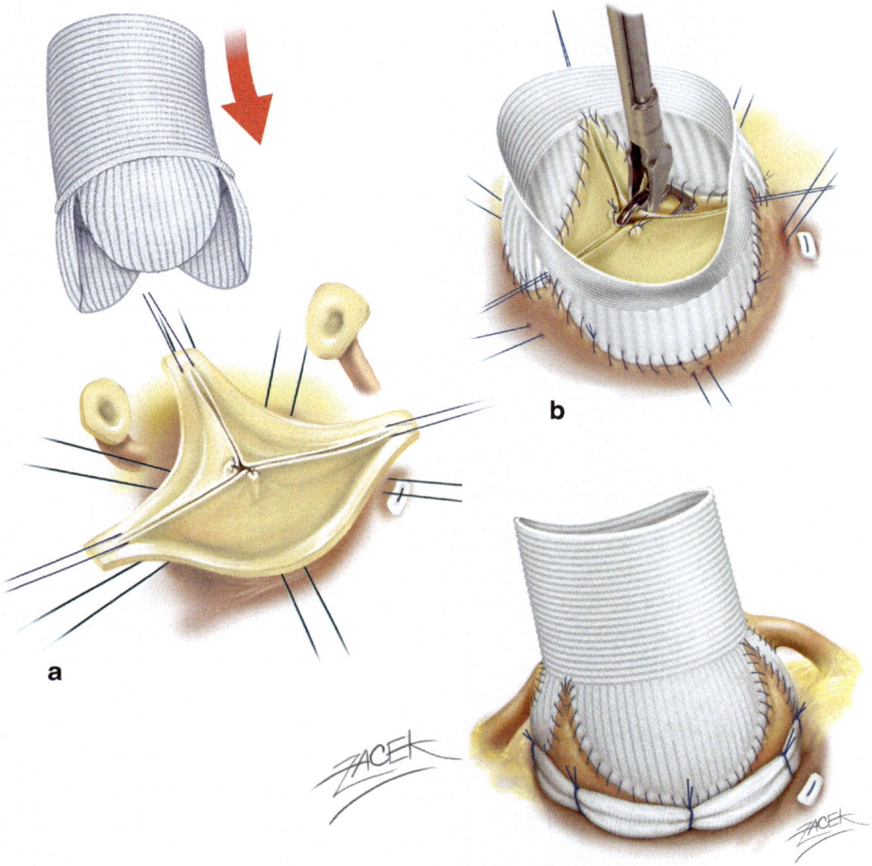

Fig. 10.6 Standardized steps in Remodeling of the aortic root associated with cusp effective height resuspension and external expansible subvalvular aortic ring annuloplasty: (**a**) five "U" stitches are circumferentially placed, inside out, in the subvalvular plane except at the level of the commissure between the non and right coronary sinuses where a sixth stitch is placed externally in order to avoid damage to the membranous septum. Remodeling of the aortic root is then performed by scalloping a bulged graft; (**b**) measure of cusp effective height with the caliper; (**c**) the anchoring "U" stitches are passed through the inner aspect of the prosthetic aortic ring and tied down externally in the subvalvular position

Intraoperative transoesophageal echocardiography (TEE) is performed in all cases. Any residual AI > grade 1 mandates re-exploration of the aortic valve.

Postoperative anticoagulation consists of aspirin (75 mg/d) administered for 2 months unless persistent atrial fibrillation presented, in which case oral anticoagulation is used.

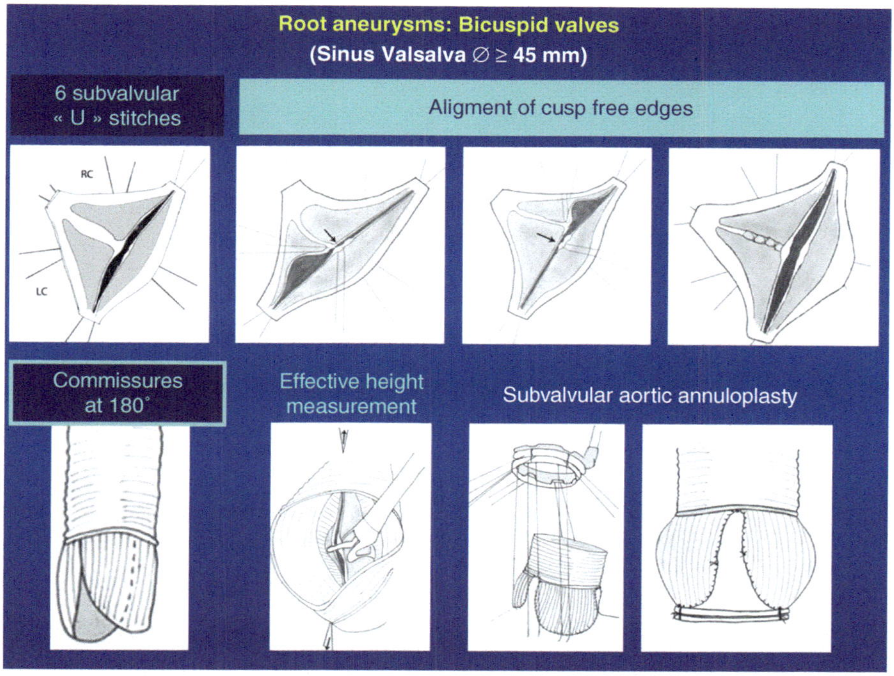

Fig. 10.7 Standardized steps in Remodeling of the aortic root associated with cusp effective height resuspension and external expansible subvalvular aortic ring annuloplasty in case of bicuspid aortic root aneurysm

10.5 Results

Results of 177 patients with Remodeling and external aortic ring annuloplasty were studied [34]. Preoperative AI ≥ grade 3 was present in 79 patients (44.7%). Valve was bicuspid in 59 patients (33.3%). External annuloplasty was performed through a homemade Dacron ring (56) or a dedicated expansible aortic ring (121).

Thirty-day mortality was 2.9% (5). Mean follow-up was 41.1 ± 36.4 months. For the whole series, freedom from valve-related reoperation, AI ≥ grade 3, AI ≥ grade 2 and MAVRE were respectively 89.5%, 90.5%, 77.4% and 86.6% at 7 years, with similar results for tricuspid and bicuspid valves. Since 2007, systematic use of calibrated expansible ring annuloplasty, followed a year later by systematic cusp effective height assessment significantly increased 7-year freedom from valve-related reoperation, AI ≥ grade 3 and MAVRE respectively up to 99.1% ± 0.9% ($p = 0.017$), 100% ($p = 0.026$), and 96.3% ± 1.8% ($p = 0.035$), while freedom from AI ≥ grade 2 remained unaffected (78.1% ± 7.6%). Calibrated annuloplasty and effective height assessment were identified as protective factors from reoperation (respectively HR 0.13 [95%CI 0.02–1.06], p = 0.057), and HR 0.11 [95%CI 0.01–0.95], p = 0.044) (Fig. 10.7).

10.6 Isolated Aortic Insufficiency: Surgical Steps of the Double Sub and Supra Valvular External Aortic Ring Annuloplasty [35, 36] (Fig. 10.8, Video 10.3)

In case of isolated AI (all ascending aorta diameter < 40 mm), surgical steps are the same, except that the root is preserved and coronary buttons are not detached from the aortic wall. A double external aortic annuloplasty is performed at annular and STJ levels.

- *Dissection of the subvalvular plane*

The aorta is completely transsected 1 cm above the sino-tubular junction. External dissection of the aortic root down to the aortic annular base is performed,

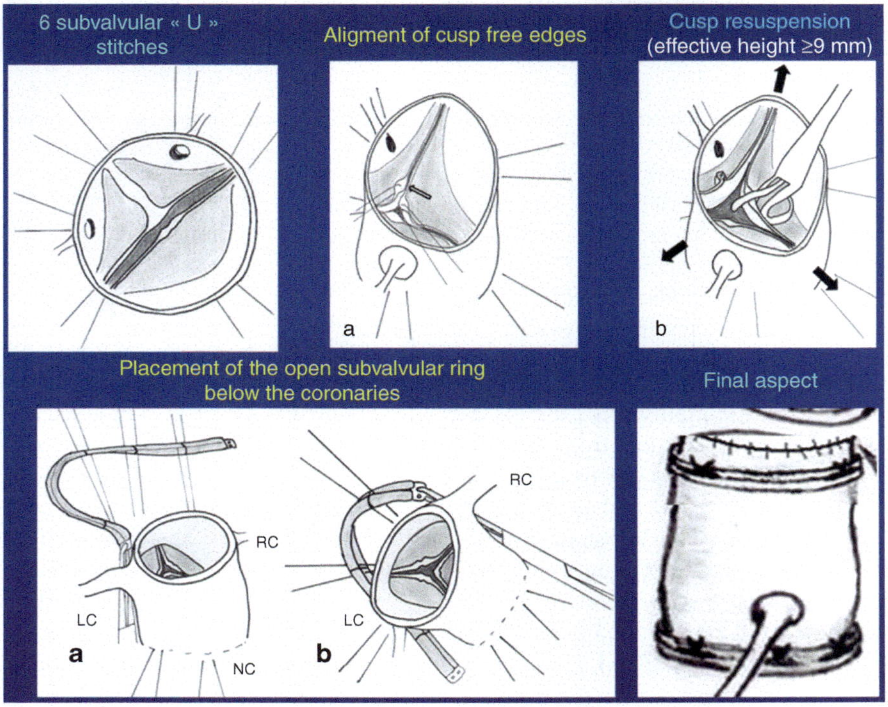

Fig. 10.8 Standardized steps in double sub and supra-valvular external aortic annuloplasty associated with cusp effective height resuspension

Table 10.2 Criteria for choice of the aortic ring diameters in case of isolated aortic insufficiency

	Aortic annular base Ø (Hegar dilators, mm)			
	25–27	28–30	31–35	>36
STJ extra-aortic ring Ø (mm)	25	27	29	31
Subvalvular extra-aortic open ring Ø (mm)	25	27	29	31

passing under the coronary arteries, without detaching them from the aortic wall. The external aspect of the aortic wall is dissected free from the pulmonary artery and infundibulum and from the roof of the left atrium, in order to reach the subvalvular plane. The internal aortic annular base diameter is measured with Hegar dilators.

Measurement of the native aortic annular base internal diameter with Hegar dilators is the sole criterion to determine the size of the expansible external subvalvular aortic ring, which is downsized by one size (CORONEO, Inc.) (Table 10.2)

Geometric height of each cusp is measured using a ruler from the aortic insertion in the nadir of the sinus to the Nodulus of Arantius. Cusps are suitable for repair if geometric height ≥ 17 mm in tricuspid aortic valves and ≥20 mm in bicuspid valves.

- *Placement of sub-valvular U-anchoring stitches for ring annuloplasty*:

Six "U" stitches (2-0 pledgeted polyester needle 25 or 26 mm) are placed circumferentially from inside-out in the subvalvular plane, below the nadir of each cusp and at the base of each interleaflet triangle, except between the right and non-coronary sinuses where the sixth stitch is placed externally on the atrium wall at the lowest level of dissection, in order to avoid potential lesion to the bundle of His or membranous septum.

- *First step of aortic cusp repair: alignment of cusp free edges*

The first step of valve repair, consists of aligning the cusp free edges and correcting any excess free margin length through central plicating stitches or cusp resection. A polypropylene 6/0 stay suture is passed through each noduli of Arantius. A grasper pulls outwards on the corresponding commissure while the two stitches at the level of the noduli of Arantia are retracted in the opposite direction. The excess length of free edge is then determined. Same step is performed for each hemi-cusp. Distance between the two stitches determines the area for the central plicating stitches to equalize each hemi-cusp free edge length (polypropylene 5 or 6/0-13)

- *Placement of the six anchoring supra-valvular U-stitches and placement of the STJ ring*

Three U stitches supra-valvular stitches (2-0 pledgeted polyester needle 25 or 26 mm) are placed 2 mm above each commissure and three stitches are placed in between commissural stitches above each coronary ostia, and the last one half way between the stitch at the level of the non coronary-left coronary commissure and the non coronary-right coronary commissure. The commissural stitches are placed at 120° for tricuspid valves and at 180° for bicuspid valves on the STJ ring (Extra-Aortic™, CORONEO, Inc., Montreal, QC, Canada)

- *Valve repair: resuspension of the cusp effective height*

After reduction of supravalvular diameter with the STJ ring, commissural traction sutures are placed to mimic a pressurized aortic root in order to measure the effective height of each cusp. A dedicated cusp caliper is used to evaluate any residual or induced cusp prolapse according to the principle of Schäfers et al. (Fehling Instruments, Karlstein, Germany) [30]. Plicating stitches are added on the free edge of the culprit leaflet until an effective height of 9 mm is obtained.

- *Placement of the aortic prosthetic ring in subvalvular position*

The 'open' subvalvular prosthetic ring, is passed below the coronary arteries. The ring is closed with a series of "U" stitches at the NC level and stitches are tightened around the ring in subvalvular position.

- *Suture of the aorta*

Transsection of the aorta is closed in standard fashion with running suture.

10.7 Tubular Aorta Aneurysm: Supra Coronary Aorta Replacement with External Subvalvular Aortic Annuloplasty (Fig. 10.9)

In case of tubular aorta aneurysm (sinuses of Valsalva <40–45 mm), surgical steps are the same as for isolated AI with preservation of the root, except that tubular aorta is replaced by a supra-coronary graft instead of STJ ring. The commissures are placed at 120° on the supra coronary tube for tricuspid valves and at 180° for bicuspid valves combined to the non Coronary sinus replacement (Valsalva graft with a single tong) in case of bicuspid right-left fusion. The 'open' subvalvular prosthetic ring, is passed below the coronary arteries. The ring is closed with a series of "U" stitches at the NC level and stitches are tightened around the ring in subvalvular position. Measurement of the native aortic annular base internal diameter with Hegar dilators is the sole criterion to determine the size of the expansible external subvalvular aortic ring, which is downsized by one size (CORONEO, Inc.) (Table 10.3)

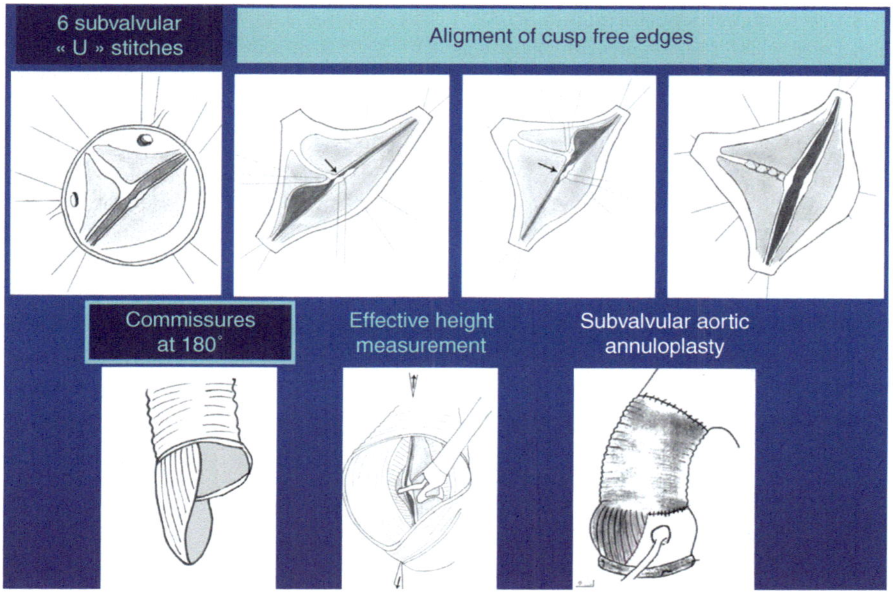

Fig. 10.9 Standardized steps in supra coronary aorta replacement with external subvalvular aortic annuloplasty

Table 10.3 Criteria for choice of the aortic ring and tube graft diameters in case of supra coronary aneurysm

	Aortic annular base Ø (Hegar dilators, mm)			
	25–27	28–30	31–35	>36
Tube graft Ø (mm)	26	28	30	32
Subvalvular aortic ring Ø (mm)	25	27	29	31

10.8 Results

We analyzed long term results of 232 consecutive patients operated on with these standardized and physiological approaches to aortic valve repair according to each phenotype of dystrophic ascending aorta [35]. Data were collected into the multicentric international AVIATOR registry (AorticValve repair InternATiOnal Registry): 149 patients with root aneurysm underwent Remodeling with external ring, 21 tubular aorta aneurysms underwent supra-coronary grafts with external open ring, 62 isolated aortic insufficiency (AI) underwent double sub and/or supravalvular external open ring. Preoperative AI ≥ grade III was present in 58.6% (133), valve was bicuspid in 37.9% (88).

Cusp repair was performed in 75.4% (175) patients. The 30-day operative mortality was 1.4% (3). Mean follow-up was 40.1 ± 37.8 months (0–145.5). Actuarial survival at 7 years was 89.9%. Freedom from reoperation at 7 years was similar among each phenotype, respectively 90.5% for root aneurysms, 100% for tubular aorta aneurysms and 97.5% for isolated AI with no difference between bicuspid and tricuspide valve. Freedom from AI ≥ grade 2 and from AI ≥ grade 3 at 7 years were respectively 76.0% and 93.1% for root aneurysms, 92.9% and 100% for tubular aorta aneurysms, 57.3% and 82.2% for isolated AI. Eye balling repair achieved suboptimal valve competency when compared to systematic cusp effective height assessment which tended to improve freedom from reoperation respectively from 85.8% ± 5.5% to 98.9% ± 1.1% and freedom from AI ≥grade 3 from 89.8% ± 4.9% to 100%. For isolated AI, an additional STJ ring (double sub and supra-valvular annuloplasty) tended to reduce recurrent AI when compared to single subvalvular annuloplasty [35].

10.9 Comments

As for mitral valve repair, aortic annuloplasty is gaining wider acceptance for aortic valve repair [4, 27, 28, 31–37, 41–55]. Long term results of a standardized approach to aortic valve repair using a systematical adjunct of an external aortic ring annuloplasty demonstrates a low rate of reoperation, regardless of ascending aorta phenotype, or type of valve [34, 35]. A dilated aortic annulus greater than 25 to 28 mm, when left untreated, has been shown as a major risk factor for failure of the valve sparing remodeling technique or isolated repair for bicuspid and tricuspid valve [4–13]. Aortic annuloplasty through an external annuloplasty ring efficiently addresses this issue, aiming at a sustained long-term outcome by reducing the dilated aortic annulus (−5 mm), increasing the coaptation height thus protecting the repair, as is the case for mitral valve repair [4, 5, 27, 28, 34, 35, 37]. These results are consistent with recent publications showing that the reimplantation technique provides more significant and durable annular reduction (−7 mm) than sub commissural annular stiches, thus enhancing that the proximal suture of a reimplantation technique not only stabilizes the aortic annulus but –most importantly- performs an aortic annuloplasty [12, 13, 38].

Ideal aortic annuloplasty should ensure good haemodynamic function, biocompatibility, stability of aortic annular base diameter reduction and be easy to implant without interference with the conduction system or cusp tissue. Although sub commissural plicating stitches are fast and easy to perform they impair valve dynamics and induce a low amount of annular reduction [11–13, 38]. Controversy remains between external and internal annuloplasty rings. Although subvalvular plane in the right coronary sinus is easier to reach with internal rings, endovascular placement may interfere with cusp mobility and increase risks for hemolytic or thromboembolic events. Advantage of a ring placed externally is to prevent these complications and avoids placing tension on the device's fixation stitches by the expanding aorta.

External circular stitch annuloplasty may be faster to perform than ring annuloplasty, however safety and reproducibility remain to be evaluated [41].

In our series, annuloplasty for isolated AI provided freedom from reoperation of 94.7% at 7 years. However, the rate of AI ≥ grade 2 remains a concern for single annuloplasty. An additional ring at STJ level (double sub and supra-valvular annuloplasty) seems to improve freedom from recurrence of AI ≥ grade 2 and AI ≥ grade 3 (respectively $p = 0.070$, $p = 0.099$) when compared to single subvalvular annuloplasty. Absence of supravalvular annuloplasty at the STJ level in combination with subvalvular annuloplasty may disturb the STJ/annulus ratio with a significantly larger STJ diameter when compared to the reduced aortic annulus diameter. The systematic adjunct of a supravalvular STJ ring to a subvalvular aortic annuloplasty ring by restoring proper STJ/annulus ratio may increase coaptation and improve stability of the repaired valve. This is consistent with Fattouch et al. findings showing that freedom from recurrent AI was significantly higher for patients who underwent David's procedure or annulus remodelling by home made prosthetic ring than those who underwent isolated (space) subcommissural plasty ($P < 0.01$) or subcommissural plasty plus ascending aortic replacement ($P = 0.02$) [39].

Furthermore, as recently mentioned in a systematic review of valve sparing root replacement series, report of valve-related events is heterogeneous, emphasizing the need for uniform standardized reporting of aortic valve-sparing and repair procedures and their outcomes [40]. In order to encourage collaboration between centers in their reporting of aortic valve-sparing and repair procedures, the Heart Valve Society initiated the multicenter, prospective AVIATOR registry which is open to all centers willing to participate (AorticValve repair InternATiOnal Registry, aviator@heartvalvesociety.org)

Conclusions

External aortic ring annuloplasty provides a reproducible technique for aortic valve repair with satisfactory long results for each ascending aorta phenotype with bicuspid or tricuspid valve. As for mitral valve repair, the standardisation through the systematical adjunct of aortic annuloplasty when the annulus is dilated above 25 mm might contribute to increase the rate of repair for dystrophic AI, reproducibility and long term stability. Multicentric longer follow-up is ongoing with AVIATOR registry.

References

1. Iung B, Baron G, Butchart EG, Delahaye F, Gohlke-Barwolf C, Levang OW, Tornos P, Vanoverschelde JL, Vermeer F, Boersma E, Ravaud P, Vahanian A. A prospective survey of patients with valvular heart disease in Europe: The Euro Heart Survey on Valvular Heart Disease. Eur Heart J. 2003;24(13):1231–43.
2. Roberts WC, Ko JM, Moore TR, Jones WH 3rd. Causes of pure aortic regurgitation in patients having isolated aortic valve replacement at a single US tertiary hospital (1993 to 2005). Circulation. 2006;114(5):422–9.

3. Roman MJ, Devereux RB, Niles NW, et al. Aortic root dilatation as a cause of isolated, severe aortic regurgitation. Prevalence, clinical and echocardiographic patterns, and relation to left ventricular hypertrophy and function. Ann Intern Med. 1987;106:800–7.
4. Lansac E, Di Centa I, Bonnet N, Leprince P, Jault F, Rama A, Acar C, Pavie P, Gandjbakhch I. Aortic prosthetic ring annuloplasty: a useful adjunct to a standardized aortic valve-sparing procedure? Eur J Cardiothorac Surg. 2006;29(4):537–44.
5. Lansac E, Di Centa I, Raoux F, Al Attar N, Acar C, Joudinaud T, Raffoul R. A lesional classification to standardize surgical management of aortic insufficiency towards valve repair. Eur J Cardiothorac Surg. 2008;33:872–80.
6. Jeanmart H, de Kerchove L, Glineur D, Goffinet JM, Rougui I, Van Dyck M, Noirhomme P, El Khoury G. Aortic valve repair: the functional approach to leaflet prolapse and valve-sparing surgery. Ann Thorac Surg. 2007;83:S746–51.
7. Lansac E, Di Centa I. From dynamic anatomy to aortic annuloplasty: the tale of the ring. In: Yankah CA, Weng Y, Hetzer R, editors. Aortic root surgery: the biological solution. Berlin Heidelberg: Springer; 2010. p. 102–32.
8. Kunihara T, Aicher D, Rodionycheva S, Groesdonk HV, Langer F, Sata F, Schäfers HJ. Preoperative aortic root geometry and postoperative cusp configuration primarily determine long-term outcome after valve-preserving aortic root repair. J Thorac Cardiovasc Surg. 2012;143(6):1389–95.
9. Luciani GB, Casali G, Tomezzoli A, Mazzucco A. Recurrence of aortic insufficiency after aortic root remodeling with valve preservation. Ann Thorac Surg. 1999;67(6):1849–52.
10. Hanke T, Charitos EI, Stierle U, Robinson D, Gorski A, Sievers HH, Misfeld M. Factors associated with the development of aortic valve regurgitation over time after two different techniques of valve-sparing aortic root surgery. J Thorac Cardiovasc Surg. 2009;137(2):314–9.
11. Fattouch K, Moscarelli M, Castrovinci S, Murana G, Dioguardi P, Guccione F, Nasso G, Speziale G, Lancellotti P. Mid-term results of bicuspid aortic valve repair guided by morphology and function assessment. Interact Cardiovasc Thorac Surg. 2017 Apr 3;25(1):83–8. https://doi.org/10.1093/icvts/ivx027.
12. de Kerchove L, Mastrobuoni S, Boodhwani M, Astarci P, Rubay J, Poncelet A, et al. The role of annular dimension and annuloplasty in tricuspid aortic valve repair. Eur J Cardiothorac Surg. 2016;49(2):428–37.
13. Navarra E, El Khoury G, Glineur D, Boodhwani M, Van Dyck M, Vanoverschelde JL, et al. Effect of annulus dimension and annuloplasty on bicuspid aortic valve repair. Eur J Cardiothorac Surg. 2013;44:316–23.
14. Khelil N, Sleilaty G, Palladino M, Fouda M, Escande R, Debauchez M, Di Centa I, Lansac E. Surgical anatomy of the aortic annulus: landmarks for external annuloplasty in aortic valve repair. Ann Thorac Surg. 2015;99(4):1220–6.
15. Sievers HH, Hemmer W, Beyersdorf F, et al. The everyday used nomenclature of the aortic root components: the tower of Babel? Eur J Cardiothorac Surg. 2012;41:478–82.
16. Anderson RH. Demolishing the tower of babel. Eur J Cardiothorac Surg. 2012;41:483–4.
17. Frater RWM, Anderson RH. How can we logically describe the components of the arterial valves? J Heart Valve Dis. 2010;19:438–40.
18. Anderson RH, Devine WA, Ho SY, Smith A, Mc KR. The myth of the aortic annulus: the anatomy of the subaortic outflow tract. Ann Thorac Surg. 1991;52:640–6.
19. Sutton JP, Ho SY, Anderson RH. The forgotten interleaflet triangles: a review of the surgical anatomy of the aortic valve. Ann Thorac Surg. 1995;95:419–27.
20. de Kerchove L, Jashari R, Boodhwani M, Duy KT, Lengelé B, Gianello P, Mozala Nezhad Z, Astarci P, Noirhomme P, El Khoury G. Surgical anatomy of the aortic root: implication for valve-sparing reimplantation and aortic valve annuloplasty. J Thorac Cardiovasc Surg. 2015;149(2):425–33.
21. Yacoub M, Fagan A, Stassano P, Radley-Smith R. Result of valve conserving operations for aortic regurgitation [abstract]. Circulation. 1983;68(suppl):III321.
22. Soncini M, Votta E, Zinicchino S, Burrone V, Mangini A, Lemma M, et al. Aortic root performance after valve sparing procedure: a comparative finite element analysis. Med Eng Phys. 2009;31:234–43.

23. Leyh RG, Schmidtke C, Sievers HH, Yacoub MH. Opening and closing characteristics of the aortic valve after different types of valve-preserving surgery. Circulation. 1999;100(21):2153–61.
24. Fries R, Graeter T, Aicher D, Reul H, Schmitz C, Böhm M, Schäfers HJ. In vitro comparison of aortic valve movement after valve-preserving aortic replacement. J Thorac Cardiovasc Surg. 2006;132(1):32–7.
25. Marom G, Haj-Ali R, Rosenfeld M, Schäfers HJ, Raanani E. Aortic root numeric model: annulus diameter prediction of effective height and coaptation in post-aortic valve repair. J Thorac Cardiovasc Surg. 2013;145:406–11.
26. le Polain de Waroux JB, Pouleur AC, Robert A, Pasquet A, Gerber BL, Noirhomme P, et al. Mechanisms of recurrent aortic regurgitation after aortic valve repair: predictive value of intraoperative transesophageal echocardiography. JACC Cardiovasc Imaging. 2009;2:931–9.
27. Lansac E, Di Centa I, Sleilaty G, Arnaud Crozat E, Bouchot O, Hacini R, Blin D, Doguet F, Bessou JP, Albat B, De Maria R, Villemot JP, Portocarrero E, Acar C, Chatel D, Lopez S, Folliguet T, Debauchez M. An aortic ring: from a physiological reconstruction of the root to a standardized approach of aortic valve repair. J Thorac Cardiovasc Surg. 2010;140:S28–35.
28. Lansac E, Di Centa I, Sleilaty G, Bouchot O, Arnaud Crozat E, Blin D, Acar C, Debauchez M. An aortic ring to standardize aortic valve repair: a preliminary results of a prospective multicentric cohort of 144 patients. Eur J Cardiothorac Surg. 2010;38:147–54.
29. Schäfers HJ, Schmied W, Marom G, Aicher D. Cusp height in aortic valves. J Thorac Cardiovasc Surg. 2013;146(2):269–74.
30. Schäfers HJ, Bierbach B, Aicher D. A new approach to the assessment of aortic cusp geometry. J Thorac Cardiovasc Surg. 2006;132:436–8.
31. Wuliya M, Sleilaty G, Di Centa I, et al. An expansible aortic ring to preserve aortic root dynamics after aortic valve repair. Eur J Cardiothorac Surg. 2014;47(3):482–90. https://doi.org/10.1093/ejcts/ezu174.
32. Lansac E, Di Centa I, Raoux F, Bulman-Fleming N, Ranga A, Abed A, Ba M, Paolitto A, Letourneur D, Meddahi Pelle A. An expansible aortic ring for a physiological approach to conservative aortic valve surgery. J Thorac Cardiovasc Surg. 2009;138:718–24.
33. Lansac E, Di Centa I, Vojacek J, Nijs J, Hlubocky J, Mecozzi G, Debauchez M. Valve sparing root replacement: the remodeling technique with external ring annuloplasty. Ann Cardiothorac Surg. 2013;2:117–23. https://doi.org/10.3978/j.issn.2225-319X.2013.01.15.
34. Lansac E, Di Centa I, Sleilaty G, Lejeune S, Berrebi A, Zacek P, Debauchez M. Remodeling root repair with an external aortic ring annuloplasty. J Thorac Cardiovasc Surg. 2017;153(5):1033–42. https://doi.org/10.1016/j.jtcvs.2016.12.031.
35. Lansac E, Di Centa I, Sleilaty G, Lejeune S, Khelil N, Berrebi A, Diakov C, Mankoubi L, Malergue MC, Noghin M, Zannis K, Salvi S, Dervanian P, Debauchez M. Long-term results of external aortic ring annuloplasty for aortic valve repair. Eur J Cardiothorac Surg. 2016;50(2):350–60.
36. Lansac E, Di Centa I, Arnaud Crozat E, Bouchot O, Doguet F, Daroca T, Nijs J. An external open ring for isolated aortic valve repair. MMCTS. 2011. https://doi.org/10.1510/mmcts.2009.004119. http://mmcts.ctsnetjournals.org/cgi/content/abstract/2011/0214/mmcts.2009.004119.
37. Basmadjian L, Basmadjian AJ, Stevens LM, Mongeon FP, Cartier R, Poirier N, El Hamamsy I. Early results of extra-aortic annuloplasty ring implantation on aortic annular dimensions. J Thorac Cardiovasc Surg. 2016;151(5):1280–5.
38. Vallabhajosyula P, Komlo C, Szeto WY, Wallen TJ, Desai N, Bavaria JE. Root stabilization of the repaired bicuspid aortic valve: subcommissural annuloplasty versus root reimplantation. Ann Thorac Surg. 2014;97(4):1227–34.
39. Fattouch K, Castrovinci S, Murana G, Nasso G, Guccione F, Dioguardi P, Salardino M, Bianco G, Speziale G. Functional annulus remodelling using a prosthetic ring in tricuspid aortic valve repair: mid-term results. Interact Cardiovasc Thorac Surg. 2014;18(1):49–54.
40. Arabkhani B, Mookhoek A, Di Centa I, Lansac E, Bekkers JA, De Lind Van Wijngaarden R, et al. Reported outcome after valve-sparing aortic root replacement for aortic root aneurysm: a systematic review and meta-analysis. Ann Thorac Surg. 2015;100(3):1126–31.

41. Aicher D, Schneider U, Schmied W, Kunihara T, Tochii M, Schäfers HJ. Early results with annular support in reconstruction of the bicuspid aortic valve. J Thorac Cardiovasc Surg. 2013;145:S30–4.
42. Izumoto H, Kawazoe K, Oka T, Ishibashi K, Yamamoto H, Yamamoto F. Leaflet suspension and subvalvular annuloplasty in aortic valve prolapse. Asian Cardiovasc Thorac Ann. 2009;17(3):278–81.
43. Hetzer R, Komoda S, Komoda T. Remodeling of aortic root by annular reconstruction and plication of sinuses of valsalva. J Card Surg. 2008;23:49–51.
44. Kollar A. Valve-sparing reconstruction within the native aortic root: integrating the Yacoub and the David methods. Ann Thorac Surg. 2007;83:2241–3.
45. Takamoto S, Nawata K, Morota T. A simple modification of 'David-V' aortic root reimplantation. Eur J Cardiothorac Surg. 2006;30:560–2.
46. Schäfers HJ. Aortic annuloplasty: a new aspect of aortic valve repair. Eur J Cardiothorac Surg. 2012;41(5):1124–5.
47. Sievers HH. Aortic annuloplasty ring: coronet or flat or not or what? Eur J Cardiothorac Surg. 2012;42(1):155–6.
48. Taylor WJ, Thrower WB, Black H, Harken DE. The surgical correction of aortic insufficiency by circumclusion. J Thorac Surg. 1958;35(2):192–205.
49. Cabrol C, Cabrol A, Guiraudon G, Bertrand M. Treatment of aortic insufficiency by means of aortic annuloplasty. Arch Mal Coeur Vaiss. 1966;59(9):1305–12.
50. de Kerchove L, Vismara R, Mangini A, Fiore GB, Price J, Noirhomme P, Antona C, El Khoury G. In vitro comparison of three techniques for ventriculo-aortic junction annuloplasty. Eur J Cardiothorac Surg. 2012;41(5):1117–23.
51. Mangini A, Lemma MG, Soncini M, Votta E, Contino M, Vismara R, Redaelli A, Antona C. The aortic interleaflet triangles annuloplasty: a multidisciplinary appraisal. Eur J Cardiothorac Surg. 2011;40(4):851–7.
52. Rankin JS, Conger JL, Tuzun E, Winkler JA, Harms KM, Beavan LA, Fossum T, Cohn WE. In vivo testing of an intra-annular aortic valve annuloplasty ring in a chronic calf model. Eur J Cardiothorac Surg. 2012;42(1):149–54.
53. Kazui T, Tsuboi J, Izumoto H, Nakajima T, Ishihara K, Kawazoe K. Aortic root remodeling with aortic annuloplasty: mid-term results. Circ J. 2007;71(2):207–10.
54. Fattouch K, Sampognaro R, Speziale G, Ruvolo G. New technique for aortic valve functional annulus reshaping using a handmade prosthetic ring. Ann Thorac Surg. 2011;91(4):1154–8.
55. Hahm SY, Choo SJ, Lee JW, Seo JB, Lim TH, Song JK, et al. Novel technique of aortic valvuloplasty. Eur J Cardiothorac Surg. 2006;29(4):530–6.

Aortic Annulus Stabilization Using Internal Rings

11

Khalil Fattouch, Tommaso Favara, Francesco Guccione, and Pietro Dioguardi

The past 20 years have seen the growing range of valve lesion etiologies turn nonvalvular conditions into the primary causes of aortic regurgitation [1]. Valves present relatively small lesions of the leaflets and concomitant dilatation of the ascending aorta with aortic regurgitation that can be explained thanks to our improved knowledge of the functional aortic annulus' role in valve function. The geometric relations and dynamic behavior of aortic root components have been seen to ensure valve competence when leaflets have no structural lesions [2].

The aortic annulus is the tightest part of the functional aortic annulus complex and is defined as a virtual ring at the level of the hinge points of the aortic valve leaflets. This hinge point plane is below the anatomic plane where the left ventricular outflow tract myocardium meets the beginning of the aorta [3].

The lesson from mitral valve showed that the annuloplasty is an important component of valve repair because serves to reduce annular dimension appropriately for leaflet coaptation and provides annular stability to prevent late annular dilatation and repair failure.

Stabilization of this anatomic structure by applying aortic valve reimplantation within a vascular graft has not uniformly resulted in adequate valve stability.

Currently established aortic annuloplasty techniques include commissural annuloplasty and stabilization by external grafts.

Each approach has its pros and cons, and the decision regarding the ideal technique is made in the context of patient related factors, valvular pathology, and the aortic root complex.

The two most widely used techniques of external graft are the remodeling technique, developed by Yacoub, and the reimplantation technique, developed by David.

K. Fattouch, Ph.D. • T. Favara, M.D. • F. Guccione, M.D. • P. Dioguardi, M.D. (✉)
GVM Care and Research, Cardiovascular Department, University of Palermo,
Viale Reggione Siciliana, Palermo, Italy
e-mail: pt.dioguardi@libero.it

K. Fattouch et al. (eds.), *Advances in Treatments for Aortic Valve and Root Diseases*, https://doi.org/10.1007/978-3-319-66483-5_11

Aortic root remodeling does not correct the dilation of the aortic annulus that can lead to the failure of the procedure and the recurrence of aortic insufficiency. As a result, many surgeons prefer the reimplantation technique. However, the classic remodeling technique provides more physiologic movements of the cusps within the three reconstructed neo-sinuses. This preserves root expansibility through the inter-leaflet triangles during the cardiac cycle [4, 5]. Moreover recent research has focused on modified remodeling techniques, such as a remodeling root reconstruction in association with an aortic annuloplasty to combine the advantages of both the remodeling and reimplantation techniques [6–8]. Different concepts of an annuloplasty approach have been proposed, i.e. external ring, internal ring or suture annuloplasty.

11.1 Internal Aortic Annuloplasty

Today, subcommissural plasty, initially described by Cabrol et al., represents the first surgical choice in aortic valve [9]. Through this type of annuloplasty, only a component of the aortic annulus (the nadir or aorto-ventricular junction) is corrected, leaving the other components (the STJ) untreated: it is probably the main reason why performing this reparative technique is still controversial. As described by Anderson et al., the AVA does not have a circular biplane shape, but it is a complex tridimensional structure composed of the nadir of the aortic leaflets, the commissures and by the STJ [10].

During the subcommisural plasty technique, is not clear how decide the exact amount of the annulus diameter reduction. The surgeon just include and fix the commissures by the sutures, always considering that their movements are fundamental to preserve valve motion and reduce the stress on the aortic leaflets. Moreover, the suture placed in the subcommissural position, between the right coronary cusp and the other cusps, is placed at the level of the interventricular septum, and so it could move down the ventricle muscle. All these situations can be considered reasons why different authors experienced failure of the subcommissural plasty especially, in patients with AI and a dilated left ventricle [11].

In last decade, other surgical techniques were attempted as a possible key to provide stabilization of the aortic annulus over time.

In 2011 **Laurent de Kerchove et al**. compared in vitro three different techniques of ventricular aortic junction (VAJ) annuloplasty: the subcommisural plasty (SCA), external ring (ER) and internal ring (IR) annuloplasty [12].

For each, they sought to quantify parameters of valve function and root morphology. Ten fresh porcine aortic valve preparations were tested in a pulsatile mock loop.

The annuloplasty techniques were then performed successively in each sample. Each technique was tested, then removed and the following technique performed. SCA was applied at 50% of interleaflet triangle height; the ER and IR were applied with a moderate reduction (15–20%) of the VAJ.

They showed that effective orifice area decreased significantly with each annuloplasty technique compared with baseline ($P < 0.001$) (Table 11.1). Mean

Table 11.1 Pooled data of ten samples

	B	SCA	ER	IR	*P*-value of the difference between treatments					
					B vs. SCA	B vs. ER	B vs. IR	SCA vs. ER	SCA vs. IR	ER vs. IR
OT, ms	35 (28–40)	25 (17–28)	21 (16–25)	31 (25–37)	<0.05	<0.05	ns	ns	<0.05	<0.05
CT, ms	67 (57–79)	57 (53–61)	51 (48–58)	52 (43–62)	ns	<0.05	<0.05	ns	ns	ns

OT opening time, *CT* closing time, *B* basal, *SCA* subcommissural annuloplasty, *ER* external ring, *IR* internal ring

transvalvular pressure drop was significantly higher in the ER and IR vs. SCA (P = 0.007) (Table 11.2). Annuloplasty reduced valve opening and closing time in comparison to baseline. Echocardiography confirmed that the VAJ experienced a greater reduction with the ER and IR vs. SCA. A narrowing of the lower third of the sinuses of Valsalva was observed after the ER, and subvalvular narrowing was observed after the IR. Valve coaptation increased with all annuloplasty techniques.

They demonstrated that the ER and IR have greater potential to reduce VAJ diameter in comparison to SCA. The IR induced a subvalvular remodeling of the VAJ, whereas the ER induced a paravalvular remodelling.

In 2013 **Fattouch et al.** published a study which was performed to evaluate 250 patients underwent aortic valve repair using an aortic valve annuloplastic system consisting of a handmade prosthetic ring [13].

11.1.1 Components of the Aortic Annuloplasty System

The new ring has two components. The first was a circular ring used to undersize the circumference of the aortic valve nadir (the aortoventricular junction; (Fig. 11.1a). The second was a three crown-like shaped ring used for the STJ remodeling (Fig. 11.1b). The circular ring was constructed by the Simplici-T band (Medtronic, Minneapolis, MN). A Dacron graft (InterVascular Inc., Montvale, NJ) was scalloped to construct the ring for the STJ.

The circular ring was sutured into the left ventricular outflow tract in the aortic subvalvular position and the STJ ring was sutured from the outside of the aortic root just at the level of the STJ. The three vertical bands of the STJ ring were fixed to the underlying circular ring to stabilize the continuity between the STJ and nadir of the aortic valve.

11.1.2 Surgical Technique

The circular ring was fixed into the left ventricular outflow tract just below the aortic valve nadir (the aortoventricular junction) and the three crown-like shaped ring was

Table 11.2 Pooled data of ten samples

	B	SCA	ER	IR	*P*-value of the difference between treatments					
					B vs. SCA	B vs. ER	B vs. IR	SCA vs. ER	SCA vs. IR	ER vs. IR
Q_{mean} (L/min)	*4.7 ± 0.2*	*4.7 ± 0.3*	*4.6 ± 0.2*	*4.6 ± 0.3*	*ns*	*ns*	*ns*	*ns*	*ns*	*ns*
p_{art} (mmHg)	*96.3 ± 3.2*	*97.2 ± 2*	*98.7 ± 3.3*	*99.4 ± 4.2*	*ns*	*ns*	*ns*	*ns*	*ns*	*ns*
Φ (mm)	21.9 ± 1.4	19.3 ± 1.1	18.1 ± 1.4	17.8 ± 1.2	0.001	0.001	0.001	0.007	0.001	ns
ΔP_{mean} (mmHg)	3.1 ± 1.2	5.0 ± 1.4	8.6 ± 2.7	7.9 ± 3.2	ns	0.001	0.001	0.001	0.007	ns
ΔP_{max} (mmHg)	24.3 ± 3.3	26.5 ± 3.2	31.3 ± 4.1	30.8 ± 4.4	ns	0.001	0.001	0.002	0.004	ns
EOA (cm^2)	3.9 ± 0.7	3.0 ± 0.4	2.3 ± 0.5	2.4 ± 0.5	0.001	0.001	0.001	0.005	0.03	ns
VLV (mL)	3.0 ± 1.6	2.9 ± 2.3	3.8 ± 2.1	4.0 ± 2.7	ns	ns	ns	ns	ns	ns

The imposed working conditions are reported in italics

B basal, *SCA* subcommissural annuloplasty, *ER* external ring, *IR* internal ring. Q_{mean} imposed flow rate, p_{art} simulated arterial blood pressure, Φ sample diameter, ΔP_{mean} mean systolic pressure drop across the sample, ΔP_{mean} maximum systolic pressure drop across the sample, *EAO* effective orifice area, *VLV* valve leakage volume

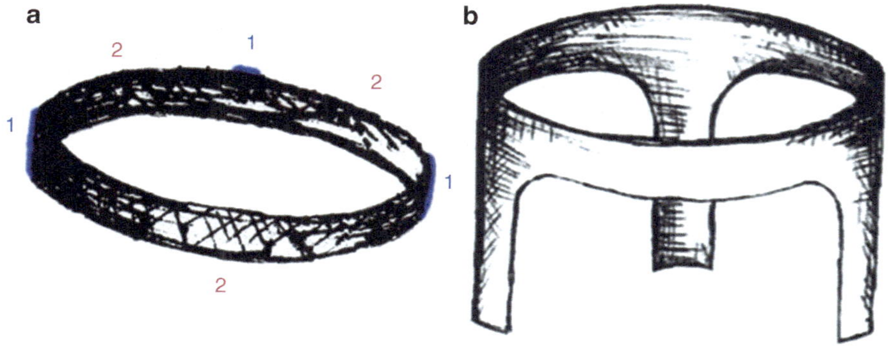

Fig. 11.1 (**a**) The first component is circular ring used to undersize the circumference of the aortic nadir. (**b**) The second was a three crown-like shaped used for STJ remodelling

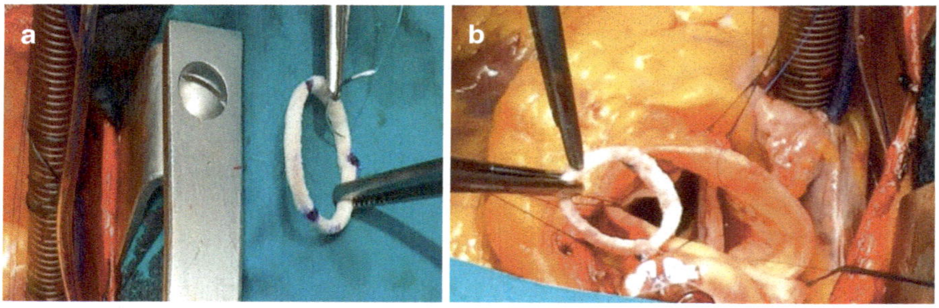

Fig. 11.2 (**a**, **b**) the circular ring is fixed into the left ventricular outflow tract just below the aortic valve nadir (the aortoventricular junction) and the three crown-like shaped ring is sutured to the STJ from the outside of the aortic root

sutured to the STJ from the outside of the aortic root (Fig. 11.2a,b). The circular ring was fixed into the left ventricular outflow tract in the subvalvular position. Ti-Cron 2-0 U stitches (Coviden, Mansfield, MA) were placed first on the prosthetic ring from inside to outside and subsequently under the aortic leaflets like in the David procedure from inside to outside.

Ti-Cron sutures were placed under the entire circumference of the aortic valve, except for the interleaflet triangles. In this way, the interleaflet triangles were above the suture line and remained free to move during the cardiac cycle, reducing leaflets stress. Under the coronaries ostia, the Ti-Cron U stitches were placed through the aortic annulus from the ventricular side to the aortic side (as in valve replacement); in this way, the author avoided the coronaries ostia mobilization that leads to easier and faster technique (Fig. 11.3a, b).

The STJ ring was sutured from outside of the aortic root just at the level of the STJ using 4-0 Prolene sutures. The ring was sutured to the aortic wall using an overandover running suture technique or by interrupted sutures. At the end of the procedure, the three vertical bands of the STJ ring were fixed to the underlying circular ring to stabilize the continuity between the STJ and the nadir of the aortic valve. The length of the three arms

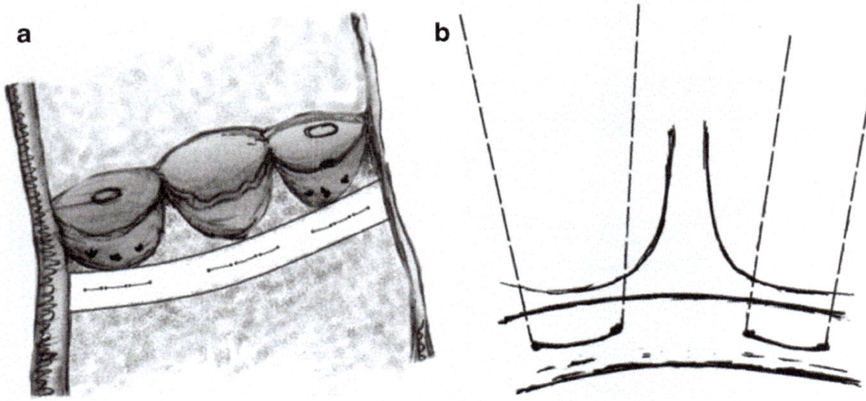

Fig. 11.3 (**a**, **b**) Ti-Cron sutures are placed under the entire circumference of the aortic valve except for the interleaflets triangles. Under the coronaries ostia the Ti-Cron-U-stiches are placed through the aortic annulus from the ventricular side to the aortic side

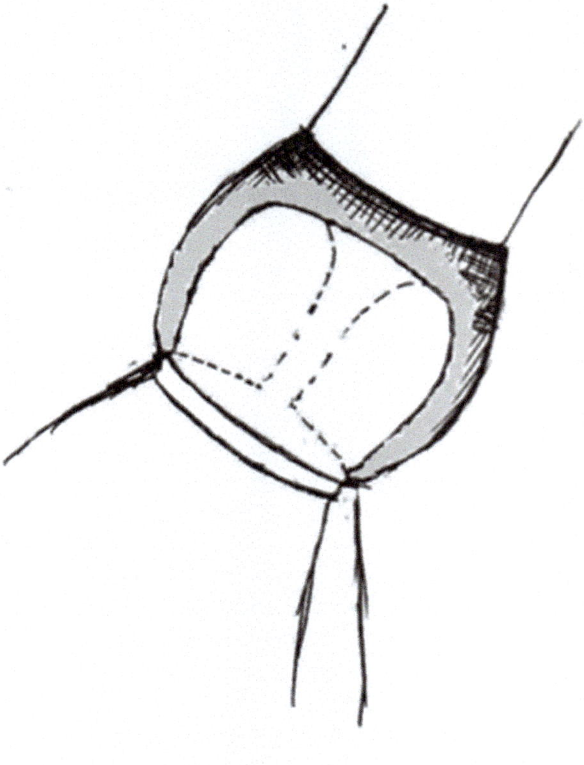

Fig. 11.4 At the end of procedure the three vertical bands of the STJ ring are fixed to the underlying circular ring to stabilize the continuity between the STJ ring and nadir of the aortic valve (to avoid upward future displacement)

coming down was determined at the end of the procedure and was selected according to the distance between the STJ ring and the circular aortic ring (Fig. 11.4).

The role of the three arms was to stabilize the distance between the aortic ring and the STJ ring and to avoid future upward displacement of the STJ in cases of ascending aorta or aortic root dilation.

11.1.3 Sizing Method

In all patients, the size (diameter) of the prosthetic circular ring was calculated according to the height of the leaflet measured from the Noduli of Arantius to the base of the cusp. The three leaflets were considered as the three triangles that cover the entire surface of a circle (the ring). Moreover, it must be left about 8 mm from the free margin of each cusp into the coaptation surface. The author preferred to select the diameter of the ring according to the height of the smallest cusp because in this way obtaining security of a good coaptation between all cusps.

The circular ring size must be calculated following the current formula Radius (r) of the ring/height of the cusp—8 mm.

The size of the STJ ring was calculated by the diameter of the native STJ plus 3–4 mm. They used the Hegar sizer to measure exactly the diameter between the tips of the three commissures, taking the aortic valve in the closing position. The STJ ring was used to stabilize the STJ to avoid future dilatation. Accuracy must be taken to avoid the use of an undersized STJ ring because it leads to inward displacement of the commissures that may lead to cusps prolapse.

11.1.4 Results

Mean length of the coaptation surface was 10 ± 2 mm. The mean clinical follow-up (100% complete) was 22 ± 16 months. All patients were free from cardiac and valve-related events, and no complications due to ring implantation occurred.

In 2013 **Mazzitelli et al.** [14] published early results of a new aortic internal ring. The design of the HAART ring ('Hemispherical' Aortic Annuloplasty Reconstructive Technology; BioStable Science and Engineering, Inc., Austin, TX, USA) was developed from anatomic studies of human cadaver valves, as well as CT angiography of normal human valvular geometry. The ring was based on the concept that the permanent restoration of normal annular circumference and elliptical shape will facilitate the quality of valve repair in tri-leaflet aortic valves, both acutely and long term. The three-dimensional rings are computer milled from one-piece Titanium blocks and covered with a thin layer of Dacron cloth to promote rapid endothelialization. Base geometry of the ring is elliptical with a 2:3 minor-to-major diameter ratio and three equidistant subcommissural posts that flare 10° outward. Aortic valves were approached through complete transverse aortotomies, 1.5 cm above the right coronary artery and commissural tops. Traction sutures were placed above each commissure for exposure. After performing an accurate valve analysis to identify leaflet pathology (Fig. 11.5a), leaflet free-edge lengths were sized with special ball sizers such that twice the leaflet free-edge length

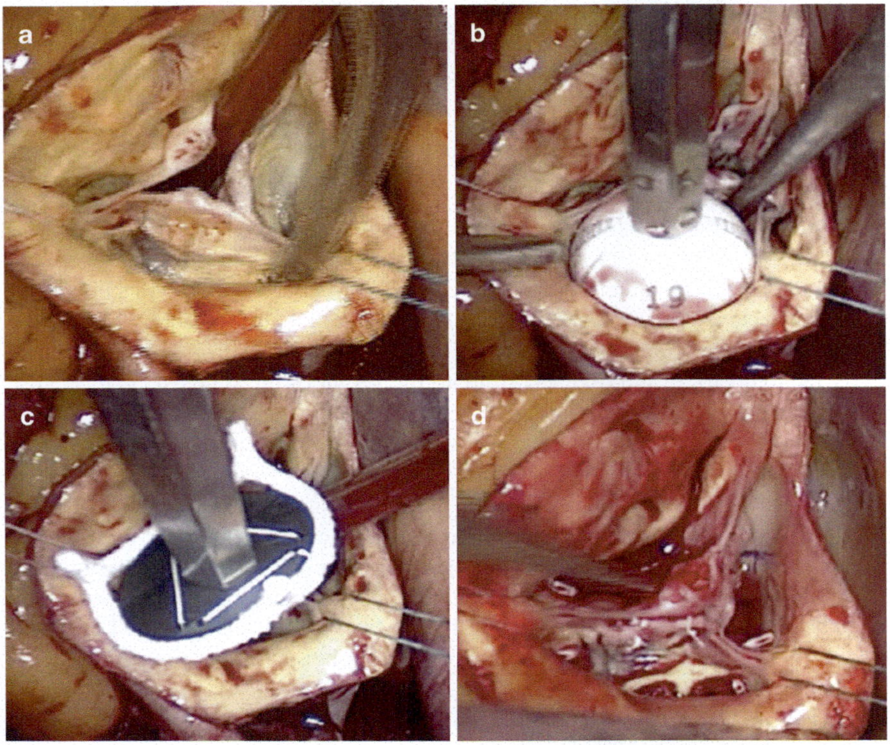

Fig. 11.5 Ring implantation technique. (**a**) Valve with Grade 3 AI due to a dilated annulus at 27 mm, central coaptation gap and scarred, retracted Noduli. (**b**) The leaflet inter-commissural free-edge length sizes to a predicted 19 mm annulus (180° stippled areas), demonstrating important annular dilatation. (**c**) A 19-mm annuloplasty ring is shown above the valve, with the minor diameter post at the posterior (left/non-coronary) commissure. (**d**) The finished result after annuloplasty, Nodular release with the CUSA device and leaflet plication

equaled the required ring circumference, as previously validated (Fig. 11.5b). The rings were sutured beneath the leaflets and commissures, and directly into the annuli, using nine transannular horizontal mattress sutures of 4-0 Prolene™ (Ethicon, Inc., Somerville, NJ, USA)—one in each post and two in the body of each sinus—supported with small supra-annular Dacron pledgets (Fig. 11.5c, d). Ring implantation time ranged from 27 to 19 mm. In 2015 they also published a new article to assess the safety and efficacy of an internal geometric annuloplasty ring in a regulatory trial of aortic valve reconstruction.

Sixty-five patients with predominant moderate-to-severe trileaflet aortic insufficiency (AI) underwent aortic valve repair with an average age of 63 ± 13 years (mean ± SD). All had initial implantation of an internal aortic annuloplasty ring. Follow-up was for a maximum of 3 years and a mean of 2 years. No in-hospital operative mortalities, major complications or early or late valve-related events occurred. The annular diameter before repair was 26.5 ± 2.3 mm, and the average ring diameter used was 21.5 ± 1.6 mm. The preoperative AI grade (0–4) was 2.9 ± 0.8 and improved after repair to 0.6 ± 0.7 ($P < 0.0001$) (Table 11.3), as did the NYHA class. The mean valve

Table 11.3 (**a**) Survival after aortic valve repair. (**b**) Reoperative aortic valve replacement over time

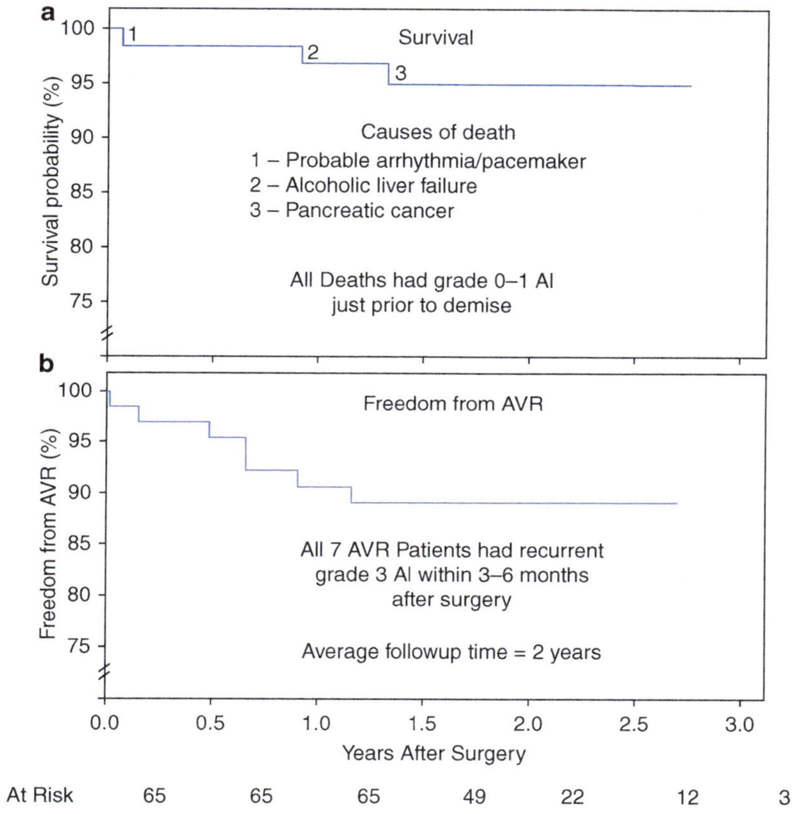

Table 11.4 Mean ± SEM AI data over time after aortic valve repair. The *P* -values are given for Friedman's tests of changes over time to 1 year of follow-up. SEM: standard error of the mean

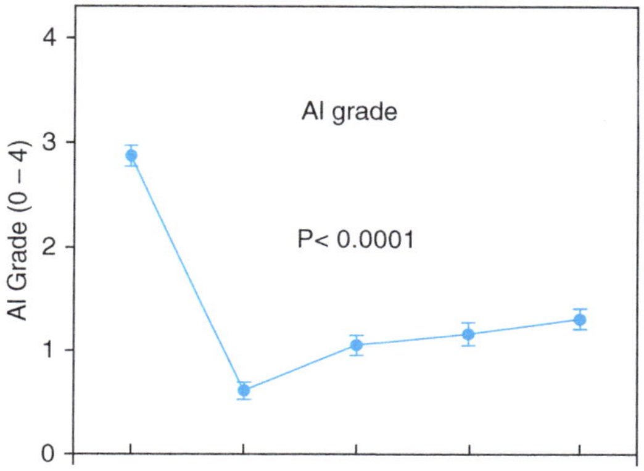

Table 11.5 Non-parametric presentation of AI data over time after aortic valve repair

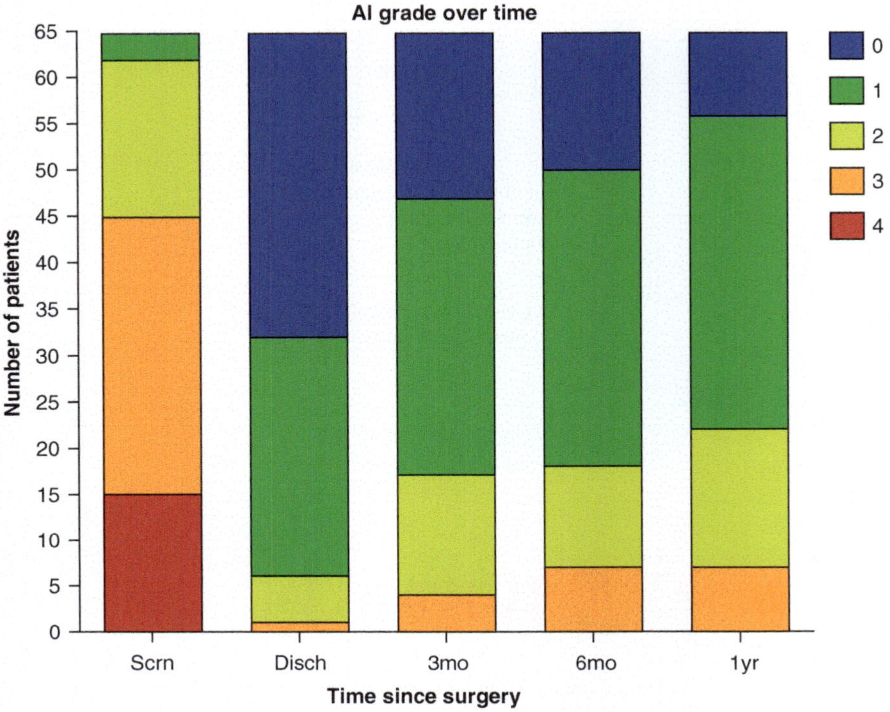

gradient was 8.6 ± 4.3 mmHg, and at 3 years, the Kaplan–Meier survival rate was 95%, with no valve-related mortality (Table 11.4). Over the 3 years, aortic valve replacement was required in seven patients (10.8%) for reasons usually related to surgical technique. Most repair failures occurred early, and results stabilized after 6 months (Table 11.5). No structural complications of the rings were observed.

They concluded that geometric ring annuloplasty was a safe and effective adjunct to aortic valve repair. Because most early repair failures were technical, increasing experience with geometric ring annuloplasty for aortic valve reconstruction has the potential to standardize and improve outcomes.

Richardt et al. in 2014 [15] described a novel rigid aortic annuloplasty ring. They tested in vitro ten fresh porcine aortic roots in a pulsatile flow simulator. The rigid prosthetic ring device had an outer diameter of 21 mm and an inner diameter of 19.5 mm and consisted of a closed, rigid metal ring that was covered with a woven Dacron layer (Figs. 11.6 and 11.7).

This size was chosen in relation to the internal anatomic diameter of the native root. In particular, the metal part of the ring device is not embedded uniformly into the Dacron layer: the upper portion of the ring consisted only of a soft Dacron layer for stitching, aiming to prevent leaflet contact after suturing.

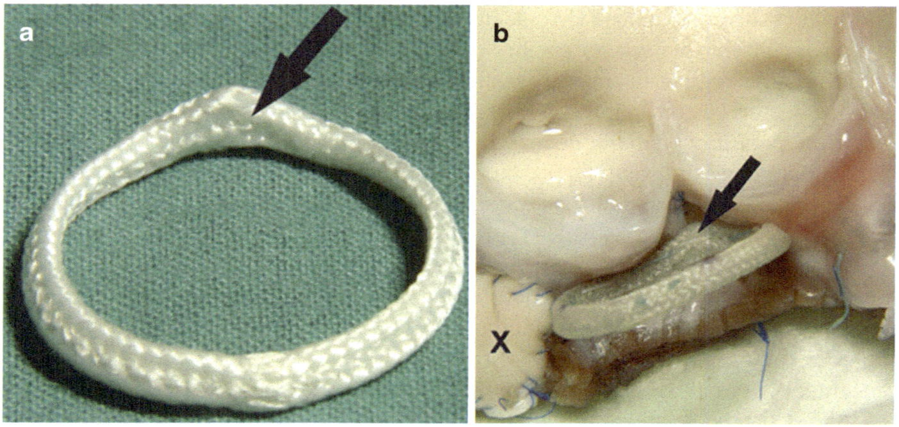

Fig. 11.6 (**a**) A novel rigid annuloplastic ring tested by Richardt in 2014. (**b**) The triangle elevation is placed at the area of the under-leaflet triangle between the right and non-coronary sinus, intending to prevent injury of their conduction bundle

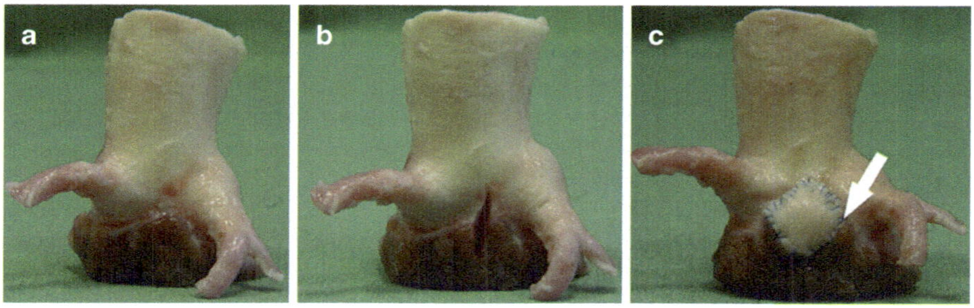

Fig. 11.7 (**a**, **b**, **c**) The aortic root was dissected from the outside the noncoronary sinus in both directions toward the coronary ostia

The advantages of this rigid novel aortic annuloplasty prosthetic ring (Genesee BioMedical, Inc., Denver, CO) were the following: (1) the suture ring prevents contact to the leaflets to avoid any leaflet contact injury, (2) there is no dependence on valve geometry, such that it can be used in bicuspid as well as in tricuspid valves, (3) it protects the area of the conduction bundle to prevent injury to the conduction system, (4) internal application facilitates implantation, and (5) rigidity assures a definite shape.

The triangle elevation (conduction triangle) was placed at the area of the under-leaflet triangle between the right and noncoronary sinus, intending to prevent injury to the conduction bundle. Suturing was accomplished after regular aortotomy through the aortic valve. The sutures (2-0 polyfilament) were placed from inside the left ventricular outflow tract to the outside of the root after dissection of this area. In the clinical setting, it is intended that the root will be dissected from outside the noncoronary sinus in both directions toward the coronary ostia. In this area the ring can be fixed with stitches from inside to outside of the root. In the opposite area it is intended that the ring will be fixed by stitches placed from inside the outflow tract into the sinus of the left and right coronary leaflets. With the annuloplasty ring, regurgitation volume decreased and coaptation height of the leaflets increased.

Mean pressure gradient increased from 2.98 ± 0.38 mm Hg (group D) to 3.72 ± 0.40 mm Hg (group R; $p < 0.0001$). Conclusions. This novel aortic annuloplasty ring has the potential for supporting aortic valve reconstruction by remodeling the subvalvular area.

In conclusion at this time, there is no evidence of the superiority of one technique or implant over another. Few annuloplasty devices have been used clinically. Thus, there is growing interest in an annuloplasty for the aortic valve and the increasing impression that it will be beneficial for aortic valve repair. At the same time, there is uncertainty as to the best mode of application of such a device (external vs. internal) and the best type of material (expansible, flexible or rigid). For clinical decisions, haemodynamic function, stability and biocompatibility will be essential. The device will have to effectively stabilize the aortoventricular junction at the desired diameter. It should not have acute or long-term interference with the conduction system and cusp mobility and structure [16].

References

1. Boodhwani M, de Kerchove L, Glineur D, et al. Repair-oriented classification of aortic insufficiency: impact on surgical techniques and clinical outcomes. J Thorac Cardiovasc Surg. 2009;137:286–94.
2. Ho SY. Structure and anatomy of the aortic root. Eur J Echocardiogr. 2009;10:i3–10.
3. Carr JA, Savage EB. Aortic valve repair for aortic insufficiency in adults: a contemporary review and comparison with replacement techniques. Eur J Cardiothorac Surg. 2004;25:6–15.
4. Minakata K, Schaff VH, Zehr JK, et al. Is repair of aortic valve regurgitation a safe alternative to valve replacement? J Thorac Cardiovasc Surg. 2004;127:645–53.
5. Álvarez-Cabo R. Sparing aortic valve techniques. J Thoracic Dis. 2017;9(Suppl 6):S526–32.
6. de Kerchove L, El Khoury G. Anatomy and pathophysiology of the ventriculo-aortic junction: implication in aortic valve repair surgery. Ann Cardiothorac Surg. 2013;2(1):57–64.
7. Erasmi AW, Sievers HH, Bechtel JF, et al. Remodeling or reimplantation for valve-sparing aortic root surgery? Ann Thorac Surg. 2007;83:S752–6. discussion S785-90.
8. Patel ND, Weiss ES, Alejo DE, et al. Aortic root operations for Marfan syndrome: a comparison of the Bentall and valve-sparing procedures. Ann Thorac Surg. 2008;85(6):2003–10.
9. Cabrol C, Cabrol A, Guiraudon G, et al. Treatment of aortic insufficiency by means of aortic annuloplasty. Arch Mal Coeur Vaiss. 1966;59:1305–12.
10. Anderson RH, Devine WA, Ho SY, Smith A, McKay R. The myth of the aortic annulus: the anatomy of the subaortic outflow tract. Ann Thorac Surg. 1991;52:640–6.
11. Fattouch K, Castrovinci S, Murana G, Nasso G, Guccione F, Dioguardi P, Salardino M, Bianco G, Speziale G. Functional annulus remodelling using a prosthetic ring in tricuspid aortic valve repair: mid-term results. Interact Cardiovasc Thorac Surg. 2014;18:49–55.
12. Kerchove L d, Vismara R, Mangini A, Fiore GB, Price J, Noirhomme P, Antona C, Khoury GE. In vitro comparison of three techniques for ventriculo-aortic junction annuloplasty. Eur J Cardiothorac Surg. 2012;41:1117–24.
13. Fattouch K, Sampognaro R, Speziale G, Ruvolo G. New technique for aortic valve functional annulus reshaping using a handmade prosthetic ring. Ann Thorac Surg. 2011;91:1154–8.

14. Mazzitelli D, Fischlein T, Scott Rankin J, Choi Y-H, Stamm C, Pfeiffer S, Pirk J, Detter C, Kroll J, Beyersdorf F, Griffin CD, Shrestha M, Nöbauer C, Crooke PS, Schreiber C, Lange R. Geometric ring annuloplasty as an adjunct to aortic valve repair: clinical investigation of the HAART 300 device. Eur J Cardiothorac Surg. 2016;49:987–93.
15. Richardt D, Bucsky B, Charitos EI, Sievers H-H, Scharfschwerdt M. A novel rigid annuloplasty ring for aortic valve reconstruction: an in vitro investigation. Ann Thorac Surg. 2014;97:811–5.
16. Schäfers H-J. Aortic annuloplasty: a new aspect of aortic valve repair (editorial comment). Eur J Cardiothorac Surg. 2012;41:1124–5.

Part IV

Aortic Root Surgery Techniques

12 Root Replacement with Biological Valved Conduits

Paolo Berretta and Marco Di Eusanio

In 1968, Bentall and De Bono introduced the surgical technique involving composite aortic valve and root replacement with reimplantation of the coronary arteries for treatment of thoracic aortic aneurysms [1]. Since its introduction, Bentall procedure has proven to be a safe and effective technique [2–4], and has been considered the gold standard in the surgical treatment of combined aortic valve and root pathologies. As initially described by Bentall and De Bono, it involved the use of a composite mechanical valved conduit. However, the use of biological aortic valve prostheses has increased noticeably over the last years [5]. This trend may be due to the raising prevalence of aortic valve diseases in the elderly population [6], the growing data proving excellent long-term durability of latest aortic prostheses [7, 8], the need for long-term anticoagulation for mechanical valves [6, 9] and the development of minimally invasive transcatheter valve-in-valve techniques [10]. Together, these data have triggered the development of alternative biological root substitutes and techniques for aortic root replacement such as biological hand-sewn composite grafts, xenograft aortic bioprosthetic root and total biological valved conduit. Compared to mechanical composite grafts, these biological valved conduits do not require lifelong oral anticoagulation and are subsequently associated with a lower thromboembolic/haemorragic risk.

The aim of this manuscript was to review the available biological valved conduits and discuss on current evidence of Bentall procedure using a biological valve prosthesis.

P. Berretta, M.D. • M. Di Eusanio, M.D., Ph.D. (✉)
Cardiac Surgery Unit, Ospedali Riuniti, Ancona, Italy
e-mail: paolo.berretta@ospedaliriuniti.marche.it; marco.dieusanio@ospedaliriuniti.marche.it

K. Fattouch et al. (eds.), *Advances in Treatments for Aortic Valve and Root Diseases*, https://doi.org/10.1007/978-3-319-66483-5_12

12.1 Surgical Indications

Different conditions may require the surgical replacement of the aortic valve and root with a biological valved conduit. These include aneurysms, aortic dissections, and infections involving the aortic root.

12.1.1 Aortic Aneurysm

Indications for aortic root repair are based primarily on aortic diameter and resulting from findings on natural history concerning the risk of complications, weighed against the risk of elective surgery. According to the current guidelines aortic root diameters of 5.0–5.5 cm or more, in asymptomatic patients without a connective tissue disorder, should be replaced to prevent aortic dissection and rupture. Furthermore, elective aortic root replacement is recommended in a less dilated aorta (4.2–5.0 cm), if the patient has a genetic or familial predisposition to aneurysm formation or dissection [11, 12]. In particular, patients with Marfan syndrome should undergo elective operation for aortic diameters ≥5 cm. An aortic diameter of 4.5 cm appears to be a reasonable threshold for prophylactic surgery in Marfan patients with family history of aortic dissection or aortic size increase >3 mm/year, severe aortic or mitral regurgitation, or desire for pregnancy [11–13]. Earlier operations have been suggested for aortic diameters of 4.2 cm or greater in patients with Loeys-Dietz syndrome or a confirmed TGFBR1 or TGFBR2 mutation [11]. A lower threshold of 5 cm should be also considered in patients with bicuspid aortic valve with additional risk factors, such as family history of aortic dissection, hypertension, coarctation of the aorta and aortic size increase >3 mm/year [12]. For patients who have an indication for aortic valve surgery, lower threshold (4.5 cm) for aortic repair can be evaluated.

Finally, patients with symptoms suggestive of expansion of an aortic aneurysm should be considered for prompt aortic repair.

12.1.2 Type A Acute Aortic Dissection

In patients with type A acute aortic dissection (TA-AAD), standard indications for aortic root replacement include extensive dissection and disruption of the aortic sinuses and the presence of a concomitant aortic root dilatation [11].

However, the optimal surgical management of the dissected aortic root is still controversial. Several groups have encouraged a systematic replacement of the dissected root to improve long-term outcomes by decreasing late aortic dilatation, re-dissection and recurrence of valve insufficiency [14, 15]. Nevertheless, this approach is perceived to carry higher operative mortality due to increased technical complexity. Therefore others surgeons suggest a conservative management involving supra-coronary ascending aorta replacement and commissural resuspension or aortic valve replacement, to minimize operative risks and improve early results [16]. In this setting, a report from the International Registry of Acute Aortic Dissection (IRAD) analysed data on 1995 patients undergoing TA-AAD surgery and stratifying results according to type of root management. Findings revealed that a complete aortic root replacement did not worsen hospital mortality compare to more conservative root treatment, in selected patients. Nevertheless, midterm survival and freedom from aortic reoperation were independent of root management type [17]. In a comparable study, Castrovinci et al. [18] demonstrated that an aggressive approach with replacement of the aortic root did not increase early mortality as well as late survival. However, in the long run, root replacement appeared to be protective against proximal aortic re-intervention. Therefore, during TA-AAD surgery, management of the aortic root should be determined by each patient's clinical and anatomical characteristics as well as by the surgical experience of the operating surgeon. Complete root replacement seems justified in patients with well-acknowledged risk factors for late aortic complications or likely need for re-operations (connective disease, bicuspid aortic valve and young age).

12.1.3 Infective Endocarditis

Aortic root replacement for native or prosthetic acute aortic valve endocarditis is a technically demanding intervention and represent a great challenge for cardiovascular surgeon. The main indications for surgery are heart failure, uncontrolled infection and prevention of embolic events [19]. Due to the patients' preoperative condition, persistent sepsis, and destructive processes at the level of left ventricular outflow tract, aortic annulus and proximal aorta, operative outcomes are still unsatisfactory, with a mortality rate ranging between 4 and 32% [20–27]. The choice of valve substitutes to replace destroyed heart valves is still a matter of controversial discussion in the surgical community. Various techniques have been suggested for reconstruction of the aortic root, involving repair with autologous or bovine pericardium and mechanical or biolgical valve replacement, and use of composite grafts, homografts, or autografts [20, 21, 28–31]. Root replacement with homograft material is frequently recommended because of its resistance to infection as well as its flexibility and pliability, which allow to construct tension-free suture lines and fill any abscess cavities [20, 29]. Several data have suggested that homograft aortic root replacement is associated with a lower mortality and a lower incidence of recurrent endocarditis compared with prosthetic material [20, 28, 29, 32, 33]. Nevertheless the majority of evidence is limited to observational studies. Moreover homografts are often of limited availability, especially during emergency procedures. In this setting, recent findings seems to indicate that mechanical and biological prostheses, may lead to comparable outcomes in terms of persistent or recurrent infection and survival, if associated with complete debridement of annular abscesses [34, 35]. Thus, aortic root replacement for active endocarditis still represents a serious concern and, with the lack of randomized studies comparing outcomes between different valve substitutes, selecting the most effective continues to be challenging.

12.2 Surgical Technique

The ascending aorta and the aortic root are approached using a standard median sternotomy or an upper J-ministernotomy extended to the right third or fourth intercostal space [36, 37]. The pericardium is opened and the ascending aorta, the proximal arch, the right atrium and the right superior pulmonary vein are adequately exposed. After systemic heparinization, cardiopulmonary bypass (CPB) is instituted by means of standard central cannulation involving distal ascending aorta and right atrium. The left side of the heart is vented through the right superior pulmonary vein. The ascending aorta is gently clamped and cardioplegic arrest is achieved as usual. The aneurysm is opened 3 cm above the right coronary ostium and the modified Bentall procedure using "button technique" is performed in the standard fashion [38]. In particular the aortic root is extensively freed from surrounding tissue and the buttons containing the coronary ostia are carefully prepared and fully mobilized for the following re-attachment. The non-coronary sinus is resected. The aortic valve is removed and the anulus debrided.

12.2.1 Biological Valved Conduits and Implantation Techniques

Currently, there are four types of biological valved conduits available on the market: (1) the so-called biological hand-sewn composite graft, (2) the Medtronic Freestyle Root (Medtronic, Irvine, CA, USA); (3) the Sorin Mitroflow Valsalva Conduit (Livanova, Saluggia, Italy) and (4) the No-React® BioConduit (BioIntegral Surgical, Inc., Ontario, Canada).

12.2.1.1 Hand-Sewn Composite Graft

Hand-sewn composite grafts are directly assembled by the operating surgeon, using all available aortic valve bio-prostheses coupled with an appropriate Dacron vascular graft;

The appropriate aortic valve bio-prosthesis is selected by measuring the aortic annulus with the dedicated sizer. Adding 5 mm to the size of the measured aortic annulus determines the Dacron vascular graft size. The bio-prosthetic valve is inserted into the vascular graft, so that the collar of the graft and the sewing ring of the prosthetic valve are in close contact. Standard 2/0 braided interrupted sutures or continuous 2/0 (or 3/0) polypropylene sutures are placed through the native aortic annulus and then passed together through the sewing ring of the aortic prosthesis and the collar of the Dacron graft in a single-step manner. The composite graft is parachuted to a sub-anular position and the sutures are tied-down and cut. A 4/0 polypropylene running suture can be used to approximate the aortic remnant to the sewing ring to improve hemostasis [39]. Appropriate holes for re-implantation of the coronary buttons are made in the Dacron graft using a cautery. First the left, and then the right coronary artery, are attached using 5/0 (or 6/0) polypropylene running sutures. The distal anastomosis between the Dacron graft and the aorta will complete the intervention (Fig. 12.1).

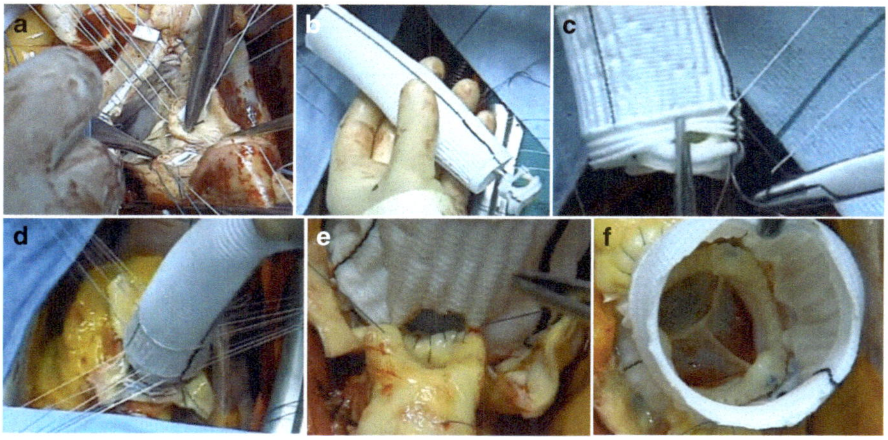

Fig. 12.1 Hand-sewn composite graft assembling and implantation techniques. Standard 2/0 braided interrupted sutures are placed through the native aortic annulus (**a**). The bio-prosthetic valve is inserted into the Dacron graft, so that the collar of the graft and the sewing ring of the prosthetic valve are in close contact (**b**). Annulus sutures are then passed through the sewing ring of the aortic prosthesis and the collar of the Dacron graft in a single-step manner (**c**). The composite graft is parachuted to a sub-anular position and the sutures are tied-down and cut (**d**). First the left (**e**), and then the right coronary artery, are re-attached (**f**)

Some groups suggest to assembly the graft by fixing the valve prosthesis inside the Dacron graft using a running suture, leaving a few millimetres rim of vascular graft below the aortic prosthesis for anastomosing to the annulus. Thus, the composite graft is implanted in a supra-annular position by passing the sutures through the end of the Dacron graft rather than through the sewing ring of the aortic prosthesis [40–42]. This technique may allow the surgeon to place a larger size valve than the annulus because the valve is seated above the aortic annulus, and to replace a degenerated bio-prosthesis within the vascular graft rather than replacing the complete conduit [43]. In-fact, during re-operation, the valve prosthesis can be easily removed from the inside of the vascular graft, and effectively replaced by a new prosthesis fixed at the native aortic annulus in the standard manner. However, this graft assembling technique is time consuming and may prolong operative times.

12.2.1.2 Medtronic Freestyle Root

Medtronic Freestyle is a xenograft stentless aortic bioprosthetic root composed by an intact porcine aortic root with ligated coronary arteries. It is preserved in a buffered 0.2% glutaraldehyde solution that is applied simultaneously to the in inflow and outflow portions of the porcine aortic root at a pressure of 40 mmHg to distend the aortic root to normal anatomical dimensions. The valve has a ring of polyester at the inflow and covering the septal myocardium that provides strength and ease of implantation [44]. Valve leaflets are treated with an alpha-amino oleic (AOA®) anti-calcification process and zero pressure leaflet fixation, aiming to preserve a natural

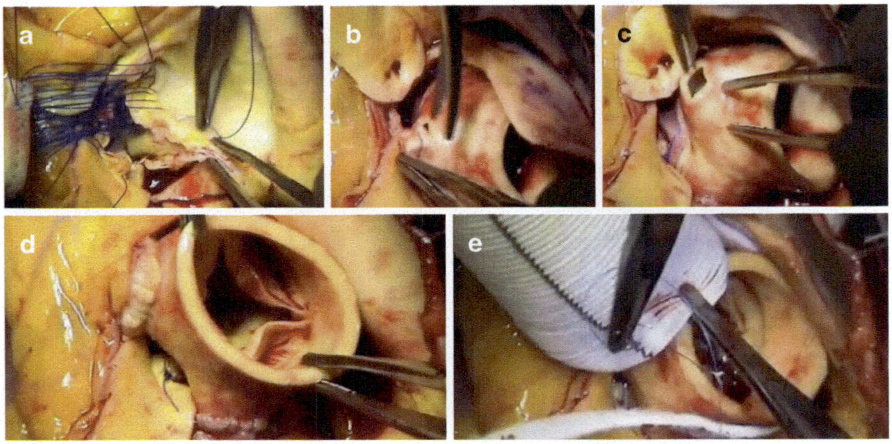

Fig. 12.2 Medtronic Freestyle Root implantation technique. The proximal anastomosis is performed using continuous polypropylene sutures (**a**). The coronary ostia of the graft are opened with scissors (**b**) and the native coronary arteries are re-attached to the corresponding sinus of Valsalva (**c–d**). Frequently, an interposition Dacron vascular graft is required to complete the distal anastomosis between the Freestyle root and the native distal aorta (**e**)

collagen crimp and thereby maintain optimal shock-absorbing capacity [45]. The Medtronic Freestyle Root is available in a wide range of sizes, from 19 to 27 mm.

The size of the annulus is measured and an appropriate Freestyle Root bio-prosthesis is chosen. The proximal anastomosis is performed using multiple braided interrupted sutures or continuous polypropylene sutures. During proximal anastomosis construction, the left coronary artery of the graft must be align with the left coronary button of the native aorta to allow for following re-attachment. The coronary ostia of the graft are opened with scissors and the native coronary arteries on their buttons of aortic wall are re-attached end to side to the corresponding sinus of Valsalva using a 5/0 (or 6/0) polypropylene running suture. Frequently, an interposition Dacron vascular graft is required to complete the distal anastomosis between the Freestyle root and the native distal aorta, due to the reduced length of the Freestyle root (Fig. 12.2).

12.2.1.3 Sorin Mitroflow Valsalva Conduit

The Mitroflow Valsalva Conduit is a vascular graft designed to be coupled directly with the Mitroflow or the Crown (Livanova, Saluggia, Italy) aortic pericardial prosthesis. The aortic valve and the conduit are simply and quickly assembled together during the operation. The proximal portion of the vascular graft mimics the sinus of Valsalva. The Mitroflow valve is composed with a single-unit stent that provides flexibility and includes a radiopaque sewing ring. The bovine pericardium is assembled outwardly the stent to maximise the flow area. The manufacturing process includes Phospholipid Reduction Treatment (PRT) to decrease valve degeneration by reducing calcium uptake in the pericardial tissue. Available sizes for the aortic valve prosthesis range between 21 and 27 mm, coupled with a 5-mm larger Valsalva conduit.

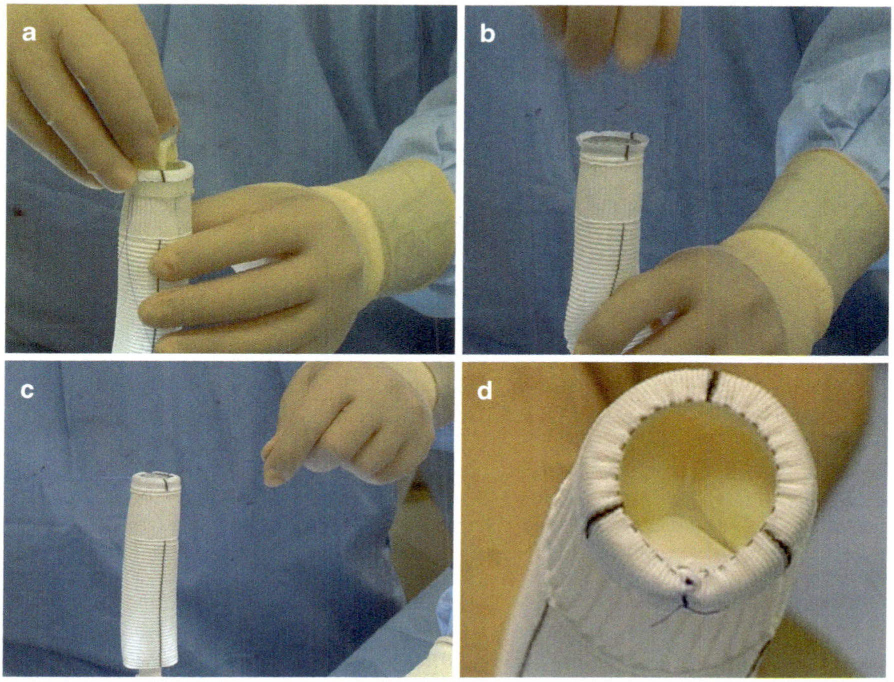

Fig. 12.3 Mitroflw Valsalva Conduit assembling process. Alignment of the valve commissure posts with the orientation guides on the conduit cuff and insertion of the valve into the conduit (**a**). Removal of the cuff unfolding ring (**b**). Folding of the conduit cuff over the sewing ring of the valve by pulling tying the suture (**c**–**d**)

For implantation, the annulus is measured using a dedicated valve sizer, and the corresponding Crown valve and a 5 mm larger Mitroflow Valsalva Conduit are selected. The valve and the Valsalva graft are quickly assembled before implantation. The assembling process involves four steps (Fig. 12.3): (1) lining up the valve commissure posts with the orientation guides on the conduit cuff and (2) inserting the valve into the conduit; (3) sliding off the graft the unfolding ring and pulling the conduit cuff up over the valve; (4) pulling the cuff suture until the conduit cuff folds down over the sewing ring of the valve and tying the suture. After the assembling, standard 2/0 braided interrupted sutures or continuous 2/0 (or 3/0) polypropylene sutures are passed through the native aortic annulus and through the sewing ring of the Mitroflow Valsalva Conduit. The graft is lowered into the aortic anulus and the sutures are tied-down and cut. The graft holder must be detached from the device only after the conduit has been sewn to the anulus. A 4–0 running suture can be used to approximate the aortic remnant to the sewing ring of the Valsalva conduit [39]. The coronary buttons are reattached to the skirted portion of the graft as usual. The distal anastomosis between the conduit and the distal aorta will complete the repair [37] (Fig. 12.4).

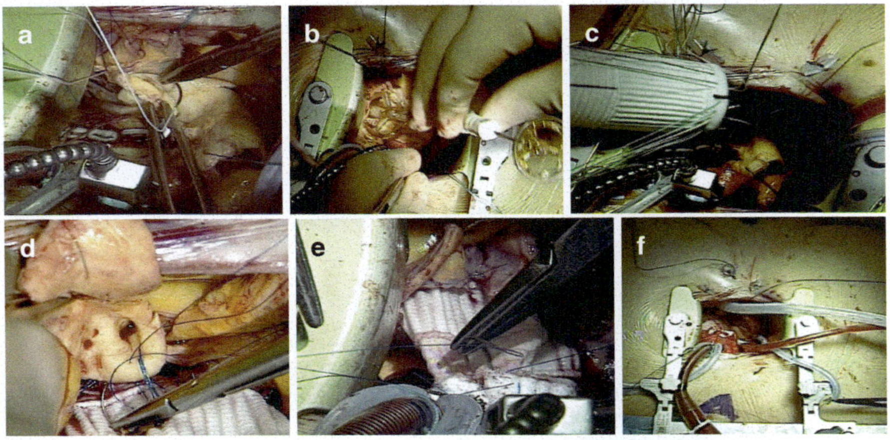

Fig. 12.4 Minimally invasive Mitroflw Valsalva Conduit implantation technique. Standard 2/0 braided interrupted sutures are passed through the native aortic annulus (**a**). The aortic annulus is measured using a dedicated valve sizer (**b**). After graft assembling (Fig. 12.3), the annulus sutures are passed through the sewing ring of the conduit (**c**), the graft is lowered into the aortic anulus and the sutures are tied-down and cut. The coronary buttons are re-attached to the skirted portion of the graft (**d**). The distal anastomosis between the conduit and the distal aorta complete the repair (**e**, **f**)

12.2.1.4 BioIntegral No-React® BioConduit

The BioIntegral No-React® BioConduit consists of a bovine straight graft (15 cm long) with an incorporated porcine stentless valve. The stentless valve is assembled using three non coronary aortic porcine cusps combined on a scallop-shaped tubular bovine pericardium. The BioConduit is glutaraldehyde cross-linked, detoxified and treated with the No-React® anticalcification and antidegenerative process, making biological tissues non-reactive and biocompatible [46]. No-React® BioConduit does not require rinsing before implantation. Six different conduit sizes are available, ranging between 21 and 31 mm.

For implantation, after the assessment of the aortic annulus with sizers provided by the company, an appropriate BioIntegral No-React® BioConduit is selected. The graft is secured to the aortic anulus using preferably a continuous 3/0 polypropylene suture or an interrupted sutures. It is important to align the suture line of the tube of the conduit with the middle of the non-coronary cusp. It avoids to perforate the suture line during re-attachment of the coronary arteries. The latter is made opening the conduit adjacent to the left and right coronary ostium with scissors. The coronary buttons are re-attached using 6–0 (or 5/0) running sutures. Then the distal anastomosis will be completed as usual (Fig. 12.5).

12.2.1.5 Biological Valved Conduits: Advantages and Drawbacks

Both the Freestyle root and the No-React® BioConduit incorporate a stentless biological valve. If this peculiarity is likely a minor issue during aortic root operations because a small aortic annulus is very rare in this patients and increased transvaluvlar gradients are rarely a concern after a biological Bentall

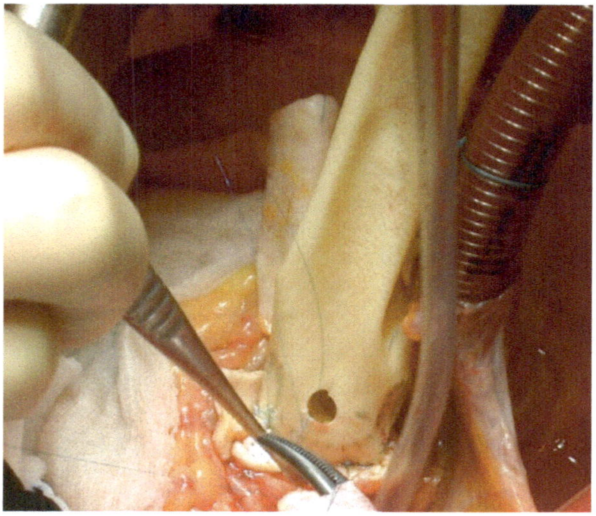

Fig. 12.5 BioIntegral No-React® BioConduit. Left coronary artery re-attachment

procedure, stentless valved conduits allow the surgeon to replace the aortic valve independently from the graft, which considerably simplify re-interventions due to structural aortic valve degeneration. Moreover, both devices may provide a valid alternative to the homograft, in patients with infective endocarditis. Both have no presence of foreign material and a great pliability which helps to adapt the prosthesis to an irregular aortic annulus [47, 48]. To date, no robust evidence is available about Freestyle root resistance to infection in active endocarditis, although several studies demonstrated excellent mid-term freedom from endocarditis in patient undergoing root replacement using Freestyle xenograft [31, 49]. While some Authors [48, 50] reported promising early results using No-React® BioConduit, in patients with and without endocarditis, other groups revealed unfavourable long term outcomes due to sudden structural valve failure, aorto-ventricular disconnection and recurrence of endocarditis [51–53]. In addition, an unusually high rate of unexplained deaths was reported al using this conduit [52].

The main drawback of the Freestyle root is the reduced length of the graft that often requires an interposition graft to connect the xenograft to the distal ascending aorta. This may prolong the operative times, increase the risk of bleeding from an additional suture-line and increase the surgery costs. The Freestyle xenografts as well as the No-React® BioConduit may severely calcify over time, thus strongly increasing the complexity of secondary root intervention.

The hand-sewn composite grafts still represent the most commonly biological valved conduits employed [54]. The main advantage of these grafts involves the possibility of combining different valve prostheses with different vascular grafts on which the operating surgeons strongly rely on. Furthermore, the aforementioned limitations of the Freestyle root and the No-React® BioConduit do not concern the hand-sewn composite grafts. Nevertheless the latter are certainly less handy, and in particular the passage of sutures through the sewing ring of the assembled graft may be uncomfortable and prolong operative times. These limitations may be overcome using the Sorin Mitroflow Valsalva Conduit. This device, thanks to a simple adjunct to a standard Valsalva graft, can be more easily and quickly assembled to a Mitroflow or a Crown valve. This allow to improve the graft handy and may reduce the operative times.

12.3 Current Evidence

The choice of valve prosthesis in an individual patient is based on consideration of several factors, including age, valve prosthesis durability, surgical risk, expected hemodynamics for a specific valve type and size, the potential need for long-term anticoagulation, and patient preferences [6, 55]. Over the last years, based on improved long term valve prostheses durability, data showing satisfactory results after secondary AVR [56], the development of transcathter valve in valve interventions, acknowledged reduced quality of life and occurrence of detrimental haemorrhagic and thromboembolic complications with long-life anticoagulation, the use of biological aortic valve prostheses has dramatically increased and represent almost 80% of all valve implants [57, 58]. Similarly, significant changes in aortic root replacement procedures have been observed [59, 60]. These involve movement away from mechanical composite grafts to aortic valve-sparing procedures in younger patients, and rise of biological valved conduits for older patients [54] and those who believe they will be candidates for valve-in-valve transcatheter procedure in the future. Data from the Society of Thoracic Surgeons (STS) database revealed that the usage of biological stented valves has approximately doubled, in patients undergoing root replacement. Conversely, stentless and homograft valves have become less common [59].

Over the last years, valve-sparing root replacement techniques, have been shown to provide excellent early and long-term outcomes, in patients with aortic root pathology [61]. However, not all patients are good candidates for valve sparing procedures due to frequent aortic leaflets disorders, increased technical complexity and longer operational duration [62]. Furthermore, the durability of biological valve prostheses may be superior to that of spared aortic valves and to the expectancy of life of aged patients. Therefore, complex valve-sparing procedures represent less appealing alternatives in elderly patients, and root replacement operations using biological composite grafts are more frequently performed in this setting.

To date, several studies have shown satisfactory outcomes for patients undergoing aortic root replacement using biological valved conduits. Etz et al. [63] reported on 275 patients who underwent Bentall operation with an hand-sewn biological composite graft. Hospital mortality was 6.2%, and the postoperative stroke rate was 1.5%. Long-term survival in men was similar to that of a normal matched control population, but was significantly lower in women. During follow up, the rate of stroke and significant haemorrhage was estimated as 0.85 and 0.3 per 100 patient/years respectively. No structural valve deterioration was found within 10 years. Reoperation for valve failure occurred in only one patient 12 years postoperatively.

A report from the Baylor College group [64] examined the early and late outcomes of aortic root replacement using stentless porcine xenografts. A graft extension for ascending aorta replacement was required in almost 98% of cases. Operative mortality was 7.6%. At a mean follow up of 3.3 ± 1.5 years, no structural valve failure occurred, with a low incidence of late valve-related complications (6.8%).

In the largest institutional study, Dapunt et al. [65]. reviewed hospital and mid-term results in 317 patients who underwent aortic root replacement using Freestyle xenograft. Overall operative mortality was 7.9% and postoperative stroke occurred in 3.1% of patients. Echocardiographic findings demonstrated excellent clinical results with low transvalvular gradients. At 5 years, no structural valve deterioration and no thromboembolic complications were described. Similarly, Kon et al. [66] reported no valve failure and outstanding hemodynamic performance (mean systolic gradient 6.7 mmHg; mean effective orifice area 1.8 cm^2) at the 8 year follow up. Long-term results (up to 12 years) for the Freestyle xenograft, have suggested excellent clinical findings, prosthesis durability, and hemodynamic performance. Nevertheless, most of the available data are focused solely on the use of the xenograft for subcoronary aortic valve replacement [49, 67–72]. Thus, strongest data are still needed to better evaluate long-term outcomes and durability of Freestyle root replacement.

Recently, in a systematic review, Castrovinci et al. [54] analysed early and late outcomes, in 3298 unselected patients underwent aortic root replacement using biological valved conduits. The mean age of patients was 67.1 years, and the main indication for surgery was degenerative aneurysm (75.1%), followed by acute aortic dissection (7.5%) and endocarditis (5.7%). Overall, average weighted mortality was satisfactory (6.4%; range 0–20%) and comparable to the pooled estimates for patients undergoing aortic root replacement using mechanical composite grafts [73]. Postoperative stroke were identified in 3.7% (range, 0–29%) of patients, and myocardial infarction in 2.9% (range 0–8%). Five and 10- years survival was 76 and 58% respectively.

Biological valved conduits have been associated with an increased risk of re-intervention, compared with mechanical composite grafts [3, 54, 73]. In this setting, Svensson et al. [60] assessed long-term outcomes on 957 patients underwent four aortic root procedures: aortic valve sparing (n = 261), composite biological graft (n = 297), composite mechanical graft (n = 156) and allograft root (n = 243). All procedures provided excellent survival and good durability. Early reoperation was more common after valve sparing and biological composite graft procedures, and allograft root replacement and biologic composite grafts had the highest risk of late reoperation. However, the increased risk of reoperation using biological valved conduits has to be weighed against the risk of life-long anticoagulation and an increased risk of thromboembolic complications related to mechanical composite grafts [3, 54, 73]. Furthermore, it has been demonstrated that re-operation on the aortic root can be performed with satisfactory outcomes, in particular when carried out on an elective basis, and has proven to be not a risk factor for mortality or morbidity in patient operated on at high volume aortic center by experienced surgeons [74, 75]. Moreover, the choice of valve prosthesis (mechanical or biological) seems to have no influence on early and long term clinical outcomes in patients undergoing root surgery [76].

Given the lengthening of life expectancy, the number of elderly patients with thoracic aorta diseases is continuously increasing. However concerns remain whether elderly patients can undergo aortic root surgery with outcomes and improvement in quality of life comparable to that obtained in younger patients. In this setting, some Authors revealed satisfactory surgical outcomes on septuagenarians [77] and octogenarians [78] undergoing aortic root replacement with biological composite grafts. In the afore-mentioned systematic review [54], no statistical correlation between mean age and mortality or incidence of postoperative stroke was identified, in patients undergoing aortic root replacement with biological valved conduits. Nevertheless, a report from STS database including patients undergoing aortic root replacement, showed that operative mortality and length of stay worsened significantly with increased patient age [59]. Recently, Sorabella et al. [78] reported on 592 patients undergoing aortic root replacement stratifying outcomes according to patients' age: patients less than 80 years old versus octogenarians. A biological composite graft was used in 88% of octogenarians. Hospital mortality was not significantly different between groups, being 5.9% in elderly patients and 2.3% in younger patients ($p = 0.2$). Moreover, the incidence of major postoperative complications was similar in the groups. Octogenarians cohort was associated with longer postoperative length of stay and decreased mid-term survival. Given the baseline frailty of the elderly population, the above-mentioned data suggested that aortic root replacement can be safely and effectively performed in selected elderly patients. Therefore a surgical approach should be considered in all patients and not should be denied on the basis of advanced age alone.

Conclusion

Aortic root replacement using biological valved conduits has being increasingly performed due to the growing prevalence of aortic valve diseases in the aging population, and rising evidence of improved long-term durability of the latest valve prostheses. Given the absence of valuable evidence demonstrating the superiority of a specific conduit, the choice of the graft is most frequently determined by surgeon's preference. Current evidence suggests favourable early and mid-term outcomes for biological root replacement. However, strongest long-term data are needed to adequately assess the durability and long-term outcomes of these conduits.

References

1. Bentall H, De Bono A. A technique for complete replacement of the ascending aorta. Thorax. 1968;23:338–9.
2. Gleason TG, David TE, Coselli JS, Hammon JW, Bavaria JE. St. Jude Medical Toronto biologic aortic root prosthesis: early FDA phase II IDE study results. Ann Thorac Surg. 2004;78:786–93.
3. Sioris T, David TE, Ivanov J, Armstrong S, Feindel CM. Clinical outcomes after separate and composite replacement of the aortic valve and ascending aorta. J Thorac Cardiovasc Surg. 2004;128:260–5.

4. Zehr KJ, Orszulak TA, Mullany CJ, Matloobi A, Daly RC, Dearani JA, Sundt TM, Puga FJ, Danielson GK, Schaff HV. Surgery for aneurysms of the aortic root: a 30-year experience. Circulation. 2004;110:1364–71.
5. Brown JM, O'Brien SM, Wu C, Sikora JA, Griffith BP, Gammie JS. Isolated aortic valve replacement in North America comprising 108,687 patients in 10 years: changes in risks, valve types, and outcomes in the Society of Thoracic Surgeons National Database. J Thorac Cardiovasc Surg. 2009;137:82–90.
6. Authors/Task Force Members, Vahanian A, Alfieri O, Andreotti F, Antunes MJ, Barón-Esquivias G, Baumgartner H, Borger MA, Carrel TP, De Bonis M, Evangelista A, Falk V, Iung B, Lancellotti P, Pierard L, Price S, Schäfers HJ, Schuler G, Stepinska J, Swedberg K, Takkenberg J, Von Oppell UO, Windecker S, Zamorano JL, Zembala M, ESC Committee for Practice Guidelines (CPG), Bax JJ, Ceconi C, Dean V, Deaton C, Fagard R, Funck-Brentano C, Hasdai D, Hoes A, Kirchhof P, Knuuti J, Kolh P, Mcdonagh T, Moulin C, Popescu BA, Reiner Z, Sechtem U, Sirnes PA, Tendera M, Torbicki A, Reviewers D, Von Segesser L, Badano LP, Bunc M, Claeys MJ, Drinkovic N, Filippatos G, Habib G, Kappetein AP, Kassab R, Lip GY, Moat N, Nickenig G, Otto CM, Pepper J, Piazza N, Pieper PG, Rosenhek R, Shuka N, Schwammenthal E, Schwitter J, Mas PT, Trindade PT, Walther T. Guidelines on the management of valvular heart disease (version 2012): the Joint Task Force on the Management of valvular Heart Disease of the European Society of Cardiology (ESC) and the European Association for Cardio-Thoracic Surgery (EACTS). Eur J Cardiothorac Surg. 2012;42:S1–S44.
7. Forcillo J, Pellerin M, Perrault LP, Cartier R, Bouchard D, Demers P, Carrier M. Carpentier-Edwards pericardial valve in the aortic position: 25-years experience. Ann Thorac Surg. 2013;96:486–93.
8. Bourguignon T, Bouquiaux-Stablo A, Candolfi P, Mirza A, Loardi C, May M, El-Khoury R, Marchand M, Aupart M. Very long-term outcomes of the Carpentier-Edwards perimount valve in aortic position. Ann Thorac Surg. 2015;99:831–7.
9. Slaughter MS, Jweied E. Managing mechanical valves with reduced anticoagulation. Expert Rev Cardiovasc Ther. 2007;5:1073–85.
10. Thomas M, Schymik G, Walther T, Himbert D, Lefèvre T, Treede H, Eggebrecht H, Rubino P, Colombo A, Lange R, Schwarz RR, Wendler O. One-year outcomes of cohort 1 in the Edwards SAPIEN Aortic Bioprosthesis European Outcome (SOURCE) registry: the European registry of transcatheter aortic valve implantation using the Edwards SAPIEN valve. Circulation. 2011;124:425–33.
11. Hiratzka LF, Bakris GL, Beckman JA, Bersin RM, Carr VF, Casey DE, Eagle KA, Hermann LK, Isselbacher EM, Kazerooni EA, Kouchoukos NT, Lytle BW, Milewicz DM, Reich DL, Sen S, Shinn JA, Svensson LG, Williams DM, Society for Vascular Medicine. 2010 ACCF/AHA/AATS/ACR/ASA/SCA/SCAI/SIR/STS/SVM guidelines for the diagnosis and management of patients with Thoracic Aortic Disease: a report of the American College of Cardiology Foundation/American Heart Association Task Force on Practice Guidelines, American Association for Thoracic Surgery, American College of Radiology, American Stroke Association, Society of Cardiovascular Anesthesiologists, Society for Cardiovascular Angiography and Interventions, Society of Interventional Radiology, Society of Thoracic Surgeons, and Society for Vascular Medicine. Circulation. 2010;121:e266–369.
12. Erbel R, Aboyans V, Boileau C, Bossone E, Bartolomeo RD, Eggebrecht H, Evangelista A, Falk V, Frank H, Gaemperli O, Grabenwöger M, Haverich A, Iung B, Manolis AJ, Meijboom F, Nienaber CA, Roffi M, Rousseau H, Sechtem U, Sirnes PA, Allmen RS, Vrints CJ, ESC Committee for Practice Guidelines. 2014 ESC Guidelines on the diagnosis and treatment of aortic diseases: document covering acute and chronic aortic diseases of the thoracic and abdominal aorta of the adult. The Task Force for the Diagnosis and Treatment of Aortic Diseases of the European Society of Cardiology (ESC). Eur Heart J. 2014;35:2873–926.
13. Jondeau G, Detaint D, Tubach F, Arnoult F, Milleron O, Raoux F, Delorme G, Mimoun L, Krapf L, Hamroun D. Aortic event rate in the Marfan population a cohort study. Circulation. 2012;125:226–32.

14. Halstead JC, Spielvogel D, Meier DM, Rinke S, Bodian C, Malekan R, Ergin MA, Griepp RB. Composite aortic root replacement in acute type A dissection: time to rethink the indications? Eur J Cardiothorac Surg. 2005;27:626–32. discussion 632-3.
15. Kallenbach K, Oelze T, Salcher R, Hagl C, Karck M, Leyh RG, Haverich A. Evolving strategies for treatment of acute aortic dissection type A. Circulation. 2004;110:II–243.
16. Westaby S, Saito S, Katsumata T. Acute type A dissection: conservative methods provide consistently low mortality. Ann Thorac Surg. 2002;73:707–13.
17. Di Eusanio M, Trimarchi S, Peterson MD, Myrmel T, Hughes GC, Korach A, Sundt TM, Di Bartolomeo R, Greason K, Khoynezhad A, Appoo JJ, Folesani G, De Vincentiis C, Montgomery DG, Isselbacher EM, Eagle KA, Nienaber CA, Patel HJ. Root replacement surgery versus more conservative management during type A acute aortic dissection repair. Ann Thorac Surg. 2014;98:2078–84.
18. Castrovinci S, Pacini D, Di Marco L, Berretta P, Cefarelli M, Murana G, Alfonsi J, Pantaleo A, Leone A, Di Eusanio M, Di Bartolomeo R. Surgical management of aortic root in type A acute aortic dissection: a propensity-score analysis†. Eur J Cardiothorac Surg. 2016;50(2):223–9.
19. Habib G, Lancellotti P, Antunes MJ, Bongiorni MG, Casalta JP, Del Zotti F, Dulgheru R, El Khoury G, Erba PA, Iung B, Miro JM, Mulder BJ, Plonska-Gosciniak E, Price S, Roos-Hesselink J, Snygg-Martin U, Thuny F, Tornos Mas P, Vilacosta I, Zamorano JL, Erol Ç, Nihoyannopoulos P, Aboyans V, Agewall S, Athanassopoulos G, Aytekin S, Benzer W, Bueno H, Broekhuizen L, Carerj S, Cosyns B, De Backer J, De Bonis M, Dimopoulos K, Donal E, Drexel H, Flachskampf FA, Hall R, Halvorsen S, Hoen B, Kirchhof P, Lainscak M, Leite-Moreira AF, Lip GY, Mestres CA, Piepoli MF, Punjabi PP, Rapezzi C, Rosenhek R, Siebens K, Tamargo J, Walker DM. 2015 ESC Guidelines for the management of infective endocarditis: the Task Force for the Management of Infective Endocarditis of the European Society of Cardiology (ESC). Endorsed by: European Association for Cardio-Thoracic Surgery (EACTS), the European Association of Nuclear Medicine (EANM). Eur Heart J. 2015;36:3075–128.
20. Knosalla C. Surgical treatment of active infective aortic valve endocarditis with associated periannular abscess—11 year results. Eur Heart J. 2000;21:490–7.
21. d'Udekem Y, David TE, Feindel CM, Armstrong S, Sun Z. Long-term results of operation for paravalvular abscess. Ann Thorac Surg. 1996;62:48–53.
22. Moon MR, Miller DC, Moore KA, Oyer PE, Mitchell RS, Robbins RC, Stinson EB, Shumway NE, Reitz BA. Treatment of endocarditis with valve replacement: the question of tissue versus mechanical prosthesis. Ann Thorac Surg. 2001;71:1164–71.
23. Perrotta S, Jeppsson A, Fröjd V, Svensson G. Surgical treatment for infective endocarditis: a single-centre experience. Thorac Cardiovasc Surg. 2016;25(3):169–73.
24. Watanabe G, Haverich A, Speier R, Dresler C, Borst HG. Surgical treatment of active infective endocarditis with paravalvular involvement. J Thorac Cardiovasc Surg. 1994;107:171–7.
25. Kirali K, Sarikaya S, Ozen Y, Sacli H, Basaran E, Yerlikhan OA, Aydin E, Rabus MB. Surgery for aortic root abscess: a 15-year experience. Tex Heart Inst J. 2016;43:20–8.
26. Dossche KM, Defauw JJ, Ernst SM, Craenen TW, De Jongh BM, de la Rivière AB. Allograft aortic root replacement in prosthetic aortic valve endocarditis: a review of 32 patients. Ann Thorac Surg. 1997;63:1644–9.
27. Glazier JJ, Verwilghen J, Donaldson RM, Ross DN. Treatment of complicated prosthetic aortic valve endocarditis with annular abscess formation by homograft aortic root replacement. J Am Coll Cardiol. 1991;17:1177–82.
28. Joyce F, Tingleff J, Aagaard J, Pettersson G. The Ross operation in the treatment of native and prosthetic aortic valve endocarditis. J Heart Valve Dis. 1994;3:371–6.
29. Niwaya K, Knott-Craig CJ, Santangelo K, Lane MM, Chandrasekaran K, Elkins RC. Advantage of autograft and homograft valve replacement for complex aortic valve endocarditis. Ann Thorac Surg. 1999;67:1603–8.
30. Aagaard J, Andersen PV. Acute endocarditis treated with radical debridement and implantation of mechanical or stented bioprosthetic devices. Ann Thorac Surg. 2001;71:100–3.

31. Aoyagi S, Fukunaga S, Tayama E, Hayashida N, Kawara T. Surgical treatment of prosthetic valve endocarditis with left ventricular-aortic discontinuity: reconstruction of the left ventricular outflow tract with a xenopericardial conduit. J Heart Valve Dis. 2001;10:367–70.
32. Musci M, Weng Y, Hübler M, Amiri A, Pasic M, Kosky S, Stein J, Siniawski H, Hetzer R. Homograft aortic root replacement in native or prosthetic active infective endocarditis: twenty-year single-center experience. J Thorac Cardiovasc Surg. 2010;139:665–73.
33. Pagano D, Allen SM, Bonser RS. Homograft aortic valve and root replacement for severe destructive native or prosthetic endocarditis. Eur J Cardiothorac Surg. 1994;8:173–6.
34. Avierinos J-F, Thuny F, Chalvignac V, Giorgi R, Tafanelli L, Casalta J-P, Raoult D, Mesana T, Collart F, Metras D. Surgical treatment of active aortic endocarditis: homografts are not the cornerstone of outcome. Ann Thorac Surg. 2007;84:1935–42.
35. David TE. Aortic valve repair for active infective endocarditis. Eur J Cardiothorac Surg. 2012;42(1):127–8. ezr283
36. Di Eusanio M, Castrovinci S, Cefarelli M, Berretta P, Alfonsi J, Murana G, Di Bartolomeo R. Minimally invasive root surgery: a Bentall procedure through a J-ministernotomy. Ann Cardiothorac Surg. 2015;4:198–200.
37. Di Eusanio M, Pucci A, and Berretta P. Mini-Bentall Procedure with Mitroflow Valsalva Conduit. CTSNet. http://www.ctsnet.org/article/mini-bentall-procedure-mitroflow-valsalva-conduit. Published April 18, 2016.
38. Kouchoukos NT, Karp RB. Resection of ascending aortic aneurysm and replacement of aortic valve. J Thorac Cardiovasc Surg. 1981;81:142–3.
39. Copeland JG, Rosado LJ, Snyder SL. New technique for improving hemostasis in aortic root replacement with composite graft. Ann Thorac Surg. 1993;55:1027–9.
40. Urbanski PP, Hacker RW. Replacement of the aortic valve and ascending aorta with a valved stentless composite graft: technical considerations and early clinical results. Ann Thorac Surg. 2000;70:17–20.
41. Tabata M, Takayama H, Bowdish ME, Smith CR, Stewart AS. Modified Bentall operation with bioprosthetic valved conduit: Columbia University experience. Ann Thorac Surg. 2009;87:1969–70.
42. Albertini A, Dell'Amore A, Zussa C, Lamarra M. Modified Bentall operation: the double sewing ring technique. Eur J Cardiothorac Surg. 2007;32:804–6.
43. Urbanski PP, Heinz N, Zhan X, Hijazi H, Zacher M, Diegeler A. Modified bio-Bentall procedure: 10-year experience. Eur J Cardiothorac Surg. 2010;37:1317–21.
44. Doty DB, Cafferty A, Kon ND, Huysmans HA, Krause AH, Westaby S. Medtronic freestyle aortic root bioprosthesis: implant techniques. J Card Surg. 1998;13:369–75.
45. Westaby S, Amarasena N, Ormerod O, Amarasena GA, Pillai R. Aortic valve replacement with the freestyle stentless xenograft. Ann Thorac Surg. 1995;60:S422–7.
46. Abolhoda A, Yu S, Oyarzun JR, Allen KR, McCormick JR, Han S, Kemp FW, Bogden JD, Lu Q, Gabbay S. No-react detoxification process: a superior anticalcification method for bioprostheses. Ann Thorac Surg. 1996;62:1724–30.
47. Müller LC, Chevtchik O, Bonatti JO, Müller S, Fille M, Laufer G. Treatment of destructive aortic valve endocarditis with the freestyle aortic root bioprosthesis. Ann Thorac Surg. 2003;75:453–6.
48. Musci M, Siniawski H, Knosalla C, Grauhan O, Weng Y, Pasic M, Meyer R, Hetzer R. Early and mid-term results of the Shelhigh stentless bioprosthesis in patients with active infective endocarditis. Clin Res Cardiol. 2006;95:247–53.
49. Doty DB, Cafferty A, Cartier P, Huysmans HA, Kon ND, Krause AH, Millar RC, Sintek CF, Westaby S. Aortic valve replacement with medtronic freestyle bioprosthesis: 5-year results. In: Seminars in thoracic and cardiovascular surgery. p. 35–41;1999.
50. Galiñanes M, Meduoye A, Ferreira I, Sosnowski A. Totally biological composite aortic stentless valved conduit for aortic root replacement: 10-year experience. J Cardiothorac Surg. 2011;6:86.

51. Carrel TP, Schoenhoff FS, Schmidli J, Stalder M, Eckstein FS, Englberger L. Deleterious outcome of no-react-treated stentless valved conduits after aortic root replacement: why were warnings ignored? J Thorac Cardiovasc Surg. 2008;136:52–7.
52. Sahin A, Müggler O, Sromicki J, Caliskan E, Reser D, Emmert MY, Alkadhi H, Maisano F, Falk V, Holubec T. Long-term follow-up after aortic root replacement with the Shelhigh® biological valved conduit: a word of caution! Eur J Cardiothorac Surg. 2016;50(6):1172–8.
53. Reineke DC, Kaya A, Heinisch PP, Oezdemir B, Winkler B, Huber C, Heijmen RH, Morshuis W, Carrel TP, Englberger L. Long-term follow-up after implantation of the Shelhigh® No-React® complete biological aortic valved conduit. Eur J Cardiothorac Surg. 2016;50:98–104.
54. Castrovinci S, Tian DH, Murana G, Cefarelli M, Berretta P, Alfonsi J, Yan TD, Di Bartolomeo R, Di Eusanio M. Aortic root replacement with biological valved conduits. Ann Thorac Surg. 2015;100:37–53.
55. Nishimura RA, Otto CM, Bonow RO, Carabello BA, Erwin JP, Guyton RA, O'Gara PT, Ruiz CE, Skubas NJ, Sorajja P, Sundt TM, Thomas JD, American College of Cardiology/American Heart Association Task Force on Practice Guidelines. 2014 AHA/ACC guideline for the management of patients with valvular heart disease: a report of the American College of Cardiology/American Heart Association Task Force on Practice Guidelines. J Am Coll Cardiol. 2014;63:e57–185.
56. Naji P, Griffin BP, Sabik JF, Kusunose K, Asfahan F, Popovic ZB, Rodriguez LL, Lytle BW, Grimm RA, Svensson LG, Desai MY. Characteristics and outcomes of patients with severe bioprosthetic aortic valve stenosis undergoing redo surgical aortic valve replacement. Circulation. 2015;132:1953–60.
57. Di Eusanio M, Fortuna D, De Palma R, Dell'Amore A, Lamarra M, Contini GA, Gherli T, Gabbieri D, Ghidoni I, Cristell D, Zussa C, Pigini F, Pugliese P, Pacini D, Di Bartolomeo R. Aortic valve replacement: results and predictors of mortality from a contemporary series of 2256 patients. J Thorac Cardiovasc Surg. 2011;141:940–7.
58. Siregar S, de Heer F, Groenwold RH, Versteegh MI, Bekkers JA, Brinkman ES, Bots ML, van der Graaf Y, van Herwerden LA. Trends and outcomes of valve surgery: 16-year results of Netherlands Cardiac Surgery National Database. Eur J Cardiothorac Surg. 2014;46:386–97. discussion 397.
59. Stamou SC, Williams ML, Gunn TM, Hagberg RC, Lobdell KW, Kouchoukos NT. Aortic root surgery in the United States: a report from the Society of Thoracic Surgeons database. J Thorac Cardiovasc Surg. 2015;149:116–22.e4.
60. Svensson LG, Pillai ST, Rajeswaran J, Desai MY, Griffin B, Grimm R, Hammer DF, Thamilarasan M, Roselli EE, Pettersson GB, Gillinov AM, Navia JL, Smedira NG, Sabik JF, Lytle BW, Blackstone EH. Long-term survival, valve durability, and reoperation for 4 aortic root procedures combined with ascending aorta replacement. J Thorac Cardiovasc Surg. 2016;151:764–774.e4.
61. David TE, Feindel CM, David CM, Manlhiot C. A quarter of a century of experience with aortic valve-sparing operations. J Thorac Cardiovasc Surg. 2014;148:872–80.
62. Oka T, Okita Y, Matsumori M, Okada K, Minami H, Munakata H, Inoue T, Tanaka A, Sakamoto T, Omura A. Aortic regurgitation after valve-sparing aortic root replacement: modes of failure. Ann Thorac Surg. 2011;92:1639–44.
63. Etz CD, Homann TM, Rane N, Bodian CA, Di Luozzo G, Plestis KA, Spielvogel D, Griepp RB. Aortic root reconstruction with a bioprosthetic valved conduit: a consecutive series of 275 procedures. J Thorac Cardiovasc Surg. 2007;133:1455–63.
64. LeMaire SA, Green SY, Sharma K, Cheung CK, Sameri A, Tsai PI, Adams G, Coselli JS. Aortic root replacement with stentless porcine xenografts: early and late outcomes in 132 patients. Ann Thorac Surg. 2009;87:503–12. discussion 512-3.
65. Dapunt OE, Easo J, Hölzl PP, Murin P, Südkamp M, Horst M, Natour E. Stentless full root bioprosthesis in surgery for complex aortic valve-ascending aortic disease: a single center experience of over 300 patients. Eur J Cardiothorac Surg. 2008;33:554–9.
66. Kon ND, Riley RD, Adair SM, Kitzman DW, Cordell AR. Eight-year results of aortic root replacement with the freestyle stentless porcine aortic root bioprosthesis. Ann Thorac Surg. 2002;73:1817–21. discussion 1821.

67. Mohammadi S, Baillot R, Voisine P, Mathieu P, Dagenais F. Structural deterioration of the freestyle aortic valve: mode of presentation and mechanisms. J Thorac Cardiovasc Surg. 2006;132:401–6.
68. Kappetein AP, Braun J, Baur LH, Prat A, Peels K, Hazekamp MG, Schoof PH, Huysmans HA. Outcome and follow-up of aortic valve replacement with the freestyle stentless bioprosthesis. Ann Thorac Surg. 2001;71:601–8.
69. Deleuze PH, Fromes Y, Khoury W, Maribas P, Lemaire S, Bical OM. Eight-year results of freestyle stentless bioprosthesis in the aortic position: a single-center study of 500 patients. J Heart Valve Dis. 2006;15:247–52.
70. Cartier PC, Dumesnil JG, Métras J, Desaulniers D, Doyle DP, Lemieux MD, Raymond G. Clinical and hemodynamic performance of the freestyle aortic root bioprosthesis. Ann Thorac Surg. 1999;67:345–9.
71. Bach DS, Metras J, Doty JR, Yun KL, Dumesnil JG, Kon ND. Freedom from structural valve deterioration among patients aged < or = 60 years undergoing freestyle stentless aortic valve replacement. J Heart Valve Dis. 2007;16:649–55. discussion 656.
72. Akar AR, Szafranek A, Alexiou C, Janas R, Jasinski MJ, Swanevelder J, Sosnowski AW. Use of stentless xenografts in the aortic position: determinants of early and late outcome. Ann Thorac Surg. 2002;74:1450–7.
73. Mookhoek A, Korteland NM, Arabkhani B, Di Centa I, Lansac E, Bekkers JA, Bogers AJ, Takkenberg JJ. Bentall procedure: a systematic review and meta-analysis. Ann Thorac Surg. 2016;101:1684–9.
74. Berretta P, Di Marco L, Pacini D, Cefarelli M, Alfonsi J, Castrovinci S, Di Eusanio M, Di Bartolomeo R. Reoperations versus primary operation on the aortic root: a propensity score analysis. Eur J Cardiothorac Surg. 2016;51(2):322–8.
75. Di Bartolomeo R, Berretta P, Petridis FD, Folesani G, Cefarelli M, Di Marco L, Di Eusanio M. Reoperative surgery on the thoracic aorta. J Thorac Cardiovasc Surg. 2013;145(3 Suppl):S78–84.
76. Etz CD, Bischoff MS, Bodian C, Roder F, Brenner R, Griepp RB, Di Luozzo G. The Bentall procedure: is it the gold standard? A series of 597 consecutive cases. J Thorac Cardiovasc Surg. 2010;140:S64–70. discussion S86–91.
77. Khaladj N, Leyh R, Shrestha M, Peterss S, Haverich A, Hagl C. Aortic root surgery in septuagenarians: impact of different surgical techniques. J Cardiothorac Surg. 2009;4:1.
78. Sorabella RA, Wu YS, Bader A, Kim MJ, Smith CR, Takayama H, Borger MA, George I. Aortic root replacement in octogenarians offers acceptable perioperative and late outcomes. Ann Thorac Surg. 2016;101:967–72.

Aortic Valve Sparing: Reimplantation Technique

13

Carmelo Mignosa and Antonino S. Rubino

13.1 Introduction

In 1992, David and Feindel firstly described a technique to preserve the aortic valve during aortic root replacement [1]. Since then, the valve sparing procedures gained widespread diffusion and stimulated the research on the treatment of aortic valve insufficiency and the physiopathology of the aortic root [2–4].

As a first step to approach any kind of valve sparing technique, the aortic root should be approached as a functional unity, built up of four different structures: (1) the functional aortic annulus (FAA), which includes the sino-tubular junction (STJ) and the ventriculo-aortic junction (VAJ); (2) the aortic leaflets; (3) the intercommissural triangles; (4) the sinuses of Valsalva [5]. Of peculiar interest is the so-called virtual basal ring, a virtual plane defined by the nadir of each cusp attachment [6]. This virtual plane plays a pivotal role in valve sparing surgery because it represents the target plane where the Dacron graft should seat proximally.

Ideally, all patients with aortic root aneurysms could be scheduled for a reimplantation technique, independently from the degree of aortic insufficiency, provided that the aortic leaflets are pliable. Therefore, the reimplantation technique should be considered an aortic valve repair procedure that: (1) corrects the dilation of the aortic root both at the level of the virtual basal ring and the sino-tubular junction; (2) achieves a firm stabilization of the functional aortic annulus; (3) increases the mobility and the coaptation surface of the aortic valve cusps [7, 8].

In this chapter, we will refer to the reimplantation technique using a straight tubular graft—also called David I procedure [4].

Electronic Supplementary Material The online version of this chapter (https://doi.org/10.1007/978-3-319-66483-5) contains supplementary material, which is available to authorized users.

C. Mignosa, M.D., F.E.T.C.S. (✉) • A.S. Rubino, M.D., Ph.D.
Centro Clinico-Diagnostico "G.B. Morgagni",
Department of Cardiology and Cardiovascular Surgery, Heart Center,
Centro Cuore, Via della Resistenza, 31, Pedara (CT) 95030, Italy
e-mail: carmignosa@tiscali.it; antonio.rubino@hotmail.com

K. Fattouch et al. (eds.), *Advances in Treatments for Aortic Valve and Root Diseases*, https://doi.org/10.1007/978-3-319-66483-5_13

13.2 Surgical Technique

Our surgical technique to perform a David I procedure using a single straight tubular Dacron graft has been already described elsewhere [9].

After aortic cross-clamping, the ascending aorta is transected at the level of the sino-tubular junction, removing the dilated aortic wall distal to the incision. The commissures are suspended on 4/0 polypropilene stay sutures and the aortic valve is inspected. If the valve anatomy is suitable to be spared (e.g. the leaflet are pliable or only moderately remodeled), the aortic root is dissected as down to the annulus as possible. However, due to the peculiar anatomy of the aortic root and the relationship with the surrounding structures, the dissection plane varies around the circumference of the aortic annulus. In particular, the dissection reaches the roof of the left atrium in correspondence of the non coronary sinus and the right half of the left coronary sinus (at the level of the nadir of the respective cusps). Differently, the dissection should be stopped a bit higher in correspondence of the right coronary sinus and left half of left coronary sinus, which anatomically includes part of the muscular septum and of the right ventricular outflow tract, to avoid a perforation of the right ventricle (Fig. 13.1).

Subsequently, the sinuses of Valsalva are excised, leaving a 3–5 mm remnant of the aortic wall for subsequent reimplantation. The coronary buttons are isolated. The stay sutures are gently pulled up until a good leaflet coaptation is reached. At this time, the diameter of the graft is chosen, measuring the distance from a commissure to the insertion of the opposite leaflet, approximating to the larger size (e.g. if 29 mm is measured, we chose a 30 mm graft).

Then, U-stitches (usually 12) of 2/0-coated polyester fibers with Teflon pledgets are placed circumferentially, inside-out and horizontally, below the nadir of the leaflets in the left ventricular outflow tract (Videos 13.1 and 13.2). The Dacron graft is trimmed for a 2–3 mm length in correspondence of the nadir of each commissure, to shape the prosthetic edge in a scalloped way that corresponds to the scalloped native annulus. Subsequently, these stitches are passed on the Dacron graft to anchor it slightly below the level of the annulus (virtual basal ring) and only gently tied to avoid any purse-string effect on the LVOT. Thereafter, the commissures are pulled

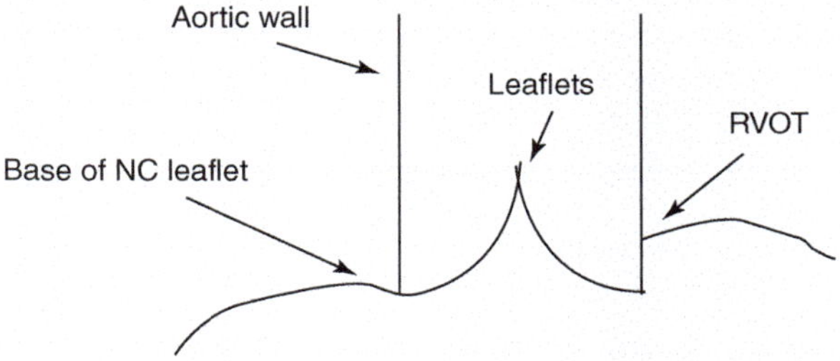

Fig. 13.1 A schematic representation of the aortic root with its external limitations. Note that at the level of the left and right sinuses, the dissection is limited by the presence of the right ventricular outflow tract (RVOT). A deeper dissection might cause the perforation of the right ventricle. *NC* non coronary. (Reprinted with permission from Jeanmart H et al. Ann Thorac Surg 2007;83:746–51.)

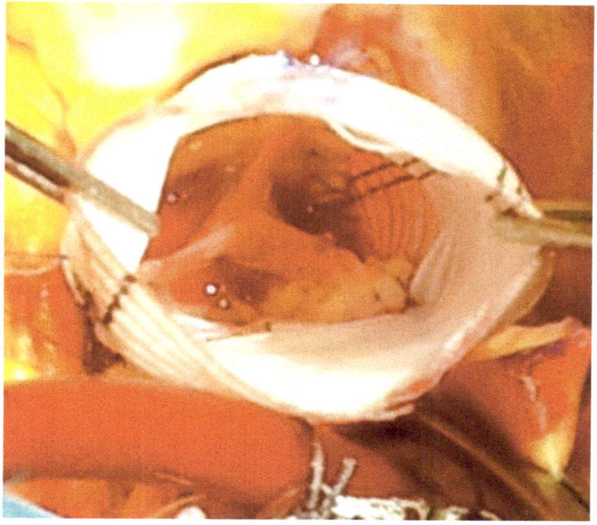

Fig. 13.2 Intraoperative view of a tricuspid aortic valve reimplanted inside a straight tubular graft

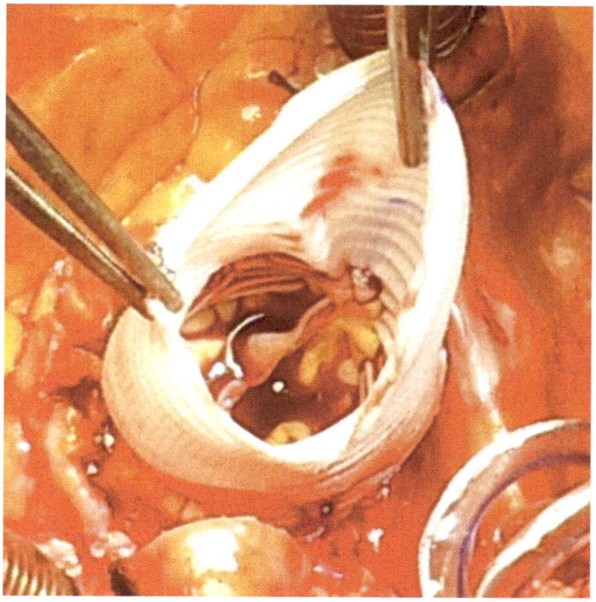

Fig. 13.3 Intraoperative view of a bicuspid aortic valve reimplanted inside a straight tubular graft

up inside the graft and fixed at the desired level to restore adequate valve competence with three running 4/0 polypropylene sutures, which act as the effective hemostatic suture lines.

When the valve has been completely reimplanted inside the graft, saline is injected to test the valve competence (Figs. 13.2 and 13.3). If necessary, adjunctive repair techniques are used accordingly to the etiology of the coaptation defect [10].

Surgeons should be advised not to perform adjunctive cusp repairs before the reimplantation is completed [11]. Accordingly, the restoration of the normal root geometry may correct a prolapse or a stretch of one or more cusps, originally due to the dilatation of the FAA itself.

David has explained that the key for long-term success relies on the level and on the length of coaptation. At the end of the procedure, coaptation must occur above the level of the nadir of the cusps, and the coaptation length must be at least 4 mm [12].

Eventually, the coronary ostia are reimplanted with the button technique with two running 5/0 polypropylene sutures. After that, cardioplegia is given directly inside the graft to test the valve competence and to check for adequate hemostasis.

13.3 Immediate Results

After more than two decades of experience, the reimplantation technique has now become a standard of care for the treatment of aortic root aneurysms. In a recent study, we have reported 0% operative mortality on 51 consecutive patients, operated electively from 2002 to 2010 [9]. This is in line with other reports, where mortality ranges from 0 to 4% [13–16]. However, in our study all the operation has been performed electively and no patient underwent a reimplantation procedure for acute aortic dissection. In this particular condition, operative mortality is often increased, more as a consequence of the underlying high-risk preoperative condition than of the procedure itself [15–17].

Beside a low operative mortality, immediate valve competence is the major result to be achieved by any valve repair procedure. Surgeons should be aware that patients' selection, along with a precise surgical technique, is the key to success in valve sparing surgery. In particular, an accurate inspection of the quality of the aortic leaflets is mandatory to approach a valve sparing procedure. In fact, severely remodeled cusps (e.g. thickening, folding, fenestrations, prolapse, elongations…) are general findings in patients with severe annular and root dilatation or chronic insufficiency. Accordingly, Thubrikar et al. showed that the increase of the length of the free edge and of the height of the leaflets parallels the dilatation of the aortic root [18]. Similarly, Grande-Allen et al. demonstrated that the increased aortic root diameters and the altered elastic properties of the aortic wall, typically documented in patients affected by the Marfan syndrome, co-operate to increase the stress and strain on the aortic leaflets, ending up in a severe remodeling of the cusps [19]. On the other hand, Badiu et al. showed that the reimplantation technique could be offered also to patients with severe preoperative aortic regurgitation [20]. Similarly, Kallenbach et al. demonstrated that preoperative severe aortic regurgitation does not impair the outcome after 3-year follow-up from a David procedure [21].

Surgeons must bear in mind that re-establishing the root geometry and achieving adequate valve competence is the main aim of a valve sparing technique. In case the root reconstruction is not sufficient *per se* to accomplish this goal, leaflet pathology should be addressed according to the etiology of the coaptation defect [10]. If, on one hand, this "*spare-and-plasty*" approach widens the treatment options to an increasing number of patients, on the other hand this methodology carries the inherent risk of failure of both procedures [11]. Accordingly, a multicenter Italian experience reported that the association of a leaflet plasty was the only independent risk factor for residual aortic valve regurgitation needing a reoperation at long-term follow-up [22]. Similarly, Oka et al. demonstrated that adjunctive cusp repair or cusp calcification were independent predictors of early failure [23]. Conversely, de Kerchove et al. reported satisfactory outcomes at discharge and at 8-year follow-up in 164 consecutive patients, 55% of them requiring adjunctive cusp repair [24].

Which role any adjunctive leaflet repair will play on the long-term freedom from aortic regurgitation is still to be determined. However, the competence of the aortic valve after a reimplantation procedure has to be considered a mandatory intraoperative result.

13.4 Long-Term Results

The excellent immediate results achieved with a reimplantation technique usually last over decades, especially in the most selected patients, such as those with a tricuspid aortic valve and less that moderate preoperative aortic insufficiency [25, 26]. Recently, David et al. reviewed all the 333 patients undergone valve sparing surgery with the reimplantation technique at their institution. At 20-year follow-up survival was 72.4%, freedom from reoperation on the aortic valve 96.9% and freedom from >2+ recurrent aortic regurgitation 96.2% [27]. Similarly, Shresta et al. reported their results in a series of 126 consecutive patients over a 17-year period, showing an overall 10-year survival of 70% and a freedom from reoperation on the aortic valve of 87%. Aortic insufficiency <2+ was observed in 89.5% of patients after a mean follow-up of 10 ± 2 years. When only elective patients are considered, excluding also Marfan patients, 10-year survival was 86%, freedom from reoperation on the aortic valve 92%; 85.8% had aortic insufficiency <2+ [15].

A recent multicenter analysis of 764 patients demonstrated that residual and progressive aortic regurgitation after the reimplantation technique is not negligible and that is influenced by aneurysm size and preoperative aortic valve competence. Interestingly, new onset aortic regurgitation after an initial valve competence more likely occurred at follow-up in case of additional cusp repair [28]. These results support two concepts: (1) patients should be operated before large aneurysms occur and aortic leaflets severely remodel; (2) accurate valve inspection and better patient selection is mandatory to achieve established valve competence in the long-term follow-up.

13.5 Performance of David I Under Stress

Several studies have clearly displayed that the sinuses of Valsava contribute actively to the opening and closing mechanisms of the aortic valve in the native root [29–31]. The benefit of recreating neo-sinuses after valve sparing operations has also been demonstrated in vitro [32] and in vivo [33]. However, the clinical superiority of techniques that recreates neo-sinuses over the original David I has never been claimed [34, 35].

Accordingly, we decided to assess the aortic valve hemodynamics during echocardiographic stress test late after David I in a selected cohort of patients from our clinical series [36]. Briefly, we enrolled only those patients undergone isolated reimplantation procedure, with preserved systolic function (left ventricular ejection fraction ≥55%) and with a follow-up ≥5 years. Patients undergone concomitant procedures (apart from adjunctive leaflet repair at the time of the David procedure), with any grade of aortic regurgitation and/or any grade of mitral regurgitation were excluded. Therefore, we selected 13 patients to undergo exercise echocardiographic stress test on a stationary cycle. Four (33.3%) patients had a bicuspid aortic valve. Additional procedures on the aortic valve were 1 subcommissural annuloplasty (7.7%), 1 patch augmentation in a bicuspid valve (7.7%), 1 plication of the free margin (7.7%), 1 reinforcement of the free edge with an over-and-over 5/0 PTFE running suture (7.7%). To ascertain the potential differences in the dynamics of the aortic valve under high workload, eight healthy volunteers were enrolled and served as Controls.

We observed that the increase of transvalvular gradients paralleled the increasing stroke volumes at incremental steps both in patients undergone David I and Controls, without reaching any clinical relevance (Peak gradient at 75 W: David I 23.8 ± 9.3 vs. Controls 11.8 ± 1.0 mmHg, $p = 0.002$; Mean gradient at 75 W: David I 13.2 ± 5.1 vs. Controls 6.4 ± 0.7 mmHg, $p = 0.002$). However, Controls increased EOAi from baseline to peak stress, whereas patients undergone David I maintained a stable valve area during the exercise (Greatest EOAi observed at 50 W: David I 1.5 ± 0.4 vs. Controls 2.0 ± 0.3 cm^2/m^2, $p = 0.001$) (Fig. 13.4).

In a similarly designed study, D'Ancona et al. showed that patients undergone David I procedure had smaller EOAi at maximal stress (David 1.4 ± 0.3 vs. Controls 1.7 ± 0.2 cm^2/m^2, $p < 0.001$), without any differences in transvalvular gradients during the stress test [37].

It is general knowledge that the lack of sinuses might reduce the opening and closing velocity of the aortic cusps [32, 33]. However the major drawback of the procedure is the reimplantation of the functional aortic annulus inside a non-compliant graft, whatever size and shape (straight vs. neo-sinuses) is considered. In such peculiar pathophysiology, both the aortoventricular junction and the sino-tubular junction are fixed to a stationary diameter. Therefore, any motion of the functional aortic annulus is prevented during the cardiac cycle, apart from the aortic leaflets, which keep their motility without any support from the other structures (e.g. the intercommissural triangles). If this will limit the lifespan of the procedure is still to be determined. The lack of sinuses plays a secondary role [38]. Interestingly, in our series we have observed that the running sutures, used to reimplant the valve, recreated a sinus-like portion along the straight tube, without either valve degeneration or impaired leaflet movements at 128-slice angio-CT scan (Fig. 13.5) [9].

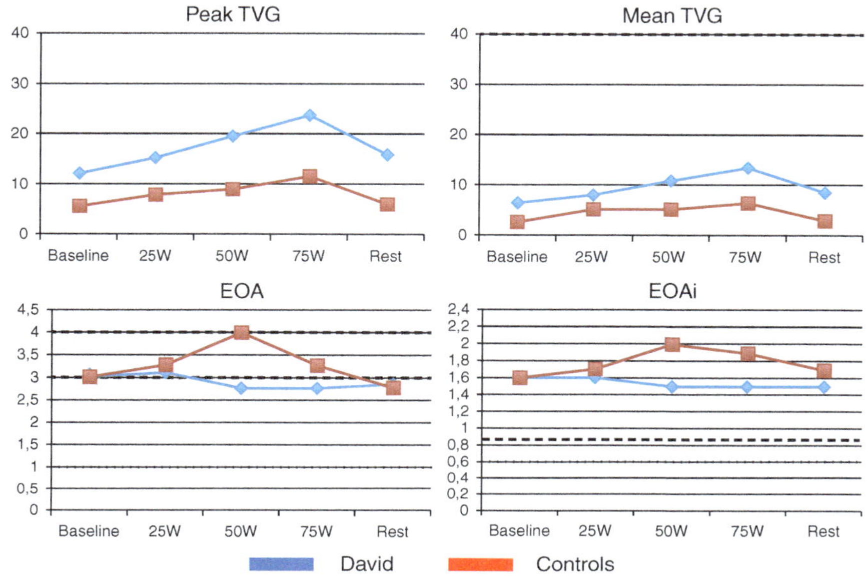

Fig. 13.4 Variation of peak and mean transvalvular gradients, effective orifice area and effective orifice area index during the test in patients undergone David I procedures and in healthy volunteers serving as controls. *Dashed lines* indicate normal reference values. *Dotted lines* indicate reference values for the diagnosis of severe aortic stenosis. (Reprinted with permission from Mignosa C et al. Semin Thorac Cardiovasc Surg 2015;27:257–63.)

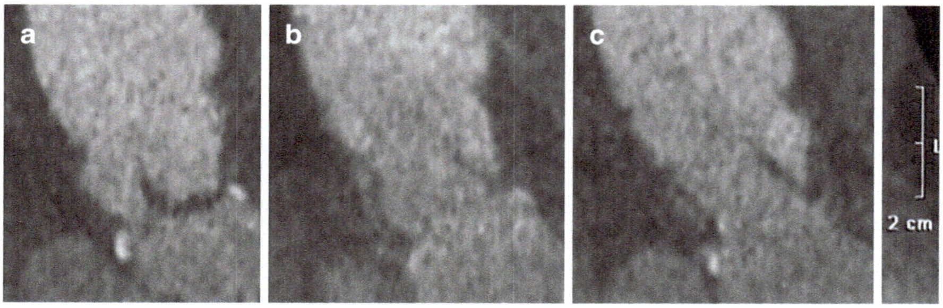

Fig. 13.5 128-slice angio-CT scan of the aortic box, showing the preserved valve motion after David I procedure during the various phases of the cardiac cycle (**a**: end diastole; **b**: early systole; **c**: complete opening at late systole). Note also the recreation of sinus-like portions, made by the running sutures used to reimplant the valve. (Reprinted with permission from Mignosa C et al. J Thorac Cardiovasc Surg 2014;148:1334–40.)

However, although smaller EOAi are frequently observed after David I, aortic valve function is maintained and its competence preserved at long-term follow-up, with sustainable results even at high workload conditions.

Conclusion

Valve-sparing procedure using a straight tubular graft (David I procedure) is safe, reproducible and delivers excellent immediate and long-term results. Reserving this technique only to patients with normal or mildly remodeled cusps will sustain long-term results. Aortic valve performance is preserved also under high flow conditions, even in absence of neo-sinuses.

References

1. David TE, Feindel CM. An aortic valve-sparing operation for patients with aortic incompetence and aneurysm of the ascending aorta. J Thorac Cardiovasc Surg. 1992;103:617–21.
2. Hopkins RA. Aortic valve leaflet sparing and salvage surgery: evolution of techniques for aortic root reconstruction. Eur J Cardiothorac Surg. 2003;24:886–97.
3. Ranga A, Bouchot O, Mongrain R, Ugolini P, Cartier R. Computational simulations of the aortic valve validated by imaging data: evaluation of valve-sparing techniques. Interact Cardiovasc Thorac Surg. 2006;5:373–8.
4. Miller DC. Valve-sparing aortic root replacement in patients with Marfan syndrome. J Thorac Cardiovasc Surg. 2003;125:773–8.
5. Sutton JP, Ho SY, Anderson RH. The forgotten interleaflet triangles: a review of the surgical anatomy of the aortic valve. Ann Thorac Surg. 1995;59:419–27.
6. Anderson RH. Defining the enigmatic annulus of the aortic valve. Eur J Cardiothorac Surg. 2016;49:101–2.
7. Boodhwani M, de Kerchove L, Glineur D, Poncelet A, Rubay J, Astarci P, Verhelst R, Noirhomme P, El Khoury G. Repair-oriented classification of aortic insufficiency: impact on surgical techniques and clinical outcomes. J Thorac Cardiovasc Surg. 2009;137:286–94.
8. Boodhwani M, El Khoury G. Principles of aortic valve repair. J Thorac Cardiovasc Surg. 2010;140:20–2.
9. Mignosa C, Di Stefano S, Mazzamuto M, Degno N, Mariani C, Romeo A, Rubino AS. Midterm follow-up of the reimplantation technique in patients with relatively normal annulus: is David I still a clinically valid option? J Thorac Cardiovasc Surg. 2014;148:1334–40.
10. El Khoury G, de Kerchove L. Principles of aortic valve repair. J Thorac Cardiovasc Surg. 2013;145:26–9.
11. De Paulis R. Aortic root surgery: from valve sparing to 'spare and plasty'. Eur J Cardiothorac Surg. 2013;38:513–4.
12. David TE. Aortic valve haemodynamics after aortic valve-sparing operations. Eur J Cardiothorac Surg. 2012;41:788–9.
13. de Oliveira NC, David TE, Ivanov J, Armstrong S, Eriksson MJ, Rakowski H, Webb G. Results of surgery for aortic root aneurysm in patients with Marfan syndrome. J Thorac Cardiovasc Surg. 2003;125:789–96.
14. Erasmi AW, Sievers HH, Bechtel JFM, Hanke T, Stierle H, Misfeld M. Remodeling or reimplantation for valve-sparing aortic root surgery? Ann Thorac Surg. 2007;83:752–6.
15. Shrestha M, Baraki H, Maeding I, Fitzner S, Sarikouch S, Khaladj N, Hagl C, Haverich A. Long-term results after aortic valve-sparing operation (David I). Eur J Cardiothorac Surg. 2012;41:56–62.
16. Leontyev S, Trommer C, Subramanian S, Lehmann S, Dmitrieva Y, Misfeld M, Mohr FW, Borger MA. The outcome after aortic valve-sparing (David) operation in 179 patients: a single-centre experience. Eur J Cardiothorac Surg. 2012;42:261–7.
17. David TE, Armstrong S, Ivanov J, Feindel CM, Omran A, Webb G. Results of aortic valve–sparing operations. J Thorac Cardiovasc Surg. 2001;122:39–46.
18. Thubrikar MJ, Labrosse MR, Zehr KJ, Robicsek F, Gong GG, Fowler BL. Aortic root dilatation may alter the dimensions of the valve leaflets. Eur J Cardiothorac Surg. 2005;28:850–6.

19. Grande-Allen KJ, Cochran RP, Reinhall PG, Kunzelman KS. Mechanisms of aortic valve incompetence: finite-element modeling of Marfan syndrome. J Thorac Cardiovasc Surg. 2001;122:946–54.
20. Badiu CC, Eichinger W, Bleiziffer S, Hermes G, Hettich I, Krane M, Bauernschmitt R. Should root replacement with aortic valve-sparing be offered to patients with bicuspid valves or severe aortic regurgitation? Eur J Cardiothorac Surg. 2010;38:515–22.
21. Kallenbach K, Karck M, Leyh RG, Hagl C, Walles T, Harringer W, Haverich A. Valve-sparing aortic root reconstruction in patients with significant aortic insufficiency. Ann Thorac Surg. 2002;74:1765–8.
22. De Paulis R, Scaffa R, Nardella S, Maselli D, Weltert L, Bertoldo F, Pacini D, Settepani F, Tarelli G, Gallotti R, Di Bartolomeo R, Chiariello L. Use of the Valsalva graft and long-term follow-up. J Thorac Cardiovasc Surg. 2010;140:S23–7.
23. Oka T, Okita Y, Matsumori M, Okada K, Minami H, Munakata H, Inoue T, Tanaka A, Sakamoto T, Omura A, Nomura T. Aortic regurgitation after valve-sparing aortic root replacement: modes of failure. Ann Thorac Surg. 2011;92:1639–44.
24. de Kerchove L, Boodhwani M, Glineur D, Poncelet A, Verhelst R, Astarci P, Lacroix V, Rubay J, Vandyck M, Vanoverschelde JL, Noirhomme P, El Khoury G. Effects of preoperative aortic insufficiency on outcome after aortic valve-sparing surgery. Circulation. 2009;120:S120–6.
25. David TE, Feindel CM, Webb GD, Colman JM, Armstrong S, Maganti M. Long-term results of aortic valve-sparing operations for aortic root aneurysm. J Thorac Cardiovasc Surg. 2006;132:347–54.
26. Ouzounian M, Rao V, Manlhiot C, Abraham N, David C, Feindel CM, David TE. Valve-sparing root replacement compared with composite valve graft procedures in patients with aortic root dilation. J Am Coll Cardiol. 2016;68:1838–47.
27. David TE, David CM, Feindel CM, Manlhiot C. Reimplantation of the aortic valve at 20 years. J Thorac Cardiovasc Surg. 2017;153:232–8. https://doi.org/10.1016/j.jtcvs.2016.10.081.
28. Kari FA, Doll KN, Hemmer W, Liebrich M, Sievers HH, Richardt D, Reichenspurner H, Detter C, Siepe M, Czerny M, Beyersdorf F. Residual and progressive aortic regurgitation after valve-sparing root replacement: a propensity-matched multi-institutional analysis in 764 patients. Ann Thorac Surg. 2016;101:1500–6.
29. Bellhouse BJ. The fluid mechanics of the aortic valve. In: Ionescu ML, Ross DN, Woller GH, editors. Biological tissue in heart valve replacement. London: Butterworth-Heinemann; 1972. p. 23–47.
30. Thubrikar MJ, Nolan SP, Aouad J, et al. Stress sharing between the sinus and leaflets of canine aortic valve. Ann Thorac Surg. 1986;42:434–40.
31. Leyh RG, Schmidtke C, Sievers HH, Yacoub MH. Opening and closing characteristics of the aortic valve after different types of valve-preserving surgery. Circulation. 1999;100:2153–60.
32. Grande-Allen KJ, Cochran RP, Reinhall PG, Kunzelman KS. Re-creation of sinuses is important for sparing the aortic valve: a finite element study. J Thorac Cardiovasc Surg. 2000;119:753–63.
33. De Paulis R, De Matteis GM, Nardi P, Scaffa R, Buratta MM, Chiariello L. Opening and closing characteristics of the aortic valve after valve-sparing procedures using a new aortic root conduit. Ann Thorac Surg. 2001;72:487–94.
34. David TE. Current readings: aortic valve-sparing operations. Semin Thorac Cardiovasc Surg. 2014;26:231–8.
35. Kari FA, Beyersdorf F, Rylski B, Stephens EH, Russe M, Siepe M. David I reimplantation procedure for aortic root replacement in Marfan patients: medium-term outcome. Interact Cardiovasc Thorac Surg. 2014;19:743–8.
36. Mignosa C, Mariani C, Deste W, Felis S, Di Stefano S, Giuffrida A, Rubino AS. Long-term hemodynamic performance of the aortic valve after David I: an echocardiographic study. Semin Thorac Cardiovasc Surg. 2015;27:257–63.
37. D'Ancona G, Ciofalo R, Biondo D, Follis M, Follis F. Midterm follow-up dynamic echocardiography evaluation after ascending aorta replacement and reimplantation of the aortic valve (David operation) in a matched control study. Eur J Cardiothorac Surg. 2012;41:785–8.
38. David TE. Back to David I. Semin Thorac Cardiovasc Surg. 2015;27:264–5.

Right Anterior Mini-Thoracotomy

14

Mauro Del Giglio and Elisa Mikus

14.1 Introduction

Minimally invasive aortic valve replacement (MIAVR) through a right mini-thoracotomy is an interesting approach witch has been introduced in 1993 [1] as an alternative to standard full sternotomy. By 1996, various techniques such as partial sternotomy and parasternal approaches have been developed [2].

Nowadays, right anterior thoracotomy and upper hemisternotomy are the mostly used minimally invasive approaches for aortic valve replacement (AVR). The right anterior mini-thoracotomy approach for aortic valve replacement involves a small, 4 to 6 cm transverse incision at the third intercostal space. While technically demanding, it offers excellent cosmetic results and no sternal or costal injury. Literature data associate the minimally invasive surgery with less bleeding, shorter duration of mechanical ventilation and reduced intensive care unit and hospital stay despite longer procedure times, together with an expected improved cosmetic result and a reduction of wound infections [3–8]. Major limitations reported for right minithoracotomy included the very tiny operating field, resulting in longer operating times compared to the standard approach, and the need for peripheral cannulation [9–11].

In order to better evaluate the potential benefits a standardization of the surgical technique itself is required.

M. Del Giglio, M.D., Ph.D. (✉) • E. Mikus, M.D.
Cardiovascular Department, Maria Cecilia Hospital, GVM Care and Research, Cotignola (RA), Italy
e-mail: maurodelgiglio@hotmail.com

K. Fattouch et al. (eds.), *Advances in Treatments for Aortic Valve and Root Diseases*, https://doi.org/10.1007/978-3-319-66483-5_14

14.2 Surgical Technique

All patients treated by a right minithoracotomy receive a totally intravenous anesthesia and a double lumen intubation.

Transesophageal echocardiography is used for monitoring heart and valve function during the operation.

A pillow is positioned under the right shoulder. A 4 to 6 cm skin incision at the third right intercostal space is performed. A soft tissue retractor (CV MICS Sorin Group, the Edwards ThruPort™ Systems or the Covidien SurgiSleeve) is used to help spreading the chest wall. The pericardium is opened far away from the phrenic nerve, over the right ventricle. Three deep stay sutures are pulled towards the operator to obtain best surgical exposure. Sutures are tightened using the Endo close, trocar site closure device (Covidien, Mansfield, MA, USA) outside the chest wall (Fig. 14.1).

At the beginning of our experience a peripheral cannulation was adopted to increase familiarity with the "new" surgical approach and to get a better operating field overview (42 patients). Nowadays, we prefer and suggest a total central cannulation avoiding the peripheral one [12].

Purse string sutures are placed before systemic heparinization treatment to avoid hematoma of ascending aorta wall and to reduce the potential blood loss. A straight arterial cannula (EOPA arterial cannula, Medtronic, Inc. Minneapolis, Minn or a Straightshot Edwards Lifesciences in a minority of cases) is positioned just below the origin of aortic arch, so that the Chitwood clamp, positioned percutaneously, did

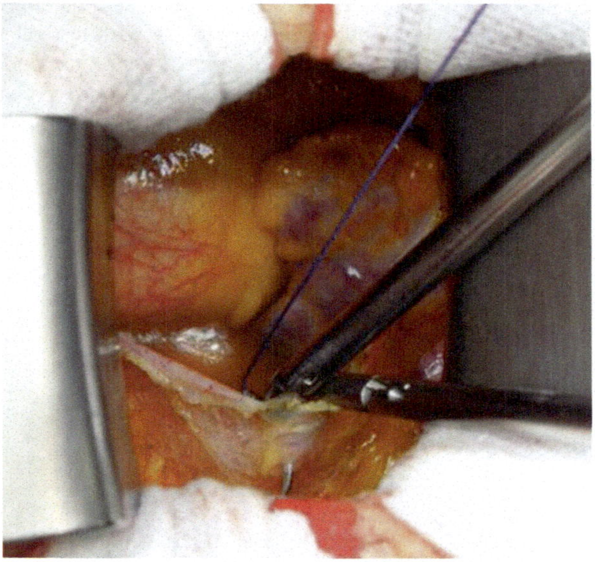

Fig. 14.1 Three pericardial stay sutures tightened using the Endo close trocar site closure device (Covidien, Mansfield, MA, USA) outside the chest wall

not hinder the operating field, while the aortic anulus is brought closer to the operator (Figs. 14.2 14.3 and 14.4). The venous purse string is placed around the left appendage and reinforced by pledgets. A three-stage MC2X venous cannula (Medtronic, Inc. Minneapolis, Minn) is inserted using the insider of left ventricle vent to facilitate the introduction. The stitch uses to fix the cannula is then pulled outside the chest using the Endo close, trocar site closure device, thus improving the exposure by moving the appendage and the right atrium away from the aortic root. The antegrade flow cannula is inserted in the ascending aorta as routinely; the ventricle is vented through the right upper pulmonary vein (DLP 20 Fr, ref. 12,002, Medtronic). The aorta is cross-clamped through a 1 cm skin incision made at the origin of the innominate vein using a Chitwood clamp. Hypothermic 6-8 °C blood cardioplegia (St Thomas with procaine) is administered in an antegrade fashion into the aortic root to stop the heart. A normothermic cardiopulmonary bypass is routinely chosen for all patients. A transverse incision of the ascending aorta is

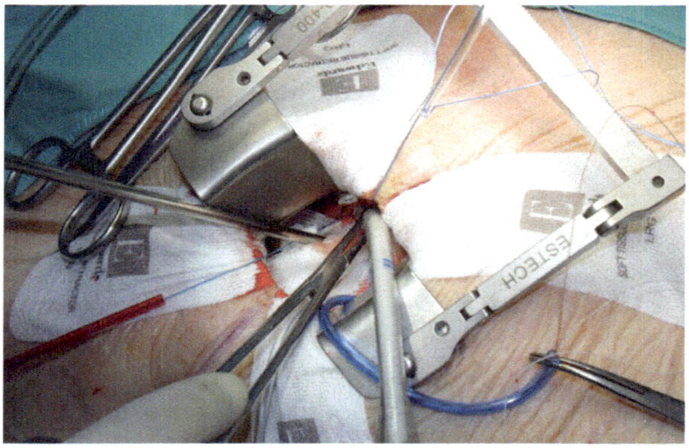

Fig. 14.2 Ascending aorta cannulation

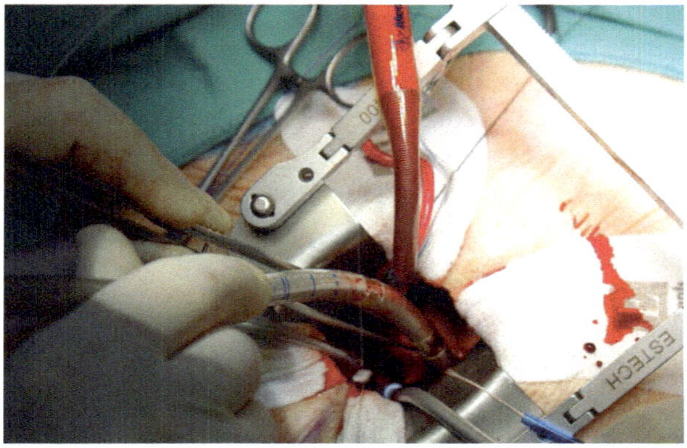

Fig. 14.3 Venous cannulation

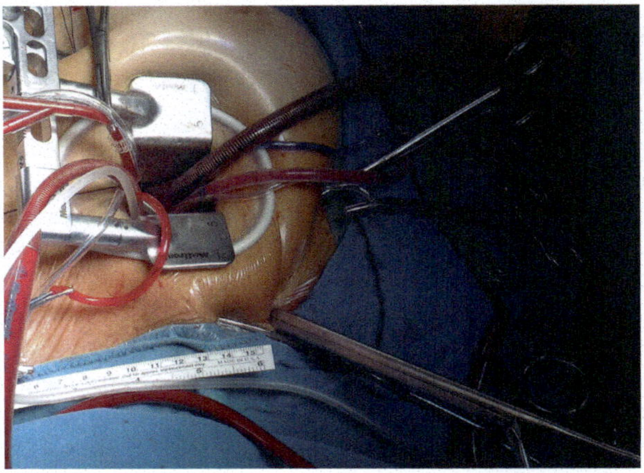

Fig. 14.4 Cross clamp insertion

performed and the aortic valve removed. Whenever possible, the native aortic valve is excised in a single step, reducing time for decalcification. The prosthesis is then sized. During the rinsing of the valve, the first stitch (4–0 polipropilene) to close the transverse aortotomy is positioned. Prosthetic valve is implanted using three running 2–0 polypropylene sutures starting from the annulus below the right coronary ostium and moving then to the annulus below the left and the non-coronary sinuses (Figs. 14.5 and 14.6).

Ascending aorta incision is sutured. Aorta is declamped, ventricular pacing wires placed on the right ventricle and patient weaned from cardiopulmonary bypass. Intraoperative transesophageal echocardiography is used to assess the correct prosthesis function and competence. Cannulas are removed and protamine administered at 1:1 ratio to heparin.

14.3 Discussion

A standardized and reproducible technique is essential to obtain good results and to teach it to next generation of cardiac surgeons. Based on these principles, we try to find a solution to all disadvantages described by literature for right minithoracotomy approach.

The first limitation reported is the need of peripheral cannulation that it is not free from complications [9–11]. After a correct learning curve using a femoral cannulation, a total central one can be easily adopted (Fig. 14.4). In addition, costal avulsion and right mammary artery interruption are avoidable, moving the retractor a little bit lateral were the intercostal space is gradually wide.

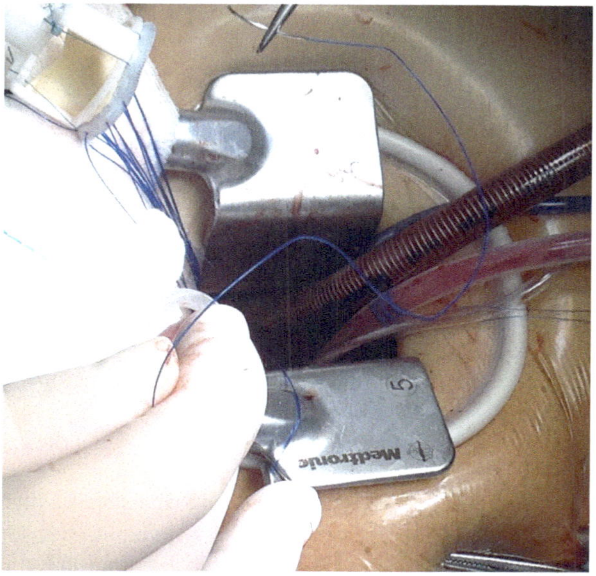

Fig. 14.5 Prosthesis implantation using tree running sutures

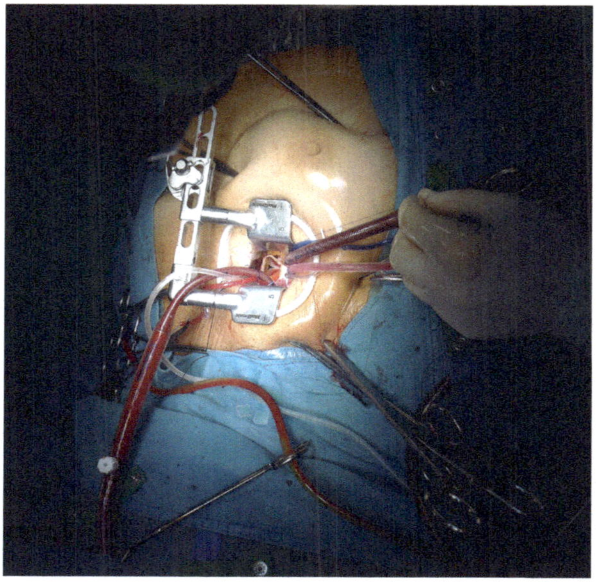

Fig. 14.6 Operative field with aortic prosthesis implanted

Moreover, the operating field is tiny but using some technical expedient such as a correct surgical exposure made with sutures tightened with the Endo close in addition to surgical experience it is possible to reach competitive cross clamping and extracorporeal times.

Many authors believe that a preoperative CT scan is essential to analyze the thoracic "architecture" and the heart anatomy [6, 13]. In our experience the ascending aorta can be easily assessed to evaluate the presence of calcified plaques in order to choose the best location for cannulation and clamp, as surgeons usually do in full sternotomy without an increase in the embolic risk as demonstrated by the low incidence of neurologic events in our experience (0.4%).

The other weak points described in literature are the need of prosthesis undersizing, which is not true in our experience, other exclusion criteria that we do not believe essential (excepted for a previous left pneumectomy) and finally the low reproducibility of this surgical technique. This can be solved thanks to a standardized technique, for which an appropriate training with the attendant learning curve is essential [14].

This surgical approach avoids the sternotomy and rib fracture, guaranteeing cosmetic, functional results and patient approval. The technical improvement achieved in more than 500 patients experience allows surgical outcomes in terms of operating times, prosthesis sizing and patients selection at least comparable to those obtained with standard full sternotomy.

Conflict of Interests Nothing to declare.

References

1. Rao PN, Kumar AS. Aortic valve replacement through right thoracotomy. Tex Heart Inst J. 1993;20:307–8.
2. Cosgrove DM III, Sabik JF. Minimally invasive approach for aortic valve operations. Ann Thorac Surg. 1996;62:596–7.
3. Murtuza B, Pepper JR, Satnbridge RD, Jone C, Rao C, Darzi A, et al. Minimal access aortic valve replacement: is it worth it? Ann Thorac Surg. 2008;85:1121–31.
4. Tabata M, Umakanthan R, Cohn L, Bolmann RM II, Shekar PS, Chen FY, et al. Early and late outcomes of 1000 minimally invasive aortic valve replacement. Eur J Cardiothorac Surg. 2008;33:537–41.
5. Gilmanov D, Bevilacqua S, Murzi M, Cerillo AG, Gasbarri T, Kallushi E, Miceli A, Glauber M. Minimally invasive and conventional aortic valve replacement: a propensity score analysis. Ann Thorac Surg. 2013;96:837–43.
6. Plass A, Scheffel H, Alkadhi H, Kaufmann P, Genoni M, Falk V, Grünenfelder J. Aortic valve replacement through a minimally invasive approach: preoperative planning, surgical technique, and outcome. Ann Thorac Surg. 2009;88:1851–6.
7. Glower DD, Desai BS, Hughes GC, Milano CA, Gaca JG. Aortic valve replacement via right minithoracotomy versus full median sterenotomy: a propensity score analysis. Innovations (Phila). 2014;9(2):75–81.
8. Phan K, Xie A, Di Eusanio M, Yan TD. A meta-analysis of minimally invasive versus conventional sternotomy for aortic valve replacement. Ann Thorac Surg. 2014;98(4):1499–511.

9. Ruttmann E, Gilhofer TS, Ulmer H, Chevtchik O, Kocher A, Schistek R, et al. Propensity score-matched analysis of aortic valve replacement by mini-thoracotomy. J Heart Valve Dis. 2010;19:606–14.
10. Glauber M, Miceli A, Gilmanov D, Ferrarini M, Bevilacqua S, Farneti M, Solinas M. Right anterior minithoracotomy versus conventional aortic valve replacement: a propensity score matched study. J Thorac Cardiovasc Surg. 2013;145:1222–6.
11. Sansone F, Punta Sansone F, Punta G, Parisi F, Dato GM, Zingarelli E, Flocco R, Forsennati PG, Bardi GL, del Ponte S, Casabona R. Right minithoracotomy versus full sternotomy for the aortic valve replacement: preliminary results. Heart Lung Circ. 2012;21:169–73.
12. Mikus E, Turci S, Calvi S, Ricci M, Dozza L, Del Giglio M. Aortic valve replacement through right minithoracotomy: is it really biologically minimally invasive? Ann Thorac Surg. 2015;99(3):826–30.
13. Glauber M, Miceli A, Bevilacqua S, Farneti PA. Minimally invasive aortic valve replacement via right anterior minithoracotomy: early outcomes and midterm follow-up. J Thorac Cardiovasc Surg. 2011;142:1577–9.
14. Murzi M, Cerillo AG, Bevilacqua S, Gilmanov D, Farneti P, Glauber M. Traversing the learning curve in minimally invasive heart valve surgery: a cumulative analysis of an individual surgeon's experience with a right minithoracotomy approach for aortic valve replacement. Eur J Cardiothorac Surg. 2012;41(6):1242–6.

15 Modified David Operation: A New Simple Method Using a Single Inflow Suture Line

Thomas Modine, Augustin Coisne, François Pontana, Khalil Fattouch, Patrizio Lancellotti, Ibrahim el Qudimat, and David Montaigne

15.1 Introduction

Composite replacement has been the standard surgical procedure for the treatment of combined aortic dilatation and aortic regurgitation [1]. Nevertheless, this intervention exposes patients to long-term risks associated with the presence of biological or mechanical prostheses, including bleeding, thromboembolic and infective events. In this context, valve sparing and repair interventions, associated with low mortality, acceptable durability and low risk valve-related events [2–4], have received increasing interest.

T. Modine, M.D., Ph.D. (✉) • F. Pontana, M.D., Ph.D. • I. el Qudimat, M.D.
Department of Cardiovascular Surgery, CHU Lille, Lille Cedex, France
e-mail: t1modine@yahoo.fr

A. Coisne, M.D. • D. Montaigne, M.D., Ph.D.
Department of Clinical Physiology and Echocardiography—Heart Valve Clinic, CHU Lille, Lille Cedex, France

European Genomic Institute for Diabetes (E.G.I.D), Lille, France

Univ Lille, Lille, France

Inserm UMR 1011, Lille, France

Institut Pasteur de Lille, Lille, France

K. Fattouch, M.D.
GVM Care and Research, Cardiovascular Department, Maria Eleonora Hospital, Palermo, Italy

P. Lancellotti, M.D., Ph.D.
Department of Cardiology, University of Liège Hospital, GIGA Cardiovascular Sciences, Heart Valve Clinic, CHU Sart Tilman, Liège, Belgium

GVM Care and Research, E.S. Health Science Foundation, Lugo, RA, Italy

K. Fattouch et al. (eds.), *Advances in Treatments for Aortic Valve and Root Diseases*, https://doi.org/10.1007/978-3-319-66483-5_15

Sarsam and Yacoub proposed the "remodeling of the aortic root" procedure [5], which preserves physiological motion of the leaflets with a better stress distribution as compared with the David's procedure [6, 7]. Because all three aortic sinuses are excised but leaving approximately 5 mm of arterial wall attached to the aortic annulus, the remodeling technique may be inappropriate in patients with Marfan Syndrome or annuloaortic ectasia. In some patients it failed to stabilize the aortic annulus and led to progressive annular and remnant aortic wall dilatation and valve incompetence [8–10].

David and Feindel proposed a procedure (David I) described as "the reimplantation technique" which provided external support of the entire aortic root complex as well as better hemostasis [11]. The original procedure consists in reimplanting the aortic valve within a Dacron tube graft.

The ideal sparing surgery aimed at building the more physiologic aortic root as possible by preserving the functional anatomy of the aortic root and valve complex. This includes the preservation of the geometry of the sinuses of Valsalva and the ratio of different components of the aortic root. De Paulis introduced a modified Dacron conduit with preformed neosinuses [12]. This conduit used in David I procedure, allows in theory to enhance leaflet closure at the end of the diastole and protects leaflets from the prosthetic wall trauma during systole.

Unfortunately, in-conduit suturing of the aortic valve annulus and a small rim of remnant sinuses to the graft is time consuming, and may lead to bleeding, and distortion of the native valve in the prosthetic root. In addition, crimping the Valsalva graft may result in its theoretical advantage loss. We here describe a modification of the previous techniques to facilitate reimplantation with a single inflow suture line. This valve reimplantation technique modification, proposed by Thomas Modine (TM), is reproducible and easy to achieve.

15.2 Methods

15.2.1 Study Population and Design

We prospectively studied patients with severe aortic dilatation referred in our cardiovascular surgery department (Dr. M Koussa—CHU Lille) for valve sparing aortic root replacement between July 2009 and October, 2015. Patients with reduced left ventricular ejection fraction (LVEF) <50%, with medical history of previous cardiac surgery, congenital heart diseases were excluded.

The local ethics committee approved the protocol and patients gave informed consent.

15.2.2 Surgical Technique

All patients were operated using the modified technique proposed by Dr. Thomas Modine and described below. After median sternotomy, a normothermic cardiopulmonary bypass was established by cannulating the distal ascending aorta, transverse aortic arch, or femoral artery, depending on the extensiveness of the aneurysm. The right atrium was also cannulated. The ascending aorta was cross-clamped just below the origin of the innominate artery and once cardiac cardioplegic arrest was obtained, the enlarged aortic root is transected starting high, above the non-coronary sinus. The valve leaflets, sinuses and annulus were examined carefully. An El Khoury approach was adopted to place the proximal suture line and to size the graft. The aortic root was externally dissected as low as possible. The height of the commissure between the non-coronary and the left coronary cusp give the size of the Valsalva graft (the height of the sinus portion of the graft is equal to its diameter) [13, 14]. The proximal suture line (2-0 Tycron contiguous sutures with pledgets) was placed along the horizontal plane formed by the base of the inter-leaflet triangles, with exception due to external limitations of root dissection at the RC/NC and RC/LC sinuses. A Valsalva graft was implanted in all these patients. The pledgeted sutures were passed through the base of the prosthesis. The collar of the Valsalva graft wall partially removed (2–3 mm are enough). Then the graft was tailored as described by Boodhwani et al. [14] to allow suspension and suturing the tailored native valve commissures to the prosthesis in the same plane, along the new sinotubular junction.

As proposed by TM, the sinuses of Valsalva were entirely removed with no arterial wall left attached to the annulus. Three rectangular commissural tabs of the aortic wall were spared for their attachment; the coronary buttons were harvested. We didn't suture the skeletalized aortic valve to the Valsalva graft wall avoiding compromising the preformed shape and size of the neoaortic sinuses.

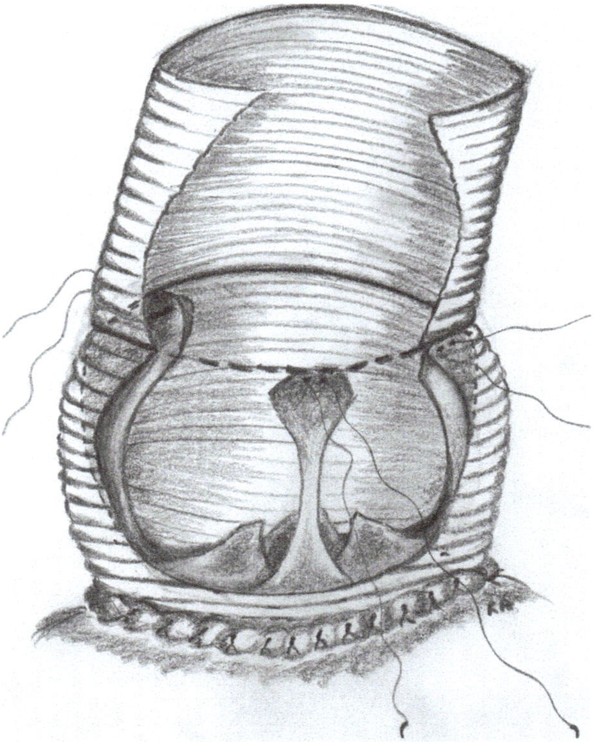

Fig. 15.1 Final aspect after reimplantation with a single inflow suture line. Each commissure is attached to the graft at the prosthetic sino-tubular junction with three polypropylene 4-0 stitches

Each commissural tabs was attached to the prosthesis, at the marked area, at the new sinotubular junction by one 4-0 polypropylene "U" pledgeted stich (Fig. 15.1). The coronary ostia were reimplanted to the corresponding sinus and the distal conduit was trimmed and sutured to the distal ascending aorta as the final step.

15.2.3 Statistical Analysis

Continuous variables were tested for normality with Shapiro test, and were given as mean ± SD. Categorical variables were given as percentages of individuals. A value of $p < 0.05$ was considered statistically significant. Statistics were performed using MedCalc v16.4 (Olstead, Belgium).

15.3 Results

Forty-one consecutive patients have been operated using this modified technique, between September 2009 and October 2015.

Characteristics of these patients are summarized in Table 15.1. Mean age was 57 ± 14 years. The population was made of 78% of male and a half has hypertension. Fifteen (36%) patients had more than a moderate aortic regurgitation (AR) and four a bicuspid aortic valve.

Pre-operative left ventricular ejection fraction (LVEF) was normal as a direct consequence of exclusion entry criteria and Valsalva sinuses were dilated as expected (50 ± 6.8 mm).

Table 15.1 Preoperative characteristics

	Operated patients (n = 41)
Clinical	
Age (years)	57 ± 14.3
Gender (male) n (%)	32 (78)
BMI (kg/m^2)	29.4 ± 6.6
Hypertension n (%)	22 (54)
Diabetes mellitus n (%)	1 (2.4)
Active smokers n (%)	5 (12.2)
Atrial fibrillation n (%)	7 (17.1)
Stroke n (%)	2 (4.9)
TTE	
LVEF (%)	58.5 ± 6.9
Aortic regurgitation	
None n (%)	17 (41.5)
Mild n (%)	9 (22)
Moderate n (%)	9 (22)
Severe n (%)	6 (14.5)
Bicuspid aortic valve n (%)	4 (10)
CT scan	
Valsalva sinuses (mm)	50 ± 6.8
Sinotubular junction (mm)	48.6 ± 8.3

Table 15.2 Surgery

	Operated patients (n = 41)
CBP time (min)	137.3 ± 27.2
Aortic clamp time (min)	118.4 ± 27.4
Bleeding (mL)	533 ± 277
Prosthesis diameter (mm)	30.9 ± 1.8
Death during surgery n (%)	0 (0)
Associated procedures n (%)	0 (0)
Postoperative AR	
None n (%)	20 (49)
Mild n (%)	20 (49)
Severe n (%)	1 (2)
Hospitalization time (days)	11 (10–13.2)

Surgery characteristics are shown in Table 15.2. The mean cardiopulmonary bypass time was 137.3 ± 27.2 min, the mean graft size was 31 ± 1.8 mm and no patient had concomitant procedure.

Transthoracic echocardiography (TTE) at discharge shown no or midl AR in 35 patients (85%).

One patient presented an acute severe aortic regurgitation, related to non-coronary/right coronary cusp commissure stitch disruption, 3 days after the surgery. This commissure was suspended using a new, pledgeted stitch and the AR corrected.

15.4 Discussion

Our initial experience with this aortic valve sparing re-implantation techniques modification is favorable. It showed to be simple, reproducible and nearly physiological technique. Indeed, although effective, aortic valve reimplantation surgery, to treat ascending aorta aneurysms is a challenging technique that requires experience and developed surgical skills. Our proposed modification showed to be easy to teach and effective. This modification allowed, in our practice, reduced CPB and cross clamping times. The pledgeted 4/0 prolene stitches are used since we observed an, delayed (day 3), acute aortic regurgitation due to commissure stitch suspension disruption. The postoperative echocardiographic control showed, unlike David 1 technique, a flow in between the commissures, confirming the motion respect of the reimplanted native valve.

15.4.1 Limits and Clinical Perspectives

We report a new aortic root sparring technique with promising short-term results. Further investigations are ongoing to analyze the long-term impact of this technique on morbimortality, reoperations and biophysical properties of the ascending aorta using transthoracic echocardiography and 4D flow cardiac magnetic resonance (CMR) (Fig. 15.2).

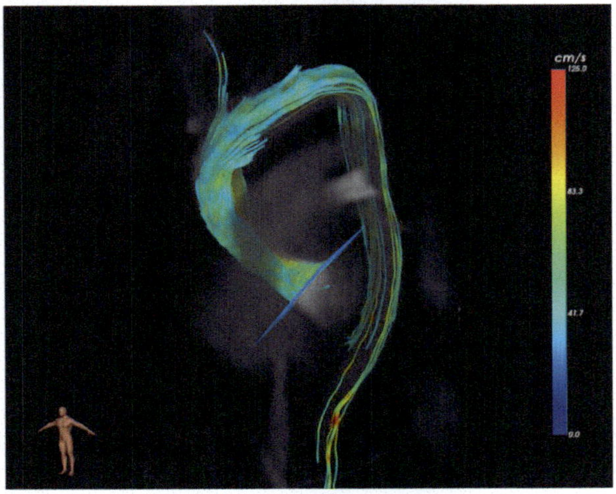

Fig. 15.2 4D flow cardiac magnetic resonance in an operated patient showing the flow formation in the ascending aorta

Conclusion

A simple technical modification using a single commissure suspension of the aortic native valve in addition to a continuous in-flow suture line to facilitate in-conduit valve reimplantation, is effective and easy to realize in daily practice with good short-term results. Further investigations are ongoing to analyze the long-term impact of this new valve sparring aortic root replacement technique.

References

1. Bentall HH, de Bono A. A technique for complete replacement of tha ascending aorta. Thorax. 1968;23:338–9.
2. Price J, De Kerchove L, Glineur D, Vanoverschelde JL, Noirhomme P, El Khoury G. Risk of valve-related events after aortic valve repair. Ann Thorac Surg. 2012;95(2):606–12.
3. Aicher D, Fries R, Rodionycheva S, Schmidt K, Langer F, Schafers HJ. Aortic valve repair lead to a low incidence of valve-related complications. Eur J Cardiothorac Surg. 2010;37(1):127–32.
4. Tourmousoglou C, Rokkas C. Is aortic valve-sparing operation or replacement with à composite graft the best option for aortic root and ascending aortic aneurysm? Interact Cardiovasc Thorac Surg. 2009;8(1):134–47. Epub 2008 Oct 21.
5. Sarsam MA, Yacoub M. Remodeling of the aortic valve annulus. J Thorac Cardiovascular Surg. 1993;105:435–8.
6. Graeter TP, Fries R, Aicher D, Reul H, Schmitz C, Schäfers HJ. In-vitro comparaison of aortic valve hemodynamics between aortic root remodeling and aortic valve reimplantation. J Heart Valve Dis. 2006;15(3):329–35.
7. Leyh RG, Schmidtke C, Sievers HH, Yacoub MH. Opening and closing characteristics of the aortic valve after different types of valve-preserving surgery. Circulation. 1999;100(21):2153–60.
8. Yacoub M, Gehle P, Chandrasekaran V, Birks EJ, Child A, Radley-Smith R. Late results of a valve preserving operation in patients with aneurysms of the ascending aorta and root. J Thorac Cardiovasc Surg. 1998;115:1080–90.

9. Birks EJ, Webb C, Child A, Radley-Smith R, Yacoub MH. Early and long-term results of a valve-sparing operation for Marfan syndrome. Circulation. 1999;100(19 Suppl):II29–35.
10. de Oliveira NC, David TE, Ivanov J, Armstrong S, Eriksson MJ, Rakowski H, Webb G. Results of surgery for aortic root aneurysm in patients with Marfan syndrome. J Thorac Cardiovasc Surg. 2003;125(4):789–96.
11. David TE, Feindel CM. An aortic valve-sparing operation for patients with aortic incompetence and aneurysm of the ascending aorta. J Thorac Cardiovasc Surg. 1992;103:617–21.
12. De Paulis R, De Matteis GM, Nardi P, Scaffa R, Colella DF, Chiarello L. A new aortic Dacron conduit for surgical treatment of aortic root pathology. Ital Heart J. 2000;1:457–63.
13. De Kerchove L, Boodhwani M, Glineur D, Noirhomme P, El Khoury G. A new simple and objective method for graft sizing in valve-sparing root replacement using the reimplantation technique. Ann Thorac Surg. 2011;92:749–51.
14. Boodhwani M, De Kerchove L, El Khoury G. Aortic root replacement using the reimplantation technique: tips and tricks. Interact Cardiovasc Thorac Surg. 2009;8(5):584–6. https://doi.org/10.1510/icvts.2008.197574.

16 Redo Surgery for Aortic Valve and Root: Demographics and Operative Options

Davide Pacini, Giacomo Murana, Luca Di Marco, Alessandro Leone, and Roberto Di Bartolomeo

16.1 Introduction

Reoperations for aortic disease are being frequent procedures. The reason is related to increasing life expectancy, numbers of people suffering from aortic stenosis and structural deterioration of a bioprosthesis. It has been estimated that in the next years redo root operations may eventually account about 10% of all ascending aorta surgical procedures [1].

Cardiac reoperations are technically more demanding than primary operations reason why they always require a meticulous surgical planning along with specific operative skills. Moreover, They are also often performed in older and functionally compromised patients who poorly tolerate complications. It is estimated that operative mortality for reoperations on the ascending thoracic aorta is ranging from 6.5 to 15%, and is always higher than the first procedure [2–4].

Nowadays, with the possibility to choose among different surgical approaches supported by advancement in perioperative care reoperations are routinely performed with significant improvement in outcomes [5–7]. Some of the technical features aimed to reduce operative invasiveness are considered the possibility to better manage different perfusion strategies (central vs. peripheral), use of hypothermia with more sophisticated cerebral and visceral monitoring and applicability of minimally invasive techniques to avoid strong adhesion and reduce operative times.

The following chapter aims to describe the basics on surgical techniques required to perform a safe reoperation on the aortic valve and root.

D. Pacini, M.D., Ph.D. (✉) • G. Murana • L. Di Marco • A. Leone • R. Di Bartolomeo
Department of Cardiac Surgery, S. Orsola Hospital, University of Bologna-Alma Mater Studiorum, Via Massarenti n. 9, 40128 Bologna, Italy
e-mail: davide.pacini@unibo.it

K. Fattouch et al. (eds.), *Advances in Treatments for Aortic Valve and Root Diseases*, https://doi.org/10.1007/978-3-319-66483-5_16

16.2 Demographics and Etiology

Over the last decades, the number of patients who require aortic valve and root replacement after prior cardiovascular surgery progressively raised [8–10]. It is estimated that in the next years aortic reoperations would became about 10% of all the surgical procedures on the ascending aorta [10]. Reasons are related to the increased incidence of aortic diseases in the ageing population, the increased use of biological aortic valves and root substitutes, and the increased use of techniques for valve-sparing aortic root reconstruction.

Structural degeneration of a bioprosthesis is the most frequent indication for reoperation in patients with tissue valves. However, the improved durability of tissue valves, as well as the availability of alternative surgical options as TAVI and sutureless valves, has led the surgeons in favor of bioprostheses in progressively younger age patients [11, 12].

In Bologna, according to what reported above, during the last decades (1990–2017) a progressive number of reintervention on the thoracic aorta was progressively observed (see Fig. 16.1). Of them, primary causes were a progression of degenerative aneurysms (35%), chronic aortic dissections (32%) and pseudoaneurysms (12%) requiring at least an intervention on the aortic root or ascending aorta.

Main indications for re-operative surgery on the aortic valve and root are (see Table 16.1):

- New onset of an aortic valve disease (stenosis/regurgitation)
- Progressive aneurysmal dilatation of the ascending aorta

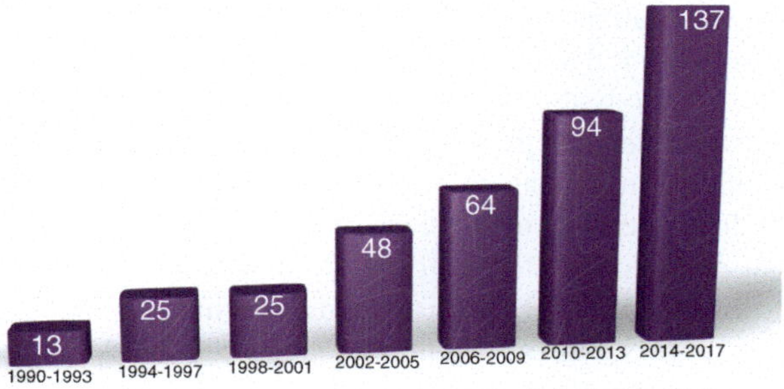

Fig. 16.1 Distribution during the years of thoracic aortic reoperations including the aortic valve in Bologna, S. Orsola Hospital

Table 16.1 Indications for redo operations of the aortic valve and root

Surgical indication	Etiology
Completely new onset	• Aortic valve disease (stenosis) • Ascending aorta and root pathologies (aneurysm, dissection) • Infective endocarditis
Progression aortic disease	• Aneurysm • Acute dissection
Surgical complications	• Mechanical (aortic regurgitation after valve sparing operation, bioprosthesis dysfunction, pseudoaneurysm) • Infective

- Dissection of the aortic root after ascending aorta replacement
- Pseudoaneurysm (usually in the suture lines) after a prior aortic surgery
- Failure of a sparing aortic root reconstruction
- Structural deterioration of a bioprosthesis
- Prosthesis aortic valve dysfunction
- Perivalvular leaks
- Infective endocarditis

16.3 Pre-Operative Planning

A meticulous attention to preoperative details is crucial to overcome any possible pitfall coming from chest re-entry. Before skin incision, a complete preoperative scheduling give the possibility to minimize the damage of heart and great vessels during re-sternotomy and it may anticipate any pitfalls coming from hostile aortic root and valve anatomy.

It always requires an adequate preoperative imaging; plain X-ray, computed tomography, magnetic resonance imaging, or angiography may be necessary to plan the most appropriate procedure. An angio-CT scan is mandatory to investigate the relationship between the anterior mediastinal structures and the posterior aspect of the sternum (see Fig. 16.2). The radiologic features that influence the re-entry strategy is a close distance (<5 mm) or a direct contact between the inner surface of the sternum and the aortic wall or the previous vascular prosthesis or the right ventricle, and also the patency and location of coronary by-pass grafts (especially LIMA). Angio-CT also guide on the choice of the most appropriate arterial cannulation site, shows root and ascending aorta anatomy (annulus size, coronary ostia location, presence of pseudoaneurysms etc.) and prove calcifications on the ascending aorta and arch.

Other important precaution to care about before surgery should be about the anticoagulation therapy. Patients who receive warfarin or other anticoagulants should stop it 5 days before surgery and, if necessary, replace it with heparin. Along with that all antiplatelet drugs such as aspirin and/or adenosine diphosphate (ADP) inhibitors, should be discontinued before the planned surgery.

It is mandatory to investigate for all the vital organs functions (lung, kidneys, brain) like in routine cardiac surgery. Lastly, is necessary to look for the operative

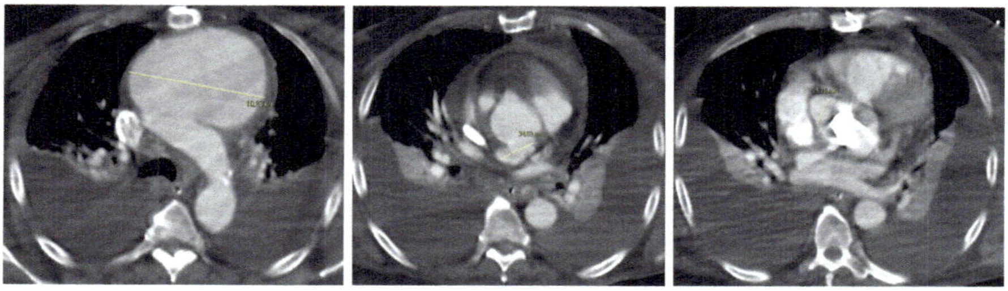

Fig. 16.2 Angio-CT scans images of high-risk chest re-entry (aorta to sternum distance <1 cm) in a patient with infective endocarditis developing pseudoaneurysms on a previous Bentall

report of prior surgery to know what kind of devices were used during the procedure, if any glue was used, if the pericardium was left open and if any complications had occurred.

16.4 Operative Strategies

Main concerns include the management of chest re-entry, CPB institution and myocardial/brain protection and specific technique for aortic repair (see Fig. 16.3).

The aorta is usually exposed through a standard sternotomy. In Bologna our technique for sternal re-opening contemplates the removal of sternal wires, use of the oscillating saw, patients kept with a systolic arterial pressure <100 mmHg, opening the pleural spaces, and cardiopulmonary bypass circuits ready on table (see Table 16.2).

Cannulation sites are carefully decided preoperatively. Vessel selection for CPB institution depends on the presence or absence of aortic dissection, atheromatous disease and degree of safety at re-entry.

In general, when surgery is limited to the root/ascending aorta and a low-risk resternotomy is anticipated, CPB arterial inflow is obtained by cannulating the extrapericardial ascending aorta or the aortic arch. On the contrary if high-risk sternal re-sternotomy is expected or in patients who required some degree of aortic

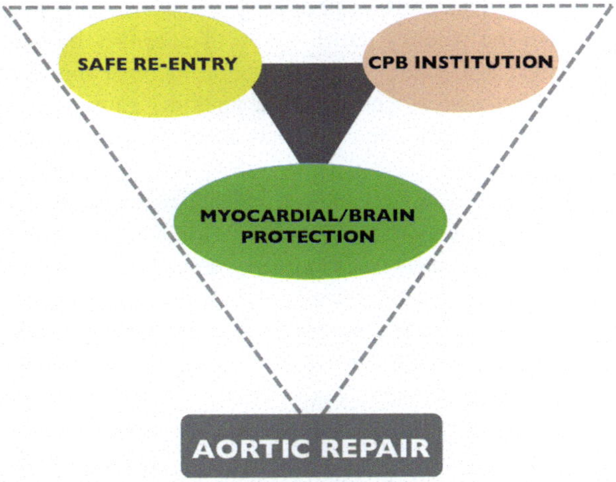

Fig. 16.3 Key points to consider during aortic valve or root redo

Table 16.2 Standard precautions to use during chest re-entry

- External defibrillation plates
- Sternal wires removal
- Use oscillating saw
- Systolic arterial pressure <100 mmHg
- Patient in anti-Trendelenburg position
- CPB circuits ready on table (including the lines to deliver cardioplegia)

arch replacement, the preferred site for arterial cannulation should be the right axillary artery or the innominate artery, mainly because they facilitate antegrade cerebral perfusion. The femoral artery is usually cannulated in patients who required CPB before resternotomy when the axillary artery is unavailable for cannulation or in unstable patients when prompt initiation of CPB became necessary.

The right atrium, the common femoral vein or both venae cavae are used for venous return.

The left heart is vented through insertion of a catheter in the right superior pulmonary vein, in the pulmonary artery trunk or in the left ventricular apex.

For myocardial protection, a retrograde or anterograde cardioplegia delivery could be selected upon surgeon preference. Obviously, the presence of aortic valve/prosthesis insufficiency or leaks from dehiscent aortic suture lines should be taken into account and selective antegrade administration of cardioplegia should be carried out. Cold crystalloid cardioplegia is recommended rather than blood-based solutions because it allows longer times of myocardial ischemia without the need to interrupt the operation.

Body and eventually myocardial temperature are constantly monitored. If the arch is not involved in the reconstruction we cool to a nasopharyngeal temperature of 32 °C, otherwise if open techniques for the distal aorta are necessary cooling is deepened to 25 °C.

In patients determined to be at high risk of chest re-entry lesion, resternotomy is performed on CPB or under deep hypothermic circulatory arrest (nasopharyngeal 18 °C). In this setting, especially in case of significant aortic insufficiency, distension of the left ventricle is avoided by venting the apex of the left ventricle through a left anterior thoracotomy.

16.5 Surgical Options for the Aortic Valve

Current treatment options for reoperative aortic valve surgery vary greatly. Options include, standard AVR with either biologic or mechanical prosthetic valves, sutureless (SU-AVR) and thanscatheter aortic valve implantation (TAVI).

It mostly depends on a patient's risk stratification and anatomic characteristics of the aortic root. Conventional aortic valve replacement still is the current gold-standard therapeutic approach for the majority of patients with severe aortic valve disease or prosthetic valve dysfunction. Improvements in cardiac anesthesia, operative techniques (including less extensive dissection), and postoperative care likely played a fundamental role to reduce mortality over time. Recent trends, have demonstrated improved outcomes for isolated reoperative AVR with an operative mortality close to a first time aortic valve replacement (<5%) [13].

To decrease the invasiveness of conventional aortic valve replacement several minimally invasive techniques using a limited surgical access (i.e., upper partial sternotomy, right anterior minithoracotomy and apex of the left ventricle) have been introduced to further improve clinical outcome. In such cases the adoption of sutureless technology may facilitate the less-invasive AVR approach.

Sutureless or rapid deployment aortic valves avoids the placement and tying of sutures and have the potential advantages over AVR to the reduce cross-clamp and cardiopulmonary bypass (CPB) duration, facilitating minimally invasive surgery and complex cardiac intervention.

There are three commercially available prostheses, including 3F Enable (Medtronic, Minneapolis, USA), Perceval S (Sorin, Saluggia, Italy), and Intuity Elite (Edward Lifesciences, Irvine, USA) [14]. All of them are tissue valves that anchor within the aortic annulus with no more than three sutures.

The 3F Enable and Perceval S sutureless prosthesis utilizes the nitinol metal frame to deploy and positions the valve within the anulus. The Intuity rapid deployment aortic valve prosthesis operates by a different mechanism, based on a balloon-expandable stainless steel and requires three sutures to ancor the valve in the appropriate annular position.

There are several similarities between sutureless aortic valves and conventional AVR. Both requires surgical incisions, cardiopulmonary bypass institution, and allow the excision of the diseased valve.

Transcatheter aortic valve implantation is the true innovative method for AVR. It is now established as the treatment of choice for patients presenting with severe aortic stenosis who are deemed inoperable or of high surgical risk. Conventional AVR still requires sternotomy, cardioplegic arrest and cardiopulmonary bypass. In contrast, when using a transcatheter technique it is feasible to implant an aortic valve prosthesis and avoid sternotomy and cardiopulmonary by-pass.

This innovative technology gives also the possibility to treat patients with a failed bioprosthesis with a valve-in-valve technique. In particular, patients with degeneration of previously surgically implanted tissue heart valves may potentially benefit from beating-heart TAVI, obviating the risks associated with using cardioplegia and cardiopulmonary bypass during redo surgery.

TAVI is a complex procedure in an elderly and frail population and therefore greater operator and institutional experience play a major role to reduced procedure times and complications.

A careful pre-operative assessment using advanced imaging of the aorta and peripheral vasculature using computed tomography and echocardiography is crucial to overcome complications during the procedure as dislocation, paravalvular leaks and coronary ostia occlusion.

General anaesthesia is required for surgical access sites (e.g., transapical or transaortic).

If the peripheral vasculature is suitable, then the transfemoral vascular approach has a number of advantages, including shorter procedure times, faster patient recovery and superior outcomes when compared to the other surgical approaches [15]. Other access sites should be considered when the transfemoral route is not thought to be suitable (e.g., minimal luminal diameter <5.5 mm, excessive tortuosity).

Transapical approach requires a small left thoracotomy and direct puncture of the left ventricular apex and avoids the requirement for large catheters to be advanced through the iliofemoral system and aortic arch. The main disadvantage is the requirement for general anaesthesia, a greater degree of myocardial injury and longer recovery times.

The use of the transaortic approach through a mini-sternotomy or right thoracotomy not only avoids the passage of large catheters through the iliofemoral system and aortic arch but also puncture of the left ventricle.

Other vascular access options with demonstrated clinical efficacy in the setting of TAVI include the transsubclavian, transaxillary and transcaval approaches for patients with anatomy that is unsuitable for the more traditional techniques.

The mortality rate associated with TAVI after previous cardiac surgery is 4.2–10%, or 7.6–17% with the valve-in-valve technique [16–19].

Contemporary TAVI devices have limitations that should be considered. Vascular complications occur in up to 25% of all patients undergoing TAVI [20]. Small vessel dimensions, moderate or severe calcification and tortuosity of the peripheral vasculature are associated with an increased incidence of complications. Acute kidney injury is a common occurrence following TAVI presumably as a consequence of numerous factors including impaired baseline renal function in this elderly comorbid patient group, contrast nephropathy, and peripheral embolization. The incidence of clinical stroke following TAVI is approximately 3–4% [21]. Anatomical features such as the presence of a severely stenotic and calcified aortic valve, use of large delivery systems, and multiple manipulations during device implantation have been associated with an increased risk of stroke.

16.6 Surgical Options for the Aortic Root

In this setting, the Bentall procedure—involving the removal of the aortic valve prosthesis and the replacement of the aortic root with a new composite graft— represents the most common surgical option for treatment [22]. However, the specific technique used to re-repair the root depend on the underlying pathology and sometimes other surgical options could be necessary. Other than the Bentall procedure only the Cabrol technique [23] and the prosthesis-sparing operation seems to be valid substitutes.

Valve sparing interventions as remodeling or reimplantation are not usually recommended or even possible because every time the aortic root is partially or completely weakened by the underlying diseased process.

A mechanical or a biological conduit can be variably used for a complete root replacement during reoperative Bentall procedures. Both have demonstrated favorable early and long-term results without showing any difference in term of late reintervention and technical complexity [24].

Among all available biological substitutes, the so-called hand-sewn composite grafts likely represent the most frequently used. This is likely related to the possibility of combining different valves with different conduits and because of stronger evidences of durability at follow-up compared to complete biological conduits.

In the context of redo bentall procedure the re-attachment of the coronary ostia is of paramount importance since torsion, kinking and inadequte mobilization are more probable than in primary interventions. They could also be involved in large aneurysms or have severe calcification that further increase the complexity of ostia reimplantation.

In 1991, Kouchoukos and coworkers [25] showed that his modification, the "open or button technique," for the reimplantation of the coronary arteries was safer in terms of a lower incidence of late false aneurysms. More than 10 years later, another innovation was represented by the introduction of a modified tube graft that incorporates pseudosinuses of Valsalva which further facilitate anatomical reconstruction of the aortic root and positively affect the coronary flow [26]. As compared to a straight tube graft, a Valsalva graft reduce the distance between the coroanry ostia and graft itself and may help decrease tension upon the sutures.

In same cases the Cabrol technique have a pivotal role. Especially in case of second or third aortic root reintervention when coronary ostia are no longer detachable. The Cabrol procedure is characterized by insertion of an ascending aortic composite graft with reimplantation of the coronary arteries by the interposition of a graft tube. In the picture is showed a case of reoperative Cabrol operation for pseudoaneurysm formation of both coronary ostia in a Loeys-Dietz patients that previously underwent a Bentall operation (see Fig. 16.4). However, Cabrol coronary

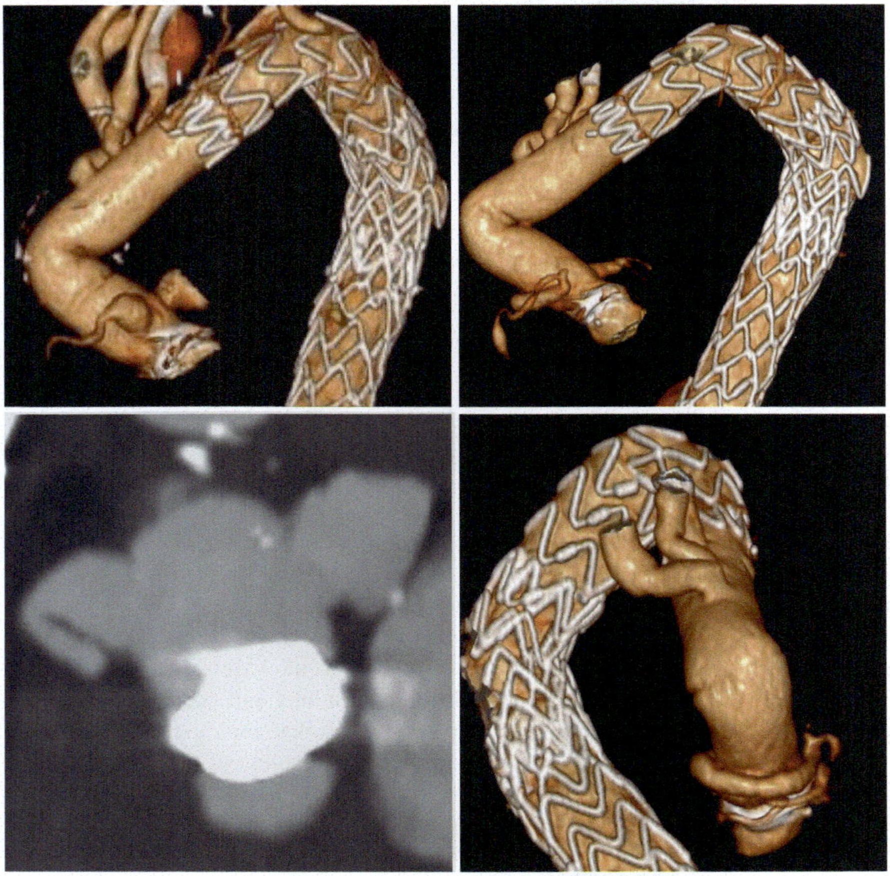

Fig. 16.4 Aortic root reoperation before and after a Cabrol procedure used to re-attach the coronary ostia after a previous Bentall operation

reimplantation should be used only in selected cases because long term patency of the coronary conduits could be disappointing which makes necessary the need for life-long anticoagulation [27].

In patients requiring aortic root reoperations and a well functioning aortic valve prosthesis it is possible to left the valve in situ and substituted only the aortic root, if necessary extending the replacement to other diseased portions of the thoracic aorta. This procedure, may facilitate surgery by reducing the operative times, avoid weakening of the aortic annulus for the removal of the previous prosthesis and reduce the risk of pseudoaneurysm formation.

This technique can be summarized as follow: after aneurysm excision is necessary to carefully inspect the prosthesis for thrombi, pannus, or reduced mobility of the leaflets. Then, the base of the aorta is trimmed to leave a 4 mm remnant. Horizontal Teflon felt-pledgeted 2–0 mattress sutures are placed from outside the aortic annulus to the sewing ring of the previously implanted valve and then to the selected conduit. The graft is parachuted, sutures knotted and root reconstruction completed in a common fashion. At follow-up, this approach in case of properly functioning mechanical prosthesis have excellent outcomes showing a 5-year freedom from re-operation of 100% and no root pseudo-aneurysms detection at imaging examination [28].

Conclusion

Over the last decade re-interventions on the aortic valve and proximal thoracic aorta have been performed with increasing frequency and with significant improvement outcomes [4, 11, 29, 30].

A meticoulous surgical planning is always necessary in order to achieve a safe re-entry.

In spite of greater operator experience and improvements in technology open aortic root reconstruction remains at high-risk for complications. Transchateter aortic valve technologies has the potential to avoid repeat sternotomy and will continue to spread among different type of etiologies but remain limited to the aortic valve and not to the root.

Of course, the limitations of current devices (and techniques) need to be recognized in order to optimize procedural and long-term outcomes.

References

1. Luciani N, De Geest R, Anselmi A, Glieca F, De Paulis S, Possati G. Results of reoperation on the aortic root and the ascending aorta. Ann Thorac Surg. 2011;92:898–903.
2. Etz CD, Plestis KA, Homann TM, et al. Reoperative aortic root and transverse arch procedures: a comparison with contemporaneous primary operations. J Thorac Cardiovasc Surg. 2008;136:860–7.
3. LeMaire SA, DiBardino DJ, Köksoy C, Coselli JS. Proximal aortic reoperations in patients with composite valve grafts. Ann Thorac Surg. 2002;74:S1777–80.
4. Malvindi PG, van Putte BP, Heijmen RH, Schepens MA, Morshuis WJ. Reoperations on the aortic root: experience in 46 patients. Ann Thorac Surg. 2010;89:81–6.
5. Jones JM, O'Kane H, Gladstone DJ, et al. Repeat heart valve surgery: risk factors for operative mortality. J Thorac Cardiovasc Surg. 2001;122:913.

6. O'Brien MF, Harrocks S, Clarke A, et al. Experiences with redo aortic valve surgery. J Card Surg. 2002;17:35.
7. Berretta P, Di Marco L, Pacini D, Cefarelli M, Alfonsi J, Castrovinci S, et al. Reoperations versus primary operation on the aortic root: a propensity score analysis. Eur J Cardiothorac Surg. 2017;51:322–8.
8. Di Bartolomeo R, Berretta P, Petridis FD, Folesani G, Cefarelli M, Di Marco L, et al. Reoperative surgery on the thoracic aorta. J Thorac Cardiovasc Surg. 2013;145(3 Suppl):S78–84.
9. Di Bartolomeo R, Berretta P, Pantaleo A, Murana G, Cefarelli M, Alfonsi J, et al. Long-term outcomes of open arch repair after a prior aortic operation: our experience in 154 patients. Ann Thorac Surg. 2017;103(5):1406–12.
10. Shrestha M, Khaladj N, Baraki H, et al. Aortic root reoperation: a technical challenge. J Heart Valve Dis. 2010;19:177–81.
11. Ohira S, Miyata H, Doi K, Motomura N, Takamoto S, Yaku H. Risk model of aortic valve replacement after cardiovascular surgery based on a National Japanese Database. Eur J Cardiothorac Surg. 2017;51:347–53.
12. Brown JM, O'Brien SM, Wu C, Sikora JA, Griffith BP, Gammie JS. Isolated aortic valve replacement in North America comprising 108,687 patients in 10 years: changes in risks, valve types, and outcomes in the Society of Thoracic Surgeons National Database. J Thorac Cardiovasc Surg. 2009;137(1):82–90.
13. Potter DD, Sundt TM 3rd, Zehr KJ, Dearani JA, Daly RC, Mullany CJ, et al. Outcomes of reoperative aortic valve replacement after previous sternotomy. J Thorac Cardiovasc Surg. 2005;129(1):94–103.
14. Di Eusanio M, Phan K. Sutureless aortic valve replacement. Ann Cardiothorac Surg. 2015;4(2):123–30.
15. Moat NE, Ludman P, de Belder MA, Bridgewater B, Cunningham AD, Young CP, et al. Long-term outcomes after transcatheter aortic valve implantation in high-risk patients with severe aortic stenosis: the U.K. TAVI (United Kingdom Transcatheter Aortic Valve Implantation) Registry. J Am Coll Cardiol. 2011;58(20):2130–8.
16. Shehada SE, Elhmidi Y, Puluca N, Öztürk Ö, Demircioglu E, Wendt D, Jakob H, Thielmann M. Impact of previous cardiac surgery in patients undergoing transcatheter aortic valve implantation: a systematic review. J Cardiovasc Surg. 2017.
17. Leshem-Rubinow E, Abramowitz Y, Steinvil A, Ben-Assa E, Chorin E, Shacham Y, et al. Outcomes of transfemoral transcatheter aortic valve implantation in patients with previous coronary bypass. Am J Cardiol. 2015;116(3):431–5.
18. Stortecky S, Brinks H, Wenaweser P, Huber C, Pilgrim T, Windecker S, et al. Transcatheter aortic valve implantation or surgical aortic valve replacement as redo procedure after prior coronary artery bypass grafting. Ann Thorac Surg. 2011;92:1324–30. discussion 1230–1.
19. Phan K, Zhao DF, Wang N, Huo YR, Di Eusanio M, Yan TD. Transcatheter valve-in-valve implantation versus reoperative conventional aortic valve replacement: a systematic review. J Thorac Dis. 2016;8:E83–93.
20. Genereux P, Webb JG, Svensson LG, Kodali SK, Satler LF, Fearon WF, et al. Vascular complications after transcatheter aortic valve replacement: insights from the PARTNER (Placement of AoRTic TraNscathetER Valve) trial. J Am Coll Cardiol. 2012;60(12):1043–52.
21. Eggebrecht H, Schmermund A, Voigtlander T, Kahlert P, Erbel R, Mehta RH. Risk of stroke after transcatheter aortic valve implantation (TAVI): a meta-analysis of 10,037 published patients. EuroIntervention. 2012;8(1):129–38.
22. Bentall H, DeBono A. A technique for complete replacement of the ascending aorta. Thorax. 1968;23:338–9.
23. Cabrol C, Pavie A, Gandjbakhch I, Villemot JP, Guiraudon G, Laughlin L, et al. Complete replacement of the ascending aorta with reimplantation of the coronary arteries: new surgical approach. J Thorac Cardiovasc Surg. 1981;81:309–15.
24. Pantaleo A, Murana G, Di Marco L, Jafrancesco G, Barberio G, Berretta P et al. Biological versus mechanical Bentall procedure for aortic root replacement: a propensity score analysis of a consecutive series of 1112 patients. Eur J Cardiothorac Surg. 2017 [Epub ahead of print].

25. Kouchoukos NT, Wareing TH, Murphy SF, Perrillo JB. Six- teen-year experience with aortic root replacement. Results of 172 operations. Ann Surg. 1991;214:308–20.
26. De Paulis R, Tomai F, Bertoldo F, Ghini AS, Scaffa R, Nardi P, et al. Coronary flow characteristics after a Bentall procedure with or without sinuses of Valsalva. Eur J Cardiothorac Surg. 2004;26:66–72.
27. Knight J, Baumüller S, Kurtcuoglu V, Turina M, Turina J, Schurr U, et al. Long-term follow-up, computed tomography, and computational fluid dynamics of the Cabrol procedure. J Thorac Cardiovasc Surg. 2010;139(6):1602–8.
28. Pacini D, Villa E, Martin-Suarez S, Bartolomeo RD. Aortic root substitution after aortic valve replacement: a prosthesis-sparing operation. Eur J Cardiothorac Surg. 2005;27(4):717–9.
29. Pacini D, Di Marco L, Loforte A, Angeli E, Dell'amore A, Bergonzini M, Di Bartolomeo R. Reoperations on the ascending aorta and aortic root. Early and late results? J Cardiovasc Surg. 2005;46(5):491–8.
30. Vassileva CM, Aranki S, Brennan JM, Kaneko T, He M, Gammie JS, et al. Evaluation of the Society of Thoracic Surgeons online risk calculator for assessment of risk in patients presenting for aortic valve replacement after prior coronary artery bypass graft: an analysis using the STS adult cardiac surgery database. Ann Thorac Surg. 2015;100(6):2109–15. discussion 2115-6.

Part V

Minimal Invasive Aortic Valve Surgery

Mini-Sternotomy

17

Alberto Albertini

Minimally-invasive cardiac surgery (MICS) approaches are becoming increasingly popular worldwide, with more and more minimally-invasive operations for valvular disease performed every year. MICS has steadily gained popularity among cardiac surgeons, cardiologists and patients due to the excellent clinical results, faster recovery time and more appealing cosmetic result. The main advantages reported with respect to conventional cardiac surgery are cosmesis, reduction of postoperative pain, blood loss and blood product transfusion, reduced ventilation time and pulmonary complications, shorter intensive care unit (ICU) and hospital stay, lower rehabilitation and hospital costs, and possibly better long-term outcomes [1, 2]. Techniques for MICS have continued to evolve rapidly in the last two decades with the scope of reducing wound size and chest trauma and potentiating the postoperative benefits. The rationale is that, in contrast to the traditional approach which requires the surgeon to saw open the sternum and spread the edges apart to gain direct access to the heart, a smaller incision in the upper part of the chest, dividing only the upper portion of the breastbone, will maintain the overall integrity of the rib cage and at the same time reduce the postoperative respiratory distress. Smaller incisions will bleed less and necessitate less tissue dissection, reducing the risk of wound infection. Moreover, by maintaining the integrity of the lower part of the sternum, particularly subjected to traction during coughing by the abdominal muscles that are involved, there is a reduced risk of sternal instability especially in elderly, obese, diabetic and chronic obstructive pulmonary disease (COPD) patients.

Minimally-invasive aortic valve replacement (MIAVR) was first described by Cosgrove and Sabik in 1996 [3]. Their pioneering approach involved a parasternal

Electronic Supplementary Material The online version of this chapter (https://doi.org/10.1007/978-3-319-66483-5_17) contains supplementary material, which is available to authorized users.

A. Albertini, M.D.
Salus Hospital GVM Care and Research, Reggio Emilia, Italy
e-mail: aalbertini@gvmnet.it

K. Fattouch et al. (eds.), *Advances in Treatments for Aortic Valve and Root Diseases*, https://doi.org/10.1007/978-3-319-66483-5_17

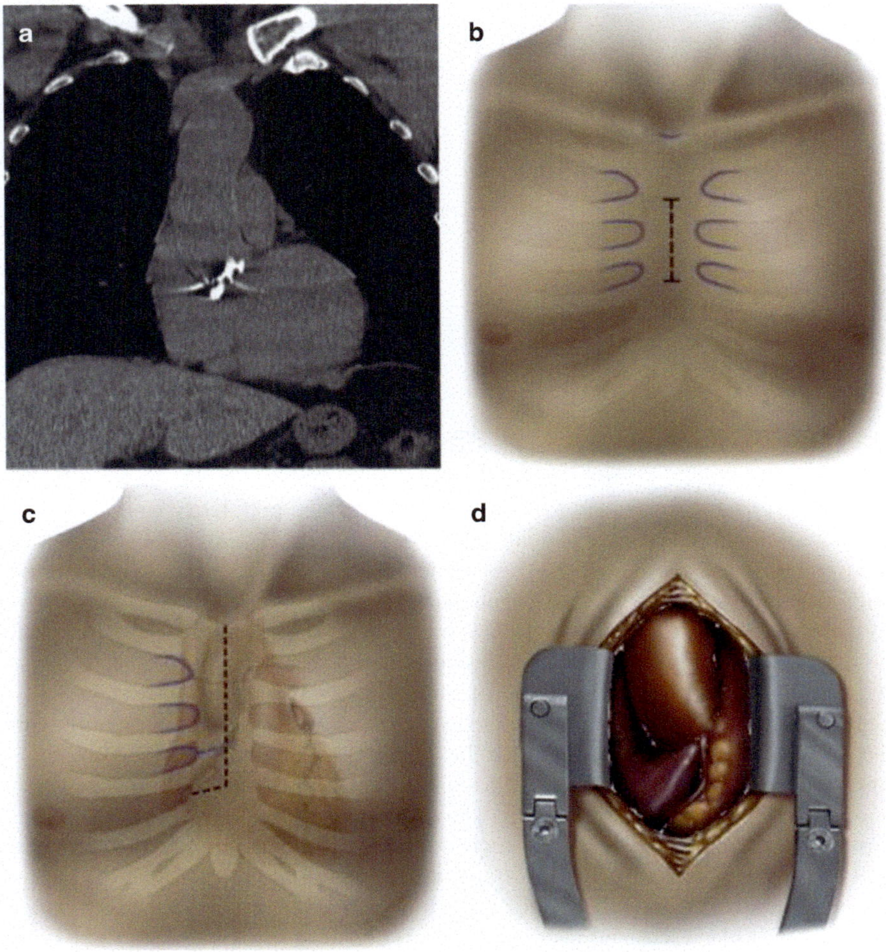

Fig. 17.1 Preoperative chest computed tomography identifying (**a**) the location of the aortic valve relative to the chest wall, (**b**) skin incision for upper hemisternotomy, (**c**) J incision into the right fourth (*black*) or third (*blue*) intercostal space, and (**d**), surgical exposure. (From Malaisrie SC et al. Current era minimally invasive aortic valve replacement: Techniques and practice. J Thorac Cardiovasc Surg. 2014;147(1):6–14. With permission)

incision of 10 cm with resection of costal cartilages and ligation of the right mammary artery and vein, utilizing cardiopulmonary bypass with peripheral arterial and vein cannulation. But this technique was soon abandoned due to the high incidence of lung herniation and rib instability, requiring often a second operation to repair the chest wall. Although many incisions were subsequently described, e.g. J, I, C, L, inverted-T and V-type approaches [4–8], further evolution has resulted in the J-shape upper ministernotomy, described by Svensson in 1997 [9, 10] (Fig. 17.1), and right anterior minithoracotomy (RAMT) as the most popular, with the upper

J-ministernotomy being currently the most widely used approach. It provides in fact a good window through which the aortic root and proximal aortic arch are freely accessible, resulting in a more 'familiar' exposure of the surgical field for the surgeon compared to RAMT. Through the upper J-ministernotomy approach, the aortic valve and ascending aorta pathologies can be treated and also complex procedures performed in almost 90% of patients.

17.1 Preoperative Evaluation

For a standard AVR via ministernotomy, if there are no contraindications such as pectum excavatum or other skeletal deformities, caudal aortic valve displacement due to aortic elongation, or pericardial calcifications, the preoperative evaluation is the same as for a full sternotomy: transthoracic echocardiography (TTE), coronary catheterization, and chest X-ray. In addition, pulmonary function testing is required in patients with COPD [11] . To determine the length of the sternotomy and to which intercostal space it should be extended, given the extreme variability of patients' body habitus, standard preoperative chest radiography usually gives enough information about the position and orientation of the aorta and aortic valve and its relation to the sternum and how the heart lies on the diaphragm. Transesophageal echocardiography (TEE) is mandatory in the operative room—a routine preoperative evaluation is performed just before skin incision to assess the valve function and morphology as well as the ascending aorta diameter and length. This information is particularly important if a sutureless valve bioprosthesis or aortic valve repair are planned. TEE is furthermore necessary in the setup of cardiopulmonary bypass (CPB) to ensure the correct positioning of the femoro-atrial venous cannula and retrograde cardioplegia catheter or endovent and, after the operation, to evaluate the valve and ventricular function and the complete de-airing of the heart.

When patients require concomitant coronary artery bypass grafting (CABG), the combined procedure is generally performed through a full median sternotomy, but nonetheless the proximal right coronary artery can be easily grafted through a ministernotomy. In elderly and high-risk patients with coronary artery stenosis favorable to treatment, percutaneous transluminal coronary angioplasty (PTCA), preferably with bare-metal stents, can be performed 4–6 weeks before a non-urgent AVR in order to make a minimally-invasive approach possible. These patients, in whom serious comorbidities increase the risk of a standard operation, would have greater benefit from a hybrid procedure. A contrast-enhanced 3D computed tomography (3D CT) of the chest, abdomen and pelvis is mandatory in the case of reoperation and of aneurisms of the ascending aorta and aortic arch [12–15]. A CT with 3D reconstruction provides valuable information about the mediastinal structures—it is fundamental for understanding the patient's anatomy and, in the case of re-surgery, assessing safety for reentry or tracking the course of the internal thoracic artery (ITA) and vein grafts in patients with previous CABG. CT also reveals the presence of calcifications on the ascending aorta and the relationship of the valve to landmarks on the bony thorax and the status of the femoral and iliac vessels if a

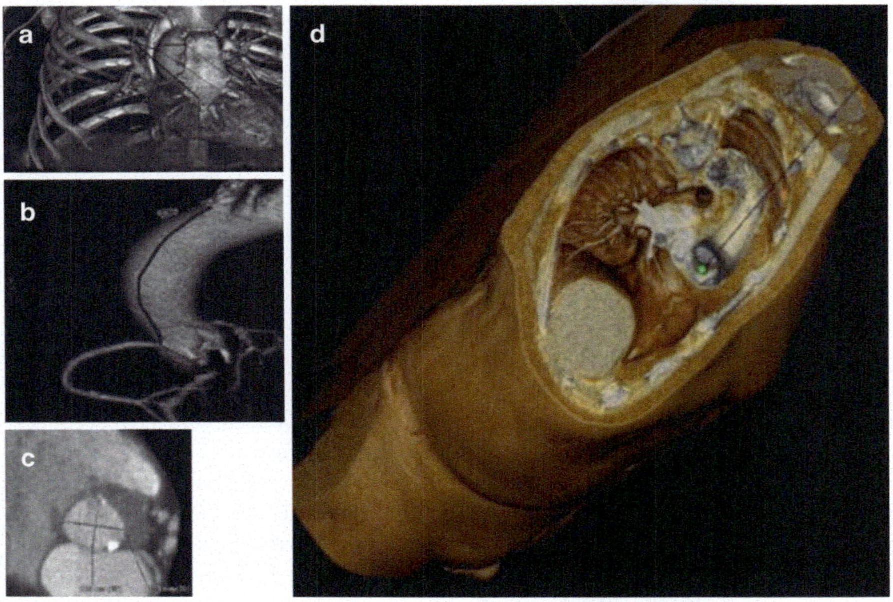

Fig. 17.2 Preoperative planning variables at multi-slice computed tomography imaging include (**a**) distance measurements from the intercostal space to the next aortic spot, aortic annulus, and right internal thoracic artery, (**b**) length of the aorta for cannulation, and (**c**) diameter evaluation for the aortic annulus. (**d**) Exact position of the aortic valve in relation to the chest wall and mediastinal structures, with high resolution enhanced 3D computed tomography with volumetric reconstruction. (From Plass A et al. Aortic valve replacement through a minimally invasive approach: preoperative planning, surgical technique, and outcome. Ann Thorac Surg. 2009;88(6):1851–6. Modified. With permission)

peripheral cannulation is planned (Fig. 17.2). Recently, contrast 3D CT has also been indicated as a tool to preoperatively evaluate the size of sutureless bioprostheses in MIAVR, similarly to transcatheter aortic valve implantation (TAVI) procedures, in order to further reduce CPB and cross-clamp time [16]. In patients with kidney failure, when other imaging methods such as chest X-ray or coronary angiograms show only aortic calcification, a non-contrast CT will suffice [17]. Once the decision is made to use a minimally-invasive approach everything must be accurately evaluated considering that is a more complex procedure with potential pitfalls, and hence requires closer cooperation with the anesthetist and pump technicians, good communication and teamwork with the assistant surgeon and scrub nurse, and adequate surgical instruments and exposition tools.

17.2 Surgical Technique: The Upper J-Ministernotomy

Conventional general anesthesia is used regardless of the surgical approach, and in patients with severe COPD a continuous thoracic epidural analgesia can be added to improve postoperative respiratory function by completely eliminating the chest pain. In the operating theatre, a triple lumen central venous line, radial artery catheter and external defibrillator pads are placed. In the case of redo operations a Swan-Ganz introducer with provision to pace the heart is added. A single lumen endotracheal tube is used and, after intubation, the TEE probe is inserted into the esophagus before incision. The surgical field is prepared so as to provide access to the whole length of the chest, with the groins and upper legs prepared as for all valve operations. The middle line is marked and landmarks identified including the sternal notch, angle of Louis and costal interspaces. A 4–8 cm midline skin incision is performed downwards from about 4 cm below the jugular notch. After making the skin incision, finger retractors are used to lift the skin and subcutaneous tissue over the length of the bone, and the interclavear ligament is resected. The sternum is cut keeping the oscillating saw in the midline and angling the cut to the third or fourth right intercostal space. Care is taken to maintain intact the ITA and vein. Careful hemostasis is maintained along the edges of the bone and bone marrow. A mini-Finocchietto or a minimally-invasive retractor is placed (Fig. 17.2). The thymus is divided and the pericardium is opened from the brachiocephalic vein to the lowest point possible below the sternal plate. Along each edge of the pericardium and at the cephalic limit of the pericardial reflection, four to five pericardial stay sutures are placed, after which the pericardial rims are lifted to skin level by charging the stay sutures under the retractor branches or pulling and attaching them to a support external to the wound (Fig. 17.3). In this way, the whole heart and especially the aorta and aortic valve are moved anteriorly, providing an effective access to the aortic root for valve repair or replacement. In cases where access needs to be extended to the distal ascending aorta or aortic arch, the brachiocephalic vein is encircled and pulled down and the brachiocephalic, left carotid and left subclavian arteries are isolated and encircled. The upper J-ministernotomy usually allows a good exposure of the proximal aortic arch, but an upper inverted-T or V-type ministernotomy can provide better exposure if a procedure involving the distal aortic arch is planned. In order to gain the advantages of antegrade perfusion during CPB, arterial cannulation is performed, whenever possible, in the distal ascending aorta or proximal aortic arch. This site is selected distal enough on the aorta to allow for placement of a cross-clamp, so a routine aortic cannula as per normal practice can be used. In all other cases, femoral or axillary arterial cannulation is required according to the status of the arteries at the groin. From the author's experience, venous central cannulation is performed with a three-stage 29 Fr flexible cannula that is placed through the right atrial appendage into the inferior vena cava. To improve exposure of the aortic root, the vein cannula can be pulled downward by fixing it to the diaphragmatic pericardium with a stay suture, or pulled laterally with a silk loop that is brought out through a parasternal hole in the chest wall at the fifth intercostal space (Fig. 17.3). This hole will be used later to pass the drain tube. The venous cannula can also be tunneled under the sternal plate to the xiphoid through the skin. Also in this case, at the end of the procedure the skin hole will be used to position the drain tube. In the case of ascending aorta dilatation, the right appendage is often hidden and displaced deeply by the aneurysm and a central venous cannulation may be difficult or impossible (Fig. 17.4). In such cases, percutaneous venous cannulation using a femoro-atrial cannula placed under TEE monitoring is

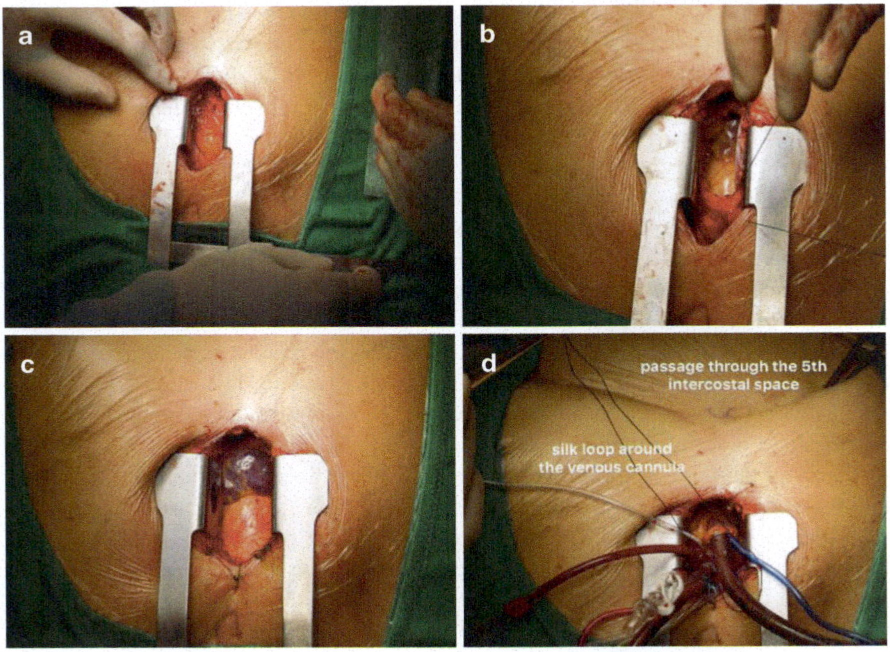

Fig. 17.3 Intraoperative view of the surgical field: (**a**) minimal invasive access via a partial upper sternotomy, (**b**) the pericardial stay sutures (**c**) the ascending aorta and right appendage exposed for cannulation, (**d**) to improve the aortic root exposure a silk loop is passed around the venous cannula and through the fifth intercostal space

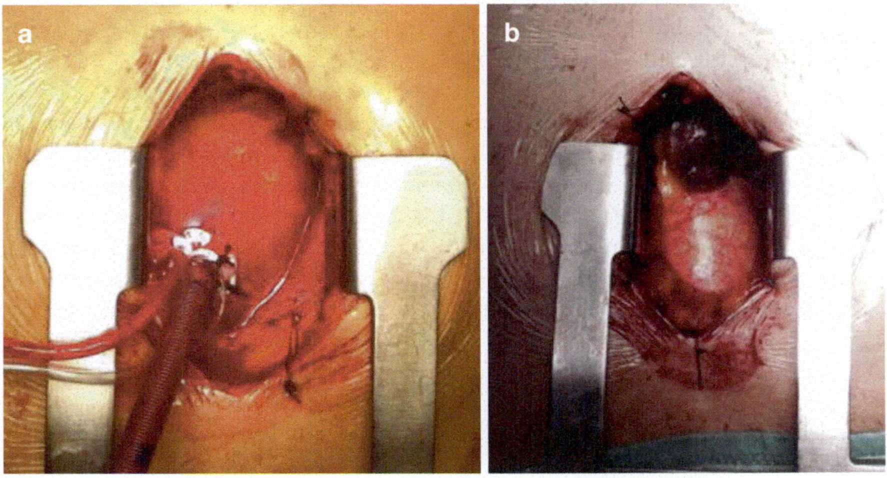

Fig. 17.4 Intraoperative view of the surgical field: (**a**) an aneurysm of the ascending aorta hides the right appendage that is displaced deeply; in this case percutaneous femoro-atrial venous cannulation is recommended, (**b**) a normal ascending aorta with good exposure of the right appendage for central cannulation

recommended, as well as in the case of reoperations. After safe cannulation and vacuum-assisted venous drainage (to improve the vein drainage), cardiopulmonary bypass is initiated and the aorta is cross-clamped directly though the incision using a standard aortic clamp or one of the several minimally invasive clamps; cardioplegia can be administered by antegrade route, injected into the ascending aorta, or with a retrograde cannula inserted either through the incision or percutaneously via the right internal jugular vein. Considering that there are many reports of conversion to full sternotomy on account of bleeding from a coronary sinus perforated by a retroplegia catheter, in the author's experience retrograde cardioplegia can be avoided; in the case of aortic insufficiency, one-half of the cardioplegia can be infused into the aortic root to arrest the heart and the remaining dose delivered directly to the coronary arteries. After administering cardioplegia, the ascending aorta is vented through the cardioplegia needle before it is transected. In this way, the aorta collapses and the heart is empty, leaving plenty of space to introduce the vent through the right superior pulmonary vein, avoiding troublesome bleeding and air embolism (Fig. 17.5). This maneuver is important especially in the case of ascending aorta aneurysms, where placing the vent before clamping may prove difficult. Left ventricular venting can alternatively be obtained by introducing the vent

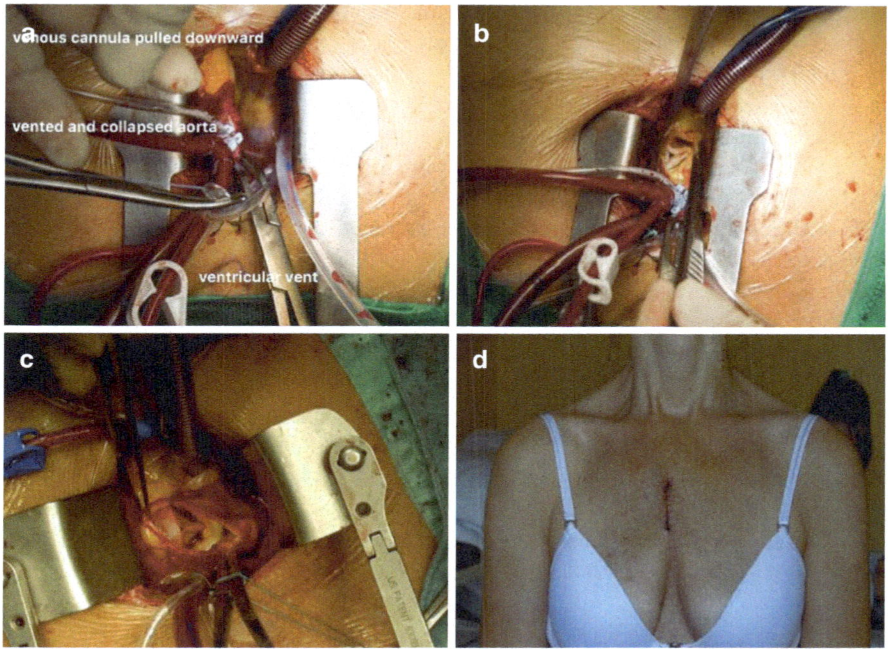

Fig. 17.5 Intraoperative view of the surgical field: (**a**) after aortic clamping and cardioplegic arrest the aorta is vented and collapsed, the venous cannula is pulled downward and the ventricular vent is easily and safely inserted through the superior right pulmonary vein; (**b**) view of aortic valve through minimal invasive access; (**c**) view of the aortic valve bioprosthesis implanted; (**d**) the skin incision

into the pulmonary artery, and directly into the left ventricle through the aortic valve, or through an endovent inserted percutaneously under TEE guidance [18]. We prefer to introduce the ventricular vent into the superior right pulmonary vein after cardiac arrest and temporary venting through the aorta—this sequence results in a safer and easier maneuver. The planned procedure on the aortic valve and or ascending aorta and arch is then performed according to the surgeon's preference using standard or minimally-invasive instruments that can make cutting, aortic valve debridement and suturing easier.

Aortotomies must be sutured with extreme care and it is worth doubling the suture, as controlling bleeding from the aorta after releasing the clamp may be very difficult due to the small space of the surgical field. Because of limited manipulation for de-airing, to prevent air embolism the surgical field is continuously flooded with carbon dioxide throughout the whole open-heart time of the operation. Then the ventricular vent is stopped while closing the aortotomy to allow the heart to fill spontaneously and, after releasing the aortic clamp, continuous venting through the ascending aorta is continued for 5–10 min and transesophageal echocardiography is assessed to control valve integrity, ventricular function, and complete de-airing. The pacing wires are placed on the right ventricle surface in cardiac arrest before releasing the aortic clamp; sometimes adiposity may impair ventricular capture and, if needed, a transvenous pacing wire can be placed. At the end of the procedure, a drain tube is positioned in the mediastinum through the skin passing under the xiphoid and the sternal plate or, alternatively, though a parasternal hole at the fifth right intercostal space, avoiding to open the pleura and damage the mammary artery and vein. After successful weaning from CPB, the cannulas are removed and protamine is administered. The aortic suture line, cannulation sites and any other potential sites are checked for bleeding and the pericardial stay sutures are released. The two halves of the sternum are then routinely sutured with steel wires.

In addition to the upper J-ministernotomy, many other incision techniques have been described. Following the initial description of a right parasternal incision, the manubrial sparing lower ministernotomy and reversed-C sternotomy were abandoned because they signified increased complexity but without providing any benefit. In the category of manubrial splitting ministernotomies, the inverted-T or the V-type sternotomies are still used in some centers, mainly for complex procedures involving the aortic arch. In these cases, the sternotomy is extended in both lateral directions in the second or third intercostal spaces—perpendicularly in the inverted-T or in a V-form in the V-type approach—these approaches allow a wider exposure of the upper mediastinum and better access to the distal aortic arch. The sternal closure is, however, more complicated than with the upper J technique, as these sternotomies sometimes require sternal plates [19, 20] and have an increased risk of sternal instability.

17.3 Minimally-Invasive Aortic Valve Reoperations

In 1997, Tam et al. [21] reported the successful application of an upper hemisternotomy in a patient with a history of AVR undergoing re-operative AVR. Since then, many reports have been published demonstrating excellent results and numerous advantages gained from reduction of the surgical trauma. Comparison to non randomized groups undergoing full sternotomy have shown that this approach, minimizing mediastinal dissection and handling of friable tissues on sternal reentry, results in shorter operative time, less risk of injury to a patent mammary artery graft or the right ventricle, reduced blood loss, reduced blood transfusion and shorter ICU stay [22, 23]. The upper J-ministernotomy approach is the one most widely used for patients undergoing re-operative AVR—the technique is similar to that previously described for primary operations with a few slight differences. In all cases, a 3D contrast enhanced CT scan is recommended to guide the operative approach. Volumetric reconstruction shows all the mediastinal structures in extremely fine detail, making it possible to identify the exact position of the aortic valve relative to the skin and mediastinal structures. This allows to plan the location and length of the incision and to which intercostal space it should be extended, considering that in redo procedures only the adherences of the ascending aorta can be debrided, leaving in most cases the whole heart fixed to the pericardium and to the sternum. For this reason it is not possible to lift the aorta with the stay sutures in order to improve the exposure of the aortic valve, as in a primary operations. 3D CT is also useful to assess the status of the femoral arteries for cannulation and to track the course of the vein and ITA grafts in patients with previous CABG [24, 25]. After making the upper J-ministernotomy, the pericardiolysis is extended only to the ascending aorta avoiding to touch the right atrium in order to limit as much as possible debridement and bleeding. Usually it is possible to directly cannulate the ascending aorta with a standard arterial cannula. If the right appendage can be easily isolated a central venous cannulation is possible but the cannula may result cumbersome in the surgical field as it cannot be moved downward. In this case, a percutaneous venous cannulation with a 22–25 Fr femoro-atrial cannula inserted under TEE guidance may be safer and simpler, and the left ventricle can be vented as in primary operations. Careful preoperative planning normally allows an optimal access to the aortic root and the aortic valve. Given that debridement can be limited to the ascending aorta, in order to prevent damage of patent internal mammary grafts in patients with previous CABG the ITA grafts are always left unclamped during cross-clamping time. Cardioplegia is administered by antegrade and/or retrograde route to arrest the heart but frequently, after a few minutes, the heart restarts beating or fibrillating. If the ventricle is well vented this generally does not interfere with the procedure. The reflow blood coming out from the coronary arteries can sometimes obscure the view of the valve; to avoid this, the coronary ostia can be temporarily occluded by means of a 3–5 mm Pruitt or Fogarty catheter. The use of blood or crystalloid cardioplegias, that can be repeated many times, may be more practical than extended-effect cardioplegias that are washed out by the blood flowing out from the patent ITAs. To protect the heart during procedures with unclamped LITA, Kaneko et al. [26] in a series of 51 consecutive patients utilized cooling of the patient to 25–30 °C and if, after administering cardioplegia, the cardiac activity restarted an additional dose of potassium was given through the pump in order to reach a serum dosage of 6.0–6.8 mEq. Ultrafiltration was used to reduce the potassium level at the end of the procedure. In our experience, as confirmed in many other reports from the literature, leaving the heart perfused by the ITAs during cross-clamp time without cooling the patient and elevating the serum potassium does not constitute a problem in terms of postoperative ventricular malperfusion.

17.4 Ministernotomy Approach for Sutureless AVR

Even if transcatheter valves can be viewed as the ultimate minimal access valve approach, the AVR technique is still open to further improvement, and this is the case with the new "sutureless" (SU) aortic bioprostheses. These prostheses are designed to allow a fast and simple deployment reducing the extracorporeal circulation (ECC) and cross-clamping time (CCT) while the absence of sutures makes these valves very versatile in MIAVR, significantly simplifying the procedure. This new generation of rapid-deployment SU bioprostheses has recently been introduced into clinical practice and their use is rapidly increasing (Video 17.1). The two models currently available in Europe and under trial at various stages in the United States are Perceval S (Livanova, London, UK) and Intuity (Edwards Life Sciences, Irvine, CA, USA). Favorable clinical outcomes have been reported with the use of both valves in several studies [27, 28] and their use in MIAVR has been demonstrated to be safe, with short postoperative times and excellent hemodynamic performance and postoperative outcomes [29–32]. The recent CADENCE–MIS randomized trial compared outcomes between 100 AVR operations involving implantation of an Edwards Intuity valve though ministernotomy and 100 AVRs in which conventional stented bioprostheses were implanted though full sternotomy. The results demonstrated significant shorter cross-clamp time for the minimally-invasive procedure associated to a lower incidence of patient-prosthesis mismatch and significantly lower transvalvular gradients [33]. Similarly, other studies have demonstrated the same advantages for the Sorin Perceval S bioprosthesis. Santarpino et al. [30] reported excellent results with implantation of Sorin Perceval S through ministernotomy in terms of mortality and hemodynamic performance with a very low rate of paravalvular leakage and also shorter CPB and CCT in high risk patients.

17.5 Potential Pitfalls and Complications

The upper J-ministernotomy approach for AVR is probably the most simple and reproducible in the scenario of minimally-invasive cardiac operations due to its relatively traditional approach to the aortic valve and ascending aorta and the use of central cannulation, which is possible in the majority of cases. However, it necessitates a specific training program on account of the increased procedural complexity which is a consequence of the restricted visualization of the surgical field and the limited manipulation of the cardiac situs. Even if the risks associated to this type of surgery are the same as those for conventional aortic valve replacement, the whole surgical team needs to be open-minded and aware of the pitfalls. AVR is the simplest and most frequent procedure performed through upper J-ministernotomy, but reoperations or more complex procedures involving the ascending aorta and arch as well as Ross procedures should be entrusted to surgeons who are highly experienced in MICS [34–37]. Conversion to full sternotomy is the most frequent complication reported in minimally-invasive aortic valve surgery (AVS), occurring in 3–4% of cases on average [38–40] although extremely rare (0.3%) in high volume centers [1]. However, in contrast to conversion from other minimally-invasive cardiac surgery procedures (e.g. RAMT-AVR, minimally-invasive mitral valve surgery, and minimally-invasive direct coronary artery bypass) conversion from MIAVR to full sternotomy is comparatively easy in that one has simply to extend the sternotomy downwards. The most frequent reasons for conversion are poor exposure of the aortic valve, uncontrolled bleeding and ventricular dysfunction, distention or fibrillation. Conversion due to poor exposure of the aortic valve can occur before or after CPB and aortic clamping, and an adequate preoperative planning and greater experience could completely eliminate this issue. To avoid uncontrolled bleeding, all surgical points such as the aortotomy and cannulation sites must be well visualized and constantly monitored. It is better to avoid blind potential bleeding points, and if there is continuous bleeding from an unidentified source full sternotomy is mandatory and should not be delayed. In minimally-invasive AVS, bleeding has been described as a result of coronary sinus rupture after insertion of a retroplegia catheter, from the right atrium, aortotomy and cannulation sites. In order to reduce the risk of bleeding and to simplify the procedure, retrograde cardioplegia can be avoided as antegrade cardioplegia may be sufficient to adequately protect the heart even in the case of severe aortic insufficiency. In the case of more complex procedures, such as Bentall operations or ascending aorta replacements with aortic valve sparing procedures, Ross operations, etc., bleeding from coronary ostia or proximal sutures at the level of the aortic annulus can be difficult to manage due to limited room in the surgical field and poor visualization. In the case of an extended hematoma of the aortic root due to tissue frailty that can occur in AVR, the pericardium must be further opened downward to avoid a distortion or a compression of the right coronary artery between the hematoma and the pericardium itself, and if there are doubts conversion to full sternotomy is recommended. Other causes of conversion are ventricular distention, dysfunction and fibrillation, while late conversion is usually due to cardiac tamponade. To avoid ventricular distention, the ventricular vent must be left in place until the complete restart of cardiac activity, then removed just before weaning from CPB. For all technical difficulties that can occur during a minimally-invasive AVS procedure due to any cause, including excessive loss of time, a timeline must be established by the surgical team to evaluate and manage the situation and to decide when to convert to full sternotomy, in order to avoid compromising the outcome of the operation. Problems and complications in the case of groin vessel cannulation and reversed flow CPB are the same as described for all cardiac operations, requiring peripheral cannulation and antegrade perfusion as the preferred solution whenever possible [41].

In expert hands, most patients with valvular disease can be offered minimally-invasive procedures with excellent results and the rate of complications and conversions has been shown to significantly decrease with experience, considering that the learning curve of an expert surgeon to achieve confidence with a minimally-invasive procedure averages 40–50 operations [42]. It is not clear how training programs should adapt to this new reality and how young surgeons should be taught and mentored in these new techniques without compromising the expected excellent clinical outcomes and high levels of safety. In this sense, the steps to build a minimally-invasive AVS program require, first, that a multidisciplinary team composed of surgeons, anesthesiologists, cardiologists, perfusionists and nurses be set up. The whole team must be trained in the knowledge and skills of minimally-invasive cardiac surgery, and visits to high-volume centers for MICS, participation in instructional courses as well as the mentorship of an expert surgeon are recommended. The learning curve will require full communication among all team members and, especially in the initial phase, longer operation times must be accepted and potential complications must be well evaluated and managed without adversely affecting patient care [43, 44], trying to avoid in the beginning older, obese and high-risk patients with multi-comorbidities in order to limit procedural and CPB duration.

17.6 Outcomes

In the mid-1990s, minimally invasive 'keyhole' approaches for mitral valve and aortic valve operations were pioneered. Currently the upper J-ministernotomy seems the most popular approach for minimally invasive AVS. It has proven to be safe and capable of providing excellent short- and long-term results in terms of mortality [2]. Despite the lack of large-scale randomized controlled studies, given that the few randomized trials published average 40 patients and are insufficiently powered for statistical significance [2, 45, 46], many observational retrospective and propensity-score matched studies as well as meta-analyses have confirmed the advantages of minimally-invasive AVS compared to traditional full sternotomy [42, 47–52] and in recent reports from high volume centers the short- and long-term mortality resulted lower in patients operated by minimally-invasive AVS [1] (Fig. 17.6). Even if cosmesis remains an unquestionable benefit of MS (Fig. 17.3), the randomized and multiple-matched cohort trials have highlighted many other advantages such as shorter ventilation time, less postoperative pain, shorter ICU and hospital stay, as well as reduced blood loss and need for transfusion [53–57] whereas other advantages such as short- and long-term mortality, the lower rate of postoperative atrial fibrillation, and less wound infections remain controversial. Johnston et al. [58] measured the value of forced expiratory volume in 1 s (FEV_1) (Fig. 17.7) on the first two postoperative days and found a significantly better value in patients operated though the minimal access approach (Fig. 17.8). This may be related to the lower trauma impact on the chest and tissue traction and to the reduced postoperative pain, which is another parameter that resulted significantly

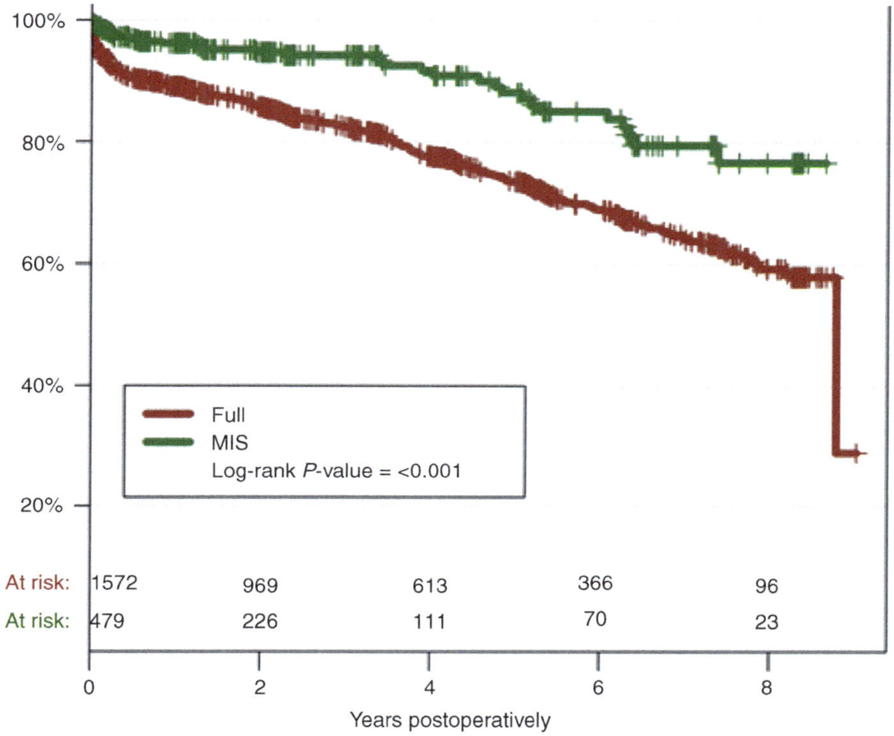

Fig. 17.6 Overall survival curves for unmatched patients. (From Merk DR, Lehmann S, Holzhey DM, Dohmen P, Candolfi P, Misfeld M, Mohr FW, Borger MA. Minimal invasive aortic valve replacement surgery is associated with improved survival: a propensity-matched comparison. Eur J Cardiothorac Surg. 2015;47(1):11–7. With permission)

lower in ministernotomy patients. The reduction of postoperative bleeding and of the need for transfusion, that has been widely reported, leads furthermore to a lower incidence of renal failure and, although some doubts have been raised about the adequacy of de-airing, no difference has been demonstrated between ministernotomy and full sternotomy in terms of neurological events. Myocardial infarctions and wound infections have the same incidence compared to full sternotomy, while sternal instability is lower in ministernotomy. In addition, the safety of MIAVR has been widely demonstrated by multiple retrospective observational series and meta-analyses [59, 60], and acceptable results have been published in specific subgroups such as octogenarians [61], obese patients [62], patients with left ventricular dysfunction, and in re-operative surgery. Furthermore, the ministernotomy approach has been reported to be safe not only for MIAVR, but also for other interventions. Shresta et al. [63] have published a series of valve-sparing aortic root replacements with results comparable to those done with conventional full sternotomy, and there are many reports of complex operations such as

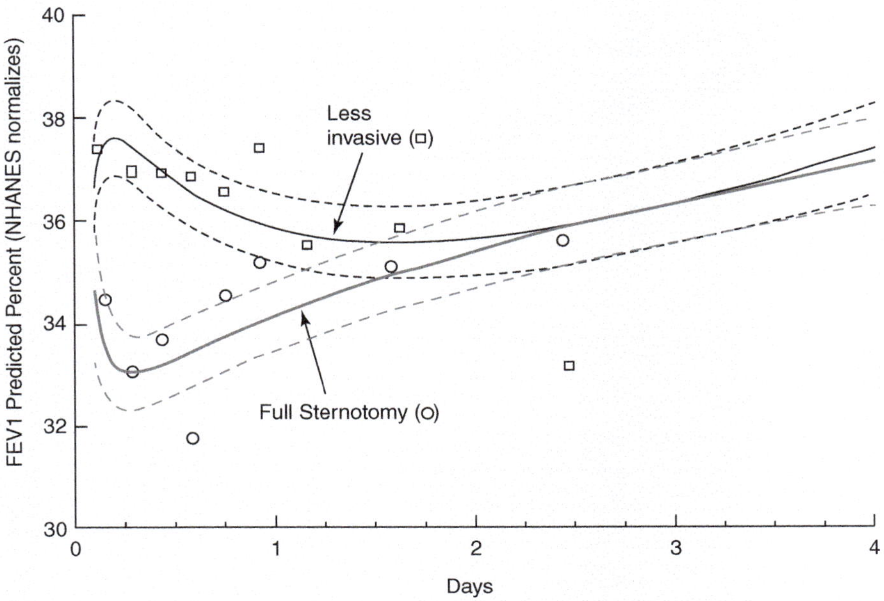

Fig. 17.7 Temporal pattern of post-extubation forced expiratory volume at 1-s (FEV_1) as percent of predicted after less invasive and full sternotomy aortic valve surgery among propensity-matched patients. *Solid lines* are parametric estimates of temporal trend enclosed within *dashed lines* 68% confidence limits (equivalent to ± 1 standard error). *Symbols* represent data grouped within time frames without regard for repeated assessment, simply to provide crude verification of model fit. (From Johnston DR, Atik FA, Rajeswaran J, Blackstone EH, Nowicki ER, Sabik JF 3rd, Mihaljevic T, Gillinov AM, Lytle BW, Svensson LG. Outcomes of less invasive J-incision approach to aortic valve surgery. J Thorac Cardiovasc Surg. 2011;144(4):852–858.e3. With permission)

ascending aorta and arch replacement or Ross operations performed through a minimally-invasive approach with equivalent results to those with conventional full sternotomy. One of the drawbacks of minimally-invasive AVS has been identified in the longer CPB and cross-clamp times linked to a more difficult operation. A recent meta-analysis by Phan et al. showed an average cross-clamp and CPB time of 8–9 min longer compared to full sternotomy—this value is considered to be insignificant in the clinical outcome of the patients and the recent introduction of the self-expandable bioprostheses for MIAVR has further reduced CPB and CCT by up to 40% [64]. Less transfusions and shorter ICU and hospital stays are expected to reduce hospital costs and there are several reports calculating and demonstrating the savings effect of the faster recovery and return to normal life in terms of reduced rehabilitation and social costs, even if there are no RCTs and few studies analyzing this economic aspect. Cohn et al. report a reduction by 20% of total charges for minimal access patients [65] and other similar studies have led to the same results with a significant cost savings in patients operated through ministernotomy [66, 67].

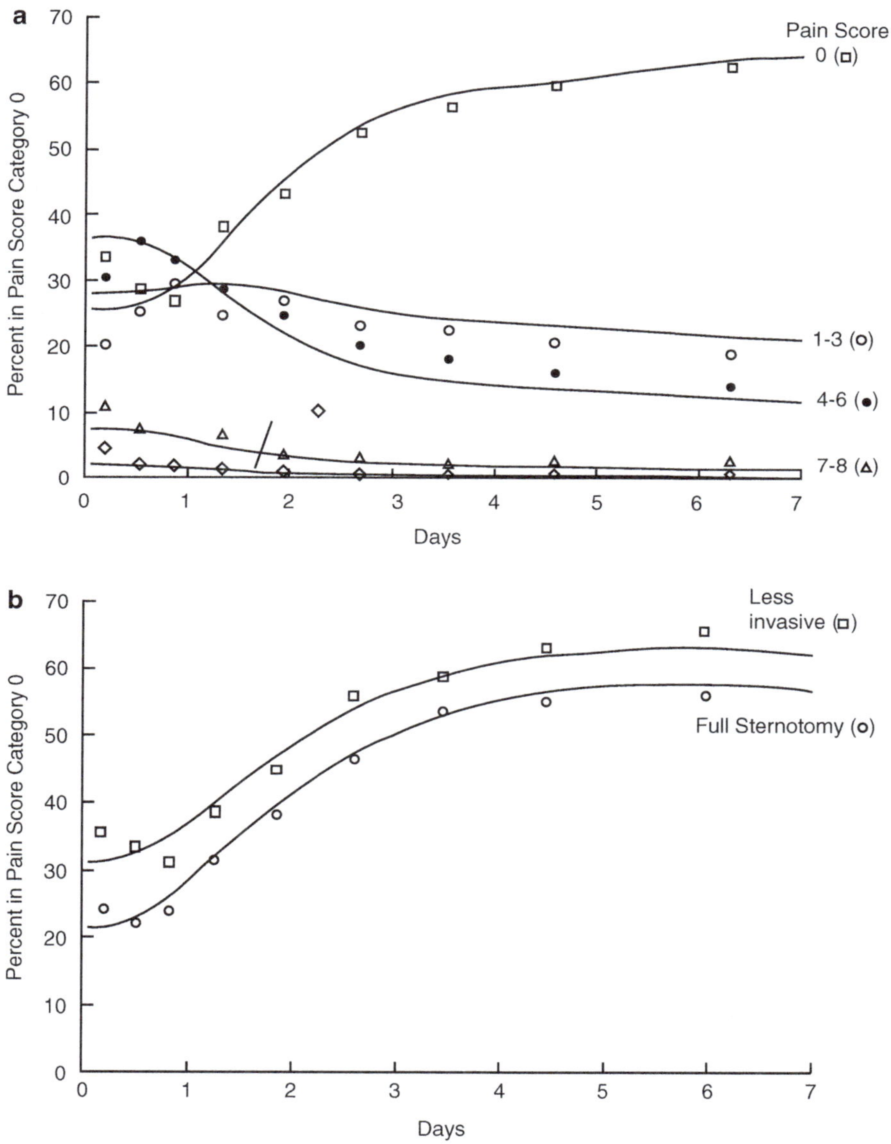

Fig. 17.8 Temporal pattern of pain score categories after less invasive versus full sternotomy aortic valve surgery among propensity-matched patients. *Symbols* represent data grouped within time frames without regard for repeated assessment, simply to provide crude verification of model fit. *Solid lines* are parametric estimates of percentage of patients in each category. (**a**) all pain score categories, (**b**), Proportion of patients without pain (category 0). (From Johnston DR, Atik FA, Rajeswaran J, Blackstone EH, Nowicki ER, Sabik JF 3rd, Mihaljevic T, Gillinov AM, Lytle BW, Svensson LG. Outcomes of less invasive J-incision approach to aortic valve surgery. J Thorac Cardiovasc Surg. 2011;144(4):852–858.e3. With permission)

17.7 Summary

Considerable progress has been made in recent years regarding the overall outcomes of surgical treatment of the aortic valve and aortic diseases. The minimally-invasive approach is becoming more and more popular and the variety of surgical strategies and adjuncts proposed to minimize the principal complications of these cardiac operations indicates that this sophisticated surgical treatment is still evolving. Ministernotomy has proven to be a safe approach for aortic valve replacement (AVR) and aortic root operations with excellent postoperative outcomes in terms of short- and long-term mortality and postoperative complications and it can be routinely used for these procedures.

References

1. Merk DR, Lehmann S, Holzhey DM, Dohmen P, Candolfi P, Misfeld M, Mohr FW, Borger MA. Minimal invasive aortic valve replacement surgery is associated with improved survival: a propensity-matched comparison. Eur J Cardiothorac Surg. 2015;47(1):11–17.; discussion 17. https://doi.org/10.1093/ejcts/ezu068.
2. Khoshbin E, Prayaga S, Kinsella J, Sutherland FW. Mini-sternotomy for aortic valve replacement reduces the length of stay in the cardiac intensive care unit: meta-analysis of randomised controlled trials. BMJ Open. 2011;1(2):e000266. https://doi.org/10.1136/bmjopen-2011-000266.
3. Cosgrove DM 3rd, Sabik JF. Minimally invasive approach for aortic valve operations. Ann Thorac Surg. 1996;62(2):596–7.
4. Karimov JH, Santarelli F, Murzi M, Glauber M. A technique of an upper V-type mini sternotomy in the second intercostal space. Interact Cardiovasc Thorac Surg. 2009;9(6):1021–2. https://doi.org/10.1510/icvts.2009.215699.
5. Aris A. Reversed "C" ministernotomy for aortice valve replacement. Ann Thorac Surg. 1999;67(6):1806–7.
6. von Segesser LK, Westaby S, Pomar J, Loisance D, Groscurth P, Turina M. Less invasive aortic valve surgery: rationale and technique. Eur J Cardiothorac Surg. 1999;15(6):781–5.
7. Concistrè G, Miceli A, Chiaramonti F, Farneti P, Bevilacqua S, Varone E, Solinas M, Glauber M. Sutureless aortic valve implantation through an upper V-type ministernotomy: an innovative approach in high-risk patients. Innovations (Phila). 2013;8(1):23–8. https://doi.org/10.1097/IMI.0b013e31828d6b03.
8. Granov N, Kacila M, Mujicic E, Hadzimehmedagic A, Custovic F, Kulic M. V-type mini sternotomy in aortic valve replacement. Med Arch. 2012;66(3):213–4.
9. Svensson LG. Minimal-access "J" or "j" sternotomy for valvular, aortic, and coronary operations or reoperations. Ann Thorac Surg. 1997;64(5):1501–3.
10. Malaisrie SC, Barnhart GR, Farivar RS, Mehall J, Hummel B, Rodriguez E, Anderson M, Lewis C, Hargrove C, Ailawadi G, Goldman S, Khan J, Moront M, Grossi E, Roselli EE, Agnihotri A, Mack MJ, Smith JM, Thourani VH, Duhay FG, Kocis MT, Ryan WH. Current era minimally invasive aortic valve replacement: techniques and practice. J Thorac Cardiovasc Surg. 2014;147(1):6–14. https://doi.org/10.1016/j.jtcvs.2013.08.086.
11. Plass A, Scheffel H, Alkadhi H, et al. Aortic valve replacement through a minimally invasive approach: preoperative planning, surgical technique and outome. Ann Thorac Surg. 2009;88:1851–6.
12. Heuts S, Maessen JG, Sardari NP. Preoperative planning of left-sided valve surgery with 3D computed tomography reconstruction models: sternotomy or aminimally invasive approach? Interact Cardiovasc Thorac Surg. 2016;22(5):587–93. https://doi.org/10.1093/icvts/ivv408.

13. Loor G, Roselli EE. Imaging and minimally invasive aortic valve replacement. Ann Cardiothorac Surg. 2015;4(1):62–6. https://doi.org/10.3978/j.issn.2225-319X.2014.11.06.
14. Stoliński J, Plicner D, Grudzień G, Kruszec P, Fijorek K, Musiał R, Andres J. Computed tomography helps to plan minimally invasive aortic valve replacement operations. Ann Thorac Surg. 2016;101(5):1745–52. https://doi.org/10.1016/j.athoracsur.2015.10.076.
15. Roselli EE. Interventions on the aortic valve and proximal thoracic aorta through a minimally invasive approach. Ann Cardiothorac Surg. 2015;4(1):81–4. https://doi.org/10.3978/j.issn.2225-319X.2014.11.02.
16. Margaryan R, Kallushi E, Gilmanov D, Micelli A, Murzi M, Solinas M, Cerillo AG, Glauber M. Sutureless Aortic Valve Prosthesis Sizing: Estimation and Prediction Using Multidetector-Row Computed Tomography. Innovations (Phila). 2015;10(4):230–235.; discussion 235. https://doi.org/10.1097/IMI.0000000000000182.
17. Ammar R, Porat E, Eisemberg DS, et al. Utility of spiral CT in minimally invasive approach for aortic valve replacement. Eur J Cardiothorac Surg. 1998;14(Suppl1):S130–3.
18. Kraidin JL, Pantin EJ, Anderson MB, Zhou BL, Solina AR. Edwards EndoVent as a pacing catheter for minimally invasive aortic valve surgery: a novel approach. Innovations (Phila). 2011;6(4):253–6. https://doi.org/10.1097/IMI.0b013e31822c9f88.
19. Lentini S, Specchia L, Nicolardi S, Mangia F, Rasovic O, Di Eusanio G, Gregorini R. Surgery of the ascending aorta with or without combined procedures through an upper ministernotomy: outcomes of a series of more than 100 patients. Ann Thorac Cardiovasc Surg. 2016;22(1):44–8. https://doi.org/10.5761/atcs.oa.15-00245.
20. Russo MJ, Gnezda J, Merlo A, Johnson EM, Hashmi M, Raman J. The arrowhead ministernotomy with rigid sternal plate fixation: a minimally invasive approach for surgery of the ascending aorta and aortic root. Minim Invasive Surg. 2014;2014:681371. https://doi.org/10.1155/2014/681371.
21. Tam RK, Garlick RB, Almeida AA. Minimally invasive redo aortic valve replacement. J Thorac Cardiovasc Surg. 1997;114(4):682–3.
22. Mikus E, Calvi S, Tripodi A, Dozza L, Lamarra M, Del Giglio M. Minimally invasive reoperative aortic valve replacement. Ann Cardiothorac Surg. 2015;4(1):67–70. https://doi.org/10.3978/j.issn.2225-319X.2014.11.09.
23. Gosev I, Neely RC, Leacche M, McGurk S, Kaneko T, Zeljko D, Loberman D, Javed Q, Cohn LH, Aranki SF. The impact of a minimally invasive approach on reoperativeaortic valve replacement. J Heart Valve Dis. 2015;24(2):181–6.
24. Gaeta R, Lentini S, Raffa G, Pellegrini C, Zattera G, Viganò M. Aortic valve replacement by ministernotomy in redo patients with previous left internalmammary artery patent grafts. Ann Thorac Cardiovasc Surg. 2010 Jun;16(3):181–6.
25. Zeitani J, Pugliese M, Mvondo CM, Chiariello G, Bellos K, Simonetti G, Chiariello L. Surgical approach to aortic valve replacement after previous bilateral internal thoracic artery grafting. Tex Heart Inst J. 2013;40(2):170–2.
26. Kaneko T, Loberman D, Gosev I, Rassam F, McGurk S, Leacche M, Cohn L. Reoperative aortic valve replacement in the octogenarians-minimally invasive technique in the era of transcatheter valve replacement. J Thorac Cardiovasc Surg. 2014;147(1):155–62. https://doi.org/10.1016/j.jtcvs.2013.08.076.
27. Fischlein T, Meuris B, Hakim-Meibodi K, Misfeld M, Carrel T, Zembala M, Gaggianesi S, Madonna F, Laborde F, Asch F, Haverich A, CAVALIER Trial Investigators. The sutureless aortic valve at 1 year: a large multicenter cohort study. J Thorac Cardiovasc Surg. 2016;151(6):1617–1626.e4. https://doi.org/10.1016/j.jtcvs.2015.12.064.
28. Dalén M, Biancari F, Rubino AS, Santarpino G, Glaser N, De Praetere H, Kasama K, Juvonen T, Deste W, Pollari F, Meuris B, Fischlein T, Mignosa C, Gatti G, Pappalardo A, Svenarud P, Sartipy U. Aortic valve replacement through fullsternotomy with a stented bioprosthesis versus minimally invasive sternotomy witha sutureless bioprosthesis. Eur J Cardiothorac Surg. 2016;49(1):220–7. https://doi.org/10.1093/ejcts/ezv014.
29. Fischlein T, Pfeiffer S, Pollari F, Sirch J, Vogt F, Santarpino G. Sutureless valve implantation via mini J-sternotomy: a single center experience with 2 years mean follow-up. Thorac Cardiovasc Surg. 2015;63(6):467–71. https://doi.org/10.1055/s-0035-1554043.

30. Santarpino G, Pfeiffer S, Jessl J, Dell'Aquila AM, Pollari F, Pauschinger M, Fischlein T. Sutureless replacement versus transcatheter valve implantation in aortic valve stenosis: a propensity-matched analysis of 2 strategies in high-riskpatients. J Thorac Cardiovasc Surg. 2014;147(2):561–7. https://doi.org/10.1016/j.jtcvs.2013.10.025.
31. Zannis K, Folliguet T, Laborde F. New sutureless aortic valve prosthesis:another tool in less invasive aortic valve replacement. Curr Opin Cardiol. 2012;27(2):125–9. https://doi.org/10.1097/HCO.0b013e3283501a11.
32. Misfeld M. Minimally invasive aortic valve replacement using the Perceval S Sutureless valve. Ann Cardiothorac Surg. 2015;4(2):203–5. https://doi.org/10.3978/j.issn.2225-319X.2015.02.07.
33. Borger MA, Moustafine V, Conradi L, Knosalla C, Richter M, Merk DR, Doenst T, Hammerschmidt R, Treede H, Dohmen P, Strauch JT. A randomized multicenter trial of minimally invasive rapid deployment versus conventional full sternotomy aortic valve replacement. Ann Thorac Surg. 2015;99(1):17–25. https://doi.org/10.1016/j.athoracsur.2014.09.022.
34. Perrotta S, Lentini S, Rinaldi M, D'armini AM, Tancredi F, Raffa G, Gaeta R, Vigano M. Treatment of ascending aorta disease with Bentall-de bono operation using a mini-invasive approach. J Cardiovasc Med (Hagerstown). 2008;9(10):1016–22. https://doi.org/10.2459/JCM.0b013e32830214a6.
35. Benedik J, Mourad F, Eißmann M, Jakob H, Perrey. Minimally invasive David reimplantation of bicuspid aortic valve. Ann Cardiothorac Surg. 2015;4(2):206–7. https://doi.org/10.3978/j.issn.2225-319X.2015.02.08.
36. Totaro P, Carlini S, Pozzi M, Pagani F, Zattera G, D'Armini AM, Vigano M. Minimally invasive approach for complex cardiac surgery procedures. Ann ThoracSurg. 2009;88(2):462–466.; discussion 467. https://doi.org/10.1016/j.athoracsur.2009.04.060.
37. Franke UF, Albert M, Rustenbach C, Baumbach H. Minimally invasive Ross procedure through partial upper sternotomy. Interact Cardiovasc Thorac Surg. 2009;9(3):545–6. https://doi.org/10.1510/icvts.2009.203067.
38. Moscoso Ludueña M, Rastan AJ. Complications and conversions in minimallyinvasive aortic valve surgery. Ann Cardiothorac Surg. 2015;4(1):94–8. https://doi.org/10.3978/j.issn.2225-319X.2014.11.14.
39. Tabata M, Umakanthan R, Khalpey Z, et al. Conversion to full sternotomy during minimal-access cardiac surgery: reasons and results during a 9.5 years experience. J Thorac Cardiovasc Surg. 2007;134:165–9.
40. Johnston DR, Atik FA, Rajeswaran J, Blackstone EH, Nowicki ER, Sabik JF 3rd, Mihaljevic T, Gillinov AM, Lytle BW, Svensson LG. Outcomes of less invasive J-incision approach to aortic valve surgery. J Thorac Cardiovasc Surg. 2012;144(4):852–858.e3. https://doi.org/10.1016/j.jtcvs.2011.12.008.
41. Murzi M, Glauber M. Central versus femoral cannulation during minimallyinvasive aortic valve replacement. Ann Cardiothorac Surg. 2015;4(1):59–61. https://doi.org/10.3978/j.issn.2225-319X.2014.10.06.
42. Brinkman WT, Hoffmann W, Dewey TM, Culica D, Prince SL, Herbert MA, Mack M, Ryan WH. Aortic valve replacement surgery: comparison of outcomes in matched sternotomy and PORT ACCESS groups. Ann Thorac Surg. 2010;90(1):131–5. https://doi.org/10.1016/j.athoracsur.2010.03.055.
43. Vohra HA, Vaja R, Iakovakis I, Bapat V, Szostek J, Young C. Starting out in minimally invasive aortic valve replacement in the UK. Interact Cardiovasc Thorac Surg. 2016;22(1):1–4. https://doi.org/10.1093/icvts/ivv279.
44. Gosev I, Kaneko T, McGurk S, McClure SR, Maloney A, Cohn LH. A 16-year experience in minimally invasive aortic valve replacement: context for the changing management of aortic valve disease. Innovations (Phila). 2014;9(2):104–110.; discussion 110. https://doi.org/10.1097/IMI.0000000000000053.
45. Phan K, Tsai YC, Niranjan N, Bouchard D, Carrel TP, Dapunt OE, Eichstaedt HC, Fischlein T, Gersak B, Glauber M, Haverich A, Misfeld M, Oberwalder PJ, Santarpino G, Shrestha ML, Solinas M, Vola M, Yan TD, Di Eusanio M. Suturelessaortic valve replacement: a

systematic review and meta-analysis. Ann Cardiothorac Surg. 2015;4(2):100–11. https://doi.org/10.3978/j.issn.2225-319X.2014.06.01.
46. Borger MA, Moustafine V, Conradi L, Knosalla C, Richter M, Merk DR, Doenst T, Hammerschmidt R, Treede H, Dohmen P, Strauch JT. A randomized multicenter trial valve replacement. Ann Thorac Surg. 2015;99(1):17–25. https://doi.org/10.1016/j.athoracsur.2014.09.022.
47. Mihaljevic T, Gillinov MA, Cosgrove DM. Minimally invasive aortic valve replacement. Multimed Man Cardiothorac Surg 2006;2006(315). https://doi.org/10.1510/mmcts.2005.001131.
48. Attia RQ, Hickey GL, Grant SW, Bridgewater B, Roxburgh JC, Kumar P, Ridley P, Bhabra M, Millner RW, Athanasiou T, Casula R, Chukwuemka A, Pillay T, Young CP. Minimally invasive versus conventional aortic valve replacement: a propensity-matched study from the UK national data. Innovations (Phila). 11(1):15–23. https://doi.org/10.1097/IMI.0000000000000236.
49. Hiraoka A, Totsugawa T, Kuinose M, Nakajima K, Chikazawa G, Tamura K, Yoshitaka H, Sakaguchi T. Propensity score-matched analysis of minimally invasiveaortic valve replacement. Circ J. 2014;78(12):2876–81.
50. Lim JY, Deo SV, Altarabsheh SE, Jung SH, Erwin PJ, Markowitz AH, Park SJ. Conventional versus minimally invasive aortic valve replacement: pooled analysis of propensity-matched data. J Card Surg. 2015;30(2):125–34. https://doi.org/10.1111/jocs.12493.
51. Furukawa N, Kuss O, Aboud A, Schönbrodt M, Renner A, Hakim Meibodi K, Becker T, Zittermann A, Gummert JF, Börgermann J. Ministernotomy versus conventional sternotomy for aortic valve replacement: matched propensity score analysis of 808patients. Eur J Cardiothorac Surg. 2014;46(2):221–226.; discussion 226-7. https://doi.org/10.1093/ejcts/ezt616.
52. Burdett CL, Lage IB, Goodwin AT, White RW, Khan KJ, Owens WA, Kendall SW, Ferguson JI, Dunning J, Akowuah EF. Manubrium-limited sternotomy decreases blood loss after aortic valve replacement surgery. Interact Cardiovasc Thorac Surg. 2014;19(4):605–10. https://doi.org/10.1093/icvts/ivu196.
53. Lehmann S, Merk DR, Etz CD, Seeburger J, Schroeter T, Oberbach A, Uhlemann M, Hoellriegel R, Haensig M, Leontyev S, Garbade J, Misfeld M, Mohr FW. Minimallyinvasive aortic valve replacement: the Leipzig experience. Ann Cardiothorac Surg. 2015;4(1):49–56. https://doi.org/10.3978/j.issn.2225-319X.2014.11.03.
54. Van der Merwe J, Casselman F, Stockman B, Van Praet F, Beelen R, Maene L, Vermeulen Y, Degrieck I. Minimally invasive primary aortic valve surgery: the OLVAalst experience. Ann Cardiothorac Surg. 2015;4(2):154–9. https://doi.org/10.3978/j.issn.2225-319X.2015.01.08.
55. Foghsgaard S, Gazi D, Bach K, Hansen H, Schmidt TA, Kjaergard HK. Minimally invasive aortic valve replacement reduces atelectasis in cardiac intensive care. Acute Card Care. 2009;11(3):169–72. https://doi.org/10.1080/17482940903082228.
56. Ariyaratnam P, Loubani M, Griffin SC. Minimally invasive aortic valver replacement: comparison of long-term outcomes. Asian Cardiovasc Thorac Ann. 2015;23(7):814–21. https://doi.org/10.1177/0218492315587606.
57. Brown ML, McKellar SH, Sundt TM, et al. Ministernotomy versus conventional sternotomy for aortic valve replacement: a systematic review and meta-analysis. J Thorac Cardiovasc Surg. 2009;137:670–9.e5.
58. Johnston DR, Roselli EE. Minimally invasive aortic valve surgery: Cleveland clinic experience. Ann Cardiothorac Surg. 2015;4(2):140–7. https://doi.org/10.3978/j.issn.2225-319X.2014.10.03.
59. Murtuza B, Pepper JR, Stanbridge RD, et al. Minimal access aortic valve replacement: is it worth it? Ann Thorac Surg. 2008;85:1121–31.
60. Neely RC, Boskovski MT, Gosev I, Kaneko T, McGurk S, Leacche M, Cohn LH. Minimally invasive aortic valve replacement versus aortic valve replacement through full sternotomy: the Brigham and Women's Hospital experience. Ann Cardiothorac Surg. 2015;4(1):38–48. https://doi.org/10.3978/j.issn.2225-319X.2014.08.13.

61. ElBardissi AW, Shekar P, Couper GS, Cohn LH. Minimally invasive aortic valve replacement in octogenarian, high-risk, transcatheter aortic valve implantation candidates. J Thorac Cardiovasc Surg. 2011;141(2):328–35. https://doi.org/10.1016/j.jtcvs.2010.08.056.
62. Santana O, Reyna J, Grana R, Buendia M, Lamas GA, Lamelas J. Outcomes of minimally invasive valve surgery versus standard sternotomy in obese patients undergoing isolated valve surgery. Ann Thorac Surg. 2011;91(2):406–10. https://doi.org/10.1016/j.athoracsur.2010.09.039.
63. Shrestha M, Krueger H, Umminger J, Koigeldiyev N, Beckmann E, Haverich A, Martens A. Minimally invasive valve sparing aortic root replacement (Davidprocedure) is safe. Ann Cardiothorac Surg. 2015;4(2):148–53. https://doi.org/10.3978/j.issn.2225-319X.2014.08.04.
64. Vola M, Campisi S, Gerbay A, Fuzellier JF, Ayari I, Favre JP, Faure M, Morel J, Anselmi A. Sutureless prostheses and less invasive aortic valve replacement: just an issue of clamping time? Ann Thorac Surg. 2015;99(5):1518–23. https://doi.org/10.1016/j.athoracsur.2014.12.072.
65. Cohn LH, Adams DH, Couper GS, et al. Minimally invasive cardiac valve surgery improuves patient satisfaction while reducing costs of cardiac valve replacement. Ann Surg. 1997;226(4):421–6. discussion 427–428.
66. Ghanta RK, Lapar DJ, Kern JA, Kron IL, Speir AM, Fonner E Jr, Quader M, Ailawadi G, et al. Minimally invasive aortic valve replacement provides equivalent outcomes and reduced cost compared with conventional aortic valve replacement: A real world multi-istitutional analysis. J Thorac Cardiovasc Surg. 2015;149(4):1060–5. https://doi.org/10.1016/j.jtcvs.2015.01.014.
67. Hassan M, Miao Y, Maraey A, Lincoln J, Brown S, Windsor J, Ricci M. Minimally invasive aortic valve replacement: cost-benefit analysis of ministernotomy versus minithoracotomy approach. J Heart Valve Dis. 2015;24(5):531–9.

18 Right Anterior Mini-Thoracotomy for Aortic Valve Replacement

Marco Solinas and Giacomo Bianchi

18.1 Clinical Background

Valvular heart disease epidemiology has been dramatically chanced over the past decades in developed nations, mainly due to the decreased prevalence of rheumatic heart disease. The rise in life expectancy along with chronic disease has been paralleled by an increased frequency of degenerative valve disease. In a population-based study from the National Heart and Blood Institute (NCBI) the overall prevalence in the USA is 2.5% with wide age-related variation from 0.7% in those aged 18–44 years to 13.3% in those over the age of 75 [1]. Since aortic valve replacement is the mainstay of degenerative aortic valve disease, the population undergoing treatment faces risks due to age and chronic health conditions. In the UK sixth National Adult Cardiac Surgical 2008 report, the mortality rate was 1.8% in nearly 5000 patients aged 60–70 years old operated in 2004–2008, while increased to 5.5% for 420 patients over the age of 85 who had isolated aortic valve surgery in the same time frame [2]. In a report from Society of Thoracic Surgeons National Database encompassing 108,687 patients in 10 years, risk adjusted mortality and stroke rate decreased progressively over the years, with a reduction of the overall mortality of 24%, and risk-adjusted mortality of 33%; as age-dependent function, mortality and stroke where low even in the 8th and 9th decade of life (2% and 2.5%, respectively), while still female patients experience a higher mortality compared to males [3]. At the time of these reports, the adoption rate of minimally invasive surgery was low and very limited data were available to assess the potential of this approach over the standard full sternotomy to treat isolated aortic valve disease. Historically, cardiac surgery was the last surgical discipline to adopt minimally invasive surgical techniques and some centers are still reluctant to embrace it. In order to avoid the postoperative respiratory dysfunction, chest instability, chronic

M. Solinas, M.D. (✉) • G. Bianchi, M.D., Ph.D.
Ospedale del Cuore—Fondazione Toscana "G. Monasterio", 54100 Massa, Italy
e-mail: marco.solinas@ftgm.it

K. Fattouch et al. (eds.), *Advances in Treatments for Aortic Valve and Root Diseases*, https://doi.org/10.1007/978-3-319-66483-5_18

pain and incidence of deep sternal wound infection associated with a median sternotomy, numerous alternative incisions were evaluated. In the late 1990's, the group from Cleveland Clinic fostered the adoption of right parasternal incision for aortic valve that necessitated resection of the third and fourth costal cartilages, burdened by many problems of the median sternotomy, e.g. chest wall instability, difficult conversion to midline approach and required transection of the right internal mammary artery [4]. Minimally invasive aortic valve surgery is now most commonly performed via a limited skin incision, with a partial upper sternotomy that extends into the third or fourth intercostal space (also known as a 'J'-sternotomy or reversed-L-shaped sternotomy) [5]. Right anterior thoracotomy (RAMT) for aortic valve replacement (AVR) was first reported by Rao et al. in 1993, but remained unadopted for many years [6] until modified into minimally invasive approach by Benetti et al. from Argentina with the report of two patients treated this way [7]; this approach was then popularized by the New York University Medical Centre surgeons since the late 1990s. In order to reduce the surgical trauma, to decrease the feared mediastinitis, sternal instability and wound infection, our group strongly encouraged the adoption of RAMT for isolated AVR. This approach came historically after a comprehensive and almost 10-years-long program of minimally invasive mitral valve surgery, from which we redeployed technical skill and technological instrumentation.

18.2 Patient Selection

18.2.1 RAMT as a Strategy for the "All Comers"?

Clinical evaluation of candidates for RAMT should start with a careful assessment of the morphological features of the chest. Since the surgical field is limited in RAMT, surgeons embracing this technique should select carefully the patients at the beginning and than, as the experience increases, move to a more liberal approach. Ideal candidate to start with is an ectomorph patient, with no chest wall abnormalities such as pectus excavatum, or previous rib fracture; patients with osteogenic disorders, i.e. osteogenesis imperfecta, should be avoided; known disease of the pleura or the lung, such as previous pleuritis, pleural calcifications or moderate-severe chronic obstructive pulmonary disease (COPD), should be considered relelative to absolute exclusion criteria at the beginning.

18.3 Imaging Tools

18.3.1 Chest X-Ray

Chest radiography is a simple yet informative tool for patients' evaluation at the beginning. In postero-anterior projection we evaluate, along with classical radiologic semeiology signs, the ascending aorta profile, calcifications of the aortic button, size of the intercostal spaces, pleural calcifications or adhesions, hilar congestion, diffuse lung disease or elevated hemidiaphragm; also ribs' abnormalities or severe deformations of the spine are evident. In lateral projection, we routinely assess the distance of the ascending aorta from the sternum, the height of the diaphragm and it is important to define the actual location of abnormalities seen at the postero-anterior view.

18.3.2 CT Scan

Computed tomography (CT scan) images are useful for preoperative planning of the surgical access. In a small series of patients, Ammar et al. found that using non-contrast CT images yield the same location of the aortic valve as found at operating table [8]. In our institution, we routinely use non-contrast 64-slice CT scan (Toshiba Aquilon ONE; Toshiba Medical System, Tokio, Japan) to evaluate the anatomic relationship between the intercostal spaces (ICS), sternum, ascending aorta and aortic valve. The patient lies on the CT scan bed with the arms resting along the body; after a deep breath, the volume is acquired. We have elaborated two CT-criteria to choose between RAMT and ministernotomy (MS): right lateral or completely retrosternal position of the ascending aorta at the level of pulmonary artery bifurcation (Fig. 18.1); a distance of the aorta from the skin at the same level above 10 cm; the retrosternal position and a deep thorax are considered unfavourable anatomic conditions for the RAMT approach (Fig. 18.2) [9]. Ascending aortic calcifications and aortic root calcifications, when found at the CT images represent a relative contraindication for RAMT, depending on their location and extension. Aortic root calcification is not considered a contraindication for RAMT, but it should be treated as a special condition: in this case sutured valves are less suitable, while sutureless valves are the ideal option [10, 11]. Three-dimensional reconstruction of non-contrast CT scan can easily visualize the morphology of calcified aortic valves,

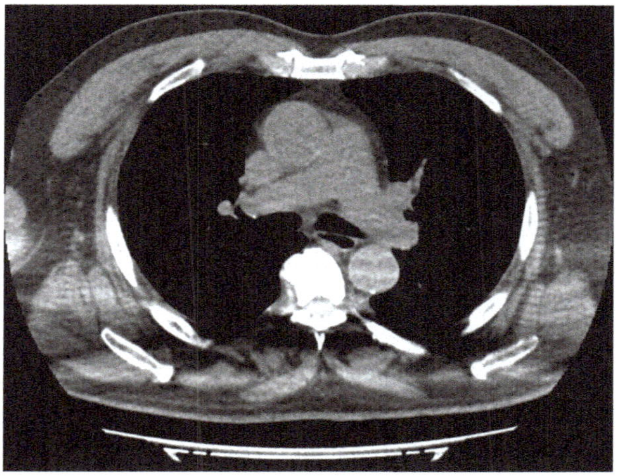

Fig. 18.1 Non contrast CT scan: rightward position of the ascending aorta at the level of pulmonary bifurcation. This anatomy is favourable for RAMT

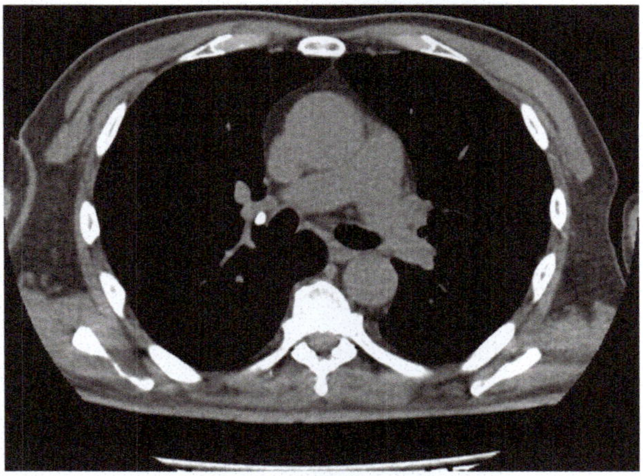

Fig. 18.2 Non contrast CT scan: the postion of the ascending aorta at the level of pulmonary artery bifurcation is completely behind the sternum; also a slight dilatation of the ascending aorta is noticeable. This anatomic conformation should not be favourable for RAMT approach

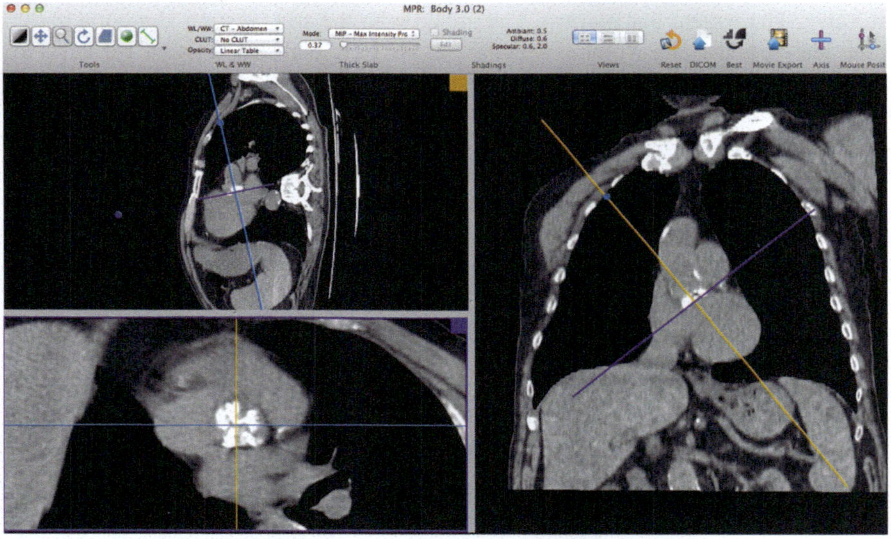

Fig. 18.3 Three-dimensional multi-planar reconstruction of tricuspid aortic valve

helping in differentiate tricuspid or bicuspid aortic valves; in Figs. 18.3 and 18.4, using 3D multi-planar reconstruction (MPR) of an open-source DICOM software (OsiriX—Pixmeo SARL), both degenerative aortic valve pathologies are illustrated. Bicuspid valve disease is not a contraindication for RAMT with sutured valves nor with sutureless; while in the first case is pretty straightforward to orientate the prosthetic valve, with sutureless valves (i.e. Livanova Perceval as the only one available on market at the time of writing) care must be taken when recreating the three nadirs that are positioned at approximatively 120 degrees; the surgeon could use commercially available sizers in order to recreate it [12]. If peripheral cannulation is

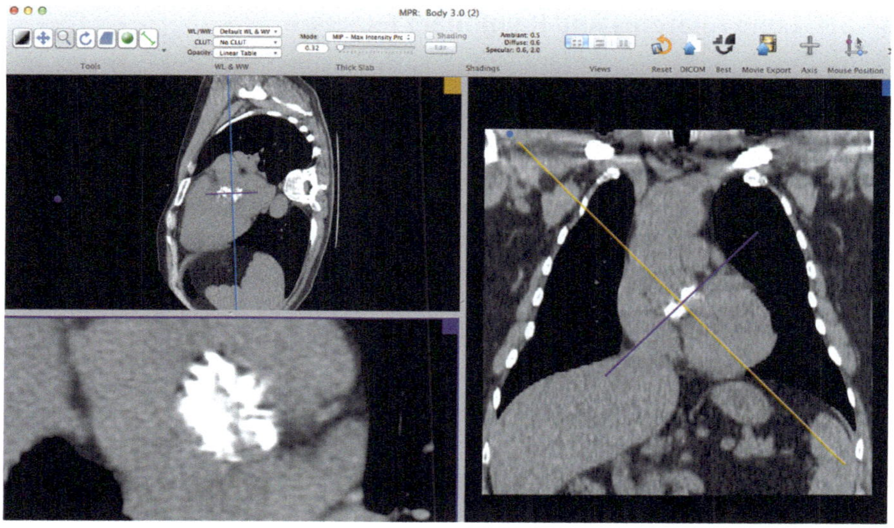

Fig. 18.4 Three-dimensional multi-planar reconstruction of a heavely calcified bicuspid aortic valve

anticipated, the CT can be extended through the entire aorta or a femoral arterial duplex may be obtained to elucidate the quality of the femoral vessels [13]. Although not routinely used in our center, with the advent of TAVI option, more patients with aortic stenosis undergo contrast-enhanced 3D CT scan, as part of the planning strategy. A proportion of them, after heart team discussion, could switch to RAMT treatment. The images can serve to estimate and predict preoperatively the size of the prosthesis, being especially true and useful in those case where sutureless valves are used [14]. Lung and pleural imaging are of utmost importance when planning an AVR through RAMT; CT scan can identify pleural adhesions, plaques, lung bullae, blebs and also lung parenchymal disease; all these features must be taken in account and not overlooked by the surgeon planning this strategy.

18.3.3 Echocardiography

Standard preoperative trans-thoracic echocardiogram is obtained for all patients, according to the current guidelines [15]. Evaluation for minimally invasive valve replacement is independent of the aortic pathology, although aortic valve stenosis is more prominent than aortic regurgitation. Echocardiography data useful for minimally invasive approach are, among others, LVOT diameter, aortic annulus, root and ascending aorta dimensions. This anatomical features are not directly related with the access, but with the aortic valve prosthesis planned for implantation; this aspect will be further discussed in the special section "sutured vs. rapid deployment vs. sutureless valve in RAMT".

18.3.4 Lung Anatomy and Pulmonary Function

In our center, RAMT approach is carried out without single lung ventilation; with mainly to avoid potential complications from lung reperfusion, atelectasis and laringo-tracheal traumatism as well. In case of severe chronic obstructive pulmonary disease (COPD), bollous emphysema, adhesions, pleural plaques or parenchymal disease, we consider these conditions as contraindication for RAMT. During the screening for an aortic patient as potential candidate for minimally invasive surgery, we recommend CT scan with lung window and pulmonary function tests, being known that pleural opening is associated with an early decrease in lung function, but with significant improvement after 3 months [16].

18.3.5 Concomitant CAD

Concomitant coronary artery disease is not considered an absolute contraindication in our center. If coronary lesions are more than 50% of the vessel lumen at angiography, but not critical and the patient did not experienced angina and has no documentation of ischemia at functional tests, the procedure could be carried on using the minimally invasive approach of choice, favoring the hybrid treatment [17].

18.4 Surgical Technique

18.4.1 Anesthesia and Patient Preparation

The procedure is performed in a standard operating room with each team member positioned according to existing protocols for conventional surgery. General anesthesia is provided according standard protocol for conventional aortic valve surgery. Cruent blood pressure monitoring is obtained through cannulation of radial artery; a standard 4-lumen IV catheter is placed in the right internal jugular vein and a percutaneous sheath (8.5 Fr) introducer is placed to secure an access for endocavitary pacemaker lead, if needed. After adequate plane of anesthesia is ensured, the patient is intubated with single lumen endotracheal tube and mechanical ventilation is started, according to standard protocol. Two defibrillator pads are placed across the chest wall with the right pad placed under the patients' right shoulder and left pad over the anterior left chest wall [18]. The patient is placed supine with arms along the flanks; differently from minimally invasive mitral valve surgery, for this procedure there is no need to tilt the patient leftward placing an inflatable balloon under the right shoulder. Then, Trans-Esophageal Echocardiography (TEE) is used for assessment of aortic valve and cardiac function, ventricular filling, aid for peripheral venous cannula insertion, de-airing manouver and for final result assessment. Afterward, the patient's skin is prepared with antiseptic solutions according to intraoperative protocol. Draping is accomplished with care to expose on the right side: superiorly the right clavicular edge, the pectoral muscle and laterally the right anterior axillary line, towards the right limb to expose the anterior superior iliac spine and the groin; on the left side the sternal notch is exposed and draping continues parallel to the left sternal edge, then laterally to include the anterior superior iliac spine and the groin. An adhesive aseptic strip is then applied to the exposed areas, thus, minimizing the possible risk of contamination.

18.4.2 Skin Incision and Soft Tissues Separation

The skin incision is extended parallel 1 cm from the sternal notch of the 2nd intercostal space for 5–6 cm. The subcutaneous tissue is divided with electrocautery towards the pectoralis major fascia that is incised (Fig. 18.5); careful spread of tissue allows respect for the muscle, less post-operative pain, ease of reconstruction and better functional recover. The intercostal muscle is then divided in the more lateral aspect; the surgeon ask for lung deflation and the pleural space is entered securely. An 8 × 10 cm gauze soaked in saline solution is placed between the lung and the chest, to allow ventilation during the next phase: right internal thoracic artery (RITA) pedicle isolation. In order to do so, the pedicle is isolated in a lateral-to-medial fashion, progressively; when identified, the endothoracic fascia is divided from underneath the vessel; the pedicle will appear mobile, but further mobilization could be accomplished detaching small intercostal branches (Fig. 18.6).

Then, a 10 cm silicon soft tissue retractor (Estech—Livanova) is placed ensuring complete isolation of the cavity from the skin and outer layers, minimizing the risk of contamination (Fig. 18.7). In our routine practice, once fully mobilized, the RITA pedicle can be displaced with the soft tissue retractor without any evident injury after the removal; at discretion of surgeon, it can be divided at the beginning of the procedure, if felt safer. I order to enhance direct vision, a surgical metallic multiuse retractor (Estech, San Ramon, CA, USA) is inserted and rib spreading is accomplished at clinical pace. Usually, surgical view is sufficient, but in special cases, as in patients with narrow intercostal spaces, 3rd rib disarticulation at costo-condral level could be an option not to overlook, especially at the beginning of the experience.

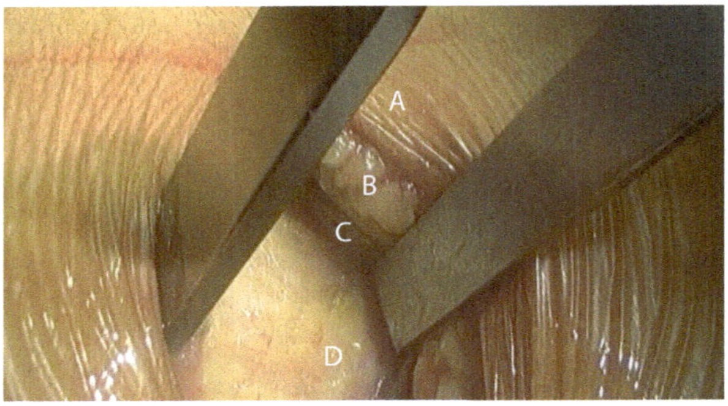

Fig. 18.5 Incision of the skin (*A*), subcutaneous layer (*B*) and pectoralis major (*C*); fat tissue covering the intercostal muscle is exposed (*D*)

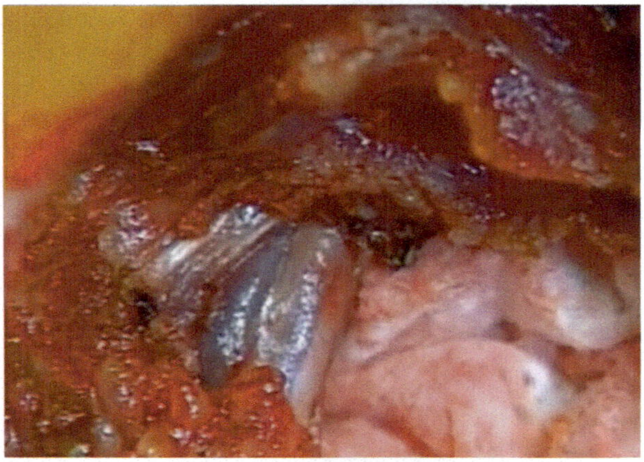

Fig. 18.6 Right internal thoracic artery pedicle exposed. The internal thoracic fascia is opened also below the pedicle to enhance mobilization

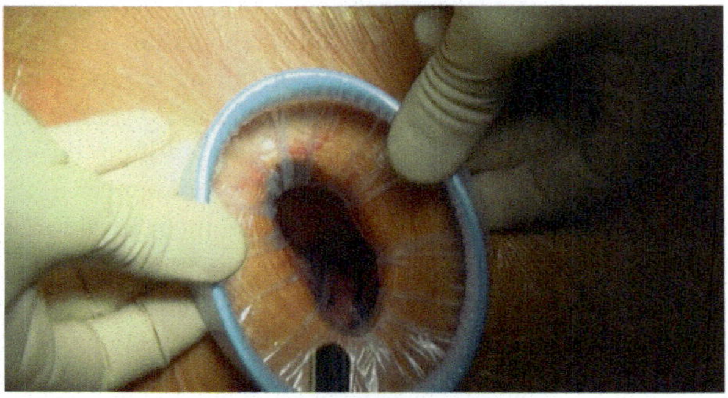

Fig. 18.7 Soft tissue retractor to enhance spreading and isolation of the surrounding tissue from the chest cavity

18.4.3 Pericardial Opening and Aorta Exposure

The pericardium along with ascending aorta bulging should be visible at this time; some mediastinal fat could be in the surgeon's view, but there is usually no need for extensive removal. The phrenic nerve course is identified and the fat/pericardial incision stars at the highest point; the pericardium is progressively opened cranially and caudally. At this point, 2/0 silk stay sutures are placed on the left side of the pericardium and, on the right side, one just above the inner reflection of the pericardium on the superior vena cava (SVC) and another near the brachiocefalic vein to SVC confluence. These stay sutures are gently retracted and the aorta is then displaced rightward to the surgeon's field. To enhance this displacement, the right stay sutures can be tunnellized to the anterior axillary line at the second intercostal space and tension secured with a small shod. The saline-soaked gauze can be removed now as the aforementioned manouvers create a tent that isolates the right lung, so bilateral lung ventilation can continue without interfering with the surgeon's work. The patient's pressure is lowered to 80 mmHg to ensure safer manipulation of the ascending aorta. With a small peanut, the pericardial reflection on the great vessels is opened, allowing more room for aortic cannulation site. A double non-adsorbable 3/0 braided suture purse-string is made beyond the Brachiocefalic artery takeoff. At this point heparin is administered and the operation continues with the preparation of the groin.

18.4.4 Percutaneous Venous Cannulation Technique

Femoral vein is percutaneously cannulated with a 7 Fr sheath for later cardiopulmonary bypass. In our center this maneuver is done before skin incision and heparin administration in order to minimize bleeding in the event of femoral artery puncture. A 260 cm guidewire is placed through the venous introducer sheath and is advanced to the right atrium and over the superior cavo-atrial junction under visualization with the TEE probe adjusted to a bicaval view (90–120°). In this particular view, the superior vena cava (SVC) is on the right and IVC on your left as you view them; at the top of the screen near the probe is the interatrial septum and left atrium. With the guidewire held in place, the introducer sheath is removed. With a n°11 blade the puncture site is enlarged and progressive dilators passed to ensure adequate space for venous cannula insertion. It is then advanced into the femoral vein and its tip should be 3–4 cm beyond the superior cavo-atrial junction. The guidewire is slowly withdrawn while holding the cannula in place. The venous cannula sheath is then removed and de-airing accomplished by partially unclamping and expelling blood and any residual air from the lumen before connecting to the venous line of the CPB circuit (Fig. 18.8). One silk stay suture is placed on the skin as a tourniquet over the cannula body to fix it in place and prevent dislodgement. This tourniquet may be easily released and refixed if we need to adjust (push or pull) the cannula

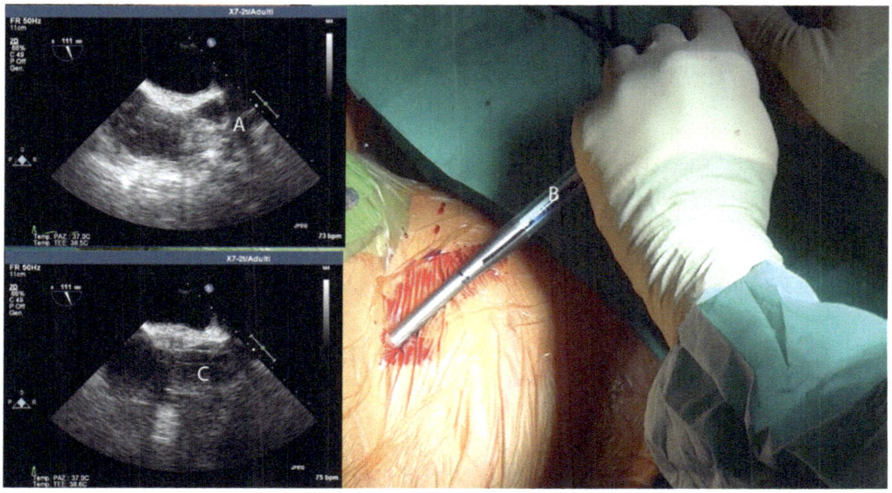

Fig. 18.8 Percutaneous femoral vein cannulation. Using Seldinger's technique (*A*: guidewire at superior cavo-atrial junction) the tip of the cannula is advanced towards the superior vena cava; the shaft is retracted (*B*) and the cannula is further advanced to allow concomitant optimal drainage of SVC and IVC (*C*)

during the procedure. The choice of venous cannula gauge is based on patients' weight and surgeons' preference; in our Institution we use a range of 22–25 Fr depending on patient's specific nomogram; rarely 19 Fr is used for small patients. Our cannula of choice is the Medtronic Biomedicus multistage cannula (Medtronic, Minneapolis, MN, USA).

18.4.5 Aortic Cannulation

Direct aortic cannulation is accomplished using an Estech Easyflow cannula (Estech, San Ramon, CA, USA) or Medtronic EOPA cannula (Medtronic, Minneapolis, MN, USA). In the first case, the aortic adventitia is opened progressively with a n°11 blade until intimal layer is exposed; at that point a small incision is made and the cannula is inserted. The Easy Flow cannula has an obturator the allows stiffening during insertion and after its removal the cannula is very pliable; also a stop ring is available to control the depth of aortic cannulation, that we set at the marker nearest the tip. When EOPA cannula is used, it is inserted using Seldinger's technique under TEE monitoring, proceeding as following: the anesthesiology is asked to visualize the descending thoracic aorta; then the center of the double purse string is punctured and a guide-wire is inserted and visualized at TEE; progressive dilatation is accomplished and then the EOPA cannula is inserted. In either way the antegrade aortic cannulation is made, the double purse strings are tightened, secured with n°2 Silk suture, the aortic cannula de-aired and connected with the arterial line of the CPB. When activated clotting time (ACT) is above 450 s, the CPB is started and lungs deflated.

18.4.6 Procedure

After CPB initiation, venous drainage is achieved with vacuum assistance set at −40 mmHg and the patient is cooled down to 34 or 35 °C if a sutureless or rapid deployment prosthesis is expected to be implanted. The right superior pulmonary vein is exposed and ventricular venting line is inserted and secured over a pledgeted 3/0 braided suture. With the electrocautery, the aorta is divided from pulmonary artery and an umbilical tape is passed around the aorta to ensure the highest clamping zone and secure total encircling within the clamp's jaws. A combined Y-shape cardioplegia/aortic vent catheter is placed into the ascending aorta, and cardioplegia lines are connected in the usual manner. The aorta is then clamped and antegrade cardioplegia is administered. The Fig. 18.9 illustrates the surgeon's view of the field at the time of aortic cross-clamp. Cardioplegic solutions are at discretion of the surgeon and according to the institutional standards of procedure; in our center we routinely use warm blood antegrade cardioplegia or cold crystalloid cardioplegia (HTK Custodiol, Koehler Chemie, Alsbach-Haenlein, Germany), depending of anticipated complexity of procedure; in most cases, and thanks to the advent of sutureless bioprosthesis, the time of a one or two shots of warm blood cardioplegia

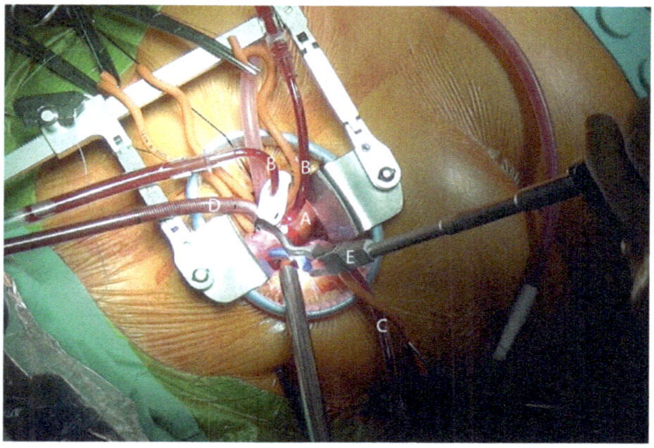

Fig. 18.9 Illustration of the surgical field: *A*, Ascending aorta; *B*, Aortic Vent and Cardioplegia line; *C*, Ventricular Vent through the right superior pulmonary vein; *D*, Arterial cannula; *E*, Aortic Clamp

are enough for the whole procedure. If RAMT is planned for severe aortic regurgitation, the aorta is cross-clamped and opened in normal fashion with active left ventricular suction to minimize blood flooding, while the heart is still beating. The coronary ostia are identified and cardioplegia is selectively infused with dedicated cannulae. Repeat cardiolegia can be avoided administering cold cristalloyd cardioplegia or, as in most of the cases, delivering additional selective shot of warm blood cardioplegia. After diastolic arrest of the hear and completion of cardioplegia delivery, the aortic root is emptied and left ventricle as weel. Aortotomy site and shape depends on the anticipated kind of prosthesis to be inserted. In case of conventional sutured prosthesis, the "S-shaped" towards the non coronary sinus incision is standard, but in case of sutureless valves e.g. Livanova Perceval we use a partial transverse aortotomy immediately below the aortic fat pad. Aortic valve removal and decalcification in case of severe degenerative disease is carried out in standard fashion. In case of sutured valve, the three commissural stitches are placed, the valve sized and implantation proceeds according to standard local operative protocol. Right anterior minithoracotomy approach could be eased by sutureless valve technology; for its characteristics of modularity, collapsibility and quick implantation, the Livanova Perceval S responds in full to this commitment. In this case we proceed as follows: after decalcification, three 4/0 Prolene sutures are placed at the nadir of each Valsalva sinus; the valve is sized according to manufacturer's protocol and prepared; the three prolene sutures are passed through the relative rings in the valve and it is deployed following the valve's specific procedure. Patient's rewarming is initiated, the left ventricular venting is reduced in order to fill the heart, de-airing maneuvers accomplished and aortotomy is closed in standard fashion with two running 4/0 Prolene sutures. The aortic cross clamp is removed and the heart is allowed to be systemically reperfused. After established a valid cardiac rhythm, the heart is filled, the de-airing carried out and TEE control of the surgical result made at half CPB support. For a brief period of time, the CPB is re-established completely allowing left ventricular venting along with aortic venting removal and subxyfoid chest tube tunnelization in the right pleura. The patient is progressively weaned from CPB and heparin reversal with protamine administered. Accurate hemostasis proceeds in standard fashion; the pericarium is closed with three interrupted stitches of 4/0 Prolene over the single chest tube; mediastinal fat can be also placed as cover in case of future surgery. The soft tissue retractor is removed and accurate hemostasis is provided to the intercostal muscle; the RITA pedicle is inspected for bleeding or hematoma; if it is the case, we recommend to divide it with vascular clips to minimize inapparent bleeding after the chest closure. The intercostal space is secured with two non adsorbable n°1 braided sutures in order to prevent the development of pneumocele. Reconstruction of the chest soft tissue layers proceeds following the local standards of operation.

18.5 Special Issues

18.5.1 Learning Curve of RAMT

Although theoretical and actual advantages of RAMT have been recognized, many surgeons are still reluctant to perform it; reasons could be multifactorial, including the lack of established training programmes, the perception that success is limited to more proficient surgeons and the fear of potential deleterious patient's outcome. Our group evaluated the learning curve of RAMT compared with standard AVR (SAVR) by the means of CUSUM method. Right anterior minithoracotomy (RAMT) group had less post-operative VAM, blood transfusion requirements, less incidence of atrial fibrillation; also ICU stay and overall hospital stay was lower than SAVR group. The analysis of the CUSUM curve revealed that even at the beginning of the RAMT program the complication rate was below the accepted failure; furthermore, no learning curve effect was observed [19]. Recently we analyzed the learning curve of RAMT approach using sutureless valve; six surgeons were analyzed: the program starter surgeon, who trained two other surgeons had a small initial learning curve; skill transfer was safe with a good preformance as shown by the CUSUM curves (Fig. 18.10). The other three surgeons were introduced to the sutureless technology (Perceval S—LivaNova, London, UK) later on, when the institutional experience was more consistent: this resulted in a lack of learning curve from a "transmitted learning" effect [20].

18.5.2 Sutured Vs. Rapid Deployment Vs. Sutureless Valve in RAMT

Conventional AVR with sutured prosthesis, based on the extraordianry short- and long-term outcomes, is the gold standard for the treatment of severe symptomatic aortic stenosis; nevertheless their use in RAMT can be cumbersome: valve exposure, decalcification and stitches placement (especially the right coronary Sinus of Valsalva) can be difficult due to the angle formed between the surgeon, the thoracotomy and the annular structures of the aortic root. This could potentially

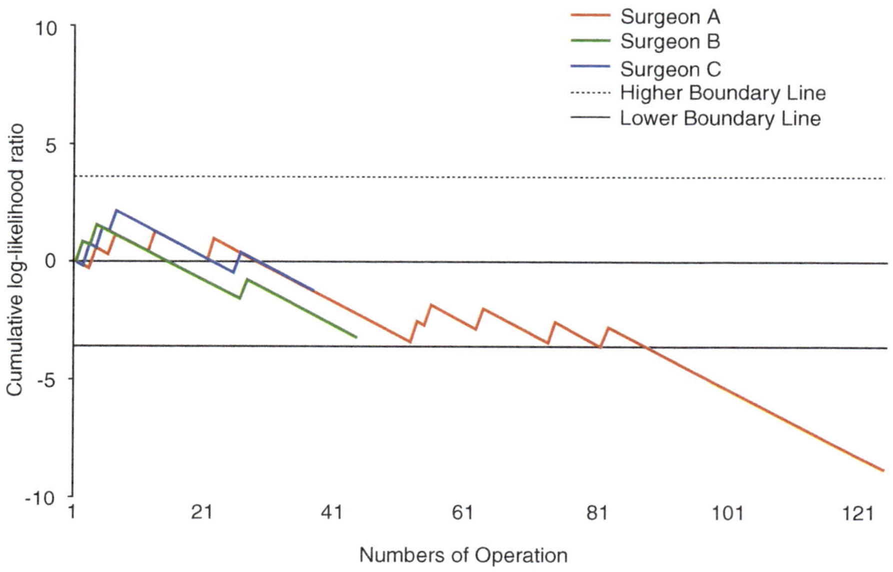

Fig. 18.10 Individual CUSUM curves for device success end point for surgeons A, B, and C. The acceptable failure rate was set at 5%. (Reprinted with permission from Murzi et al. J Thorac Cardiovasc Surg. 2016; https://doi.org/10.1016/j.jtcvs.2016.04.094.)

eliminates all the benefits of the minimally invasive surgery as reduction of cross clamp time, CPB time and overall surgical time. Recent technological developments have led to an alternative to conventional bioprostheses, which avoids the placement and tying of sutures, i.e. the "sutureless" and the rapid deployment aortic valves. Currently there are two commercially available prostheses, since the 3F Enable (Medtronic, Minneapolis, USA) is no longer available, i.e. Perceval S (LivaNova PLC, London, UK) and Intuity Elite (Edward Lifesciences, Irvine, USA). The first prosthesis utilizes a nitinol core that allows the valve to be collapsed and deployed even in small surgical access; after deployment, the nitinol radial force holds the valve in place with no need of sutures for the Perceval S. The Intuity elite operates on a different mechanism based on a balloon-expandable stainless steel and cloth-covered frame which is implanted with the aid of a balloon catheter delivery system and expands the frame within the appropriate annular position. Three sutures are required in the case of the Edwards Intuity valve. The MIAVR have shown to produce similar outcomes of the conventional AVR, but with some important improvements, such as decreased hospitalization, reduction in sternal wound complications, reduced surgical trauma and improved cosmesis [21]. However, the minimally invasive approach is not generally adopted, since is more technically demanding, with a different learning curve compared to standard AVR, and initially reported longer cross clamping and CPB time. Recent meta-analysis of MIAVR with standard bioprostheses have demonstrated such conclusions along with no clear survival advantage or marked reduction of major complications of MIVAR compared to standard

AVR [22, 23, 24]. The advent of sutureless or rapid deployment AVR (SU-RD AVR), led to a reduction in cross-clamp time and CPB duration as reported in a recent meta-analysis by the International Valvular Surgery Study Group (IVSSG): from 12 observational reports, the pooled cross-clamp tome and CPB duration for isolated AVR were 56.7 and 33 min, respectively, half of that reported by the Society of Thoracic Surgeons (STS) National Database for isolated conventional AVR [22]. As alternative to the conventional bioprosthesis, sutureless and rapid deployment valves demonstrated excellent hemodynamic performances. In a recent randomized trial, the Edwards Intuity showed significantly lower mean transvalvular gradient (8.5 vs. 10.3 mmHg) and lower PPM (0% vs. 15%) over the conventional bioprosthesis [25]. The PPM occurrence is associated with failure to symptoms regression, lesser left ventricular remodeling and reduced event-free late survival [26, 27]; its incidence is higher in patients with smaller annulus, obese, elderly females [28]. In a recent report from Hannover group, sutureless valves demonstrated a greater effective orefice area (EOA) for any given size and lower gradients at follow-up when compared to conventional AVR in a geriatric population (≥75 years) with small aortic annulus [29]. Furthermore, paravalvular leaks (PVL) occurrence is reduced when compared to TAVI technology: in a recent papers [30], the PVL can occur in TAVI up to 12%, while for sutureless and rapid deployment valves the pooled rate was 2–4%; the study also showed that paravalvular leak complications appeared to be a function of the SU-AVR learning curve, with significant reduction over time [24].

References

1. Nkomo VT, et al. Burden of valvular heart diseases: a population-based study. Lancet. 2006;368:1005–11.
2. Casula RP. Minimal access aortic valve surgery. In: Inderbitzi, editor. Minimally invasive thoracic and cardiac surgery. Berlin: Springer; 2012.
3. Brown JM, et al. Isolated aortic valve replacement in north america comprising 108,687 patients in 10 years: changes in risks, valve types, and outcomes in the society of thoracic surgeons national database. J Thorac Cardiovasc Surg. 2009;137:82–90.
4. Cosgrove DM 3rd, Sabik JF, Navia JL. Minimally invasive valve operations. Ann Thorac Surg. 1998;65:1535–1538.; discussion 1538–9.
5. Svensson LG, D'Agostino RS. "j" incision minimal-access valve operations. Ann Thorac Surg. 1998;66:1110–2.
6. Rao PN, Kumar AS. Aortic valve replacement through right thoracotomy. Tex Heart Inst J. 1993;20:307–8.
7. Benetti FJ, Mariani MA, Rizzardi JL, Benetti I. Minimally invasive aortic valve replacement. J Thorac Cardiovasc Surg. 1997;113:806–7.
8. Ammar R, Porat E, Eisenberg DS, Uretzky G. Utility of spiral ct in minimally invasive approach for aortic valve replacement. Eur J Cardiothorac Surg. 1998;14(Suppl 1):S130–3.
9. Gilmanov D, et al. Minimally invasive aortic valve replacement: 12-year single center experience. Ann Cardiothorac Surg. 2015;4:160–9.
10. Concistrè G, Farneti P, Miceli A, Glauber M. Sutureless aortic bioprosthesis in severe aortic root calcification: an innovative approach. Interact Cardiovasc Thorac Surg. 2012;14:670–2.
11. Lio A, Scafuri A, Nicolò F, Chiariello L. Valve replacement with a sutureless aortic prosthesis in a patient with concomitant mitral valve disease and severe aortic root calcification. Tex Heart Inst J. 2016;43:186–8.

12. Nguyen A, et al. Sutureless aortic valve replacement in patients who have bicuspid aortic valve. J Thorac Cardiovasc Surg. 2015;150:851–7.
13. Loor G, Roselli EE. Imaging and minimally invasive aortic valve replacement. Ann Cardiothorac Surg. 2015;4:62–6.
14. Margaryan R, et al. Sutureless aortic valve prosthesis sizing: estimation and prediction using multidetector-row computed tomography. Innovations (Phila). 2015;10:230–5. discussion 235.
15. Wharton G, et al. A minimum dataset for a standard adult transthoracic echocardiogram: a guideline protocol from the british society of echocardiography. Echo Res Pract. 2015;2:G9–G24.
16. Stoliński J, et al. Respiratory system function in patients after aortic valve replacement through right anterior minithoracotomy. Thorac Cardiovasc Surg. 2016;65(3):182–90.
17. Gilmanov DS, et al. Hybrid treatment for aortic stenosis and cad: minimally invasive sutureless aortic valve replacement and delayed pci. In: 10th International Congress of Update in Cardiology and Cardiovascular Surgery; 2014. p. S61.
18. Saroul C, Keller G, Benaissa M, Lehot JJ. Anesthesia for minimally invasive cardiac procedure. Ann Fr Anesth Reanim. 2011;30(Suppl 1):S38–43.
19. Murzi M, et al. Traversing the learning curve in minimally invasive heart valve surgery: a cumulative analysis of an individual surgeon's experience with a right minithoracotomy approach for aortic valve replacement. Eur J Cardiothorac Surg. 2012;41:1242–6.
20. Murzi M, et al. Exploring the learning curve for minimally invasive sutureless aortic valve replacement. J Thorac Cardiovasc Surg. 2016;152(6):1537–1546.e1.
21. Brown ML, McKellar SH, Sundt TM, Schaff HV. Ministernotomy versus conventional sternotomy for aortic valve replacement: a systematic review and meta-analysis. J Thorac Cardiovasc Surg. 2009;137:670–679.e5.
22. Phan K, Xie A, Di Eusanio M, Yan TD. A meta-analysis of minimally invasive versus conventional sternotomy for aortic valve replacement. Ann Thorac Surg. 2014;98:1499–511.
23. Lim JY, et al. Conventional versus minimally invasive aortic valve replacement: pooled analysis of propensity-matched data. J Card Surg. 2015;30:125–34.
24. Phan K, Zhou JJ, Niranjan N, Di Eusanio M, Yan TD. Minimally invasive reoperative aortic valve replacement: a systematic review and meta-analysis. Ann Cardiothorac Surg. 2015;4:15–25.
25. Borger MA, et al. A randomized multicenter trial of minimally invasive rapid deployment versus conventional full sternotomy aortic valve replacement. Ann Thorac Surg. 2015;99:17–25.
26. Pibarot P, Dumesnil JG. Prosthesis-patient mismatch: definition, clinical impact, and prevention. Heart. 2006;92:1022–9.
27. Head SJ, et al. The impact of prosthesis-patient mismatch on long-term survival after aortic valve replacement: a systematic review and meta-analysis of 34 observational studies comprising 27 186 patients with 133 141 patient-years. Eur Heart J. 2012;33:1518–29.
28. Wilbring M, Alexiou K, Schumann E, Matschke K, Tugtekin SM. Isolated aortic valve replacement in patients with small aortic annulus-a high-risk group on long-term follow-up. Thorac Cardiovasc Surg. 2013;61:379–85.
29. Shrestha M, et al. Aortic valve replacement in geriatric patients with small aortic roots: are sutureless valves the future? Interact Cardiovasc Thorac Surg. 2013;17:778–82. discussion 782.
30. Athappan G, et al. Incidence, predictors, and outcomes of aortic regurgitation after transcatheter aortic valve replacement: meta-analysis and systematic review of literature. J Am Coll Cardiol. 2013;61:1585–95.

19 Totally Endoscopic Aortic Valve Replacement (TEAVR)

Marco Vola

19.1 Introduction

Modern treatment of Aortic valve stenosis is nowadays highly encouraged towards transcatheter valve replacement (TAVR) [1, 2]. Although several studies confirm the interest of this therapeutic option, before to routinely extend TAVR indications into younger intermediate and low risk patients, some issues should be addressed: in TAVR long term durability is not yet assessed. Second, a certain amount of mild paravalvular leakages (PVL) still persists, which has been recently proven to be an independent factor of higher mortality at multivariate analysis [3, 4]. Conductive blocks are still frequent [5], even if incidence is lower as compared with the first generation of prosthesis.

On the other hand, despite requiring a cardiopulmonary by-pass (CPB) and longer operative times when employing sutured valves, surgery of the aortic valve has evolved over the last two decades from full sternotomy to ministernotomy and minithoracotomy. Such minimally invasive approaches have shown to reduce the wall chest trauma, the post-operative ventilator usage [6] and blood transfusions [7]. The group of Leipzig showed even a tendency to a higher survival [6].

It is also known that a further degree of reduction of the wall chest trauma has been described in the field of coronary artery surgery (TECAB, per totally endoscopic coronary by-pass Graft) and atrial septal defect repair, and it has been associated to a higher early post-operative life quality [8, 9] as compared to open mini approaches.

It is thus logic to safely pursuit the effort in reducing the invasiveness of SAVR and to target the thoracoscopic approach: in this way the aortotomy of the ascending aorta, the aortic valve ablation, valve sizing, prosthesis delivery and ascending aorta

M. Vola, M.D., Ph.D.
Adult Cardiac Surgery Unit, University Hospital of Lyon, Boulevard Pinel, Bron, France
e-mail: marc.vola@chu-lyon.fr

K. Fattouch et al. (eds.), *Advances in Treatments for Aortic Valve and Root Diseases*, https://doi.org/10.1007/978-3-319-66483-5_19

closure have to be performed by the exclusive guidance of endoscopic images. Only a few micro incisions admitting the insertion of the endoscopic instruments, of the valvular prosthesis, and of the camera are performed in the chest with no costal spreading.

The first human totally endoscopic aortic valve replacement has been performed and published in 2014 [10]. The technique acronym has been defined as TEAVR (totally endoscopic aortic valve replacement). TEAVR, as compared with other minimally invasive techniques, should be a further step in maximizing the potential of the early post-operative comfort and life quality, while continuing to provide a radical therapy as surgery is, with the potential advantages of the complete ablation of the diseased valvular tissue [11].

19.2 Description of the Technique

TEAVR can be achieved with use of sutureless (SU) valves [12]. Such prosthesis are pericardial bioprostheses mounted into an expandable metallic stent; the anchoring mechanism into the native annulus is guaranteed exclusively by the radial force of the stent. In that way stitches and knots are avoided, resulting in a major simplification of any minimally invasive approach [13, 14]. Moreover, two models of SU valve allow a compression of the stent that is a key element in reducing the global diameter of the prosthesis. In that way, the prosthesis can be inserted into a micro incision (20 mm) through the thoracic wall, and without any costal divarication. These prostheses are the Medtronic Enable (Medtronic, Minneapolis, MIN., Fig. 19.1, left), and the Livanova Perceval (Livanova, London, UK, Fig. 19.1, right).

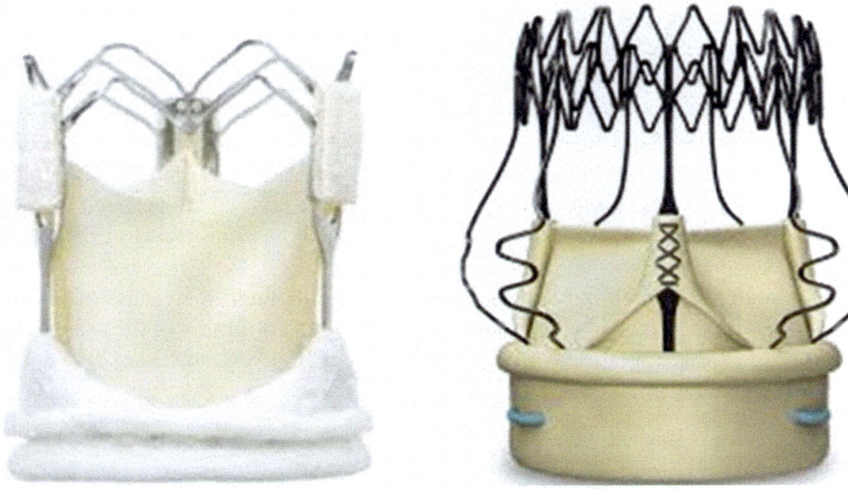

Fig. 19.1 Nitinol stented and compressible SU bioprostheses: *left*: The Medtronic Enable (Medtronic, Minneapolis). *Right*: the Livanova Perceval (Livanova, London, UK)

We used the Enable valve along the feasibility cohort of TEAVR [15], but this prosthesis was withdrawn from the marked in 2015, and we are now continuing the experience with use of the Perceval prosthesis, which is simpler in the sequence of delivery.

19.3 Patient Selection

Anatomical criteria: A preoperative CT scan is performed in all patients in order to check the permeability of the iliac and femoral arteries in view of a femoro-femoral cardiopulmonary bypass (CPB). A 3D reconstruction of the costal grill (Fig. 19.2) and of the thorax cutaneous plan (Fig. 19.3) is performed in each patient in order to plan the ideal site of penetration of surgical trocars.

The patient is selected according to the anatomical criteria on chest computed tomography previously followed in 2014 [10]: periaortic working space (distance between the inferior margin of the sternum and the aortic anterior wall) >2 cm, and

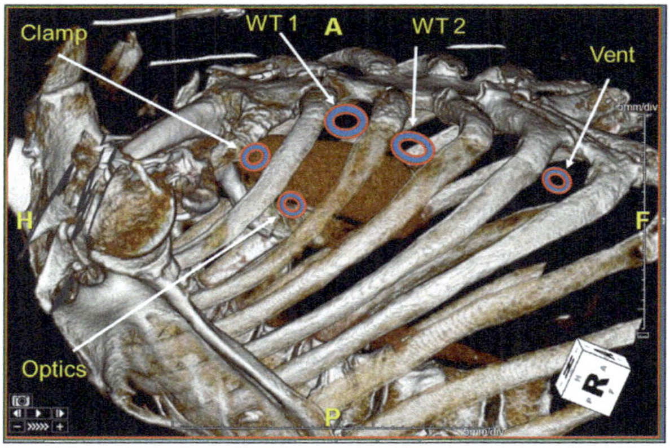

Fig. 19.2 3D reconstruction of the costal grill

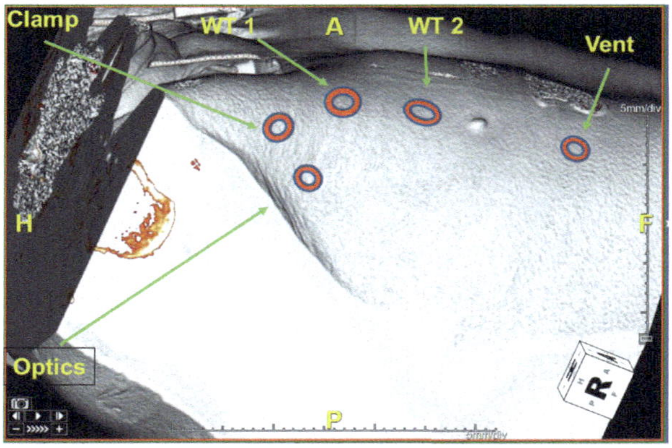

Fig. 19.3 Superficial volume rendering and trocar war map with a projection over the skin of the sites of the incisions

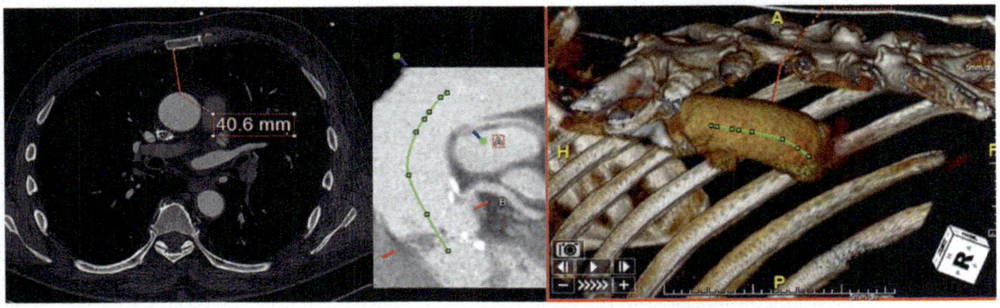

Fig. 19.4 CT scan anatomical criteria for patient election to TEAVR. *Left*: distance between the sternum and the anterior margin of the ascending aorta has to be minimum of 20 mm. *Middle and right* (3D reconstruction): the central line of the intrapericardial ascending aorta has to be measured at least of 5 cm

length of the intrapericardial ascending aorta >5 cm (Fig. 19.4). Heavily calcifications of the ascending aorta are a formal contraindication to this approach. All these aforementioned criteria have to be respected in order to select patients for whom the ascending aorta running suture can be easily performed in the endoscopic setting. It has to be considered that during TEAVR the aortotomy should be more vertical and right sided as compared with open surgery, and that it is limited superiorly by the aortic transcutaneous clamp and inferiorly by the Ninitol stent of the SU valve. This is why short ascending aortas may be problematic.

Other criteria: since TEAVR requires, in the actual state of development of the procedure, longer cross clamp and CPB times as compared with open approaches, patients that well tolerate such operative durations (usually intermediate and low risk), with a non-compromised left ventricle contractility and no renal impairment, should be preferred. Moreover, these patients, usually younger and active, not only are supposed to better overcome this surgical procedure, but also to profit in the every-day activities of the non-aggression of the thoracic wall, since they still have an active life style. The rapid restitution to car driving and professional activities is likely to have, in this subset, an economic impact.

19.4 Surgical Setting

The operation is performed under general anesthesia and with use of a transesophageal echocardiography. This echographic monitoring is mandatory to assess the proper positioning of the guidewires inserted with a Seldinger technique into the common femoral vessels (short horizontal surgical access in our experience, but possible in the next future with a percutaneous access) in the descending aorta and in the vena cava, since the ascension of the CPB cannulas, arterial and venous, is performed over those wires.

Several thoracic micro incisions are necessary to manage the TEAVR procedure: The intervention is performed with selective lung ventilation. Two working trocars (Flaxipath, Ethicon, Fig. Inc., Somerville, NJ) of 20 mm diameter (main) and

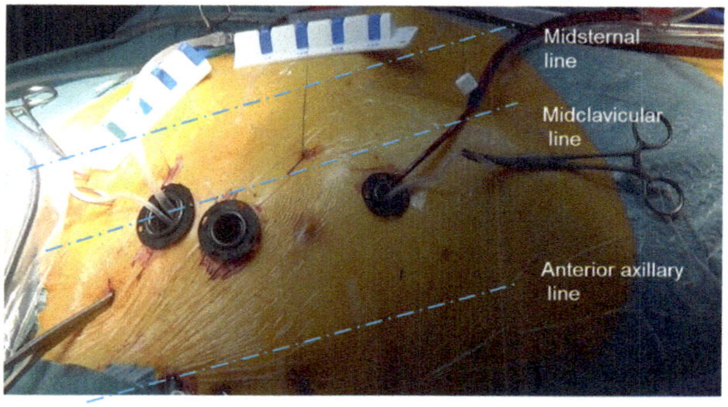

Fig. 19.5 Trocar disposition in the operative field

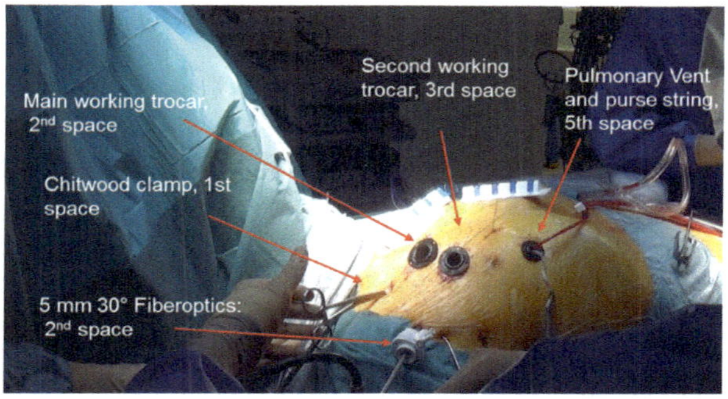

Fig. 19.6 Trocar disposition in the operative field

15 mm diameter (secondary) are positioned in the second and third right intercostal spaces (Fig. 19.5) respectively, between the midclavicular and the anterior axillary line. The main working port has to be inserted in the axis of the aortic root in order to allow the insertion of the holder of the SU valve and of the surgical instruments (see image reconstruction at the CT scan) as aligned as possible with the root. The position of this trocar is thus critical. In theory, the camera (5 mm, 30°) and the second working port can have alternative positions (e.g., the camera could be medial as compared to the main working port; the second working port could be more median or lateral depending on the dimensions and curvature of the ascending aorta). A 7 mm trocar is inserted in the fifth intercostal space to host a venting line (16 French, DLP 12001, Medtronic, Minneapolis, Min.), the purse string and tourniquet, and a carbon dioxide line (Fig. 19.6).

The following operative steps are: deflation of the right lung, partial right thymectomy (to enhance the working space), opening of the pericardium anteriorly to the phrenic nerve, transcutaneous suspension of its merges by four prolene 4/0 stitches, and start of the femoro-femoral CPB. Once the heart cavities decompressed by the active venous drainage, it is possible to prepare a U-double patched purse string (prolene 4/0, 16 mm needle) at the right inferior pulmonary vein, for the vent. After aortic cross clamping (transcutaneous Chitwood clamp, first intercostal space), cardioplegia is delivered directly into the aortic root (histidine- tryptophan ketoglutarate cardioplegic solution; Kohler Chemie, Alsbach-Hahnlein, Germany).

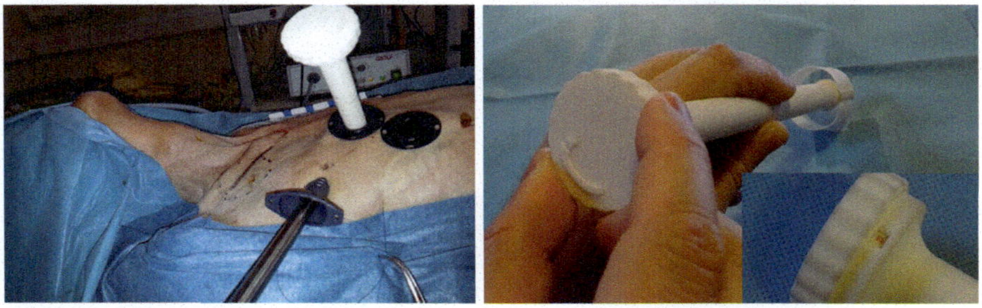

Fig. 19.7 Vola's calibrator prototype in a cadaveric study. The calibrator is inserted through the main working trocar (*left*); expansion of the tape (*right top*) and external indication of the measured diameter (*right, bottom*)

Once the aortic calcified leaflets removed and the aortic annulus decalcified, sizing may be performed. In the first phase of our experience [15], we used to size the prosthesis pre operatively with a CT scan image-based method, similarly to TAVR procedures. Although we didn't register in these few cases any paravalvular leakage, it is our opinion that since the anatomy is changed by surgery with the ablation of the diseased tissues and annular calcium, the value of imaging in predicting the ideal SU prosthetic diameter is relative, because the native annulus without calcium acquires a variable degree of compliance. In that case, a physical and dynamic annular sizer, with or without a flexible shaft, able to go by its non-expanded configuration through a thoracic trocar or a very narrow port, and afterwards capable to expand into the decalcified aortic annulus, is the only safe solution for a reliable prosthesis size determination. This issue has been addressed conceiving a specific thoracoscopic annular calibrator for SU valves [16]. The device should be soon ready for human applications in 2018 (Vola expansible sizer, Fig. 19.7).

19.5 The Technique of Implantation of the Perceval Bioprosthesis

Once the native valve removed, three Prolene guiding sutures are inserted in the Nadir of each segment (non-coronary, left coronary, right coronary) of the native decalcified annulus, then extracted out of the thorax through the main trocar and symmetrically passed through the eyelets in the prosthetic flange of the collapsed prosthesis, as performed per the open technique.

Before insertion of the holder into the trocar, three tourniquets are used to keep the two arms of each guiding suture matched and to avoid twisting around the holder (Fig. 19.8) [17]. Once the prosthesis positioned at the level of the native annulus (Fig. 19.9, left), the correct orientation of the tourniquets and the prosthetic flange position is confirmed with the 5-mm camera, and the tourniquets are removed. The expansion of the Perceval valve is performed according to the standard technique, and checked with the camera upper (Fig. 19.9, right).

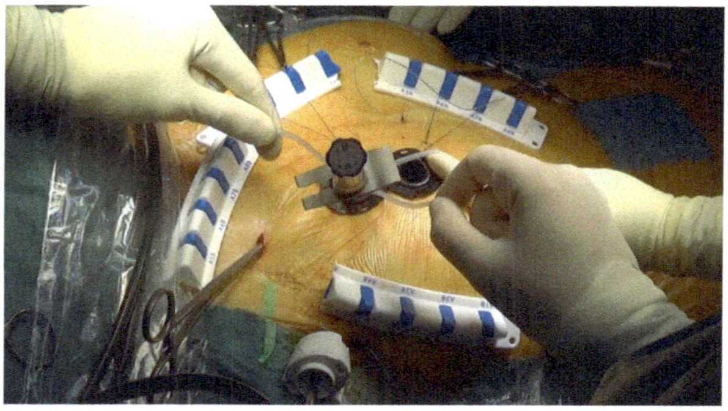

Fig. 19.8 Passage into the main working trocar of the collapsed Livanova Perceval. Note that the guiding sutures are included into plastic tourniquets

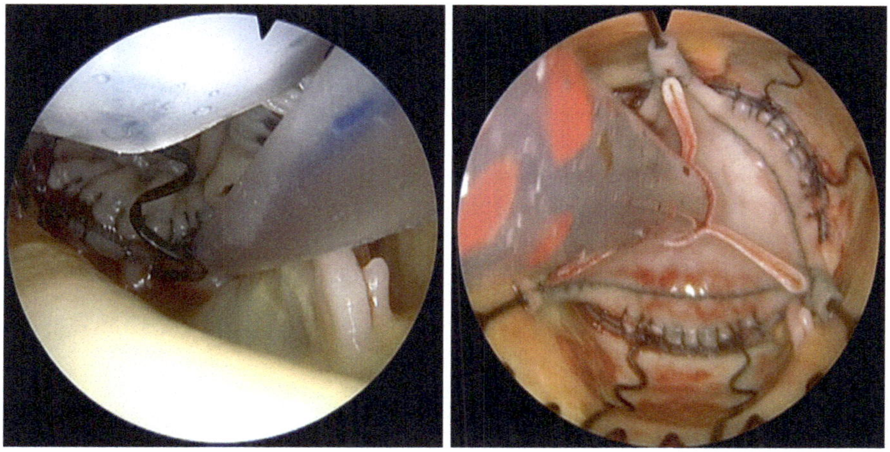

Fig. 19.9 *Left*: Endoscopic assessment of the correct position of the Perceval prosthesis into the native annulus. *Right*: correct deployment of the prosthesis and coaptation test by vacuum induction into the LV by insertion of a sucker cannula through the leaflets

De airing is then performed under TEE, monitoring the micro bubbles into left cavities and their progressive dispersion before to enable the complete physiological ejection.

19.6 Results

The actual TEAVR experience is limited in numbers, since patients are still strongly selected according to the aforementioned criteria. We are waiting the achievement of some devices (e.g. endoscopic calibrator) that should allow extension of indications to a broader population. Meanwhile an Endoscopic AVR Collaborative Group has been founded, with a first objective to train several teams experienced in minimally invasive surgery to the practice of the SU video assisted AVR. This procedure

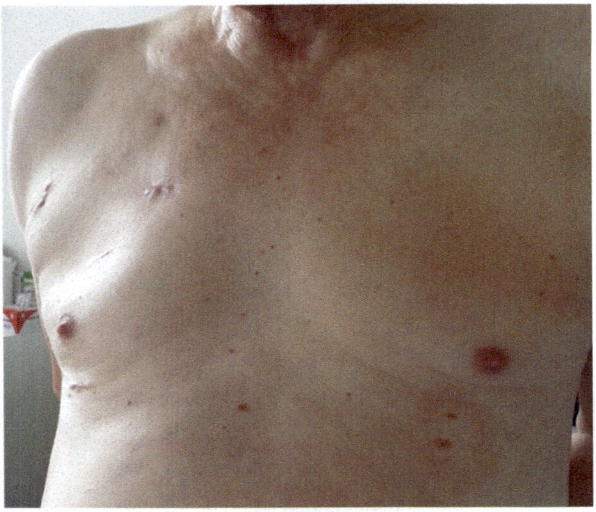

Fig. 19.10 Cosmetic aspect of TEAVR 3 months after the procedure

consists in SAVR using the endoscope guidance, but via an open limited minithoracotomy. This practice should prepare the Collaborative group teams to the switch towards the thoracoscopic setting [18].

At the state of the art we have performed more than 20 TEAVR procedures in intermediate and low risk patients, with no early mortality, no PVL, one pace-maker post-operative implant and a cross clamp time ranging between 84 and 145 min. In the Perceval subgroup as compared with the previous Enable experience, cross clamp times were lower (range 80–102 min). Life quality (SF-36) scores 1 month after the procedure was encouraging [15]. Finally the post procedural cosmetic aspect (Fig. 19.10) was scored very satisfactory by patients.

19.7 Actual Limits of Robotic TEAVR and Instrumental Perspectives: Beyond Scissors and Graspers?

Endoscopic surgery of the aortic valve has to face more narrow working spaces as compared to mitral endoscopic settings, so the triangulation between the operative instruments and the optics is more critical. After some cadaveric robotic essays with the Intuitive Si [19] model, in torsos where the aortic valve were non calcified, the aortic valve could be resected. Nevertheless, independently from the triangulation, the scissors and graspers movements inside the aortic root were possible but often problematic due to the lack of working space. In theory, in a clinical valvular and annular calcified setting, dedicated devices for surgical minimally invasive decalcification, able to cut rapidly the leaflets and simultaneously suction the debris, should be the most reliable solution for a realistic reproducibility of the technique. Robots could although play a major role in facilitating ascending aorta closure, but before to make conclusions several models (Intuitive Inc., VERB Surgical Inc., Covidien-Medtronic, Transenterix Surgical, Inc) should be tested in cadavers.

Sizing with conventional rigid sizers is a physical limit to use of trocars and to the practice of a thoracoscopic procedure. The problem should be overcome by the development of the aforementioned expandable sizers.

The most realist perspective seems then to set-up a Robotic TEAVR procedure mixing specific devices for tissue removal, annulus decalcification and sizing, SU valve as a prosthetic substitute, and articulated or robotic instruments for closing the aorta.

Disclosures Dr. Vola has been a proctor and performed lectures for Medtronic.

Bibliography

1. Zhou Y, et al. Transcatheter versus surgical aortic valve replacement in low to intermediate risk patients: a meta-analysis of randomized and observational studies. Int J Cardiol. 2017;228:723–8.
2. Praz F, et al. Latest evidence on transcatheter aortic valve implantation vs. surgical aortic valve replacement for the treatment of aortic stenosis in high and intermediate-risk patients. Curr Opin Cardiol. 2017;32(2):117–22.
3. Kodali S, et al. Paravalvular regurgitation after transcatheter aortic valve replacement with the Edwards sapien valve in the PARTNER trial: characterizing patients and impact on outcomes. Eur Heart J. 2015;36(7):449–56.
4. Maisano F, Taramasso M, Nietlispach F. Prognostic influence of paravalvular leak following TAVI: is aortic regurgitation an active incremental risk factor or just a mere indicator? Eur Heart J. 2015;36(7):413–5.
5. Nishiyama T, et al. Predictive factor and clinical consequence of left bundle-branch block after a transcatheter aortic valve implantation. Int J Cardiol. 2017;227:25–9.
6. Merk DR, et al. Minimal invasive aortic valve replacement surgery is associated with improved survival: a propensity-matched comparison. Eur J Cardiothorac Surg. 2014;47(1):11–7. discussion 17
7. Malaisrie SC, et al. Current era minimally invasive aortic valve replacement: techniques and practice. J Thorac Cardiovasc Surg. 2014;147(1):6–14.
8. Kopp M, et al. Psychomotor car-driving abilities after robotically assisted totally endoscopic coronary artery bypass grafting. Thorac Cardiovasc Surg. 2012;60(7):462–7.
9. Morgan JA, et al. Robotic techniques improve quality of life in patients undergoing atrial septal defect repair. Ann Thorac Surg. 2004;77(4):1328–33.
10. Vola M, et al. First human totally endoscopic aortic valve replacement: an early report. J Thorac Cardiovasc Surg. 2014;147(3):1091–3.
11. Vahidkhah K, et al. Valve thrombosis following transcatheter aortic valve replacement: significance of blood stasis on the leaflets. Eur J Cardiothorac Surg. 2017;51(5):927–35.
12. Karangelis D, et al. What is the role of sutureless aortic valves in today's armamentarium? Expert Rev Cardiovasc Ther. 2017;15(2):83–91.
13. Concistre G, et al. Sutureless aortic valve implantation through an upper v-type ministernotomy: an innovative approach in high-risk patients. Innovations (Phila). 2013;8(1):23–8.

14. Gilmanov D, et al. Perceval S sutureless aortic valve prosthesis implantation via a right anterior minithoracotomy. Multimed Man Cardiothorac Surg. 2013;2013:mmt012.
15. Vola M, et al. Closed chest human aortic valve removal and replacement: technical feasibility and one year follow-up. Int J Cardiol. 2016;211:71–8.
16. Vola M, et al. Proof of concept of an endoscopic sutureless valve sizer. Innovations (Phila). 2016;11(5):337–41.
17. Vola M, et al. First in human totally endoscopic perceval valve implantation. Ann Thorac Surg. 2016;102(4):e299–301.
18. Vola M, et al. Video-assisted minithoracotomy approach: technical developments towards totally endoscopic sutureless aortic valve replacement. J Card Surg. 2014;29(4):494–6.
19. Vola M, et al. Robotic total endoscopic sutureless aortic valve replacement: proof of concept for a future surgical setting. Int J Med Robot. 2015;12(3):370–4.

Sutureless Aortic Valve Implantation 20

Theodor Fischlein and Giuseppe Santarpino

It was recently reported an increase in the prevalence of patients with valvular heart disease eligible for aortic valve replacement (AVR) due to the increase in life expectancy of the general population [1]. However, the wide spectrum of patients with older age and comorbidities is associated with increased surgical risk and stimulated the development of minimally invasive aortic valve procedures that can reduce the mortality and morbidity risk even in elderly patients. Transcatheter aortic valve implantation (TAVI) procedures have been developed and extensively used in high-risk patients considered to be not eligible for standard surgery using cardiopulmonary bypass [2]. To the same extent, older patients pose significant challenge to modern cardiac surgery, even in the absence of specific high-risk features: in these patients less invasive procedures are desirable to achieve a reduction in the global risk profile and a better surgical outcome [3]. In this population, a patient-oriented assessment is usually performed since standardized guidelines on the use of a "minimally-invasive" approaches are not available, and there is substantial inter-center heterogeneity in the clinical implementation of this approach.

Since the introduction of the sutureless Perceval (Livanova Group, Saluggia, Italy, Fig. 20.1) in Europe after CE mark in 2012, the "sutureless approach" is becoming more and more popular. Sutureless implantation in general is easy, fast and safe.

Minimally invasive surgery for aortic valve replacement (AVR) has been demonstrated to be associated with positive outcomes [4] and has become an increasingly used option for managing patients with aortic stenosis, thus challenging the primacy

T. Fischlein
Paracelsus Medical University, Nuremberg, Germany

G. Santarpino (✉)
Paracelsus Medical University, Nuremberg, Germany

Città di Lecce Hospital, GVM Care and Research, Lecce, Italy
e-mail: g.santarpino@libero.it

K. Fattouch et al. (eds.), *Advances in Treatments for Aortic Valve and Root Diseases*, https://doi.org/10.1007/978-3-319-66483-5_20

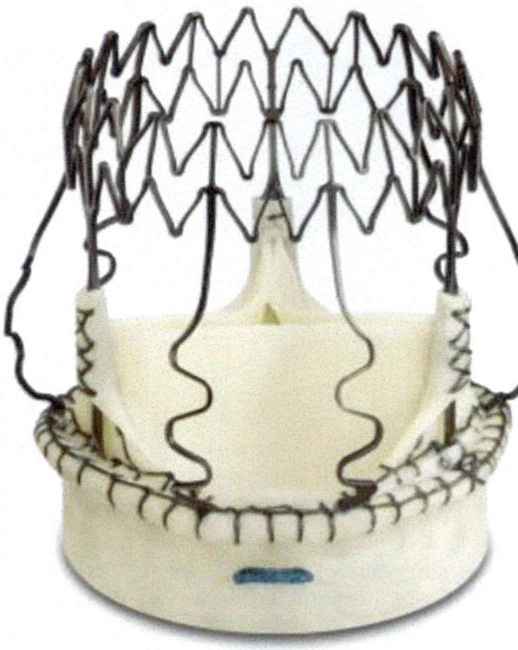

Fig. 20.1 Perceval sutureless bioprosthesis

of conventional open-heart AVR. With the development of sutureless aortic bioprostheses, the treatment of aortic valve disease has entered a new era through the use of a fast and safe implantation technique that makes minimally invasive procedures easier [5]. However, as with any new device, several decision-making and surgical problems have been reported, which may account for the occurrence of paravalvular leakage [6], device dislodgement or malpositioning requiring re-replacement [7], or for the high rates of pacemaker implantation [8].

20.1 Technical Implantation

The Perceval S aortic valve bioprosthesis (Sorin Group, Saluggia, Italy) requires a presurgical transthoracic and transesophageal echocardiography to check aortic root anatomical characteristics: the implant is in fact not recommended for bicuspid valves with asymmetrical sinuses of Valsalva, or in presence of enlarged aortic roots; available sizes allow treatment of patients with annulus up to 27 mm. For the minimal invasive surgery the patients need a intraoperatively monitoring with transesophageal echocardiography for the management of cardiopulmonary bypass and the evaluation of the prosthesis.

Under general anesthesia and orotracheal intubation, the patients undergoing AVR on cardiopulmonary bypass after partial "J" sternotomy at the third/fifth intercostal space (evaluated with chest X-ray in the presurgical screening) and minimal

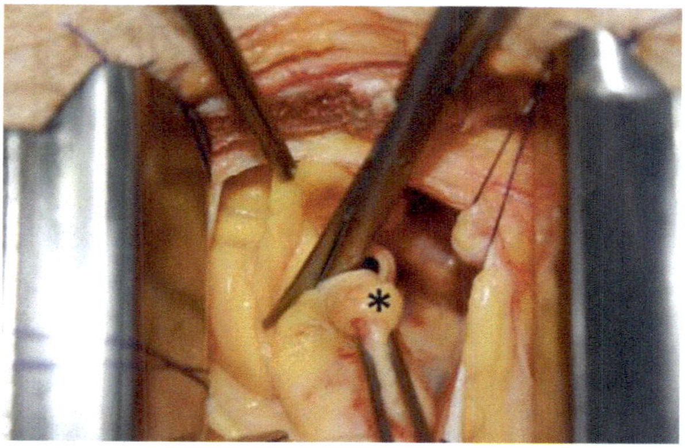

Fig. 20.2 Aortotomy and fat pad (*)

coetaneous incision (8–10 cm). Cardiopulmonary bypass was established using a straight arterial cannula in the ascending aorta or a two-stage venous cannula in the right atrial appendage (when possible) or femoral vein. The procedures were always performed during aortic cross-clamping with DeBakey or flexible or Glauber clamp and continuous infusion of cardioplegia (warm cardioplegia, Calafiore protocol) antegrade.

If a second infusion of cardioplegia was necessary, we cannulated directly the ostia and we infused the cardioplegia antegrade. The transverse aortotomy was localized in a higher position compared to an ordinary aortotomy for AVR: the reference point was the inferior margin of the "Concato preaortic rim" (fat pad), 3–4 cm from the aortic annulus (Fig. 20.2).

After excision of the diseased valve, the aortic annulus should be decalcified. After applying limited decalcification at the beginning, the technique in the meantime does not differ from the technique we apply during traditional AVR. This means meticulous removal of all, especially into the lumen reaching calcium, which might prevent sealing of the pericardial cloth to the annulus. Utmost care has to be taken, that the aorto mitral curtain remains intact. If it is injured, the Perceval will not—as will a traditional sutured valve—be able to cover this leak and prevent bleeding into the anterior mitral leaflet. If an injury is detected, we repair it with a running 5-0 Polypropylene suture, avoiding narrowing of the annulus. The presence of aortic root calcifications, which may render implantation of a traditional valve difficult, does not affect Perceval implantation. Quite the contrary is the case; it avoids manipulation of the calcific root, which is a risk factor for perioperative stroke. In endocarditic patients, we very often find involvement of the annulus and roots with abscesses or even perforations into structures that have to be patched. An intact annulus, especially located in the acoronary sinus at the aorto-mitral curtain is a condition sine qua non for Perceval implantation.

Sizers are provided as reusable tools from the company. We always pack them with the plate, which houses the collapsing device. Every sizer consists of a smaller, transparent and a larger, solid white phantom. They represent the lower and upper limits o the respective size. The transparent phantom of the larger size reflects the size of the

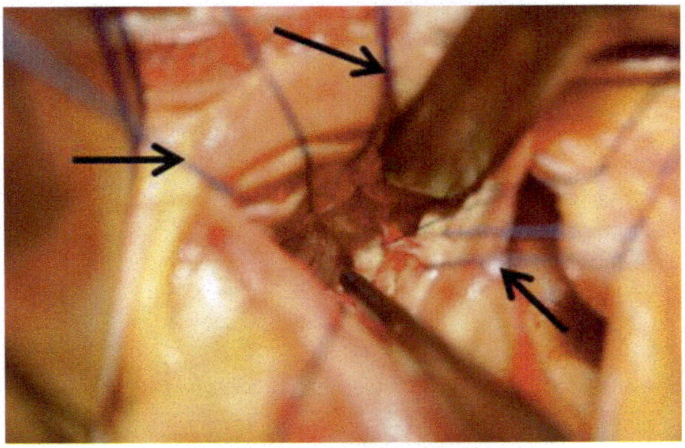

Fig. 20.3 Aortic annulus with guiding sutures (→)

white sizer from the next smaller size. Usually, we start with the smallest sizer available testing, whether the annular size of the patient is suited for Perceval implantation in general. Sizing is then repeated using the next larger phantom, until a solid colored sizer will no longer pass the annulus. The appropriate size of the prosthesis is established when the valve sizer end marked with a "V" passes easily through the aortic annulus into the left ventricle, and the one marked with a "X" remains stable above the aortic annulus. Sizing may be challenging in patients with narrow ST-junctions or high calcium load in the root. It has to be assured, that the sizer reaches the annulus. The resistance encountered may prevent a deeper introduction of the valve sizer towards where the annular diameter is larger, thus leading to an underestimation of its dimensions. Guiding sutures will help us to position the device at the exact level we want it to be. After defining the nadir of the respective sinus of valsalva, we place the suture (4–0 Polypropylene,) 1–2 mm below the annulus, across the annulus in a 90 ° angle—deep enough—and exit the aortal wall 1–2 mm above the annular line (Fig. 20.3).

This assures the following: The bite has to be big enough to hold the traction that we will apply during implantation of the device. Secondly, being at the right level below the annulus, it will be impossible to anchor the Perceval too low in the LVOT. Thirdly, before deployment of the device, we check, whether we see the exit point of the suture from the aortic wall. Since the upper pericardial curtain of the Perceval is about 2 mm thick, we assure exact seating of the valve prior to deployment.

After the lower needle of the guiding suture has been passed through the eyelets of the device, the stick with the loaded valve is guided down to the annular level. At this point, gentle traction is applied to the guiding sutures by the assistant to assure counter traction during positioning. During implantation, commissural stay sutures are released and left in place without applying traction. Before the actual deployment is carried out, exit points of the sutures are visualized. Care has to be taken, that the sutures are not tangled around the stent posts, which could interfere with the proper seating of the device. The three sutures are held firmly to guide the descent of the prosthesis with controlled traction perpendicular to the annular plane, parallel to the holder (Fig. 20.4). After this is assured for all three sutures, deployment is

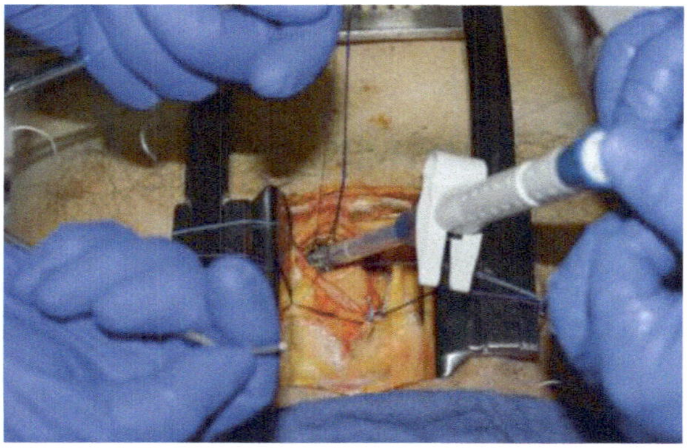

Fig. 20.4 Valve implantation

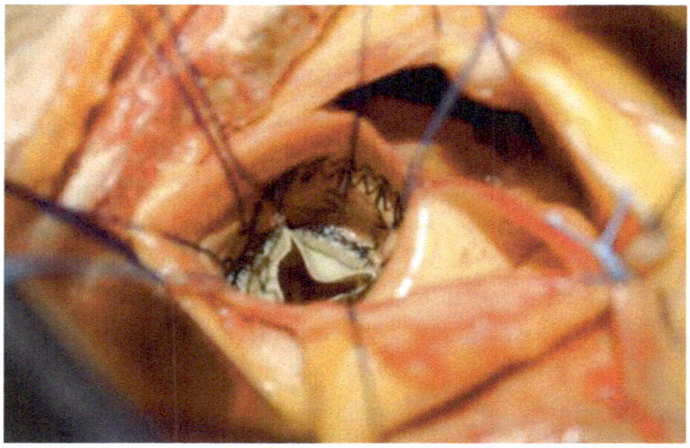

Fig. 20.5 Implanted Perceval with guiding sutures and commissural stay sutures

started with the screw on the tip of the implanting device, which unscrews the inflow portion of the valve. After that, the safety clip is removed and the sheath is pulled back to deploy the outflow part of the cage.

Again, the implanting surgeon should take care that he applies a gentle push on the implantation device to assure stable positioning at the annular level, while his assistants apply traction on the guiding sutures in the direction of the aortic axis. The inflow and outflow portions are released sequentially. During this phase, as the left ventricle is vented through the aortic valve, complete emptying of the ventricle is performed, and cardiopulmonary bypass flow is transiently reduced to allow better operative visualization. After deployment is complete, the stick is removed from the LVOT with gentle rotating movements, avoiding the device to get tangled in the prosthesis. If commissural stay sutures are used, they should be released during valvuloplasty.

After this, accurate position of the valve is again reconfirmed (Fig. 20.5). Post ballooning is carried out with the size-dedicated balloon being inserted into the prosthesis with the blue ring being at the level of the upper edge of the leaflets. The balloon will be inflated to 4 atm for the duration of 30 s. After release, the balloon is removed from the LVOT, so are the guiding and stay sutures.

It very often happens that during implantation, the upper ends of the stent posts will reach a level above the aortotomy. This will be reversed after terminating traction on the stay sutures.

Malposition of the prosthesis, which occurs if the valve is deployed too high in relation to the aortic annulus, can be identified by direct inspection of the aortic annulus. The technique used to correct prosthesis malposition has been described previously [7].

The surgical procedure was completed with the closure of the transverse aortotomy or with the other possible associated procedures. In case of associated coronary artery bypass grafting (CABG), the distal anastomosis preceded the implantation of the prosthesis but followed aortotomy and annulus sizing. Transesophageal echocardiography was performed during the procedure to assess the positioning and functioning of the prosthesis.

20.2 Literature Results

The earliest experience with the sutureless Perceval aortic bioprosthesis was aimed at establishing the safety of the device. At the time of the first implants performed in 16 high-risk patients in Germany, the primary question was whether a sutureless aortic valve would result in increased risk of device migration or dislodgement and paravalvular leakage. Intraoperative and postoperative echocardiography revealed neither aortic insufficiency nor paravalvular leakage in any patients [9].

Definitive evidence of shorter operative times using the sutureless Perceval aortic valve as compared with conventional prostheses was later provided by a study from our group that included 100 patients undergoing minimally invasive isolated aortic valve replacement (AVR) by J-sternotomy. Of these, 50 patients received a Perceval bioprosthesis and 50 patients received a stented valve. Our results did not cast any doubt: aortic cross-clamp and cardiopulmonary bypass times were 39.4 and 34% shorter in the Perceval group than in the stented group [10].

An additional single-center study that deserves mentioning for its topicality has compared hospital costs of sutureless vs. stented AVR [11]. Although the cost of the Perceval aortic valve has decreased substantially since its introduction into the market, it remains higher than that of conventional prostheses.

The development of this device for use in clinical practice was also aimed at making the minimally invasive approach easier. In particular, sutureless AVR is most commonly performed via mini J-sternotomy and right lateral minithoracotomy. The Perceval bioprosthetic valve showed optimal performance with both approaches, allowing for shorter cross-clamp times, though somewhat longer if the right lateral minithoracotomy is used [12–14]. The main contribution of sutureless valves to AVR through right lateral minithoracotomy consists in making implantation feasible also when the anatomical position of the aorta is unfavorable to the use of conventional prostheses that would be difficult to suture.

At present, the most convincing evidence regarding ease of implantation with a minimally invasive approach derives from two European multicenter studies conducted by Dalén et al. In the first study, 267 consecutive patients underwent isolated AVR with the sutureless Perceval bioprosthesis at six European centers; of these, 189 were performed through ministernotomy and 78 through a full sternotomy. Aortic cross-clamp and cardiopulmonary bypass times did not differ between groups [15]. In the second study, sutureless AVR via ministernotmy was associated with shorter operative times than stented AVR via full sternotomy (aortic cross-clamp time: 40 vs. 65 min, $p < 0.001$; cardiopulmonary bypass time: 69 vs. 87 min, $p < 0.001$) [16].

The pre-marketing Cavalier trial investigated the 30-day clinical and hemodynamic outcome from the largest study cohort, including 658 patients undergoing sutureless AVR at 25 European centers [17]. In this study, the Perceval valve proved to be safe and could be implanted with a fast and reproducible technique after a short learning curve period. In another study by the same multicenter group, 731 consecutive patients were enrolled, with a cumulative follow-up of 729 patients-years. Overall survival rates were 92.1 and 74.7% at 1 and 5 years, respectively [18]. In the post-marketing phase, a retrospective analysis of 314 patients enrolled at five European centers [19] and a Canadian study including 215 patients from six centers provided additional outcome data on AVR with the Perceval aortic valve [20]. In both studies, reproducibility of the procedure was satisfactory also for routine clinical practice and use of the Perceval prosthesis resulted in improved survival, good hemodynamic performance and favorable follow-up outcomes.

Finally, started in 2016 the international multicenter randomized PERSIST-AVR (Perceval Sutureless Implant vs. Standard Aortic Valve Replacement) trial is going to test the safety and efficacyof the Perceval bioprosthesis vs. conventional sutured valves among patients undergoing aortic valve replacement as isolated or combined procedure with CABG. If definitive evidence will be obtained to show that shorter implantation times are associated with improved clinical outcomes—along with device durability—, it is likely that the sutureless approach will become the first-line treatment strategy for AVR in patients with suitable anatomy.

An interesting opportunity provided by the Perceval aortic valve is the possibility of performing redo procedures. At present, the majority of elderly and high-risk patients are referred for TAVI or a valve-in-valve procedure in degenerated bioprostheses. However, redo patients at low risk, or included in the previously mentioned "grey zone", may benefit from surgical AVR: shorter operative times in a procedure already prolonged by tissue preparation may result in improved postoperative outcomes. In this respect, an initial experience from our group reported on 13 patients who had previously undergone cardiac surgery (coronary artery bypass grafting in seven and conventional AVR in six with an indication for valve replacement because of a degenerated bioprosthesis). The results were encouraging in terms of clinical outcome (0% mortality) and technical feasibility (prevention of graft injury due to the higher aortotomy without the need of manipulation of the root). Additionally, the stentless profile of the Perceval aortic valve made it possible to replace the previously implanted stented valve with a prosthesis of greater effective orifice area [21]. Even in patients who previously received a stentless or homograft aortic valve, the Perceval bioprosthesis may be useful in removing only the valve leaflets, so that it can be positioned on the neo-aortic root of the previously implanted prosthesis [22, 23]. In patients with degenerated homografts, the Perceval sutureless valve may be particularly useful in the presence of aortic root calcification, which may render the placement of suture stitches to secure a conventional prosthetic valve challenging. In this patient population, therefore, the Perceval aortic valve is the ideal device.

The use of the Perceval bioprosthesis has also been expanded to particular conditions and clinical situations that deserve further investigation. For instance, acute aortic regurgitation after Perceval implantation can be due to different factors, but in most cases it is due to valve malpositioning following suboptimal deployment, severe oversizing or inappropriate indication. We already know from experience, however, that a valve-in-valve procedure in a Perceval sutureless aortic bioprosthesis can be performed successfully [24]. In addition, when a malposition occurs, and the decision is made to reposition the device during the same surgery, the Perceval valve can be safely removed using the 'X movement' technique, as previously described [7].

Another condition that would benefit from more comprehensive enquiry in the future is the indication for Perceval implantation in the setting of concomitant mitral valve surgery. Although concomitant mitral disease has been shown not to be a contraindication for sutureless AVR [25, 26], we suggest to implant the Perceval bioprosthesis after mitral valve replacement has been completed, so as to assess and measure the aortic annulus after prosthetic valve deployment and mitral annular stabilization.

Finally, in particular conditions with extensive calcification of the ascending aorta (porcelain aorta), the Perceval bioprosthesis could be implanted in an intra-annular position and could be accommodated with its stent in the outflow tract even in a segment of the ascending aorta that was replaced with a tubular prosthesis [27].

20.3 Comparison with TAVI

The advent of transcatheter aortic valve implantation (TAVI), which does not require cardiopulmonary bypass (CPB), has produced a real revolution in the management of valvular heart disease [28], providing new hope and an alternative treatment option to patients who were previously considered too high risk for conventional surgery [29].

Cardiac surgeons and cardiologists can carefully consider the strengths and weaknesses of each management strategy so as to identify the most appropriate treatment option for their individual patients.

It is worth noting that, in the most important multicenter clinical studies conducted up to date, the TAVI approach has always been compared with surgical AVR using conventional prosthetic aortic valves through a full sternotomy [29]. Basically, it means that the greatest innovation in cardiology (TAVI) has been compared with an "ancient" or otherwise "remote" surgical procedure (sutured AVR, full sternotomy) considered as the standard treatment in experienced centers that are at the forefront of cardiac surgery.

Catheter based techniques have found widespread acceptance amongst patients needing an aortic valve intervention. The perception of having done the procedure through "a little whole in the groin" as compared to having the "whole chest cracked" by a surgeon depicts a patients' likewise choice of TAVI over open surgery. How can surgery gain back the faith in a very well established, long-term durable technique with very predictable results? The aortic valve surgery has recently undergone a second revolution with the introduction of sutureless aortic bioprosthetic valves into clinical practice, which has the potential to be a "game changer": The new devices possess the potential for easy and fast implantation in symptomatic patients even with a high surgical risk profile [30]. Moreover, specifically in the setting of minimally invasive surgery, the use of sutureless valves can result in a significant reduction in crossclamp and CPB times, which were reported to be 39.4% shorter than those obtained with other types of bioprosthetic valves [10].

From a technical standpoint, sutureless AVR—as does traditional AVR—reflects the curative treatment with removal of the diseased leaflets and annular calcium. The concept of sutureless implantation and fixation of the devices has been proven by the two major studies conducted by the only two competitors on the market. More than 700 patients have been followed up to 5 years in the Cavalier trial with the Perceval [18].

A clear benefit of sutureless over traditional sutured AVR could not be demonstrated, but the adoption of any mini invasive technique was higher in institutions, when the sutureless technique was available. They concluded, that sutureless valves facilitate mini invasive AVR.

Another aspect that deserves mentioning is that the TAVI technology is more expensive than open-heart surgery, with a non-negligible impact on overall hospital and healthcare costs [31]. This aspect will have to be decided also by the healthcare providers and was not meant to be a focus of this editorial.

In our opinion, in the TAVI era, AVR still has to be considered as the true curative treatment alternative, TAVI does not allow for decalcification of the aortic annulus and removal of the diseased native valve; therefore it can be used as a "palliative procedure", which however is associated with a high risk of postoperative cerebral embolism and a higher incidence of paravalvular leakage significantly affecting survival [31]. TAVI represents an extremely effective treatment option for high-risk patients who cannot undergo surgery, but its use remains questionable in low- and intermediate-risk patients because of the very limited evidence available [32].

20.4 In Conclusion...

The sutureless Perceval aortic valve is a device increasingly used in many European cardiac surgery centers. Since the first reports evaluating implantation feasibility and valve safety in humans in 2007, an increasing amount of data have become available, including pre-marketing clinical results and experience in particular conditions. Overall, excellent performances have been demonstrated in terms of hemodynamic outcomes, safety and versatility of use. However, several questions remain unanswered, especially with regard to long-term durability, risk for endocarditis, and the need for postoperative pacemaker implantation. This new valve shares with the new generation bioprosthesis valve models the transcatheter delivery modality, which allows a more tailored approach for these patients.

In high-risk patients undergoing combined or REDO surgery with prolonged surgical time as well as in patients undergoing reintervention, the use of sutureless bioprostheses is particularly valuable for the considerable reduction in the implantation time.

It is also important to mention that during minimally invasive surgery, the reduction in the working space for the passage of prosthetic sutures can be technically challenging, and this issue can be easily solved with the use of the sutureless Perceval S prosthesis. In patients with a critically small annulus, this valve allows maximization of the bioprosthetic diameter. In addition, it may reduce the rate of paravalvular leakage, which is commonly related to suboptimal suturing of the bioprosthesis fixation ring in this clinical setting.

The Perceval S sutureless aortic valve represents an easy and useful instrument for AVR. Sutureless AVR allows maintenance of physiological balances through a minimally invasive approach that should guide future innovations in cardiac surgery.

References

1. Bridgewater B, Gummert J, Kinsman R, Walton P. Towards global benchmarking: the fourth EACTS adult cardiac surgical database report. Henley-on-Thames: Dendrite Clinical Systems; 2010.
2. Zahn R, Gerckens U, Grube E, Linke A, Sievert H, Eggebrecht H, et al. German transcatheter aortic valve interventions-registry investigators. Transcatheter aortic valve implantation: first results from a multi-centre real-world registry. Eur Heart J. 2011;32:198–204.
3. Ruttmann E, Gilhofer TS, Ulmer H, Chevtchik O, Kocher A, Schistek R, et al. Propensity score matched analysis of aortic valve replacement by mini-thoracotomy. J Heart Valve Dis. 2010;19:606–14.
4. Phan K, Xie A, Di Eusanio M, Yan TD. A meta-analysis of minimally invasive versus conventional sternotomy for aortic valve replacement. Ann Thorac Surg. 2014;98:1499–511.
5. Santarpino G, Pfeiffer S, Concistré G, Fischlein T. Perceval S aortic valve implantation in mini-invasive surgery: the simple sutureless solution. Interact Cardiovasc Thorac Surg. 2012;15:357–60.
6. D'Onofrio A, Messina A, Lorusso R, Alfieri OR, Fusari M, Rubino P, et al. Sutureless aortic valve replacement as an alternative treatment for patients belonging to the "gray zone" between transcatheter aortic valve implantation and conventional surgery: a propensity-matched, multicenter analysis. J Thorac Cardiovasc Surg. 2012;144:1010–6.
7. Santarpino G, Pfeiffer S, Concistré G, Fischlein T. A supra-annular malposition of the Perceval S sutureless aortic valve: the 'χ-movement' removal technique and subsequent reimplantation. Interact Cardiovasc Thorac Surg. 2012;15:280–1.
8. Santarpino G, Pfeiffer S, Jessl J, Dell'Aquila AM, Pollari F, Pauschinger M, et al. Sutureless replacement versus transcatheter valve implantation in aortic valve stenosis: a propensity-matched analysis of 2 strategies in high-risk patients. J Thorac Cardiovasc Surg. 2014;147:561–7.

9. Shrestha M, Khaladj N, Bara C, Hoeffler K, Hagl C, Haverich A. A staged approach towards interventional aortic valve implantation with a sutureless valve: initial human implants. Thorac Cardiovasc Surg. 2008;56:398–400.
10. Santarpino G, Pfeiffer S, Concistré G, Grossmann I, Hinzmann M, Fischlein T. The Perceval S aortic valve has the potential of shortening surgical time: does it also result in improved outcome? Ann Thorac Surg. 2013;96:77–81; discussion 81-2.
11. Pollari F, Santarpino G, Dell'Aquila AM, Gazdag L, Alnahas H, Vogt F, Pfeiffer S, Fischlein T. Better short-term outcome by using sutureless valves: a propensity-matched score analysis. Ann Thorac Surg. 2014;98:611–6; discussion 616-7.
12. Fischlein T, Pfeiffer S, Pollari F, Sirch J, Vogt F, Santarpino G. Sutureless valve implantation via mini J-sternotomy: a single center experience with 2 years mean follow-up. Thorac Cardiovasc Surg. 2015;63:467–71.
13. Gilmanov D, Miceli A, Ferrarini M, Farneti P, Murzi M, Solinas M, Glauber M. Aortic valve replacement through right anterior minithoracotomy: can sutureless technology improve clinical outcomes? Ann Thorac Surg. 2014;98:1585–92.
14. Miceli A, Santarpino G, Pfeiffer S, Murzi M, Gilmanov D, Concistré G, Quaini E, Solinas M, Fischlein T, Glauber M. Minimally invasive aortic valve replacement with Perceval S sutureless valve: early outcomes and one-year survival from two European centers. J Thorac Cardiovasc Surg. 2014;148:2838–43.
15. Dalén M, Biancari F, Rubino AS, Santarpino G, De Praetere H, Kasama K, Juvonen T, Deste W, Pollari F, Meuris B, Fischlein T, Mignosa C, Gatti G, Pappalardo A, Sartipy U, Svenarud P. Ministernotomy versus full sternotomy aortic valve replacement with a sutureless bioprosthesis: a multicenter study. Ann Thorac Surg. 2015;99:524–30.
16. Dalén M, Biancari F, Rubino AS, Santarpino G, Glaser N, De Praetere H, Kasama K, Juvonen T, Deste W, Pollari F, Meuris B, Fischlein T, Mignosa C, Gatti G, Pappalardo A, Svenarud P, Sartipy U. Aortic valve replacement through full sternotomy with a stented bioprosthesis versus minimally invasive sternotomy with a sutureless bioprosthesis. Eur J Cardiothorac Surg. 2015.; pii: ezv014. [Epub ahead of print].
17. Laborde F, Fischlein T, Hakim-Meibodi K, Misfeld M, Carrel T, Zembala M, Madonna F, Meuris B, Haverich A, Shrestha M, Cavalier Trial Investigators. Clinical and haemodynamic outcomes in 658 patients receiving the Perceval sutureless aortic valve: early results from a prospective European multicentre study (the Cavalier Trial). Eur J Cardiothorac Surg. 2015;49(3):978–86.
18. Shrestha M, Fischlein T, Meuris B, Flameng W, Carrel T, Madonna F, Misfeld M, Folliguet T, Haverich A, Laborde F. European multicentre experience with the sutureless Perceval valve: clinical and haemodynamic outcomes up to 5 years in over 700 patients. Eur J Cardiothorac Surg. 2015;49(1):234–41.
19. Rubino AS, Santarpino G, De Praetere H, Kasama K, Dalén M, Sartipy U, Lahtinen J, Heikkinen J, Deste W, Pollari F, Svenarud P, Meuris B, Fischlein T, Mignosa C, Biancari F. Early and intermediate outcome after aortic valve replacement with a sutureless bioprosthesis: results of a multicenter study. J Thorac Cardiovasc Surg. 2014;148:865–71.
20. Mazine A, Teoh K, Bouhout I, Bhatnagar G, Pelletier M, Voisine P, Demers P, Carrier M, Bouchard D. Sutureless aortic valve replacement: a Canadian multicentre study. Can J Cardiol. 2015;31:63–8.
21. Santarpino G, Pfeiffer S, Concistrè G, Fischlein T. REDO aortic valve replacement: the sutureless approach. J Heart Valve Dis. 2013;22:615–20.
22. Folliguet TA, Laborde F. Sutureless Perceval aortic valve replacement in aortic homograft. Ann Thorac Surg. 2013;96:1866–8.
23. Villa E, Messina A, Cirillo M, Brunelli F, Mhagna Z, Dalla Tomba M, Troise G. Perceval sutureless valve in freestyle root: new surgical valve-in-valve therapy. Ann Thorac Surg. 2013;96:e155–7.
24. Durand E, Tron C, Eltchaninoff H. Emergency transcatheter aortic valve implantation for acute and early failure of sutureless Perceval aortic valve. Can J Cardiol. 2015;31:1204.e13–5.

25. Moriggia S, Trumello C, Buzzatti N, Iaci G, Di Giannuario G, Alfieri O. Aortic sutureless Perceval valve for small root in concomitant mitral valve replacement. J Heart Valve Dis. 2015;24:187–9.
26. Minh TH, Mazine A, Bouhout I, El-Hamamsy I, Carrier M, Bouchard D, Demers P. Expanding the indication for sutureless aortic valve replacement to patients with mitral disease. J Thorac Cardiovasc Surg. 2014;148:1354–9.
27. Santarpino G, Pfeiffer S, Fischlein T. Perceval sutureless approach in a patient with porcelain aorta unsuitable for transcatheter aortic valve implantation. Int J Cardiol. 2012;155:168–70.
28. Cribier A, Eltchaninoff H, Bash A, Borenstein N, Tron C, Bauer F, et al. Percutaneous transcatheter implantation of an aortic valve prosthesis for calcific aortic stenosis: first human case description. Circulation. 2002;106:3006–8.
29. Leon MB, Smith CR, Mack M, Miller DC, Moses JW, Svensson LG, et al. Transcatheter aortic-valve implantation for aortic stenosis in patients who cannot undergo surgery. N Engl J Med. 2010;21:1597–607.
30. Flameng W, Herregods MC, Hermans H, Van der Mieren G, Vercalsteren M, Poortmans G, et al. Effect of sutureless implantation of the Perceval S aortic valve bioprosthesis on intraoperative and early postoperative outcomes. J Thorac Cardiovasc Surg. 2011;142:1453–7.
31. Santarpino G, Pfeiffer S, Jessl J, Dell'Aquila A, Vogt F, von Wardenburg C, et al. Clinical outcome and cost analysis of sutureless versus transcatheter aortic valve implantation with propensity score matching analysis. Am J Cardiol. 2015;116:1737–43.
32. Santarpino G, Fischlein T, Pfeiffer S. 1-Year results from the NOTION randomized clinical trial: no news is good news? J Am Coll Cardiol. 2015;66:979.

Part VI

Transcatheter Aortic Valve Implantation

21 Trans-Catheter Aortic Valve Replacement: Procedure Planning and Guidance

Eric Brochet, Christopher Meduri, Vivek Rajagopal, and Sarah Rinehart

The role of non-invasive imaging for trans-catheter implant (TAVI) has increasingly been in procedure planning rather than peri-procedural imaging. With maturation of TAVI, there is movement to avoid general anaesthesia during the procedure, and rely mostly on fluoroscopy or a combination of trans-thoracic Echocardiography (TTE) and fluoroscopy. Accordingly, the emphasis is on optimal procedural planning to prevent peri-valvular leak (PVL) and complications such as annular rupture, and to establish the options for procedural access by evaluation of the vasculature. Thus, the following section will describe the role of imaging for TAVI planning followed by key steps for intra-procedural imaging.

21.1 Imaging for TAVI Planning

21.1.1 Aortic Valve Morphology and Function

TTE is the method of choice for initial evaluation of AV morphology and function. Usually it allows for adequate imaging of the number of aortic valve leaflets and its motion, the size and extent of calcification, and annular size. Furthermore, other morphological abnormalities which may be relevant to TAVI such as mobile calcium, endocarditis, sub-aortic membrane among others can be evaluated by TTE. However, additional imaging with multi-detector computed tomography (MDCT) or TEE may be necessary to further delineate these anatomical abnormalities [1]. Also, MDCT or TEE may be necessary when TTE is suboptimal and

E. Brochet, M.D. (✉)
Cardiology Department, Hôpital BICHAT, Paris, France
e-mail: eric.brochet@aphp.fr

C. Meduri, M.D. • V. Rajagopal, M.D. • S. Rinehart, M.D.
Marcus Heart Valve Center, Piedmont Heart Institute, Atlanta, GA, USA

K. Fattouch et al. (eds.), *Advances in Treatments for Aortic Valve and Root Diseases*, https://doi.org/10.1007/978-3-319-66483-5_21

does not provide the essential information of leaflet morphology especially if TAVI is being done for the primary indication of aortic regurgitation (AR). In the case of the latter, cardiac magnetic resonance imaging (CMR) may be selectively used to quantify AR, and assess the aortic leaflet and root morphology. But, CT may be still necessary to size the annulus (see below) so the use of CMR as the primary technique to plan TAVI is very rare. TTE is also the preferred method to assess the severity of AS severity which should be evaluated according to the EAE/ASE Recommendations for Evaluation of Valvular Stenosis and staged according to the AHA/ACC or the ESC/EAE Guideline for the Management of Patients with Valvular Heart Disease [2, 3]. Stress TTE may be necessary to elucidate the severity of AS in specific circumstances [4]. A detailed description of assessment of severity of AS including stress Echo can be found elsewhere in other chapters in this book. CMR may be alternative to Doppler Echocardiography to measure AV gradient in AS but has several limitations and is not recommended unless there is no other alternative [5]. When the severity of AS cannot be clarified with TTE, an alternative may be stress Echocardiography or the assessment of anatomic AVA by TEE or MDCT. Additionally, quantification of the AV calcium burden by MDCT may provide clarification of severity of AS in selected cases as described below in this chapter [6]. Parameters to assess before TAVI are summarized in Table 21.1.

Table 21.1 Parameters to be assessed before TAVI: Planning and Procedure Guidance

Aortic valve (AV)
• AV morphology (biplane 2DTEE/3DTEE)
• Severity of AS (2-D TTE/TEE, Doppler, MDCT)
• Extent and distribution of calcifications (MDCT)
• Annulus size (MDCT, biplane 2DTEE/3DTEE)
• Degree of baseline AR (2-D TEE)
Aortic root (MDCT, 3-D TEE)
• Aortic root morphology and dimensions
• Coronary ostia
Left ventricle (LV)—(2-D TTE/TEE, Doppler)
• LV global and regional function
• Presence of subaortic septal hypertrophy (septal bulge)
• Présence of LVOT obstruction
Mitral valve (MV)—(2-D TTE/TEE, Doppler)
• MV morphology
• Mechanism and severity of mitral regurgitation (MR)
Right ventricle (RV)—(2-D TTE/TEE, Doppler)
• RV dimensions and function
• Severity of tricuspid regurgitation (TR)
• Presence of pericardial effusion
Aorta—(MDCT, 2-D TEE)
• Descending aorta and aortic arch
• Aortic atheroma and thrombus
Peripheral Vessels (MDCT)
• Size, tortuosity
• Calcification
• Plaques, atheroma, hematoma
• Grafts

21.1.2 LVOT and Other Cardiac Findings

TTE is the recommended as initial test for evaluation of the LVOT size and morphology. When TTE is not optimal, MDCT or TEE can aid in the assessment. Also, TTE useful for the assessment of estimation of pulmonary pressures, and identification of other significant valve abnormalities. Lastly, left and right heart size and function can be assessed by TTE.

21.1.3 Annular Sizing and Calcium

The annulus is an elliptical virtual ring formed by the joining of basal attachments of the aortic valvular leaflets. Hence, measurements of the annulus by 2-D TTE or TEE are not accurate for sizing the TAVI prosthesis. The preferred method to measure the annulus for TAVI planning is MDCT since it allows planning of vascular access as well. The 3D dataset of MDCT avoids the systematic underestimation of the major axis of the annulus by 2-D TTE or TEE [7]. With gated MDCT, the annulus is measured during systole (typically 30–40% of the R-R interval). This accounts for the phasic changes in the annular shape and size and avoids under sizing of the prosthesis and the consequent occurrence of para-valvular leak (PVL). Reconstruction of the 3-D data in MDCT to orient the annulus orthogonal to the center-axis of the LVOT allows for the measurement of minimal and maximal diameter, annular circumference, and annular area (Fig. 21.1a). Typically, a small degree of prosthesis oversizing (~14%) is recommended; however, severe oversizing increases the risk of annular rupture [7, 8]. When contrast MDCT is contraindicated as in patients with renal dysfunction, 3-D TEE is a good alternative for TAVI planning (Fig. 21.1b) [9]. CMR may be used to size the annulus it is less validated and is less patient friendly for this purpose [10]. Although 3-D TEE requires

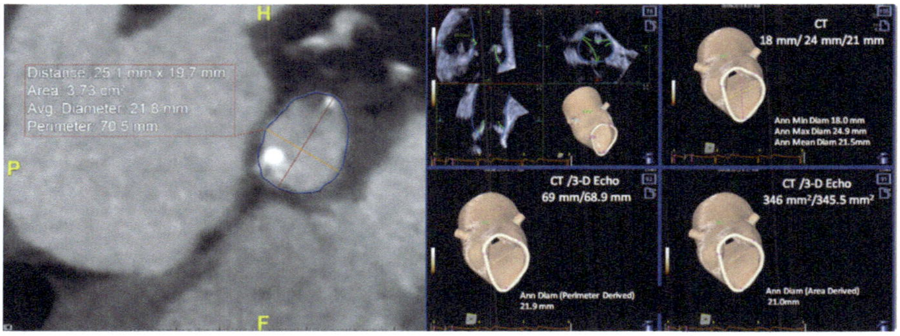

Fig. 21.1 On the left are shown standard measurements of annulus made by MDCT. Similar measurements can be made by 3-D TEE (on the right) using automated algorithm to model the aortic root. The 3-D TEE measurements of the annulus show good agreement with those made by MDCT in the example shown in the figure

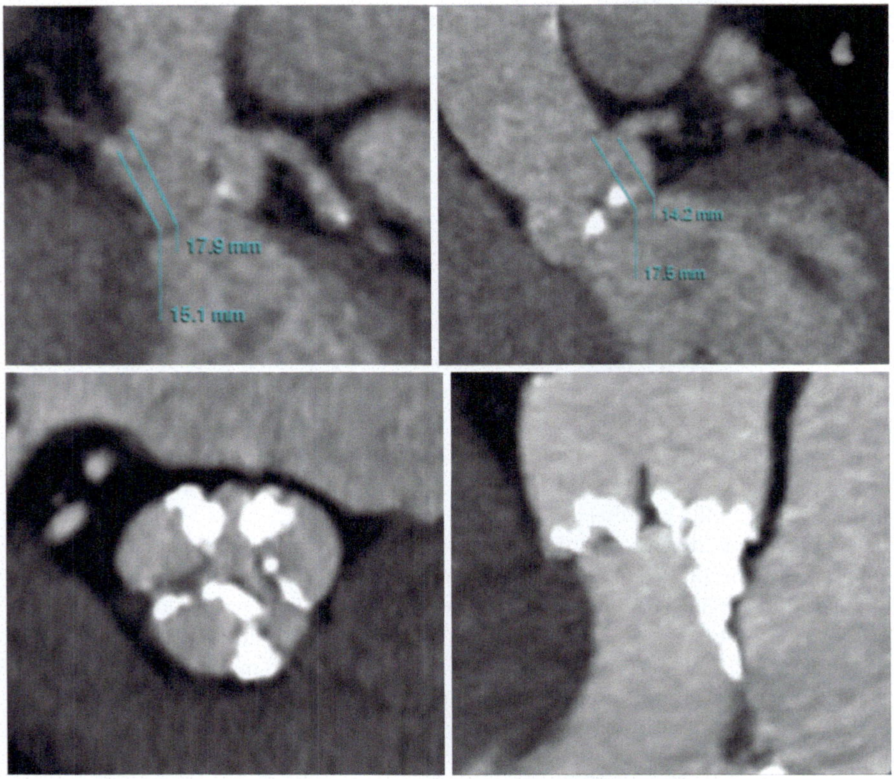

Fig. 21.2 The top panel shows the measurements of the coronary ostia (*right* and *left*) height made by MDCT. Below is shown an example of extreme calcification of the annulus with protrusion into the LVOT

sedation, it take far less time for the same information and is has been validated specifically for TAVI planning when compared to CMR. The degree of prosthesis oversizing may be higher than that by MDCT given that 3-D TEE measurements may be smaller than those made by MDCT. In AR, the degree of oversizing by MDCT and 3-D TEE may need to higher than those established for AS, since the annulus is usually dilated and the lack of significant calcium means anchoring the prosthesis will need sufficient radial force. The degree and extent of calcification of the annulus is severe AS is an important determinant of potential for annulus rupture during the procedure and the occurrence of PVL after deployment of the valve (Fig. 21.2a). MDCT is the preferred method to assess the geometry, density and the extent of the annular and aortic calcification. Moreover, the 3D data from MDCT can be used for 3-D printing to study and predict the potential for significant PVL (Fig. 21.3) [11, 12].

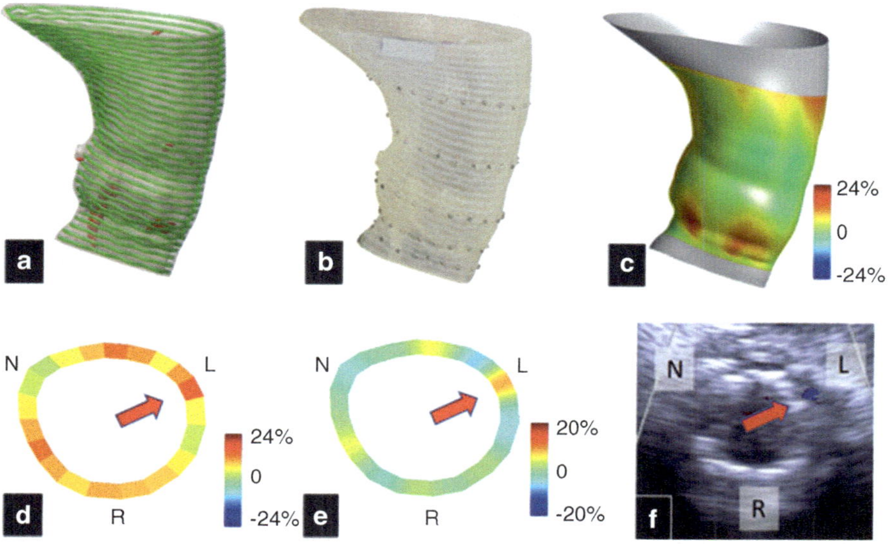

Fig. 21.3 Annular strain unevenness, which is derived from the in-vitro TAVI simulation based on the 3D printed tissue-mimicking phantom, is predictive of post-TAVI PVL. (**a**) 3D model reconstructed from the pre-TAVI contrast-enhanced CT images. (**b**) 3D printed tissue-mimicking phantom. (**c**) Circumferential strain map of the aortic root post-TAVI in vitro. (**d**) Annular strain distribution. The red arrow indicates the site of the highest strain. (**e**) Annular bulge index which describes the strain unevenness in the annulus. The red arrow indicates the most uneven site. (**f**) Post-TAVI transesophageal echocardiography with color Doppler. The red arrow indicates the PVL site, which coincides with the most uneven site in **e**. (Reproduced with permission from: Qian Z, Lancellotti P, Vannan MA. Aortic root calcium burden and post-transcatheter aortic valve implantation paravalvular leak: Can't Live Without It, Can't Live With It. Eur Heart J Cardiovasc Imaging. 2017;18:654–6)

21.1.4 Assessment of the Aortic Root

The size of sinus of Valsalva (SoV), the sino-tubular junction (STJ) and the ascending aorta (AA) are important measurements which may influence the type and size of the TAVI prosthesis. The annulus to coronary ostia distance (Fig. 21.2b) and presence of aortic calcium are also key morphological assessments in TAVI planning. MDCT is the preferred technique for evaluation of the aortic root although 2-D/3-D TEE is an alternative when contrast MDCT cannot be performed. CMR may also be used to evaluate the aortic root although the location and extent of aortic calcification may not be evaluable.

MDCT also allows assessment of the coronary arteries although the presence of significant coronary calcification in the TAVI populations may necessitate coronary angiography. The orientation of the LVOT to the aortic root, identification of coronary bypass graft location, evaluation of the proximity of the aorta, RV and LV apex to the chest wall position may all be important information for procedural planning depending on the procedural approach (trans-femoral Vs. trans-apical Vs. direct aortic). Again, MDCT is the preferred method for these assessments although CMR offers an alternative when MDCT cannot be done [10, 13].

21.1.5 Vascular Imaging

MDCT is again the test of choice to assess the thoraco-abdominal vasculature including the aorta, and the ilio-femoral vasculature. It is also useful to assess the carotids, although ultrasound may often be necessary for the latter. This evaluation allows planning the vascular access route for TAVI and assess stroke risk. Small luminal diameters, dense calcification, tortuosity and dissection of the ilio-femoral vessels increase the risk of access site complications. The presence of mobile atherosclerotic plaques in the ascending aorta, extensive aortic atheroma, intramural hematoma and ulcerated plaques increase the risk of stroke and vascular complications during TAVI. In cases with challenging vascular access, MDCT can guide alternative access approaches such as a surgical side-graft on the iliac arteries, trans-axillary, trans-apical, direct aortic, carotid, or trans-venous access approaches. Occasionally, contrast abdominal aortogram may be useful to assess the ilio-femoral vessels, especially in those whose renal functions precludes the use of contrast for MDCT. Alternatively, vascular calcification, tortuosity and size can be assessed with non-contrast CT but luminal abnormalities such as dissection, stenosis and plaques may require intravascular ultrasound or magnetic resonance angiography. The latter may also be selectively used to assess neck vessels for stroke risk assessment if there MDCT and ultrasound do not provide the necessary information.

Table 21.1 summarizes the imaging methods used for procedure planning.

21.2 Imaging for TAVI Guidance

The goal of imaging during TAVI is to guide proper deployment of the aortic transcatheter valve (THV), assess its position and function after implantation and identify immediate post-procedure complications.

Although fluoroscopy and angiography remain the primary imaging tools during TAVI the important role of transoesophageal echocardiography (TEE) monitoring has been demonstrated since the introduction of the TAVI procedure [14]. Advantages of TEE include the assessment of aortic valve and root anatomy, assessment of valve leaflet behaviour during balloon aortic valvuloplasty (BAV), precise positioning of the valve, immediate assessment of prosthetic valve function and early identification of complications [14–17]. Recently, the need for systematic use of intra-procedural TEE during TAVI has been questioned due to the fact that most large volume centres now perform most TAVI procedures under conscious sedation, without general anaesthesia. Thus, the role of echocardiography is now often reduced to transthoracic echocardiographic (TTE) assessment of the result at the end of the procedure, or in case of suspicion of complications [18]. Despite this trend, recently published guidelines continue to advocate the use of TEE as a critically important component of the intra-procedural and immediate post-procedural success of TAVI, especially when the primary indication is AR. In addition, TEE is still used during TAVI procedures with surgical approach, in case of complications, and is very useful during the early experience of centres. Moreover, it is important that Echocardiographers involved in TAVI monitoring should remain familiar with the specificities of TEE monitoring for each valve procedure, and well trained for the early detection of complications. Other echocardiographic modalities such as micro TEE probe, or intra-cardiac echocardiographic (ICE) monitoring [19], have been proposed as an alternative to TEE in patients undergoing TAVI under conscious sedation. However, these techniques have so far not gained wide acceptance.

21.2.1 Pre-Procedural Imaging

At baseline, TEE should be used to assess aortic valve (AV) morphology, number of cusps (tricuspid or bicuspid valve), symmetry or asymmetry of valve opening, extent and distribution of calcifications of the leaflets and of the annulus. The presence and location of protruding calcifications ("bulky" calcifications) should be noted. Longitudinal TEE view provides aortic root dimensions (SoV, STJ, and AA) diameters. TEE allows to redo the aortic annulus measurements and check consistency with the selected prosthetic size. Echocardiographic measurements of the AV annulus is typically performed in the longitudinal TEE plane. The correct alignment of the long axis may be improved by using biplane or X-plane imaging, providing simultaneous longitudinal and transverse images of the aortic valve. 3D TEE measurements of the AV annulus, using multiplane reconstruction of a 3D data set have been shown to provide more accurate measurements of annulus diameter than 2D TEE alone, and to compare favourably with MDCT measurements [20]. 3D TEE also allows accurate measurement of the height of coronary ostia. The degree of baseline AR should be evaluated as a reference because it can worsen after BAV. In addition, TEE is useful at the beginning of trans-apical procedures to identify the location of the apical puncture. Table 21.1 summarizes the assessments made at baseline during TAVI.

21.2.2 Peri-Procedural Imaging

The standard parameters to assess during TAVI are summarized in Table 21.2. Before valve implantation TEE, and more specifically biplane imaging, may be used to assess the correct positioning of the stiff wire in the left ventricle. During trans-apical procedures, TEE imaging, especially using real time 3D imaging can facilitate visualisation of the guidewire as it is advanced from the LV apex toward the aortic root [15, 21]. During BAV, TEE long axis view or biplane mode is

Table 21.2 Parameters to be assessed during TAVI

Before valve implantation
• AV crossing and stiff wire location (biplane/3DTEE)
• Stiff wire coaxiality (3DTEE)
During and immediately after balloon aortic valvuloplasty (BAV)
• Adequate location of the balloon
• Behaviour of the leaflets and displacement of calcifications during inflation
• Imaging of coronary ostia to assess risk of coronary obstruction
• Detection of severe AR post-BAV
During implantation of the valve
• Appropriate positioning (3D TEE for balloon expandable valves)
• Deployment of the valve (long loop recording)
After implantation of the valve
• Valve position, shape, leaflet motion, aortic regurgitation (AR) (intra or paraprosthetic AR)
• Doppler gradient
• LV function
• Patency of coronary arteries
• MV function

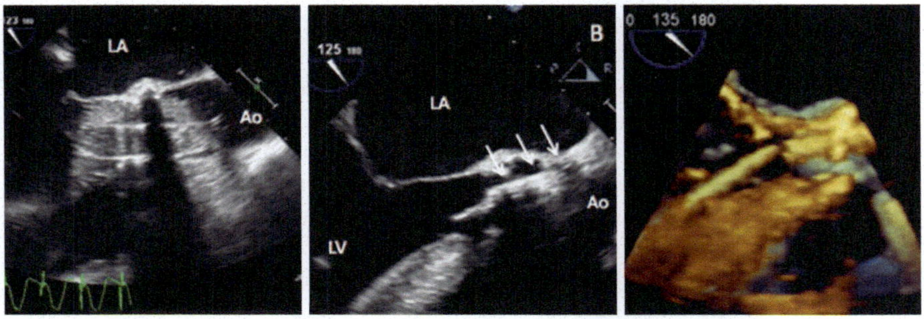

Fig. 21.4 TEE monitoring during trans apical TAVR. (**a**) Long axis 2D TEE view showing the behavior of the leaflets during balloon valvuloplasty. (**b**) Positioning of the Sapien valve. Identification of the valve before deployment with 2D TEE guidance. (**c**) Real time 3D TEE imaging

typically used to identify the proper positioning and inflation of the balloon during rapid pacing, to assess how the balloon fits into the valve annulus, and to assess potential complications, especially acute severe aortic regurgitation, which can be poorly tolerated and may require rapid deployment of the TAVI prosthesis. An important point is to assess the behaviour of the leaflets during BAV, especially when the aortic root is narrow and the height of coronary ostia is small (Fig. 21.4a).

Positioning of the valve is generally performed under fluoroscopic and angiographic guidance according to the recommendations of each prosthesis type. TEE imaging can be used in addition to fluoroscopy to provide more precise positioning of the valve. Although 2D TEE long axis view is most frequently used, real time 3D imaging may provide a more global view of the device. Specific information should be provided according to the type of prosthesis used. For balloon expandable valves, the use of high frequency 2D TEE or 3D TEE and appropriate gain settings may help to distinguish the valve from the balloon, which it is sometimes difficult (Fig. 21.4b, c). Positioning should also account for the potential valve shortening that differs depending on the generation of the valve used. For example, third generation balloon expandable valves shorten from the ventricular side. Thus, positioning of the valve should focus primarily on the aortic end of the valve. In addition, 3D TEE in short axis view may be useful to confirm co-axiality of the delivery system to the left outflow tract. Self- expanding valve deployment is generally performed under fluoroscopic guidance alone. However, TEE may be useful to identify the proper deployment of the ventricular end of the prosthesis, especially to ensure that the ventricular edge is not too high, which risks the prosthesis "jumping" into the aorta.

21.2.3 Immediate Post-Procedural Imaging

Parameters to assess immediately after TAVI are summarized in Table 21.3.

Although precise valve placement can be performed safely with fluoroscopic and angiographic imaging alone, echocardiographic imaging may be particularly useful immediately after implantation. Immediately after valve deployment, TEE in longitudinal and transverse views allows rapid assessment of valve position, shape, leaflet motion, and presence of aortic regurgitation. In the presence of significant AR, TEE plays a crucial role in specifying its mechanism and severity (Fig. 21.5a, b). Other important features to assess are presence of pericardial effusion, Doppler gradient, and LV function as well as patency of both coronary arteries and mitral valve function. When TTE is used is used to assess the procedural outcome, the same parameters are assessed although it may be difficult to obtain reliable data with patients in supine position and limitations in acoustic window.

Table 21.3 Complications during TAVI

Pericardial effusion and tamponade
Aortic regurgitation • Intra prosthetic AR (stiff wire interaction or leaflet dysfunction) • Paravalvular AR (2D LAX and SAX views, transgastric views, 3DTEE)
Mitral regurgitation • Interaction with the LVOT part of the prosthesis • LVOT obstruction (SAM) • MV damage (transapical route)
LV dynamic obstruction
Global or segmental LV dysfunction (check coronary ostia patency)
Coronary occlusion
Prosthesis malpositioning or displacement
Aortic rupture
Aortic dissection

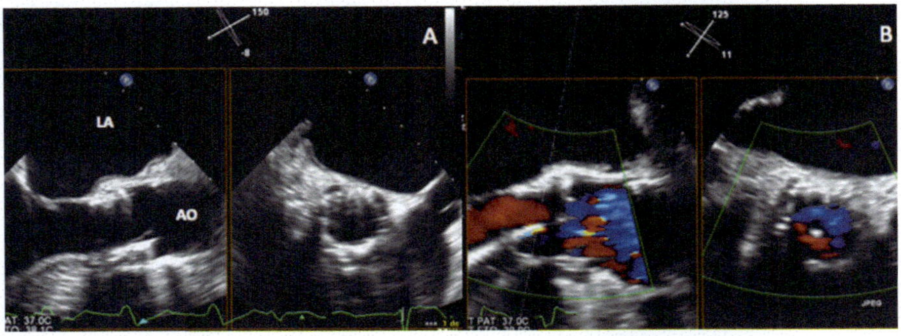

Fig. 21.5 TEE monitoring during trans apical TAVR. (**a**) Immediate assessment of result after valve deployment using simultaneous TEE longitudinal and transverse planes (X-plane imaging). (**b**) X-plane 2DTEE imaging with color Doppler showing no significant aortic regurgitation. (*LA* left atrium, *Ao* aorta)

21.2.4 Imaging TAVI Complications

Complications which can occur during TVAI are summarized in Table 21.3 and can be assessed by TEE or TTE [22]. Before valve deployment, pericardial effusion and tamponade can occur secondary to perforation of the RV by the pacing wire, perforation of the LV by the stiff guide wire or partial aortic root rupture (Fig. 21.6a). Rapid diagnosis is crucial because pericardial effusions are poorly tolerated by patients with left ventricular dysfunction and or stiffened ventricles. Multiple TEE views, including trans-gastric images should be performed if hypotension occurs without any other identified cause. In case of tamponade, TTE is also useful to guide pericardiocentesis. The presence of a new wall motion abnormality or severe global left ventricular dysfunction should raise the possibility of coronary occlusion or myocardial ischemia. Worsening of MR may occur due to interference or entrapment of the guidewire in the subvalvular apparatus or erroneous crossing of the mitral valve by the guide wire toward the left atrium during trans-apical approach, easily recognized with TEE (Fig. 21.6b). Acute severe AR may occur after BAV, and require rapid implantation of the valve (Fig. 21.6c).

After valve implantation, the assessment of the mechanisms and severity of AR should be performed rapidly and plays an important role in guiding management. Significant AR may occur due to incomplete expansion, incorrect positioning, restricted cusp motion, or inappropriate prosthetic size [23]. Intra prosthetic AR (Fig. 21.7a) is frequent, most often related to the presence of stiff wire and generally resolved rapidly after mobilisation of the wire [24]. PVL jets are often multiple and eccentric and difficult to visualize due to acoustic shadowing of the prosthesis. Assessment of the position and shape of the THV or presence of calcifications may help to understand the mechanism of AR. The use of multiple views is mandatory. TEE long-axis view is generally used first, followed by multiple SAX views at different levels, at the annulus and below the ventricular end of the THV prosthesis. Low oesophageal SAX views and deep gastric view are particularly useful as they

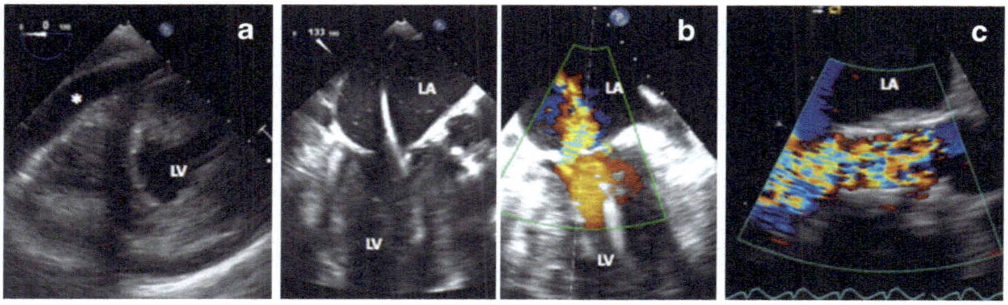

Fig. 21.6 Complications during TAVR. (**a**) Trans-gastric view showing pericardial effusion and tamponade due to perforation of the right ventricle by the pacing wire. (**b**) Mitral regurgitation due to erroneous crossing of the mitral valve by the guide wire during trans-apical approach (**c**) Severe aortic regurgitation due to cusp rupture after balloon valvuloplasty. (*LA* left atrium, *LV* left ventricle)

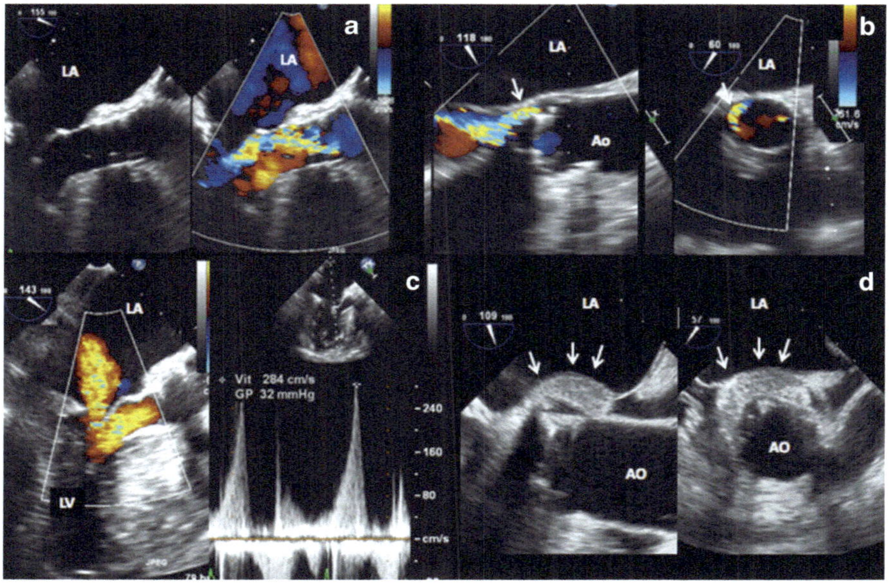

Fig. 21.7 Complications during TAVR. (**a**) intra-prosthetic aortic regurgitation due to the position of the guide wire. (**b**) Peri-prosthetic aortic regurgitation assessed with longitudinal and transverse TEE views. (**c**) Left ventricular outflow tract dynamic obstruction after valve implantation. CW Doppler showing the late systolic acceleration of the outflow jet. (**d**) TEE long axis and transverse views showing a marked echo-dense thickening of the posterior annulus after valve implantation (*arrows*) due to partial artial annulus rupture. (*LA* left atrium, *LV* left ventricle, *Ao* aorta)

allow imaging of the LVOT without acoustic shadowing. The use of multiple echocardiographic views is essential. Severity of PVL is often difficult to assess with TEE or TTE and relies on the combination of multiple parameters. The circumferential extent of the PVL jet(s) relative to the valve ring estimated in the parasternal short-axis view is the main quantitative parameter that has been proposed in the guidelines (<10% of the total circumferential extent corresponds to mild AR, and severe PV AR if >30%, Fig. 21.7b) [25, 26]. Comprehensive assessment of the degree of PVL, including cineangiography, invasive hemodynamic parameters and echocardiography (TEE or TTE) are generally required [27] before considering corrective procedures such as balloon inflation, second valve implantation or valve repositioning. It is important to know that with self-expanding prostheses, the severity of AR typically lessens over the next 30 min after implantation.

Mitral regurgitation may be due to interference of the LV outflow tract component of the THV with anterior mitral leaflet, especially in patients with small LV cavity. Another cause of acute worsening of MR is LVOT obstruction, which may occur in patients with severe septal hypertrophy. Annular rupture is a rare, but catastrophic complication of the TAVI procedure. It should be systematically suspected in any hypotension or pericardial effusion occurring without other explanation. TEE is usually the modality of choice to detect and evaluate this complication. In the case of contained rupture, peri-aortic annular hematoma may be observed as a tissue-density mass around the annulus of variable thickness, without flow. Partial rupture may result in abnormal flow with Colour Doppler toward the left or right ventricle [28, 29].

References

1. Jabbour A, Ismail TF, Moat N, et al. Multimodality imaging in transcatheter aortic valve implantation and post-procedural aortic regurgitation: comparison among cardiovascular magnetic resonance, cardiac computed tomography, and echocardiography. J Am Coll Cardiol. 2011;58:2165–73.
2. Nishimura RA, Otto CM, Bonow RO, et al. 2014 AHA/ACC guideline for the management of patients with valvular heart disease: executive summary: a report of the American College of Cardiology/American Heart Association Task Force on Practice Guidelines. Circulation. 2014;129:2440–92.
3. Joint Task Force on the Management of Valvular Heart Disease of the European Society of Cardiology (ESC); European Association for Cardio-Thoracic Surgery (EACTS), Vahanian A, Alfieri O, Andreotti F, et al. Guidelines on the management of valvular heart disease (version 2012). Eur Heart J. 2012;33:2451–96.
4. Garbi M, Chambers J, Vannan MA, Lancellotti P. Valve stress echocardiography: a practical guide for referral, procedure, reporting, and clinical implementation of results from the HAVEC Group. JACC Cardiovasc Imaging. 2015;8:724–36.
5. Garcia J, Capoulade R, Le VF, et al. Discrepancies between cardiovascular magnetic resonance and Doppler echocardiography in the measurement of transvalvular gradient in aortic stenosis: the effect of flow vorticity. J Cardiovasc Magn Reson. 2013;15:84.
6. Dulgheru R, Pibarot P, Sengupta PP, et al. Multimodality imaging strategies for the assessment of aortic stenosis: viewpoint of the Heart Valve Clinic International Database (HAVEC) Group. Circ Cardiovasc Imaging. 2016;9:e004352. https://doi.org/10.1161/CIRCIMAGING.115.004352.
7. Schoenhagen P, Tuzcu EM, Kapadia SR, et al. Three-dimensional imaging of the aortic valve and aortic root with computed tomography: new standards in an era of transcatheter valve repair/implantation. Eur Heart J. 2009;30:2079–86.
8. Hahn RT. Transcathether valve replacement and valve repair: review of procedures and intraprocedural echocardiographic imaging. Circ Res. 2016;119:341–56.

9. Calleja A, Thavendiranathan P, Ionasec RI, et al. Automated quantitative 3-dimensional modeling of the aortic valve and root by 3-dimensional transesophageal echocardiography in normals, aortic regurgitation, and aortic stenosis: comparison to computed tomography in normals and clinical implications. Circ Cardiovasc Imaging. 2013;6:99–108.
10. Kasel AM, Cassese S, Bleiziffer S, et al. Standardized imaging for aortic annular sizing: implications for transcatheter valve selection. JACC Cardiovasc Imaging. 2013;6:249–62.
11. Hansson NC, Norgaard BL, Barbanti M, et al. The impact of calcium volume and distribution in aortic root injury related to balloon-expandable transcatheter aortic valve replacement. J Cardiovasc Comput Tomogr. 2015;9:382–92.
12. Qian Z, Lancellotti P, Vannan MA. Aortic root calcium burden and post-transcatheter aortic valve implantation paravalvular leak: Can't Live Without It, Can't Live With It. Eur Heart J Cardiovasc Imaging. 2017;18:654–6.
13. Binder RK, Leipsic J, Wood D, et al. Prediction of optimal deployment projection for transcatheter aortic valve replacement: angiographic 3-dimensional reconstruction of the aortic root versus multidetector computed tomography. Circ Cardiovasc Interv. 2012;5:247–52.
14. Zamorano JL, Badano LP, Bruce C, Chan KL, Goncalves A, Hahn RT, et al. EAE/ASE recommendations for the use of echocardiography in new transcatheter interventions for valvular heart disease. Eur Heart J. 2011;32:2189–214.
15. Zamorano J, Gonçalves A, Lancellotti P, et al. The use of imaging in new transcatheter interventions: an EACVI review paper. Eur Heart J Cardiovasc Imaging. 2016;17(8):835–835af. pii: jew043.
16. Bloomfield GS, Gillam LD, Hahn RT, Kapadia S, Leipsic J, Lerakis S, et al. A practical-guide to multimodality imaging of transcatheter aortic valve replacement. JACC Cardiovasc Imaging. 2012;5:441–55.
17. Hahn RT, Little S, Monaghan MJ, et al. Recommendations for comprehensive intraprocedural echocardiographic imaging during TAVR. JACC Cardiovasc Imaging. 2015;8:261–87.
18. Sengupta P, Wiley B, Basnet S, et al. Transthoracicechocardiography guidance for TAVR under monitored anesthesia care. JACC Cardiovasc Imaging. 2015;8:379–80.
19. Bartel T, Edris A, Velik-Salchner C, Müller S. Intracardiac echocardiography for guidance of transcatheter aortic valve implantation under monitored sedation: a solution to a dilemma? Eur Heart J Cardiovasc Imaging. 2016;17:1–8.
20. Ng AC, Delgado V, van der Kley F, et al. Comparison of aortic root dimensions and geometriesbefore and after transcatheter aortic valveimplantation by 2- and 3-dimensional transesophageal echocardiography and multislicecomputed tomography. Circ Cardiovasc Imaging. 2010;3:94–102.
21. Bagur R, Rodés-Cabau J, Doyle D, et al. Usefulness of TEE as the primary imaging technique to guide transcatheter transapical aortic valve implantation. JACC Cardiovasc Imaging. 2011;4:115–24.
22. Hahn RT, Gillam LD, Little SH, et al. Echocardiographic imaging of procedural complications during self-expandable transcatheter aortic valve replacement. JACC Cardiovasc Imaging. 2015;8:319–36.
23. Détaint D, Lepage L, Himbert D, et al. Determinants of significant paravalvular regurgitation after transcatheter aorticvalve implantation: impact of device and annulus discongruence. JACC Cardiovasc Interv. 2009;2:821–7.
24. Eggebrecht H, Doss M, Schmermund A, Nowak B, Krissel J, Voigtlander T. Interventional options for severe aortic regurgitation aftertranscatheter aortic valve implantation: balloons, snares, valve-in-valve. Clin Res Cardiol. 2012;101:503–7.
25. Kappetein AP, Head SJ, Genereux P, Piazza N, van Mieghem NM, et al. Updated standardized endpoint definitions for transcatheter aortic valve implantation: the Valve Academic Research Consortium-2 consensus document. J Am Coll Cardiol. 2012;60:1438–54.
26. Pibarot P, Hahn RT, Weissman NJ, Monaghan MJ. Assessment of paravalvular regurgitationfollowing TAVR: a proposal of unifying grading scheme. JACC Cardiovasc Imaging. 2015;8:340–60.

27. Sinning JM, et al. Aortic regurgitation index defines severity of peri-prostheticregurgitation and predicts outcomein patients after transcatheter aorticvalve implantation. J Am Coll Cardiol. 2012;59:1134–41.
28. Pasic M, Unbehaun A, Buz S, Drews T, Hetzer R. Annular rupture during transcatheter aortic valve replacement: classification, pathophysiology, diagnostics, treatment approaches, and prevention. JACC Cardiovasc Interv. 2015;8:1–9.
29. Genereux P, Reiss GR, Kodali SK, et al. Periaortic hematoma after transcatheter aortic valve replacement: description of a newcomplication. Catheter Cardiovasc Interv. 2012;79:766–76.

22 Transfemoral TAVI: Devices and Techniques

Thomas Modine and Khalil Fattouch

22.1 Introduction

Trans-catheter aortic valve implantation (TAVI) has first been described with a trans-venous and trans-septal pathway by Cribier et al. [1], but it really expanded when the transfemoral arterial retrograde approach was described [2]. Ever since it has generated a tremendous enthusiasm in the interventional cardiology community and the industry. New prostheses, delivery systems, pathways, equipment, software and guidelines stemmed from this enthusiasm. Transfemoral TAVI has been favoured because of its low invasiveness and remains the first-choice pathway. In this chapter we will review the currently existing devices and techniques used for transfemoral TAVI, before reviewing some recent advances and results of this technique.

22.2 Transfemoral Access

22.2.1 Percutaneous Transfemoral Access

Before the procedure patient's anatomy will be thoroughly investigated by means of the pre-operative CT-scan (Computerized Tomography) notably for choosing valve type and size, confirm vascular access eligibility (minimum diameter sufficient, no excessive tortuosity), and coronary angiography to rule out patent obstructive coronary artery disease.

TAVI is usually performed in a hybrid operating room designed and equipped to perform both open surgical and interventional procedures. In particular, fluoroscope is

T. Modine (✉)
Centre Hospitalier Régional Universitaire de Lille, Lille 59000, France
e-mail: t1modine@yahoo.fr

K. Fattouch
GVM Care and Research, Cardiovascular Department, Maria Eleonora Hospital, Palermo, Italy

K. Fattouch et al. (eds.), *Advances in Treatments for Aortic Valve and Root Diseases*, https://doi.org/10.1007/978-3-319-66483-5_22

mandatory to guide operators' movements throughout the procedure. Transfemoral TAVI (TF TAVI) is often performed by a multi-disciplinary team including an interventional cardiologist, a cardiac surgeon, a cardiac anaesthesiologist, a radiology technician and two interventional assistants. At least one member of the team must be trained in preparation and loading of the valve device, which is performed on the ancillary table while the main operators access the aortic valve. Some teams use transesophageal echocardiography during de procedure, performed by a trained cardiologist. Make sure the patches are installed and connected to the defibrillator before scrubbing. Preference for sedation with local anaesthesia or general anaesthesia is team-dependant.

The technical steps to perform a percutaneous transfemoral TAVI are as follows (the steps are often performed at the same time by the different operators):

- 5Fr femoral vein sheath is inserted for transvenous pacemaker insertion (usually the left femoral vein). The pacemaker wire will be placed in the right ventricle and its capture will be checked by stimulating at a frequency over the rest heart rate (120/min)
- 6Fr femoral arterial sheath is inserted in the femoral artery (usually the right common femoral artery) to constitute the secondary arterial access. A 7F catheter can be warranted if invasive blood pressure is to be monitored through the same access. An echographic guidance can be used to guide the appropriate location for puncture (avoiding calcifications and tortuosity). Radial access for secondary arterial access has been described [3, 4]. A 0,035″ J-tipped soft guidewire (GuideRight™ 0.035″ × 260 cm length, tip 3 mm J-FS) is inserted to guide the pigtail catheter placed into the noncoronary cusp for procedural aortography.
- Puncture the controlateral femoral artery (usually the right common femoral artery) is performed with standard percutaneous vascular sheath-kit needle and a 7Fr sheath is inserted to consitute the primary access. Echography-guided or angiography-guided puncture is chosen according to team preferences. To perform an angiography-guided puncture position a catheter from the contralateral side inject small volumes of contrast to visualize the common femoral artery
- Pre-closure sutures are deployed using a percutaneous closure device (Perclose ProGlide® or Prostar®, Abbott, Inc., Santa Clara, CA, USA) and threads are marked with pliers
- Intravenous unfractionated heparin is administered to achieve an activated clotting time of 250 s
- A 14-F 30-cm standard sheath was advanced into the patient. This access was used to cross the aortic valve, followed by positioning of a pre-shaped stiff support wire in the LV
- A 0,035″ J-tipped soft guidewire (GuideRight™ 0.035″ × 260 cm length, tip 3 mm J-FS) is used to guide the advance of a pigtail catheter (AL1 or JR4 catheters can be switched to, according to crossing difficulties). Switch the J-tipped guidewire for a straight-tip guidewire to cross the aortic valve. The crossing step can be difficult and demand persistance.
- When the crossing is achieved push the catheter into the left ventricle then switch the straight soft guidewire for a stiff guidewire (SAFARI pre-shaped TAVI guidewire 0.035 in. × 300 cm, Boston Scientific Marlborough, MA, USA or Amplatz extra stiff 0.035-in. guidewire, Cook, Inc., Bloomington, Indiana)

- If deemed appropriate (severely calcified aortic valve) aortic balloon valvuloplasty is performed using a balloon (Nucleus™ 20 mm diameter), filled with contrast diluted with saline (1:2 ratio) during rapid ventricular pacing 160–180/min rate (RVP)
- The prosthesis implantation procedure is specific to each device (see next section)
- After the prosthesis implantation delivery system is retrieved
- The femoral access site is closed percutaneously using the pre-installed sutures (ProGlide® or Prostar®)
- Verifying angiographycally that the main vascular access for absence of vascular leak and vessel patency is not mandatory but routine for some teams
- The temporary pacemaker is retrieved immediately whenever possible unless there is a high risk for post-operative complete atrio-ventricular block (keep 24–48 h to revaluate) or the patient is stimulo-dependent to wait for a permanent pacemaker implantation

Uncomplicated procedures last a mean 45 min. Immediate extubation is warranted in the operating room if the patient is haemodynamically stable. Post-operative care involves monitoring in the intensive care unit for 24 h which includes echocardiographic evaluation looking for tamponade and prosthesis dysfunction.

22.2.2 Specific Features of the Surgical Transfemoral Access

In certain cases, percutaneous femoral main access can be difficult in case of severe frontal calcifications, severe tortuosity, very obese patients, presence of femoral graft or stent. Spot the femoral artery by feeling the pulse. A transverse incision (approximatively 3–5 cm length) is made above and parallel to the inguinal ligament. The common femoral artery is accessed in a standard fashion. When the artery is cleared puncture and the rest of the procedure is performed as a percutaneous procedure. After the valve is successfully deployed, the sheath and guidewire are removed while compressing the femoral artery above the access, and the edges of the vessel are debrided. Then the vessel is seamed and the surgical access is close in a standard fashion. Upon access vessel closure, conclusion peripheral angiography is sometimes performed to assess for any vascular complications including stenosis, dissection, or perforation.

22.3 Devices

Six CE-marked valves available for transfemoral TAVI are currently used:

- Sapien 3™
- CoreValve Evolut R™
- Acurate TF™
- Lotus™
- Direct Flow Medical™
- Portico™

Numerous other devices are under development. In this section, we will focus on the CE-approved devices. Two percutaneous main percutaneous closure devices (Prolide® and Prostar®) and neuroprotection are also presented.

22.3.1 Edwards Sapien 3

The latest valve from the Edwards Sapien™ (Edwards Lifesciences) family is the Sapien 3, which is the fourth generation in this family of balloon-expandable transcatheter heart valves. For transfemoral approach it is implanted by use of the Commander™ delivery system (Edwards Lifesciences). Bovine pericardial tissue is affixed to a radiopaque stainless steel stent frame. One of the main additional features of the Sapien 3 when compared to its predecessors is the outer PET (polyethylene terephthalate) sealing cuff intended to reduce paravalvular regurgitation. Three valve sizes are available (23 mm, 26 mm and 29 mm) to cover area-derived aortic diameter 20.7–29.5 mm and area 338–683 mm^2 The delivery system requires a 14F expandable introducer sheath (eSheath, Edwards Lifesciences, Inc.) size (5.5 mm diameter vessel) for the 23 and 26 mm prostheses, and 16F (6 mm diameter vessel) for the 29 mm valve.

The implantation of the Sapien 3 prosthesis is rather simple:

- The prosthesis is compressed before being inserted in the delivery catheter with specifically dedicated material and positioned on a valvuloplasty balloon
- Pre-dilation with a valvuloplasty balloon can be warranted according to certain operator
- The delivery system inserted through the femoral artery sheath. The prosthesis is loaded onto the balloon in the abdominal aorta. Then the delivery system crosses the aortic valve being guided by the superstiff guidewire and the Sapien 3 prosthesis is positioned with help from the balloon central radiopaque marker. When the position of the prosthesis is deemed optimal and under mandatory rapid ventricular pacing (RVP) the prosthesis is decompressed by inflating the balloon it is on. Full inflation is preserved for 5 s (to prevent later recoil). RVP is mandatory because the balloon obstructs the left ventricle outflow tract.

The CE mark of Sapien 3 was obtains in 2014 and it is extensively used in various centres worldwide (Fig. 22.1).

22.3.2 CoreValve Evolut R

The CoreValve® EvolutR™ device (Medtronic, Minneapolis, MN, USA) consists of a trileaflet porcine pericardial valve sewn in a supravalvular position in a nitinol self-expanding framework. This prosthesis is implanted through the EnVeo™ delivery system integrated 14 Fr InLine™ sheath (Medtronic). The valve leaflets are in a

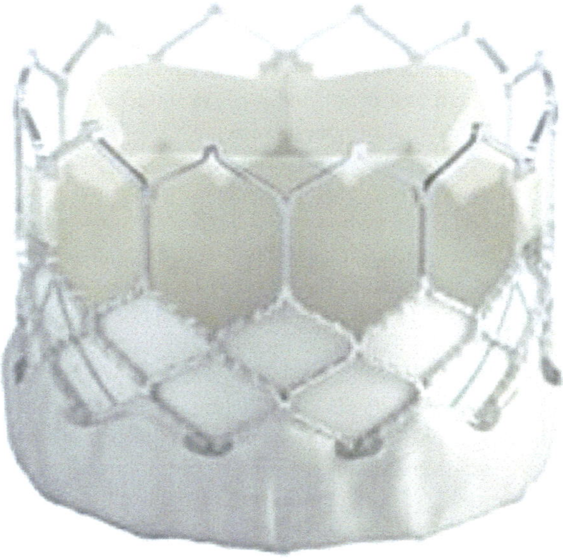

Fig. 22.1 Edwards Sapien 3™ prosthesis

supra-annular position aiming at maximising the effective orifice area. The frame is smaller than the previous CoreValve (45 mm height). A 12 mm porcine pericardium skirt is present around the inflow segment designed to protect against paravalvular leakage. The valve is fully repositionable and retrievable up to approximately 90% of total deployment. Three valve sizes are currently available (23, 26 and 29 mm) covering a range of aortic annular diameters from 18 to 28 mm according to manufacturer's instructions. The 14 Fr InLine™ sheath (true outer 18 Fr) is compatible with vessel sizes >5 mm ("sheathless" insertion).

CoreValve Evolut R implantation specific steps are as follows:

- Predilation can be performed prior to prosthesis implantation (recommended by the manufacturer)
- The 14-F sheath used for aortic valve crossing and predilatation is removed, taking care of maintaining stiffwire position in the left ventricle. The EnVeo delivery system with the InLine sheath is advanced, with the Evolut R valve loaded, into the patient. When in the aorta check by mean of fluroscopy with zoom that the prosthesis is appropriately mounted. Then advance the delivery system through the aortic valve and position the prosthesis for deployment
- An implant depth between 1 and 5 mm was recommended. Proceed with deployment from distal to proximal by progressively retrieving the prosthesis sheath in an anterograde fashion while slightly pushing the delivery system so the prosthesis maintains position. Resheath the prosthesis if you need to reposition, it is possible up until release. Retrieve the pigtail when you are halfway through the deployment.

- When the prosthesis is fully deployed perform aortic angiogram to confirm coronary artery patency and look for prosthetic leaks. If a moderate to severe periprosthetic leak is present, consider post-dilation.
- When the result is optimal retrieve the EnVeo delivery system and inLine sheath and perform percutaneous closure.

The CoreValve Evolut R received the CE mark in 2015.

ACURATE TF Symetis: ACURATE-neo aortic bioprosthesis is a second generation implanted through the ACURATE-TF transfemoral delivery system, composed of a porcine pericardial tissue valve sewn into a self-expanding Nitinol™ stent covered on the inside and outside, and a skirt of porcine pericardial which aims at prevent periprosthetic leaks. The stent is composed of two main segments: the valve segment and the "stabilisation arches". The body of the stent includes an "upper crown" of the prosthesis which is the distal part of the valve segment, it is meant to embrace the native calcified leaflets while providing supra-annular anchoring, as well as "tactile feedback" during deployment. The "lower crown" is the stent edge that minimally resides within the left ventricular outflow tract. The three "stabilisation arches" at the distal edge of the stent aim at preventing tilting of the prosthesis during final deployment. Three sizes (23, 25, 27 mm) are currently available to cover perimeter from 66 to 79, and area 346 to 573 mm^2. ACURATE neo obtained CE mark in 2014.

Implantation steps:

- After the insertion of a transfemoral introducer sheath (15F balloon-expandable or 18F rigid sheath), the ACURATE-TF delivery catheter is advanced across the aortic valve. The prosthesis-loader is usually placed 4–6 mm below the aortic annulus.
- First step: the upper-crown is opened to towards the native aortic leaflets deflecting them downward (away from the coronary ostia). With the pigtail catheter placed in the noncoronary cusp an aortography will guide the positioning.
- Second: the stabilization arches are released to contact the aortic root to prevent the tilting of the prosthesis during the final deployment.
- Finally: release the lower-crown and the valve self-expands. This transcatheter prosthesis theoretically does not require rapid ventricular pacing for its deployment. Perform aortic root angiography to confirm coronary artery patency look for paravalvular leak. In case of moderate or severe paravalvular leak consider post-dilation.

22.3.3 Lotus and Lotus Edge

The Lotus™ valve system (Boston Scientific, Marlborough, MA, USA) is trileaflet bovine pericardial valve sewn on a braided nitinol framework, mechanically expanded. Gradually decreasing in size during expansion it is measured 70 mm when fully sheathed, 35 mm upon unsheathing and 19 mm at release. A central tantanium radiopaque marker facilitating the positioning of the prosthesis within the aortic root. The inflow segment is covered with a polymeric outer adaptive seal aiming at reducing paravalvular leaks. The valve is connected to the inner catheter by three coupling fingers, ending with a connecting collar and buckles, and interacting with posts related to the commissures of the tissue valve. The design makes possible to assess the valve function, coronary artery patency, look for paravalvular leakage after the valve is positioned but before being released. The Lotus valve can be fully repositioned or retrieved at any moment until the final release of the three coupling fingers. Rapid pacing is not required during implantation, and the valve functions early in deployment. The Lotus valve comes in three sizes (23, 25 and 27 mm), covering a range of annular diameters from 19 to 27 mm. The delivery system has an 18–20 Fr profile, requiring a vessel size >6 mm, and is covered with hydrophilic coating. The Lotus prosthesis received CE-mark in 2013. The Lotus Edge™ is its very recently (2016) CE-marked upgrade.

The implantation steps are as follows:

- Pre-dilation before Lotus valve implantation is possible.
- Appropriate valve positioning is achieved by positioning the posts (distal part of the locking mechanism) over the predetermined aortic valve landing plane. An aortogram will confirm the coronary artery patency and absence of paravalvular leak.
- Before final release perform stability tests to confirm stable anchoring in the annulus (Fig. 22.2).

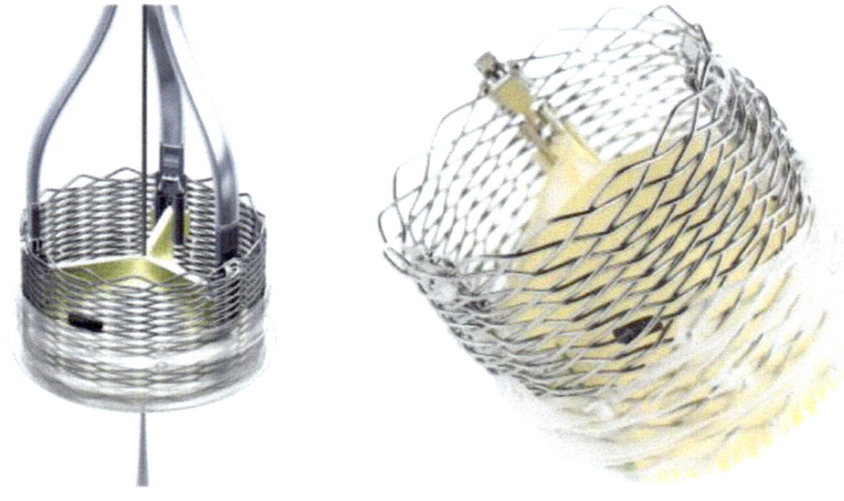

Fig. 22.2 (**a**) Lotus™ valve, (**b**) Lotus Edge™ valve

22.3.4 Direct Flow Medical

The Direct Flow Medical™ (Direct Flow Medical, Santa Rosa, California) consists in bovine pericardial tissue attached to a non-metallic polymer frame with Dacron polyester cuff. The frame is made up from flexible vertical tubular pillars connecting two inflatable polyester rings (one aortic and one ventricular). The rings are deflable for repositioning. The Direct Flow Medical valve comes in four sizes (23, 25, 27 and 29 mm), covering annular diameters from 21 to 29 mm. The prosthesis is inserted through a 18-Fr catheter-based, three-armed delivery system. No rapid ventricular pacing is required.

The implantation follows these main steps [5]:

- The system is unsheathed in the left ventricle followed by inflation of the ventricular ring with radiopaque solution and retraction of the device into the aortic root until the ventricular ring anchors below the aortic annulus.
- The aortic ring is positioned above the aortic leaflets and below the coronary ostia. Three positioning wires allow prosthesis manipulation before inflation of the aortic ring. An aortogram allows patency control of the coronary arteries and absence of paravalvular leakage.
- The device can be repositioned or retrieved by deflating both rings if device depth is unsatisfactory. For retrieval both ring balloons are deflated and the valve is pulled into a Nitinol basket (Direct Flow Medical, Santa Rosa, California) in the abdominal aorta and retrieved through the introducer sheath.
- Once the correct device position is confirmed, a quick curing polymer is instilled (instead of the radiopaque solution) to allow permanent implantation. Then the valve is released by detaching the positioning wires.

The Direct Flow Medical valve received CE-mark approval in 2013 (Fig. 22.3).

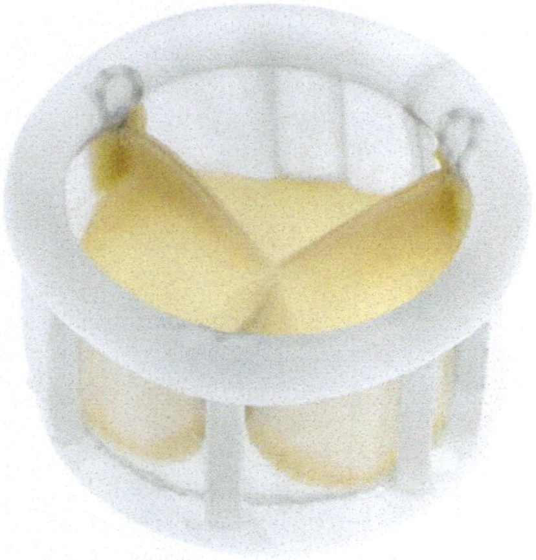

Fig. 22.3 Direct Flow Medical™ prosthesis

22.3.5 Portico

The Portico™ prosthesis (St. Jude Medical, St. Paul, MN, USA) is an intra-annular trileaflet bovine pericardial valve mounted inside a nitinol self-expanding stent. The tubular inflow portion has a porcine pericardial sealing cuff aiming at reducing peri-prosthetic leakage. The outflow segment consists of a large open cell that extends towards the ascending aorta to provide stability. The Portico is repositionable and retrievable up to 85% of deployment. Four sizes are available (23, 25, 27 and 29 mm, measuring from 49 to 53 mm height) but only the 23 and 25 mm valves have been clinically tested so far. These sizes mean to cover annular diameters ranging from 19 to 27 mm. The transfemoral delivery system is a 18 Fr (for the two smaller sizes) or 19 Fr catheter (for the two larger sizes). The valve can also be implanted using a 19 Fr SoloPath™ sheath (Terumo Europe NV, Leuven, Belgium). No rapid ventricular pacing is required.

After positioning the delivery sheath in the aortic valve deploy the Portico valve by progressively retrieving the sheath in an anterograde fashion with the expansion and sealing of the inflow segment. The valve is designed have a sub-annular placement with an intended depth of implant (1–9 mm) without extending more than 6 mm into the left ventricle outflow tract. When the 80% deployment mark is reached, confirmation is needed before pursuing. The Portico valve received CE-mark successively for its different sizes from 2012 to 2015. Today all four sizes are marked (Fig. 22.4).

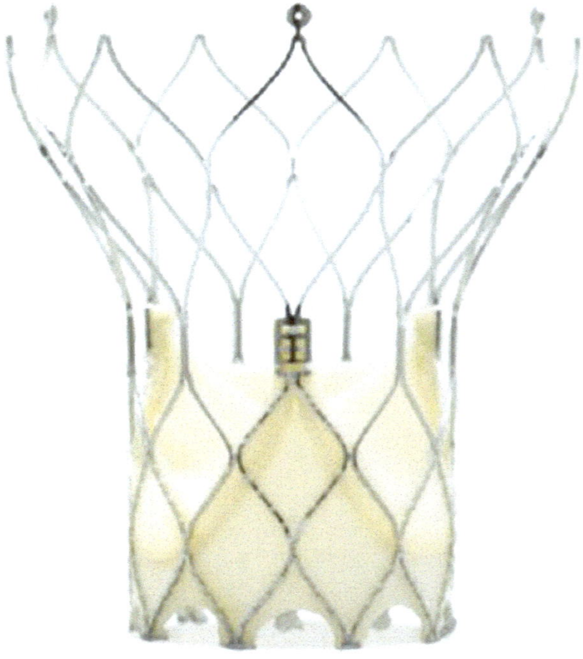

Fig. 22.4 Portico™ prosthesis

22.3.6 Percutaneous Closure Devices

Superiority of one over the other between Proglide® and Prostar® (Abbott, Inc., Santa Clara, CA, USA) is subject to debate in terms of effectiveness, safety, cost. Both devices are effective in closing the vascular access and the two-Proglide® versus one Prostar® seems to have a small advantage [6] but blindly testing the two approaches in a randomised controlled trial would be difficult.

The Proglide closure device is a 6 Fr, two nitinol needle-guided suture-mediated closure system designed for closing the femoral artery access site in patients undergoing catheterisation procedures using sheaths under 21 Fr. For sheath sizes >8 Fr, a double Proglide technique is recommended. The Prostar closure device is a 10 Fr, four nitinol needle-guided device designed for artery access-site closure following procedures using 8.5–24 Fr sheaths.

To percutaneously close a TAVI main arterial access with the Proglide device it is advanced over the guidewire with a 45° angle until passing the vessel wall (a jolt is felt) with the dedicated marker lumen showing blood marking. Unlock the anchor and slightly retrieve the device to the vascular wall. The first suture is then deployed. After removing the anchor retrieve the device and gather the sutures and mark them with pliers. Guidewire access is maintained, and a second Proglide device is inserted and deployed. After the valve implantation, the introducer sheath is slowly removed, with manual compression if needed, but the guidewire is left to maintain access. The sutures are tightened. In case of sufficient haemostasis, the guidewire can be removed and the sutures are further tightened using the knot pusher. Should haemostasis fail, it is possible to implant a third (or fourth) Proglide over the guidewire.

To perform a percutaneous closure the 10-F Prostar device is advanced over the guidewire until the dedicated marker lumen shows blood marking indicating that the sutures and needles are within the vessel lumen. The four needles are pulled back with metallic pliers while maintaining the position and entry angle of the Prostar device. The sutures are removed from the hub. Identify the upper and lower sets of sutures with pliers. The device is retracted, and the guidewire is reinserted. Then the device is removed. The sutures are tied with a sliding knot (Fig. 22.5).

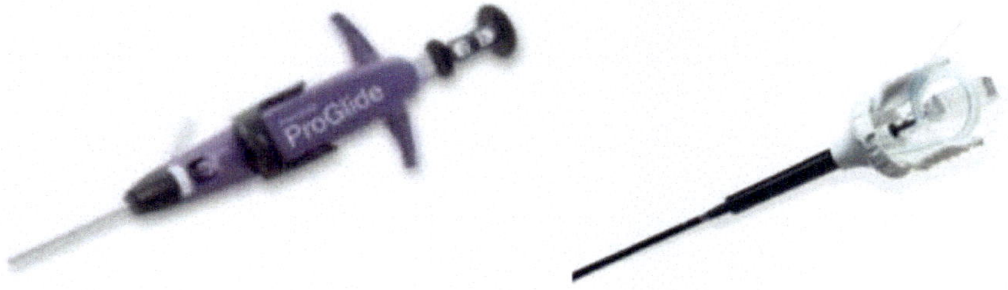

Fig. 22.5 (**a**) Proglide®, (**b**) Prostar®

22.3.7 Neuroprotection

No neuroprotection device used during the procedures has so far provided evidence of better clinical outcomes (clinical stroke) with cerebral protection devices despite surrogate endpoints (cerebral imaging) to be in favour of these devices [7–9].

Embrella Embolic Deflector® system (Edwards Lifesciences, Irvine, California) consists of an oval-shaped nitinol frame covered with a porous polyurethane membrane that is positioned at the level of the aortic arch.

Sentinel® transcatheter cerebral embolic protection device (Claret Medical, Santa Rosa, CA, USA). The Sentinel device consists of two filters within a single 6 Fr delivery catheter percutaneously placed from the right radial or brachial artery over a 0.014″ guide wire. The filters are positioned in the brachiocephalic and the left common carotid arteries before TAVI and removed after the procedure.

TriGuard HDH® embolic deflection device (Keystone Heart Ltd., Caesarea, IL, USA) is a biocompatible filter made of fine nitinol (nickel titanium alloy) wires, which is delivered transfemorally via a 9 Fr Mullins introducer sheath, positioned in the aortic arch, and anchored in position by an atraumatic stabilizer in the ostium of the innominate artery. The filter portion of the device covers the brachiocephalic, left common carotid, and subclavian arteries, maintaining blood flow to the cerebral vessels through 130 μm pores while deflecting larger emboli to the descending aorta. The filter is coated with an anti-thrombotic coating (SurModics, Inc. Eden Prairie, MN, USA) (Fig. 22.6).

22.4 Complications

Complications of transfemoral TAVI are numerous and can be related to the prosthesis, the procedure, the vascular access, contrast media, irradiation, anaesthesia, post-operative and intensive care.

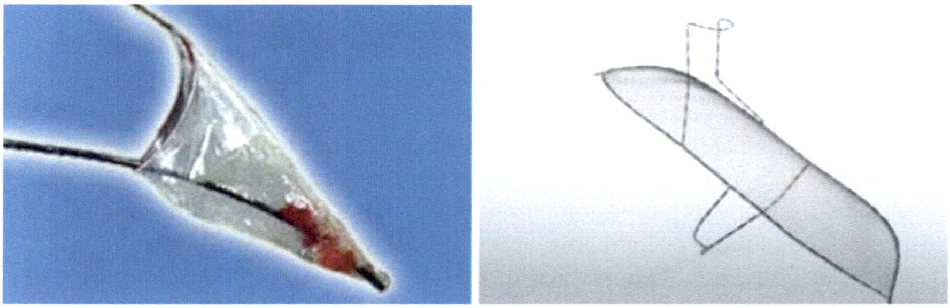

Fig. 22.6 (**a**) Sentinel®, (**b**) TriGuard®

Peri-procedural and 30-day mortality is less and less observed in recent trials probably due to a better selection of patients (low and intermediate surgical risk instead of inoperable and high risk patients), improvement in devices and operator skills, up to 1% in the most recent studies [10]. Improvement must be further pursued to enhance this major safety outcome.

Peri-procedural strokes are another major issue with TAVI. During the procedure valve fragments of tissue and calcification are detached because of the primitive valve manipulation. These fragments can embolize into the brain.

Pacemaker rates are prosthesis-dependant. Predictive factors for pacemaker use during long-term follow-up are not clearly elucidated yet. Pre-existing right bundle branch block is a pre-operative predictor of complete atrio-ventricular block after TAVI and the majority of post-TAVI complete atrio-ventricular blocks appeared with one week in a meta-analysis published in 2012 with the first-generation valves [11].

Although primary prosthesis dysfunction is rare (special attention is warranted with new devices that have not yet been extensively used) but paravalvular leaks are a major concern for patients and a concurrence topic for the industry. Multiple studies associated moderate to severe leaks to long term increased mortality [10, 11] but constant progress of the devices reduced the rate of significant post-procedural leaks. Kodali et al. reported a 3.4% rate of moderate post-TAVI leaks (without any severe leak) with Sapien 3 in a recent cohort [12]. Long-term function of the TAVI bioprostheses also seem to be favourable with stable prosthesis haemodynamic parameters 5 years after Sapien and CoreValve prostheses in two cohorts [13, 14].

Infective endocarditis is rare but real with TAVI devices with an approximative rate of 1% per person-year with a median time to event of 5.3 month after the procedure but is associated with a poor prognosis. Enterococci species and Staphylococcus aureus were the most frequently isolated microorganisms [15].

22.5 Indications and Patient Selection

TAVI has been developed to treat severe symptomatic aortic stenosis which remains its main indication. The last European Society of Cardiology guidelines on the treatment of aortic valve diseases were published in 2012 and recommended the use of TAVI in high risk patients with severe aortic stenosis (class IIaB) with life-expectancy of more than 1 year, with indication validated by the "Heart Team". More recently the American Heart Association and American College of Cardiology recommended in 2014 in patients who meet an indication for AVR for AS who have a prohibitive surgical risk and a predicted post-TAVR survival superior to 1 year (class IB) and as an alternative to surgical replacement in high-risk patients (class IIaB). Recent data from PARTNER-2 trial and others provided arguments to extend indications to intermediate surgical risk patients and ongoing trials will reliably test TAVI in low risk patients (disposable literature is encouraging). New guidelines are eagerly awaited in 2017.

Guidelines do not address the question of the appropriate approach for TAVI. Although trans-femoral access provides the best results (in terms of mortality, vascular access complications, bleeding) than other, more invasive, approaches, some patients cannot benefit from the optimal trans-femoral approach. This may be due to vessel diameter < 5 mm, heavily calcified vessels, tortuosity and significant abdominal and thoracic aortic disease. Up to 35% of patients eligible for TAVI have an unsuitable peripheral artery anatomy [16].

When a patient is considered eligible to TAVI he shall undergo pre-operative evaluation to validate feasibility:

- Coronary artery angiography: to look for frequent concomitant coronary artery disease. When warranted percutaneous coronary intervention is recommended prior to TAVI because of the risk of an impossible (or complex) access to coronary arteries after the prosthesis is implanted [17]. Other valuable information can be gathered: the ascending aorta can be measured (looking for aortic aneurysm), transaortic hemodynamic gradient, and the ilio-femoral vessels are evaluated for diameter, tortuosity, calcification to contemplate trans-femoral access.
- Cervico-thoraco-abdomino-pelvic and proximal lower limbs CT-scan with contrast injection: is nowadays mandatory, unless contraindicated. It provides important information for valve sizing (usually treated with dedicated software), calcification assessment, ascending aorta measurements, and peripheral vessel anatomy to choose the appropriate approach (iliofemoral, carotid, subclavian). Carotid anatomy is also to be considered because of frequent (up to 33%) [18] concomitant severe lesions that need to be addressed before cardiac procedures.
- Echocardiography: to exclude significant associated valvulopathy requiring intervention. Concomitant mitral valvulopathy (regurgitation or stenosis) is frequently present in elderly patients with severe aortic stenosis, but unless it is severe should not be considered as a contraindication to aortic valve implantation. If the mitral valvulopathy is severe, surgical replacement under cardiopulmonary bypass should be reconsidered by the "Heart Team".

In conclusion, eligible patients to transfemoral TAVI regroup one or several of the following criteria:

- High risk and inoperable patients with severe symptomatic aortic stenosis should be considered for TAVI according to currently used guidelines. Intermediate risk patients shall be discussed for aortic valve replacement with the "Heart Team".
- With a suitable anatomy for trans-femoral access: common femoral artery diameter >5 mm, no heavily calcified vessels, no excessive tortuosity or significant abdominal and thoracic aortic disease

22.6 Results of Transfemoral TAVI

22.6.1 Sapien Family and CoreValve

TAVI has been found to be non-inferior to surgical aortic valve replacement (SAVR) of severe aortic stenosis in PARTNER 1 high risk trial, superior to standard treatment including aortic valvuloplastyin inoperable patients. Transfemoral (TF) TAVI was superior to SAVR in intermediate risk patients in the PARTNER 2 trial. A meta-analysis of all-risk patients considering four randomised controlled studies (PARTNER 1A, US CoreValve High Risk, NOTION, PARTNER 2) found a significant 13% relative risk reduction of 2-year all-cause death in favour of TAVI regarding SAVR (HR 95%CI: 0.87 (0.76–0.99), p = 0.038 that was all-the-more pronounced in the TF TAVI (excluding the complex surgical pathways) with a 20% relative risk reduction (HR 0.80 (0.69–0.93), p = 0.04). The same meta-analysis on the other hand showed no difference in terms of stroke, and more new pacemaker implantations and paravalvular regurgitations with TAVI [19–23].

Thourani et al. recently found superiority of TAVI with the Sapien 3 prosthesis over SAVR in intermediate risk patients in terms of 1-year all-cause death (−5.2%, −8.0 to −2.4; p = 0.0003) and stroke (−3.5%, −5.9 to −1.1; p = 0.0038). But SAVR was still superior to TAVR for moderate or severe aortic regurgitation (1.2%, 0.2 to 2.2; p = 0.0149).

Never-the-less 5-year all-cause mortality after the Sapien valve has been reported to be as high as 67.8% [14] and 55% after CoreValve [13] in high risk patients thus further progress must be pursued to enhance long term survival.

Some results have emerged regarding treatment of pure severe aortic regurgitation with CoreValve with mitigated results [24]. New devices are trying to respond to the challenge [25].

22.6.2 Second-Generation Valves

So far only registries have been published regarding the second-generation prostheses but randomised trials are ongoing for some of them.

A registry of twenty patients intermediate risk patients treated for severe aortic stenosis transfemoral ACURATE Neo reported favourable short term (30-day) outcomes with no mortality, no significant leaks, and one newly implanted pacemaker [26].

The REPRISE II prospective of 120 patients treated with the Lotus prosthesis showed a 30-day mortality rate of 4.2%, stroke of 5.9%, a high rate of new pacemaker implantations 28.6%, but a low rate of post-procedural significant leaks (only 1 moderate regurgitation). One-year mortality was 10.9% and strokes were observed in 9.2% of cases [27]. A randomised trial comparing the Lotus valve to the CoreValve is ongoing (NCT02202434).

A 102-patient prospective cohort treated with the Portico prosthesis showed a 2.9% rate of 30-day mortality, 7.8% rate of ischemic cerebral events (strokes and transient ischemic attacks) and 9.8% rate of new pacemakers [28].

Lefevre et al. recently published results observed on their prospective registry of 100 high risk patients. At 30 days mortality rate was low (1%), but the stroke rate was high (7%), same for the rate of implanted pacemakers (17%). One-year mortality and stroke were both 10%. No 1-year periprosthetic leaks were observed but one third of the patients were lost to follow-up [29].

Conclusion

Transfemoral TAVI has become over the years the new standard of care to treat severe aortic stenosis. Numerous technological advances have favoured this technique's positioning in the standard practice. These advances will further push the limits of the percutaneous aortic valve replacement procedures and probably its indications. New guidelines are warranted to address intermediate and low risk patients. But a recent survey reported that 45% of centres across Europe have already extended their TAVI practice to intermediate risk patients [30]. Nevertheless, some issues must be addressed including the high rate of pacemaker implantations, periprosthetic leaks, valve durability, bicuspid patients, anti-thrombotic regimen, TAVI-in-TAVI procedures. Luckily when time comes to talk about TAVI research has been particularly active and numerous studies are ongoing to address all these questions that will soon find answers.

References

1. Cribier A, Eltchaninoff H, Bash A, Borenstein N, Tron C, Bauer F, et al. Percutaneous transcatheter implantation of an aortic valve prosthesis for calcific aortic stenosis. Circulation. 2002;106(24):3006–8.
2. Webb JG, Chandavimol M, Thompson CR, Ricci DR, Carere RG, Munt BI, et al. Percutaneous aortic valve implantation retrograde from the femoral artery. Circulation. 2006;113(6):842–50.
3. Wynne DG, Rampat R, Trivedi U, de Belder A, Hill A, Hutchinson N, et al. Transradial Secondary Arterial Access for Transcatheter Aortic Valve Implantation: Experience and Limitations. Heart Lung Circ. 2015;24(7):682–5.
4. Allende R, Urena M, Cordoba JG, Ribeiro HB, Amat-Santos I, DeLarochellière R, et al. Impact of the use of transradial versus transfemoral approach as secondary access in transcatheter aortic valve implantation procedures. Am J Cardiol. 2014;114(11):1729–34.
5. Schofer J, Colombo A, Klugmann S, Fajadet J, DeMarco F, Tchétché D, et al. Prospective multicenter evaluation of the direct flow medical transcatheter aortic valve. J Am Coll Cardiol. 2014;63(8):763–8.
6. Mehilli J, Jochheim D, Abdel-Wahab M, Rizas KD, Theiss H, Spenkuch N, et al. One-year outcomes with two suture-mediated closure devices to achieve access-site haemostasis following transfemoral transcatheter aortic valve implantation. EuroIntervention. 2016;12(10): 1298–304.
7. Kapadia SR, Kodali S, Makkar R, Mehran R, Lazar RM, Zivadinov R, et al. Protection against cerebral embolism during transcatheter aortic valve replacement. J Am Coll Cardiol. 2017;69(4):367–77.
8. Rodés-Cabau J, Kahlert P, Neumann F-J, Schymik G, Webb JG, Amarenco P, et al. Feasibility and exploratory efficacy evaluation of the Embrella Embolic Deflector system for the prevention of cerebral emboli in patients undergoing transcatheter aortic valve replacement: the PROTAVI-C pilot study. JACC Cardiovasc Interv. 2014;7(10):1146–55.
9. Haussig S, Mangner N, Dwyer MG, Lehmkuhl L, Lücke C, Woitek F, et al. Effect of a cerebral protection device on brain lesions following transcatheter aortic valve implantation in patients with severe aortic stenosis: the CLEAN-TAVI randomized clinical trial. JAMA. 2016;316(6):592–601.
10. Vahanian A, Urena M, Walther T, Treede H, Wendler O, Lefèvre T, et al. Thirty-day outcomes in patients at intermediate risk for surgery from the SAPIEN 3 European approval trial. EuroIntervention. 2016;12(2):e235–43.

11. Erkapic D, De Rosa S, Kelava A, Lehmann R, Fichtlscherer S, Hohnloser SH. Risk for permanent pacemaker after transcatheter aortic valve implantation: a comprehensive analysis of the literature. J Cardiovasc Electrophysiol. 2012;23(4):391–7.
12. Kodali S, Thourani VH, White J, Malaisrie SC, Lim S, Greason KL, et al. Early clinical and echocardiographic outcomes after SAPIEN 3 transcatheter aortic valve replacement in inoperable, high-risk and intermediate-risk patients with aortic stenosis. Eur Heart J. 2016;37(28):2252–62.
13. Barbanti M, Petronio AS, Ettori F, Latib A, Bedogni F, De Marco F, et al. 5-year outcomes after transcatheter aortic valve implantation with corevalve prosthesis. JACC Cardiovasc Interv. 2015;8(8):1084–91.
14. Mack MJ, Leon MB, Smith CR, Miller DC, Moses JW, Tuzcu EM, et al. 5-year outcomes of transcatheter aortic valve replacement or surgical aortic valve replacement for high surgical risk patients with aortic stenosis (PARTNER 1): a randomised controlled trial. Lancet. 2015;385(9986):2477–84.
15. Regueiro A, Linke A, Latib A, Ihlemann N, Urena M, Walther T, et al. Association between transcatheter aortic valve replacement and subsequent infective endocarditis and in-hospital death. JAMA. 2016;316(10):1083–92.
16. Kurra V, Schoenhagen P, Roselli EE, Kapadia SR, Tuzcu EM, Greenberg R, et al. Prevalence of significant peripheral artery disease in patients evaluated for percutaneous aortic valve insertion: preprocedural assessment with multidetector computed tomography. J Thorac Cardiovasc Surg. 2009;137(5):1258–64.
17. Blumenstein J, Kim W-K, Liebetrau C, Gaede L, Kempfert J, Walther T, et al. Challenges of coronary angiography and intervention in patients previously treated by TAVI. Clin Res Cardiol. 2015;104(8):632–9.
18. Fusini L, Mirea O, Tamborini G, Muratori M, Gripari P, Cefalù C, et al. Incidence and severity of atherosclerotic cardiovascular artery disease in patients undergoing TAVI. Int J Cardiovasc Imaging. 2015;31(5):975–85.
19. Siontis GCM, Praz F, Pilgrim T, Mavridis D, Verma S, Salanti G, et al. Transcatheter aortic valve implantation vs. surgical aortic valve replacement for treatment of severe aortic stenosis: a meta-analysis of randomized trials. Eur Heart J. 2016;37(47):3503–12.
20. Thyregod HGH, Steinbrüchel DA, Ihlemann N, Nissen H, Kjeldsen BJ, Petursson P, et al. Transcatheter versus surgical aortic valve replacement in patients with severe aortic valve stenosis: 1-year results from the all-comers NOTION randomized clinical trial. J Am Coll Cardiol. 2015;65(20):2184–94.
21. Leon MB, Smith CR, Mack MJ, Makkar RR, Svensson LG, Kodali SK, et al. Transcatheter or surgical aortic-valve replacement in intermediate-risk patients. N Engl J Med. 2016;374(17):1609–20.
22. Leon MB, Smith CR, Mack M, Miller DC, Moses JW, Svensson LG, et al. Transcatheter aortic-valve implantation for aortic stenosis in patients who cannot undergo surgery. N Engl J Med. 2010;363(17):1597–607.
23. Adams DH, Popma JJ, Reardon MJ, Yakubov SJ, Coselli JS, Deeb GM, et al. Transcatheter aortic-valve replacement with a self-expanding prosthesis. N Engl J Med. 2014;370(19):1790–8.
24. Roy DA, Schaefer U, Guetta V, Hildick-Smith D, Möllmann H, Dumonteil N, et al. Transcatheter aortic valve implantation for pure severe native aortic valve regurgitation. J Am Coll Cardiol. 2013;61(15):1577–84.
25. Seiffert M, Bader R, Kappert U, Rastan A, Krapf S, Bleiziffer S, et al. Initial German experience with transapical implantation of a second-generation transcatheter heart valve for the treatment of aortic regurgitation. JACC Cardiovasc Interv. 2014;7(10):1168–74.
26. Bagur R, Teefy PJ, Kiaii B, Diamantouros P, Chu MWA. First North American experience with the transfemoral ACURATE-neoTM self-expanding transcatheter aortic bioprosthesis. Catheter Cardiovasc Interv. 2016;90(1):130–8.
27. Meredith IT, Walters DL, Dumonteil N, Worthley SG, Tchétché D, Manoharan G, et al. 1-year outcomes with the fully repositionable and retrievable lotus transcatheter aortic replacement

valve in 120 high-risk surgical patients with severe aortic stenosis: results of the REPRISE II Study. JACC Cardiovasc Interv. 2016;9(4):376–84.
28. Manoharan G, Linke A, Moellmann H, Redwood S, Frerker C, Kovac J, et al. Multicentre clinical study evaluating a novel resheathable annular functioning self-expanding transcatheter aortic valve system: safety and performance results at 30 days with the Portico system. EuroIntervention. 2016;12(6):768–74.
29. Lefèvre T, Colombo A, Tchétché D, Latib A, Klugmann S, Fajadet J, et al. Prospective multicenter evaluation of the direct flow medical transcatheter aortic valve system: 12-month outcomes of the evaluation of the direct flow medical percutaneous aortic valve 18F system for the treatment of patients with severe aortic stenosis (DISCOVER) Study. JACC Cardiovasc Interv. 2016;9(1):68–75.
30. Petronio AS, Capranzano P, Barbato E, Piazza N, Baumbach A, Haude M, et al. Current status of transcatheter valve therapy in Europe: results from an EAPCI survey. EuroIntervention. 2016;12(7):890–5.

23 Transcatheter Aortic Valve Implantation (TAVI) Using the Transapical Approach

Pavel Overtchouk and Thomas Modine

23.1 Introduction

After being initially developed in animals, trans-catheter aortic valve implantation or replacement (TAVI or TAVR) was performed for the first time in human by Alain Cribier, interventional cardiologist at Rouen Teaching Hospital via trans-femoral venous approach using trans-septal (through the inter-atrial septum) pathway to implant a percutaneous three bovine pericardial leaflet 23 mm of diameter heart valve, to treat a severe calcified aortic stenosis responsible for a cardiogenic shock in an inoperable patient [1]. Ever since TAVI has been a fast-growing technique of interventional treatment of the most frequent valvulopathy in the elderly patients.

TAVI has been evolving in very numerous ways: aortic bioprosthesis devices, catheters, guides, sheaths (sized in French equals to 1/3 mm), pathways, paved the way for hybrid rooms to be created for surgeons and interventional cardiologists working together, and even inspired technologies aiming to lower irradiation and contrast media injected.

It this chapter we will focus on the transapical approach, after a brief presentation of the devices used that will be extensively described in the next chapter.

P. Overtchouk
Pôle de Reanimation, Hôpital Roger Salengro, Centre Hospitalier et Universitaire, Lille 59037, France

T. Modine (✉)
Centre Hospitalier Régional Universitaire de Lille, Lille 59000, France
e-mail: t1modine@yahoo.fr

K. Fattouch et al. (eds.), *Advances in Treatments for Aortic Valve and Root Diseases*, https://doi.org/10.1007/978-3-319-66483-5_23

23.2 Surgical Transapical Access: Technical Aspects

The two main advantages of transapical TAVI when compared to the surgical aortic valve replacement is the avoidance of the cardiopulmonary bypass (CPB) and sternotomy, with a beating-heart left transthoracic approach. Nevertheless transapical (TA) TAVI remains a surgical procedure since it requires anterolateral minithoracotomy. Transfemoral access is the less optimal access for TAVI, but a significant number of patients have poor vascular access due to small, severely tortuous vessels, or severe peripheral vascular disease and are only amenable to treatment with some more invasive surgical procedures.

Before the procedure patient's anatomy will be thoroughly investigated by means of the pre-operative CT-scan (Computerized Tomography) notably for choosing valve type and size, forecast the transapical approach, and coronary angiography to rule out patent obstructive coronary artery disease.

TAVI is usually performed in a hybrid operating room designed and equipped to perform both open surgical and interventional procedures. In particular, fluoroscope is mandatory to guide operators' movements throughout the procedure. TA TAVI is often performed by a multi-disciplinary team including a cardiac surgeon, an interventional cardiologist, a cardiac anaesthesiologist, a perfusionist, a surgical scrub nurse trained in transcatheter equipment handling, a radiology technician and a surgical assistant. At least one member of the team must be trained in preparation and loading of the valve device, which is performed on the ancillary table while the main operators access the aortic valve. Some teams use transoesophageal echocardiography during de procedure, performed by a trained cardiologist. Make sure the patches are installed and connected to the defibrillator before scrubbing.

The technical steps are as follows (the steps are often performed at the same time by the different operators) [2–5]:

- 5Fr femoral vein sheath is inserted for transvenous pacemaker insertion. The pacemaker wire will be placed in the right ventricle and its capture will be checked. An epicardial pacing has also been described [2]
- 6Fr femoral arterial sheath is inserted in the femoral artery to constitute the secondary arterial access. A 7F catheter can be warranted if invasive blood pressure is to be monitored through the same access. An echographic guidance can be used to guide the appropriate location for puncture (avoiding calcifications and tortuosity). This sheath also enables rapid cannulation for CPB using the Seldinger technique in case of cardiac arrest.
- Anterolateral mini-thoracotomy (approximatively 5 cm wide) is performed in the left fifth or sixth intercostal space in the submammary fold to obtain a straight access to the left ventricular apex. Use of soft tissue retractor can optimize exposure and minimize rib spreading.
- The valve is loaded on the delivery system in a sterile fashion. It will be checked for proper orientation and seating.
- Pericardiotomy is performed longitudinally over the left ventricular apex, and stay sutures allow for good exposure of the apex. The usual location for puncture is lateral to the distal part of the left anterior descending artery and slightly anterior from the "true apex".

- Heparin is administered at 100 U/kg to achieve an ACT >300 s.
- Two concentric 2–0 or 3–0 Prolene polypropylene purse string sutures reinforced by 4–5 interrupted Teflon Pledgets (Ethicon Inc., Somerville, NJ) are placed at the left ventricular apex large enough for the delivery catheter to pass through (inner diameter of approximately 2 cm). A "ring pledget" technique has also been described using continuous Teflon pledget ring [6].
- The left ventricle apex is punctured at the centre of the purse string sutures (straight access, direction to the right shoulder) with a standard access hollow needle.
- Soft guide access wire (GuideRight™ 0.035″ × 260 cm length, tip 3 mm J-FS) is inserted in the left ventricle through the needle towards the aortic valve. A 12 or 14Fr sheath (30 cm long and with a soft tip; Cook Medical Inc., Bloomington, IN) is delivered into the LV apex to maintain intraventricular access. The soft guidewire will be replaced by a stiff guidewire (Amplatz™ Super-Stiff 0.035″ × 260 cm length × 7 cm J Tip Length, Boston Scientific Corporation, Natick, MA, USA). After crossing the aortic valve the stiff guidewire will be positioned in the descending aorta.
- The delivery catheter of the prosthesis will be positioned over the stiff wire.
- If deemed appropriate (severely calcified aortic valve) aortic balloon valvuloplasty is performed using a Nucleus™ balloon (20 mm diameter, filled with contrast diluted with saline, 1:2 ratio) during rapid ventricular pacing 160/min rate (RVP)
- The valve is then implanted according to the specific procedure of each valve. These will be discussed in the next section. Coaxial positioning is important, it can be achieved by manipulations with the stiff guidewire.
- After full deployment, aortic root angiography identifies paravalvular (or central) regurgitation. If the leak is significant a post-dilation with a valvuloplasty balloon can complete full prosthesis deployment and correct the leak, taking care of not overinflating because of the risk of annulus rupture.
- Once the result is optimal, the apical sheath and guidewire are simultaneously retrieved and the purse string sutures are tied to secure haemostasis. In case of persistent bleeding additional Teflon-reinforced sutures should be used until complete haemostasis is achieved.
- Protamine is administered.
- The pericardium is closed at the apex (over resorbable collagen gauze).
- Left pleural soft drain is installed and standard closure of the mini-thoracotomy is performed.

Uncomplicated procedures last 40 min to 1 h. Immediate extubation is warranted in the operating room if the patient remains haemodynamically stable. The temporary pacemaker wire is kept for 24–48 h in those patients who may be at risk of late atrio-ventricular (AV) conduction block.

Post-operative care involves monitoring in the intensive care unit for at least 24 h which includes echocardiographic evaluation looking for bleeding and prosthesis dysfunction. Fast-track protocol has been described with discharge from the intensive care unit on the same day as the procedure in high surgical risk patients (successively in 83% of cases) without increase in 30-day mortality (8%) [7]. In our centre, we also perform systematic echocardiography between day 5 and 7, before discharge to obtain baseline hemodynamic measures for the follow-up.

In certain cases, additional surgical procedures are performed during the same anaesthesia: coronary angioplasty, carotid thrombectomy, endovascular graft for abdominal aortic aneurysm for example. Additional procedures usually worsen vital prognosis so must be carefully evaluated.

Tips and pitfalls:

The apex is favoured to the free wall because of a reduced wall stress with a reduced risk of breakdown of suture line, favouring better tissue healing, and avoiding the mitral valve apparatus. It is in general better for the incision to be a bit low rather than too high, since the apex can be distracted downward with pericardial traction sutures. The position of the left anterior descending coronary artery should be noticed. Foresee an appropriate size of myocardium for your apical access depending on the width of the delivery catheter and make sure you puncture the apex with the access needle precisely at the central point within the sutures to reduce the likelihood of extending the enlarging myocardial defect beyond the control sutures. Take sufficiently deep bites in the myocardium (approximately 3–5 mm), without penetrating the left ventricular cavity. Avoid regions with epicardial fat. Hemodynamic stability must be achieved before proceeding with prosthesis implantation: crystalloids, vasopressors and/or inotropes should be administered if necessary aiming at maintain mean blood pressure above 70 mmHg. Also, hypertension must be avoided when closing the apical myocardial access, to minimize blood loss. Avoid repeated RVPs in patients with reduced left ventricle ejection fraction: it can lead to haemodynamic deterioration.

Finally, optimal communication and coordination between operating team, anaesthesiology team and paramedical team lead to efficient procedure with optimal results (Fig. 23.1).

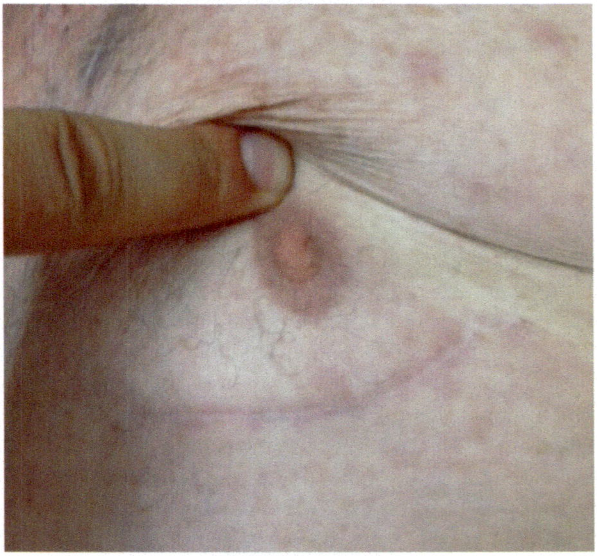

Fig. 23.1 Scar after anterolateral minithoracotomy

23.3 Complications of Transapical TAVI

Complications of imprecise valve positioning:

- Embolization: into the left ventricle in the valve is positioned too deeply or in the aorta if it is too high. In case the prosthesis embolizes in the aorta anchor it to the thoracic descending aorta, distal to the surpa-aortic axes to avoid cerebral and limb ischemia.
- Coronary occlusion: may occur when a tissue-carrying portion of the prosthesis is deployed towards a coronary ostium. When coronary artery occlusion occurs it usually leads to cardiac arrest by myocardial infarction and urgent manoeuvres have to be made by experienced interventional cardiologists to try to reopen the ostium with angioplasty.

Complications of imprecise prosthesis size choice:

- Prosthesis mismatch: the size chosen is too small with residual hemodynamically significant stenosis
- Paravalvular leak: is in certain cases due to a smaller than needed prosthesis

Rupture of the aortic annulus: is one of the most feared complications since it is often associated with immediate and definitive cardiac arrest (near 100% of cases). Aggressive overdilation of the aortic annulus and prosthesis oversizing in patients with small heavily calcified aortic annulus is forbidden.

Preserve the mitral valve and its apparatus: when navigating in the left ventricle always orientate your guidewire towards the aortic valve. If the guidewire forms an odd angle it may be due to a crossing of mitral chordae and pillars.

Other post-operative complications can worsen outcomes: stroke, acute renal failure, thromboembolic events. On a long term left ventricle pseudo-aneurysm can occur.

23.4 Devices

The aortic bioprosthesis is composed of three biological leaflets anchored on a metallic framework. Multiple bioprosthesis exist and other are being developed. Nowadays, several valves and their delivery systems exist for transapical approach. We will focus on the ones that obtained the CE-mark:

- Edwards Sapien 3™,
- Medtronik Engager™
- Acurate TA™
- JenaValve™

The J-Valve system (JieCheng Medical Technology Co., Ltd., Suzhou, China) is under development for aortic regurgitation but to date it has not been approved by regulatory bodies [8].

23.4.1 Edwards Sapien 3

The latest valve from the Edwards Sapien™ (Edwards Lifesciences) family is the Sapien 3, which is the fourth generation in this family of balloon-expandable trans-catheter heart valves. For transapical approach it is implanted by use of the Edwards Certitude™ delivery system (Edwards Lifesciences). Bovine pericardial tissue is affixed to a radiopaque stainless steel stent frame. One of the main additional features of the Sapien 3 when compared to its predecessors is the outer PET (polyethylene terephthalate) sealing cuff intended to reduce paravalvular regurgitation. Three valve sizes are available (23, 26, and 29 mm). The delivery system is still rather large (although smaller than the previous 23 Fr catheter): 18 Fr (for Sapien 3 23–26 mm) and 21 Fr (Sapien 3 29 mm) profiles.

The implantation of the Sapien 3 prosthesis through the Certitude delivery system is performed as follows:

- The prosthesis is compressed before being inserted in the delivery catheter and positioned on a valvuloplasty balloon
- Pre-dilation with a valvuloplasty balloon can be warranted according to certain operator
- When the position of the prosthesis is deemed optimal and under mandatory rapid ventricular pacing (RVP), because the balloon obstructs the left ventricle outflow tract, the prosthesis is decompressed by inflating the balloon it is on. Full inflation is preserved for 5 s (to prevent later recoil).

The CE mark of Sapien 3 was obtains in 2014 and it is extensively used in various centres worldwide (Figs. 23.2 and 23.3).

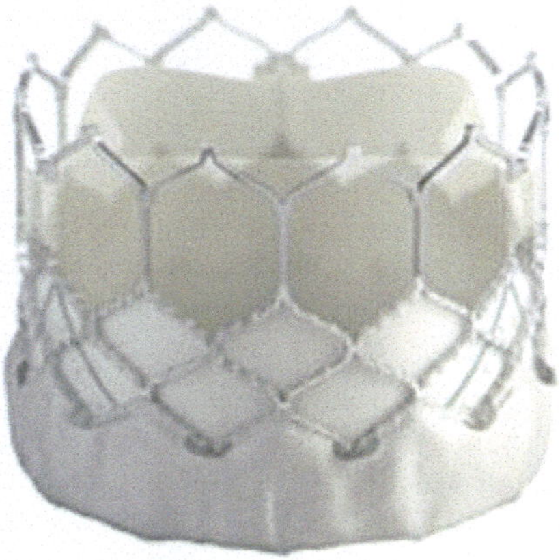

Fig. 23.2 Edwards Sapien 3™ prosthesis

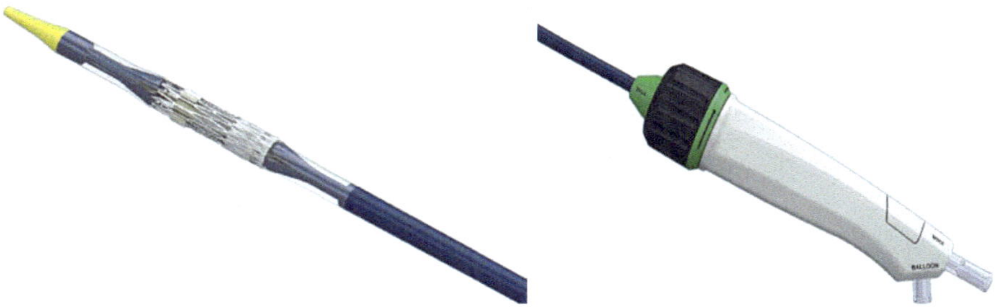

Fig. 23.3 Edwards Certitude™ delivery system (Edwards Lifesciences) [9]

23.4.2 Medtronic Engager™

The Medtronic Engager™ (Medtronic 3F Therapeutics, Inc., Santa Ana, CA) is a self-expanding nitinol stent frame and a bovine trileaflet valve. The stent frame has two components: a central frame housing the leaflets and a support frame with three control arms that aim to stabilise the device in the sinuses of Valsalva. The Engager valve is designed to minimising the risk of coronary obstruction by fitting the aortic root anatomy while respecting the coronary ostia. A polyester sleeve is sutured to the central frame aimed at reducing the risk of paravalvular regurgitation. The leaflets are in a supra-annular position to maintain circular configuration and coaptation to preserve haemodynamic properties irrespective of the calcified aortic valve anatomy. The Engager is available in two sizes, 23 and 26 mm, for an annulus range between 21 and 26.7 mm. Procedures can be performed via transapical (or direct aortic) route. The delivery system combines a 29 Fr introducer and a flexible delivery catheter creating one integral unit. A pre-dilation with a valvuloplasty balloon can be performed before prosthesis implantation if necessary.

The Engager valve is implanted through a transapical pathway according to a three-step release of the prosthesis:

- First: the control frame arms are released by pulling the sheath in a retrograde fashion (direction opposite to the delivery catheter). The prosthesis is descended in the sinuses of Valsalva. It can be rotated while in the sheath if the arms are not properly positioned. Angiographic control can confirm the correct position of the arms in the cusps.
- Second: unlocking the safety button release the commissural posts. Note that repositioning can be performed until unlocking the safety button.
- Final step: release of the self-expanding valve. The final deployment is ideally performed under rapid ventricular pacing for stability and accuracy of positioning.

The Medtronik Engager™ is CE marked since 2013 (Fig. 23.4).

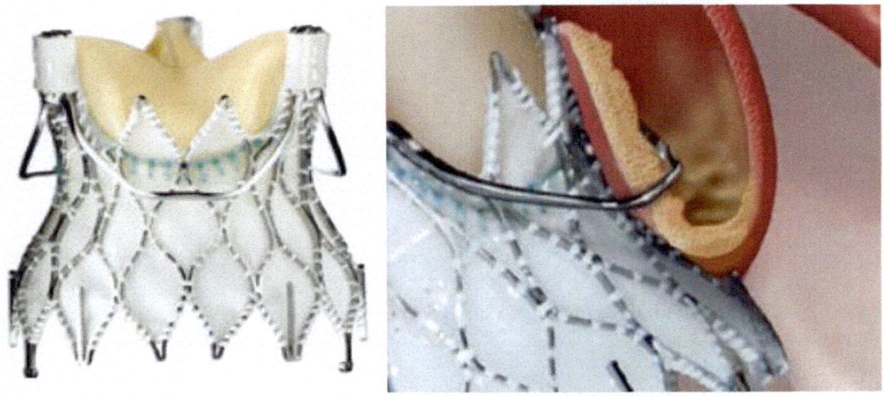

Fig. 23.4 Medtronik Engager™ (Medtronic 3F Therapeutics, Inc., Santa Ana, CA) [10]

23.4.3 ACURATE TA™

The ACURATE TA (Symetis SA, Ecublens, Switzerland) has been specifically developed for the antegrade transapical approach but a transfemoral device has also been developed (ACURATE TF™). Porcine tissue is mounted within a self-expanding nitinol stent covered by an anti-paravalvular leak skirt. The stent is composed of two main segments: the valve segment and the "stabilisation arches". The body of the stent includes an "upper crown" of the prosthesis which is the distal part of the valve segment, it is meant to embrace the native calcified leaflets while providing supra-annular anchoring, as well as "tactile feedback" during deployment. The "lower crown" is the stent edge that minimally resides within the left ventricular outflow tract. The three "stabilisation arches" at the distal edge of the stent aim at preventing tilting of the prosthesis during final deployment. A PET (polyethylene terephthalate) sealing skirt is mounted around the intra-annular part of the stent to mitigate paravalvular regurgitation. The stent commissures are another component of the valve segment, well visible under fluoroscopy with a radiopaque appearance that help the depth of positioning. The delivery catheter is 28 Fr wide with the prosthesis being fully "loaded" inside. Three markers at its distal handle aim at helping commissural alignment and anatomical rotation during the implantation.

Transapical aortic valve replacement with ACURATE TA follows a two-step protocol:

- The "stabilisation arches" are released by pulling the sheath in a anterograde fashion (direction towards the delivery catheter) followed by the "upper crown". By pulling gently on the delivery catheter with fluoroscopic visual control the operator will feel a resistance when the "upper crown" presses against the aortic valve. Radiopaque appearances will help prosthesis positioning.

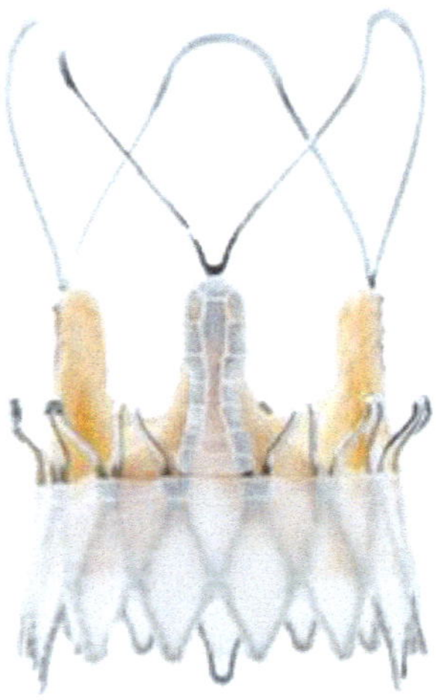

Fig. 23.5 ACURATE TA (Symetis SA, Ecublens, Switzerland) [11]

– The position is deemed optimal the operator can proceed by removing the safety pin and the valve is ready for final deployment. Final deployment is optimally performed under rapid ventricular pacing (RVP) but deployment is possible without RVP. Until final release the prosthesis is recapturable and repositionable.

It has obtained the CE mark in 2011 (Fig. 23.5).

23.4.4 JenaValve™

JenaValve™ (JenaValve Technology GmbH, Munich, Germany) is a self-expandable, partially repositionable and retrievable prosthesis. Three leaflets and a skirt manufactured from porcine pericardial tissue are attached onto a self-expanding crown-shaped nitinol stent frame. The prosthesis also includes three integral locators that engage with the native valve cusps and leaflets and provide tactile feedback for appropriate positioning. The JenaClip™ (JenaValve Technology GmbH) is an intrinsic mechanism to clip the JenaValve prosthesis onto the native valve leaflets for active fixation and to prevent migration while eliminating great radial forces on cardiac and aortic structures with the aim to avoiding atrioventricular block. Three sizes are available (23, 25, and 27 mm) to cover annulus sizes from 21 to 27 mm.

The device is implanted through a 32 Fr sheathless delivery catheter (Cathlete; JenaValve Technology GmbH). JenaClip™ (JenaValve Technology GmbH) is an intrinsic mechanism to clip the JenaValve prosthesis onto the native valve leaflets for active fixation and to prevent migration.

The implantation follows a three-step procedure (after potential aortic pre-dilation):

- After introduction of the delivery system with the loaded JenaValve into the ascending aorta, the positioning locators are released. The correct anatomical orientation of the respective feelers regarding the native cusps is confirmed with fluoroscopy. The catheter is pulled back up until a tactile feedback indicates the contact of the feelers with the proper cusps.
- Then release the lower stent frame, thereby clipping and anchoring the bioprosthesis onto the native leaflets. At this point the bioprosthesis is competent and functioning but still repositionable and retrievable.
- Finally release the upper part of the nitinol frame and retrieve the delivery catheter.

JenaValve™ obtained CE mark for treatment of severe aortic stenosis in 2011. Furthermore in September 2013, this bioprosthesis received CE-mark approval for the treatment of pure aortic regurgitation (Fig. 23.6).

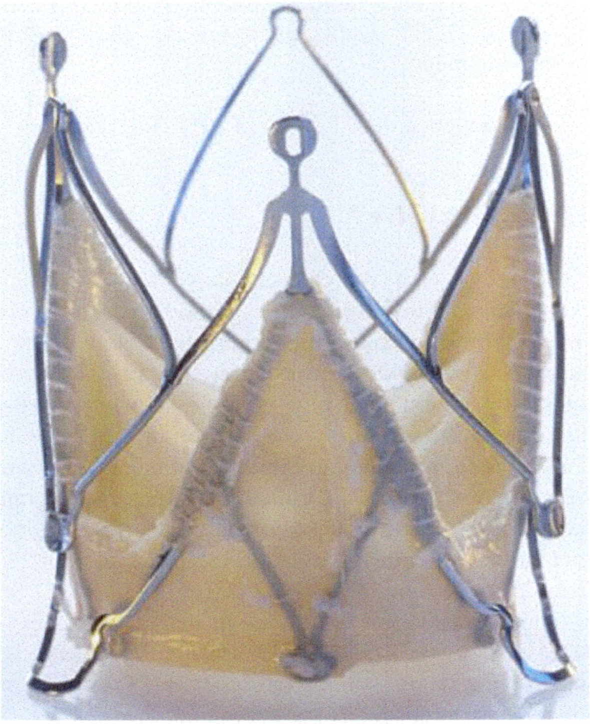

Fig. 23.6 JenaValve™ [12]

23.5 Indications and Patient Selection

TAVI has been developed to treat severe symptomatic aortic stenosis which remains its main indication. But treatment by TAVI of severe aortic regurgitation has been reported as feasible [13].

The last European Society of Cardiology guidelines on the treatment of aortic valve diseases were published in 2012 and recommended the use of TAVI in high risk patients with severe aortic stenosis (class IIaB) with life-expectancy of more than 1 year, with indication validated by the "Heart Team". More recently the American Heart Association and American College of Cardiology recommended in 2014 in patients who meet an indication for AVR for AS who have a prohibitive surgical risk and a predicted post-TAVR survival superior to 1 year (class IB) and as an alternative to surgical replacement in high-risk patients (class IIaB). Recent data from PARTNER-2 trial and others provided arguments to extend indications to intermediate surgical risk patients and ongoing trials will reliably test TAVI in low risk patients (disposable literature is encouraging). New guidelines are eagerly awaited in 2017.

Guidelines do not address the question of the appropriate approach for TAVI. Although trans-femoral access provides the best results (in terms of mortality, vascular access complications, bleeding) than other, more invasive, approaches, some patients cannot benefit from the optimal trans-femoral approach. This may be due to vessel diameter <5 mm, heavily calcified vessels, tortuosity and significant abdominal and thoracic aortic disease. Up to 35% of patients eligible for TAVI have an unsuitable peripheral artery anatomy [14], these patients are good candidates for TA TAVI.

Patient's eligible for surgical aortic valve replacement but in whom sternotomy is compromised (history of multiple sternotomies, coronary grafts, thoracic irradiation, porcelain aorta) can also benefit from TA TAVI.

Since TA TAVI needs a surgical approach the patient must be able to tolerate general anaesthesia, mechanical ventilation, do not suffer from severe haemostatic disorder, haemodynamic instability.

When a patient is considered to have high surgical risk (or inoperable), he shall undergo pre-operative evaluation of eligibility for TAVI:

- Coronary artery angiography: to look for frequent concomitant coronary artery disease. If multiple vessel disease is revealed the "Heart Team" must state on the possibility of sternotomy with coronary bypass surgery associated with aortic valve replacement versus angioplasty and TAVI, or otherwise combined minimally invasive direct coronary artery bypass with TA TAVI. When warranted percutaneous coronary intervention is recommended prior to TAVI because of the risk of an impossible (or complex) access to coronary arteries after the prosthesis is implanted [15]. Other valuable information can be gathered: the ascending aorta can be measured (looking for aortic aneurysm), transaortic hemodynamic gradient, and the ilio-femoral vessels are evaluated for diameter, tortuosity, calcification to contemplate trans-femoral access.

- Cervico-thoraco-abdomino-pelvic and proximal lower limbs CT-scan with contrast injection: is nowadays mandatory, unless contraindicated. It provides important information for valve sizing (usually treated with dedicated software), calcification assessment, ascending aorta measurements, and peripheral vessel anatomy in order to choose the appropriate approach (iliofemoral, carotid, subclavian). Carotid anatomy is also to be considered because of frequent concomitant severe (up to 33%) [16] lesions that need to be addressed before cardiac procedures.
- Echocardiography: to exclude significant associated valvulopathy requiring intervention. Concomitant mitral valvulopathy (regurgitation or stenosis) is frequently present in elderly patients with severe aortic stenosis, but unless it is severe should not be considered as a contraindication to aortic valve implantation. If severe surgical replacement under cardiopulmonary bypass should be reconsidered by the "Heart Team".
- Pulmonary function studies: pulmonary disease, which often coincides with aortic stenosis in high-risk patients. A forced expiratory volume (FEV) <1 L can contraindicate mechanical ventilation which is mandatory for TA TAVI.

In conclusion, eligible patients to TA TAVI regroup one or several of the following criteria:

- Inoperable or high surgical risk: EuroScore II calculated risk of mortality >7%, the Society of Thoracic Surgeons' score risk of mortality >8% [17], with the caveat that risk scores are helpful but not completely adapted to TAVI procedures.
- Comorbidities rendering conventional aortic valve surgery difficult: as a porcelain aorta, coronary artery grafts, previous history multiple sternotomies, radiation therapy, liver cirrhosis
- Patients unsuitable for trans-femoral TAVI: common femoral artery diameter <5 mm, heavily calcified vessels, tortuosity and significant abdominal and thoracic aortic disease
- No contra-indication: notably the patient must able to support general anaesthesia, mechanical ventilation, do not suffer from severe haemostasis disorder

23.6 Results of Transapical TAVI

Like any interventional procedure results depend on the interventional risk of the patient. TA TAVI is no exception: results are better in intermediate and low risk patients than inoperable and high risk patients (which is subject to the fact that surgical risk scores like logistic EuroScore I, EuroScore II, STS score are not sufficiently accurate to predict mortality for TAVI [18]). Comparisons between TA and transfemoral (TF) TAVI or surgical aortic valve replacement (SAVR) are based on observational prospective studies, mostly with Edwards Sapien valve, but some recent publications address results with JenaValve [19], ACURATE TA [20] and

Engager valves [21]. Besides, complication rates are continuously throughout the years. Thereafter we first discuss the results of transapically implanted Sapien 3 prosthesis versus mostly Sapien family and CoreValve transfemorally implanted prostheses. Then we site recent results for JenaValve, ACURATE TA and the Engager.

23.6.1 TA versus TF TAVI

In inoperable and high risk patients: 30-day mortality with TA TAVI is close to 5% [22, 23] compared to 1.6% via TF approach in the latest registry [23]. The rates of stroke and pacemaker implantations is similar with both pathways (around 2% and 12% respectively). Logically vascular complications are two-fold less frequent with TA approach but it is the opposite for the rate of major bleedings [23]. 30-day mortality is particularly higher in nonagerians treated with TA versus TF TAVI in a recent meta-analysis of three studies (14.2 versus 6.5%, HR 2.56 95% CI 1.63–4.01) [24–26]. In a recent cohort of 49 patients treated with Sapien 3 prosthesis 30-day mortality of TA TAVI was 14.8%, and the incidence of stroke was 5.6% [27].

Intermediate and low risk patients: outcomes were similar in both groups in terms of 30-day mortality, stroke, pacemaker implantation (close to 1.5%, 3.5% and 10% respectively) in a recent cohort [23].

23.6.2 TA TAVI vs SAVR

Inoperable and high risk patients: a retrospective study with pair matching and 164 very high risk patients (mean logistic EuroScore >29%) reported no advantage of TA TAVI over SAVR in terms of 1-year mortality (81 vs 76%, $p = 0.66$), stroke, pacemaker and indexes of physical and mental quality of life that were all similar [28]. But 5-year follow-up of PARTNER 1 high risk patients rather favoured (but without statistically significant difference) SAVR to TA TAVI (HR 1.37 95% CI: 0.98–1.92) [29].

Intermediate and low risk patients: in the PARTNER 2A randomised controlled trial study transthoracic TAVI (polled TA and transaortic TAVI) was not significantly different from SAVR in terms of composite primary outcome of all-cause death and stroke (HR 1.21 (95% CI: 0.84–1.94) [30].

One cohort reported a 5 year similar (non-significantly different, $p = 0.66$) good survival rates in low risk patients of 86% after SAVR and 76% after TA-TAVI without difference in 5 year health related physical or mental quality of life [31].

A randomised controlled trial (STACCATO) was early terminated after including 72 patients because of excessive adverse events in the TA TAVI group: five patients in a-TAVI group (14.7%: 2 deaths, 2 strokes, 1 severe acute renal failure), versus 1 stroke in SAVR group (2.8%). Besides more moderate to severe paravalvular leakages were observed in TA TAVI group (13% versus 0%) [32].

All-risk patients combined; A meta-analysis pooled the results from four randomised controlled trails with 3179 (PARTNER 2A, STACCATO, NOTION, US CoreValve High Risk) and no significant difference at 2 years (but a tendency of inferiority of TA TAVI) between TA TAVI and SAVR regarding mortality (HR 1.34, 95% CI: 0.91–1.97), stroke RR (1.67, 95% CI: 0.97–2.87), acute kidney injury (RR 1.54, 95% CI: 0.77–3.07). Life threatening or disabling bleeding were less frequently observed with TA TAVI: RR 0.53 (95% CI: 0.42 to 0.67) [30, 32–34]. Similar results were found by Siontis et al. when replacing the STACCATO trial by PARTNER 1A in terms of absence of survival benefit with TA TAVI (HR 1.17 95% CI: 0.88–1.56) [35].

23.6.3 Recent Transapical Valves

JenaValve, ACURATE TA and Engager are often described as "second-generation" transapically implanted prostheses.

A 180-patient recent registry reported outcomes with JenaValve in high risk patients (logistic EuroScore I 21%) showing a 95% success rate of the procedures, a relatively high rate of 30-day mortality (11%), more "standard" 1-year mortality (23%), a low 1.1% rate of 1-year major stroke, a low risk of moderate to severe paravalvular leaks (3.2%), a comparable risk of pacemaker implantation (14%) [19] than Sapien 3 and the latest CoreValve Evolut R (both around 12% [23, 36]).

Unlike with any other transapical prosthesis a registry of 31 patients treated for severe pure aortic regurgitation has been reported. Results are rather favourable since the procedure was successfully performed in all but one patient who required a valve-in-valve procedure (Sapien XT). The 30-day mortality rate was 12.9% (4 patients), two permanent pacemakers were implanted. 6-month mortality was 19.3%. No cerebrovascular events were noted [37].

The ACURATE TA prosthesis for TAVI via transapical pathway use in 250 high risk (logistic Euroscore I 22%, STS score 8%) patients was reported in a registry with a good 98% rate of implantation success, a similarly to JenaValve relatively high 30-day mortality rate of 6.8%, but similarly to the Sapien 3 prosthesis risk of stroke (2.8%), moderate to severe leak (2.3%) and rate of pacemaker implantation (10%) [20].

A registry of 60 patients treated with Engager prosthesis (successful procedure in all but one patient; the mean logistic EuroScore I of the cohort was 19%). The 30-day mortality was close to 10% with a 6-month mortality of 17%. One 30-day major stroke was reported and a high rate of 27% were implanted a permanent pacemaker [38].

A German registry reported similar outcomes of these three second-generation valves in 200 patients in terms of 30-day mortality (8%, 10.2%, 6.5% respectively for Engager, JenaValve, Symetis Acurate TA, $p = 0.681$), major stroke, permanent pacemaker implantation, but lower cumulative 1-year mortality with the Acurate TA valve ($p = 0.047$). Successful implantation was achieved in around 90% for all three valves. This is a small registry and some sensible differences may become significant with a larger sample size: the rate of pacemaker implantation was sensitively higher with the Engager (30%) than with the JenaValve and Acurate TA (14.8% and 21% respectively) [39].

Conclusion

Transapical TAVI was developed in late 2000 to overcome the impossibility of transfemoral access to treat severe symptomatic aortic stenosis. Initially performed with Edwards Sapien family prostheses results have been comparable to surgical aortic valve replacement in high surgical risk patient but less efficient than transfemoral TAVI. Since then second-generation valves have been developed with interesting results especially regarding treatment of pure aortic regurgitation. More data on these new valves are required to estimate their rightful position in the strategy of treatment of severe aortic diseases. Nevertheless, great progress has been achieved in miniaturising the devices and ineligibility to transfemoral access is becoming less and less problematic. Besides, other non-femoral approaches [40] have shown promising results and could further restrict indications for the transapical approach.

References

1. Cribier A, Eltchaninoff H, Bash A, Borenstein N, Tron C, Bauer F, et al. Percutaneous transcatheter implantation of an aortic valve prosthesis for calcific aortic stenosis. Circulation. 2002;106(24):3006–8.
2. Walther T, Möllmann H, van Linden A, Kempfert J. Transcatheter aortic valve implantation transapical: step by step. Semin Thorac Cardiovasc Surg. 2011;23(1):55–61.
3. Walther T, Dewey T, Borger MA, Kempfert J, Linke A, Becht R, et al. Transapical aortic valve implantation: step by step. Ann Thorac Surg. 2009;87(1):276–83.
4. Walther T, Falk V, Borger MA, Dewey T, Wimmer-Greinecker G, Schuler G, et al. Minimally invasive transapical beating heart aortic valve implantation—proof of concept. Eur J Cardiothorac Surg. 2007;31(1):9–15.
5. Albacker T, Ramankutty R, Roselli E. Transapical transcatheter aortic valve implantation [Internet]. CTSNet. 2012. http://www.ctsnet.org/article/transapical-transcatheter-aortic-valve-implantation
6. Astarci P, El Khoury G, David G, Kefer J, Renkin J, Vanoverschelde J-L. "Ring Pledget": a new concept for secure apex closure during transapical aortic valve implantation. Innovations. 2010;5(2):136–7. http://journals.lww.com/innovjournal/Fulltext/2010/03000/_Ring_Pledget___A_New_Concept_for_Secure_Apex.15.aspx.
7. Papadopoulos N, El-Sayed Ahmad A, Thudt M, Fichtlscherer S, Meybohm P, Reyher C, et al. Successful fast track protocol implementation for patients undergoing transapical transcatheter aortic valve implantation. J Cardiothorac Surg. 2016;11:55.
8. Wei L, Liu H, Zhu L, Yang Y, Zheng J, Guo K, et al. A new transcatheter aortic valve replacement system for predominant aortic regurgitation implantation of the j-valve and early outcome. JACC Cardiovasc Interv. 2015;8(14):1831–41.
9. Edwards SAPIEN 3 transcatheter heart valve [Internet]. http://www.edwards.com/eu/Products/TranscatheterValves/Pages/sapien3.aspx?WT.ac=S3campaignprod. Accessed 26 Nov 2016.
10. Transcatheter Aortic Valve Replacement—TAVR|Medtronic Engager [Internet]. http://www.medtronic-engager.com/home/transcatheter-aortic-valve-replacement/index.htm. Accessed 26 Nov 2016.

11. ACURATE TA|Symetis [Internet]. https://www.symetis.com/products/acurate-ta. Accessed 26 Nov 2016.
12. About JenaValve—JENAVALVE [Internet]. http://www.jenavalve.de/about/. Accessed 26 Nov 2016.
13. Roy DA, Schaefer U, Guetta V, Hildick-Smith D, Möllmann H, Dumonteil N, et al. Transcatheter aortic valve implantation for pure severe native aortic valve regurgitation. J Am Coll Cardiol. 2013;61(15):1577–84.
14. Kurra V, Schoenhagen P, Roselli EE, Kapadia SR, Tuzcu EM, Greenberg R, et al. Prevalence of significant peripheral artery disease in patients evaluated for percutaneous aortic valve insertion: preprocedural assessment with multidetector computed tomography. J Thorac Cardiovasc Surg. 2009;137(5):1258–64.
15. Blumenstein J, Kim W-K, Liebetrau C, Gaede L, Kempfert J, Walther T, et al. Challenges of coronary angiography and intervention in patients previously treated by TAVI. Clin Res Cardiol. 2015;104(8):632–9.
16. Fusini L, Mirea O, Tamborini G, Muratori M, Gripari P, Cefalù C, et al. Incidence and severity of atherosclerotic cardiovascular artery disease in patients undergoing TAVI. Int J Cardiovasc Imaging. 2015;31(5):975–85.
17. Nishimura RA, Otto CM, Bonow RO, Carabello BA, Erwin I, John P, Guyton RA, et al. 2014 AHA/ACC guideline for the management of patients with valvular heart disease: a report of the American College of Cardiology/American Heart Association Task Force on Practice Guidelines. J Am Coll Cardiol. 2014;63(22):e57–185.
18. Silaschi M, Conradi L, Seiffert M, Schnabel R, Schön G, Blankenberg S, et al. Predicting risk in transcatheter aortic valve implantation: comparative analysis of EuroSCORE II and established risk stratification tools. Thorac Cardiovasc Surg. 2015;63(06):472–8.
19. Silaschi M, Treede H, Rastan AJ, Baumbach H, Beyersdorf F, Kappert U, et al. The JUPITER registry: 1-year results of transapical aortic valve implantation using a second-generation transcatheter heart valve in patients with aortic stenosis. Eur J Cardiothorac Surg. 2016;50(5):874–81.
20. Kempfert J, Holzhey D, Hofmann S, Girdauskas E, Treede H, Schröfel H, et al. First registry results from the newly approved ACURATE TA™ TAVI system. Eur J Cardiothorac Surg. 2015;48(1):137–41.
21. Bagur R, Kiaii B, Teefy PJ, Diamantouros P, Lavi R, Harle C, et al. First North American experience with the engager self-expanding transcatheter aortic valve: insights from the London Health Sciences Centre Heart Team. Ann Thorac Surg. 2016 Aug 1;102(2):e167–71.
22. Gaede L, Kim W-K, Blumenstein J, Liebetrau C, Dörr O, Nef H, et al. Temporal trends in transcatheter and surgical aortic valve replacement: an analysis of aortic valve replacements in Germany during 2012–2014. Herz. 2016;42(3):316–24.
23. Kodali S, Thourani VH, White J, Malaisrie SC, Lim S, Greason KL, et al. Early clinical and echocardiographic outcomes after SAPIEN 3 transcatheter aortic valve replacement in inoperable, high-risk and intermediate-risk patients with aortic stenosis. Eur Heart J. 2016;37(28):2252–62.
24. Yamamoto M, Mouillet G, Meguro K, Gilard M, Laskar M, Eltchaninoff H, et al. Clinical results of transcatheter aortic valve implantation in octogenarians and nonagenarians: insights from the FRANCE-2 registry. Ann Thorac Surg. 2014 Jan;97(1):29–36.
25. Thourani VH, Jensen HA, Babaliaros V, Kodali SK, Rajeswaran J, Ehrlinger J, et al. Outcomes in nonagenarians undergoing transcatheter aortic valve replacement in the PARTNER-I trial. Ann Thorac Surg. 2015;100(3):785–93.
26. Biancari F, D'Errigo P, Rosato S, Pol M, Tamburino C, Ranucci M, et al. Transcatheter aortic valve replacement in nonagenarians: early and intermediate outcome from the OBSERVANT study and meta-analysis of the literature. Heart Vessel. 2016;1:1–9.
27. Webb J, Gerosa G, Lefèvre T, Leipsic J, Spence M, Thomas M, et al. Multicenter evaluation of a next-generation balloon-expandable transcatheter aortic valve. J Am Coll Cardiol. 2014;64(21):2235–43.

28. Baumbach H, Ahad S, Rustenbach C, Hill S, Schäufele T, Wachter K, et al. Conventional versus transapical aortic valve replacement: is it time for shift in indications? Thorac Cardiovasc Surg. 2017;65(3):212–7.
29. Mack MJ, Leon MB, Smith CR, Miller DC, Moses JW, Tuzcu EM, et al. 5-year outcomes of transcatheter aortic valve replacement or surgical aortic valve replacement for high surgical risk patients with aortic stenosis (PARTNER 1): a randomised controlled trial. Lancet. 2015;385(9986):2477–84.
30. Leon MB, Smith CR, Mack MJ, Makkar RR, Svensson LG, Kodali SK, et al. Transcatheter or surgical aortic-valve replacement in intermediate-risk patients. N Engl J Med. 2016;374(17):1609–20.
31. Rex CE, Hjortdal VE, Heiberg J, Klaaborg K-E. Health-related quality-of-life after transapical transcatheter aortic valve implantation. Scand Cardiovasc J. 50(5–6):377–82. http://www.tandfonline.com.doc-distant.univ-lille2.fr/doi/full/10.1080/14017431.2016.1235725
32. Nielsen HHM, Klaaborg KE, Nissen H, Terp K, Mortensen PE, Kjeldsen BJ, et al. A prospective, randomised trial of transapical transcatheter aortic valve implantation vs. surgical aortic valve replacement in operable elderly patients with aortic stenosis: the STACCATO trial. EuroIntervention. 2012;8(3):383–9.
33. Thyregod HGH, Steinbrüchel DA, Ihlemann N, Nissen H, Kjeldsen BJ, Petursson P, et al. Transcatheter versus surgical aortic valve replacement in patients with severe aortic valve stenosis: 1-year results from the all-comers NOTION randomized clinical trial. J Am Coll Cardiol. 2015;65(20):2184–94.
34. Adams DH, Popma JJ, Reardon MJ, Yakubov SJ, Coselli JS, Deeb GM, et al. Transcatheter aortic-valve replacement with a self-expanding prosthesis. N Engl J Med. 2014;370(19):1790–8.
35. Siontis GCM, Praz F, Pilgrim T, Mavridis D, Verma S, Salanti G, et al. Transcatheter aortic valve implantation vs. surgical aortic valve replacement for treatment of severe aortic stenosis: a meta-analysis of randomized trials. Eur Heart J. 2016;37(47):3503–12.
36. Manoharan G, Walton AS, Brecker SJ, Pasupati S, Blackman DJ, Qiao H, et al. Treatment of symptomatic severe aortic stenosis with a novel resheathable supra-annular self-expanding transcatheter aortic valve system. JACC Cardiovasc Interv. 2015;8(10):1359–67.
37. Seiffert M, Bader R, Kappert U, Rastan A, Krapf S, Bleiziffer S, et al. Initial German experience with transapical implantation of a second-generation transcatheter heart valve for the treatment of aortic regurgitation. JACC Cardiovasc Interv. 2014;7(10):1168–74.
38. Holzhey D, Linke A, Treede H, Baldus S, Bleiziffer S, Wagner A, et al. Intermediate follow-up results from the multicenter engager European pivotal trial. Ann Thorac Surg. 2013;96(6):2095–100.
39. Seiffert M, Conradi L, Kloth B, Koschyk D, Schirmer J, Schnabel RB, et al. Single-centre experience with next-generation devices for transapical aortic valve implantation. Eur J Cardio-Thorac. 2015;47(1):39–45; discussion 45.
40. Mylotte D, Sudre A, Teiger E, Obadia JF, Lee M, Spence M, et al. Transcarotid transcatheter aortic valve replacement: feasibility and safety. JACC Cardiovasc Interv. 2016;9(5):472–80.

24 Hot Topics in TAVI: Paravalvular Leak, Thrombosis, PM Implantation, Stroke, Durability

Caterina Gandolfo and Amerigo Stabile

Transcatheter aortic valve implantation (TAVI) is a rapidly evolving technique providing robust treatment of severe aortic valve stenosis, at least in high and intermediate risk patient cohorts [1]. However, different important limitations, having a potential impact on patient outcome, still need to be resolved. Indeed, with several first-generation balloon-expandable or self-expanding TAVI prostheses, residual paravalvular aortic regurgitation (PVL) after TAVI has been identified as a significant independent major predictor of acute and long-term mortality. Moreover, conduction disorders requiring pacemaker implantation and also concerns about early (leaflet thrombosis/decreased leaflet motion) and late valve durability, need to be resolved before applying TAVI to lower-risk patient cohorts [2].

These limitations appear to be partially patient, but certainly also TAVI system specific.

24.1 PVL

Many studies have shown an increase in the incidence of PVL among patients undergoing TAVI compared with surgical aortic valve replacement and a significant increase in mortality among those patients with moderate or severe aortic regurgitation (AR) after TAVI [3–5]. However, the impact of milder forms of AR after TAVI has been less clear [6, 7].

The impact of mild aortic regurgitation has been less clear, possibly because of the broad categories that have been used in clinical trials, but holds increasing

C. Gandolfo (✉)
Mediterranean Institute for Transplantation and Advanced Specialized Therapies (ISMETT), IRCSS UPMC ITALY, Palermo, PA 90127, Italy
e-mail: cgandolfo@ismett.edu

A. Stabile
Maria Eleonora Hospital, GVM, Palermo, Italy

K. Fattouch et al. (eds.), *Advances in Treatments for Aortic Valve and Root Diseases*, https://doi.org/10.1007/978-3-319-66483-5_24

importance in the study of next-generation devices in low- and intermediate-risk cohorts.

A more granular scheme, which is common in clinical practice and proposed for future trials, may add prognostic value.

In a recent retrospective study by Jones and coll [8], the value of a 9-grade system of aortic regurgitation was evaluated in 237 patients.

The authors report a unit hazard ratio of 2.26 (95% confidence interval, 1.48–3.43; P <0.001) for 1-year mortality for each 1+ increase in AR after TAVR, ranging from no 1-year mortality for patients with no AR to 50% in those patients with 2 to 3+ AR.

Although a 9-point grading system may be a little too granular, as data are limited with the more severe grades, this analysis does support movement toward the more expanded grading system proposed by Pibarot and colleagues in PARTNER II [9].

It is to be hoped that these data will be considered with the next iteration of VARC [10].

Recent data from the PARTNER 2 [1] and S3 High Risk Cohort [11] trials have demonstrated extremely low rates of moderate or severe AR after TAVI and failed to show a difference in 1-year mortality between patients with no or trivial AR compared with mild AR.

Certainly, a more comprehensive understanding of the spectrum of trivial to mild AR now takes on increasing importance, with the significant reductions in moderate to severe PVL among the current generation of TAVI devices and as studies extend to low-risk populations.

24.2 PPM

Post-procedural new or worsened conduction abnormalities (CA) and permanent pacemaker implantation (PPI) after TAVI remain a serious concern.

The incidence of new or worsened CA, in particular complete left bundle branch block (LBBB) and PPI with balloon-expandable valves has been reported to be between 8 and 30% [12, 13, 14, 15] and 5 and 12% [16, 17], respectively and higher is the incidence with self expandable valve [18].

Although PPI does not seem to affect survival [19, 20], overall costs and hospital stay are increased [21] and symptomatic benefit may be limited [22]. New or worsened CA may negatively affect left ventricular function recovery and increase the risk for PPI during follow-up [12, 13].

The occurrence of conduction disturbances and, therefore, need for PPMI after TAVI is explained by the close proximity of the aortic valve and the LVOT to the conduction system. The atrioventricular node is located close to the subaortic region and membranous septum, the left bundle branch runs at the base of the interleaflet triangle separating the RCC and the NCC [23]. Assumed mechanisms of post TAVI conduction disturbances are compression of the conduction system by calcium, the stent frame of the valve or hematoma [24–26]. With preexisting conduction delays within the atrioventricular node or the right bundle branch additional damage of the left bundle branch is, therefore, the plausible explanation for the high rate of PPMI in these cases, since the pressure originating from the device comes from the left ventricular side. The close relation of the left bundle branch to the aortic valve in particular results in a frequent occurrence of new-onset LBBB after TAVI.

Therefore, identification of predictors for PPI after TAVI is an important issue in the modern treatment of patients with symptomatic severe aortic stenosis. As reported in previous studies [27] and in a recent meta-analysis [28], pre-existing RBBB is a strong predictor for PPI after TAVI.

This was also observed in a recent study, by Husser O et al., where baseline ECG parameters were most important for the prediction of PPI [29] Moreover, it was found a strong, clear relationship to implantation depth and extreme oversizing.

An adjustment of implantation height and careful adherence to the sizing algorithms may result in a reduction of new or worsened CA or PPI [29].

24.3 Durability/Thrombosis

Long-term valve durability concerns have remained a limitation in the expansion of TAVI to lower-risk patients. The 5-year follow-up data from PARTNER [30–34] is reassuring, in that no episodes of structural deterioration requiring replacement were observed, and valve hemodynamics (gradient and effective orifice areas) remained stable and the gap in terms of paravalvular regurgitation has narrowed considerably with newer-generation TAVI devices [35].

Joint data from early adopting TAVI centres in Rouen and Vancouver presented by Dvir et al. at EuroPCR in May 2016 [36] suggested relatively high rates of structural degeneration of first-generation TAVI devices implanted five to 14 years previously, particularly in subjects with renal failure.

However, these preliminary unpublished data were criticised on account of methodological considerations, the novel endpoint chosen, the lack of clinical correlations (particularly symptomatic status), and failure to appreciate the hazards of presenting long-term Kaplan-Meier survival analysis based upon such small numbers at follow-up. Moreover, senior co-investigators from Rouen and Vancouver have subsequently presented refined independent analyses of the same datasets at TVT in June 2016 using different study endpoints with reassuring outcomes [37, 38]. To date, there are no robust data to signal that the durability of transcatheter heart valves is a cause for concern.

Nevertheless, additional follow-up data in transcatheter valves will be required in the future to declare equivalence with the most durable surgical bioprosthetic valves [39]. Perhaps the uncertainty of long-term durability becomes less concerning with the possibility of transcatheter valve-in-valve therapy to extend the duration of nonsurgical valve treatment.

The recent findings of aortic bioprosthetic leaflet dysfunction with leaflet immobility, thrombosis, or both are the focus of increasing interest [40–56]. Leaflet immobility and valve thrombosis have been reported with both transcatheter and surgical aortic valve bioprostheses. The relationships between these abnormalities and their incidence, time course, clinical significance, predisposing factors, optimal imaging modality, and current therapeutic options remain uncertain but are rapidly evolving. Four-dimensional computerized tomographic imaging has been determined to have the highest sensitivity in studies evaluating leaflet immobility and valve thrombosis. Echocardiography is also used during surveillance, but it appears to be less sensitive. The definitive diagnosis of valve thrombosis is based on a combination of diagnostic 4-dimensional computerized tomographic imaging findings, resolution of imaging abnormalities, and elevated transcatheter gradients with anticoagulation or surgical or pathological confirmation. Uncertainty about the incidence and clinical significance of the findings is the basis of 2 US Food and Drug Administration–approved studies comparing transcatheter and surgical aortic valve replacement with a subset undergoing surveillance 4-dimensional computerized tomographic imaging. Given the expansion of transcatheter aortic valve procedures, including potentially lower-risk patients, the resolution of these uncertainties is critical.

24.4 Stroke

In parallel with TAVI technology developments, advanced imaging systems and accessory devices have been—and will continue to be—dramatically enhanced.

Sophisticated CT image work stations for pre-procedure case planning will help to guide correct selection of valve sizes and types. Intraprocedural imaging with new wide-angle 3-dimensional intracardiac echocardiography and multimodality coregistration capabilities will improve case-based decision making without adding undo complexity.

Although the frequency of periprocedural major clinical neurological events after TAVI has decreased, lingering questions remain regarding minor neurological events and neurocognitive functional changes. Several cerebral protection devices have been developed to capture or deflect liberated embolic debris during TAVI procedures, and neuroimaging studies have already shown improvements suggesting increased cerebral perfusion with cerebral protection in early randomized clinical trials. Decisions of systematic versus selective use of such devices in high-risk patients during TAVI remain controversial and await further clinical outcomes data from ongoing randomized clinical trials.

In a recent clinical event meta-analysis including the totality of RCT on this subject to date [57], embolic protection (EP) was associated with a significantly lower risk in death or stroke, which corresponded to 4.0% absolute risk reduction and NNT of 22 (i.e., for every 22 patients assigned to an EP device, 1 death or stroke event may be averted). These findings suggest that EP may be a clinically relevant adjunctive strategy in patients undergoing TAVI. It is plausible that the magnitude of the benefit may be accentuated in patients at high risk for cerebrovascular complications. Additionally, because subclinical ischemic brain injury is associated with both cognitive and functional neurological impairment over time, prevention of subclinical embolization may be particularly important when treating younger and lower risk patients with severe aortic stenosis.

Conclusion

In conclusion, over the past decade, TAVI has evolved as an important and mature alternative to SAVR for patients with high or prohibitive surgical risk. Patient screening and procedural techniques have been effectively modified by using a heart team approach, and technical advances were introduced in a rapid fashion to simplify the procedure and reduce complications.

Further expansion of TAVI to intermediate-risk patients was in the pipeline after several observational propensity score-matching studies showing comparable survival rates at one year with TAVI and surgical valve replacement [58–61]. The indication was recently validated by the FDA after the positive results of the randomised PARTNER 2 study with the Edwards SAPIEN XT valve [1]. This study showed comparable benefit of TAVI on the primary endpoint of death and disabling stroke at two years compared to SAVR, and better results when the femoral approach was used. The superiority of TAVI versus SAVR was even enhanced in the PARTNER 2 S3i propensity score analysis study [35] using the latest generation of Edwards valves (SAPIEN 3). With similar endpoints at two years, the recent report of the SURTAVI trial with the Medtronic CoreValve at the 2017 American College of Cardiology sessions also confirmed the non-inferiority of TAVI compared to surgery in this subset of patients [18]. Of note, TAVI for intermediate-risk patients appears in the updated 2017 AHA/ACC guidelines, with a Class IIb indication. Finally, after the promising results of a first small-size randomised trial published in 2015 (NOTION trial) [62], three major randomised trials are currently ongoing in "all-comers", the upcoming results of which might lead to a broad expansion of TAVI to low-risk patients in the near future.

The modern-day medical adventure of TAVI has thus transformed clinical practice and is on the way to becoming the default strategy for the treatment of aortic stenosis. It can be predicted that within five years the indication for SAVR will be limited to patients who are not optimal candidates for TAVI.

References

1. Leon MB, Smith CR, Mack MJ, Makkar RR, Svensson LG, Kodali SK, Thourani VH, Tuzcu EM, Miller DC, Herrmann HC, Doshi D, Cohen DJ, Pichard AD, Kapadia S, Dewey T, Babaliaros V, Szeto WY, Williams MR, Kereiakes D, Zajarias A, Greason KL, Whisenant BK, Hodson RW, Moses JW, Trento A, Brown DL, Fearon WF, Pibarot P, Hahn RT, Jaber WA, Anderson WN, Alu MC, Webb JG, PARTNER 2 Investigators. Transcatheter or surgical aortic-valve replacement in intermediate-risk patients. N Engl J Med. 2016;374:1609–20.
2. Bosmans J, Paelinck B. Transcatheter aortic valve replacement: a further step towards a patient-tailored therapy. EuroIntervention. 2016;12:695–7.

3. Abdel-Wahab M, Zahn R, Horack M, Gerckens U, Schuler G, Sievert H, et al. Aortic regurgitation after transcatheter aortic valve implantation: incidence and early outcome. Results from the German Transcatheter Aortic Valve Interventions Registry. Heart. 2011;97:899–906.
4. Moat NE, Ludman P, de Belder MA, Bridgewater B, Cunningham AD, Young CP, et al. Long-term outcomes after transcatheter aortic valve implantation in high-risk patients with severe aortic stenosis: the U.K. TAVI (United Kingdom Transcatheter Aortic Valve Implantation) registry. J Am Coll Cardiol. 2011;58:2130–8.
5. Hahn RT, Pibarot P, Stewart WJ, Weissman NJ, Gopalakrishnan D, Keane MG, et al. Comparison of transcatheter and surgical aortic valve replacement in severe aortic stenosis: a longitudinal study of echocardiography parameters in cohort a of the PARTNER trial (placement of aortic transcatheter valves). J Am Coll Cardiol. 2013;61:2514–21.
6. Jerez-Valero M, Urena M, Webb JG, Tamburino C, Munoz-Garcia AJ, Cheema A, et al. Clinical impact of aortic regurgitation after transcatheter aortic valve replacement: insights into the degree and acuteness of presentation. JACC Cardiovasc Interv. 2014;7:1022–32.
7. Kodali S, Pibarot P, Douglas PS, Williams M, Xu K, Thourani V, et al. Paravalvular regurgitation after transcatheter aortic valve replacement with the Edwards Sapien valve in the PARTNER trial: characterizing patients and impact on outcomes. Eur Heart J. 2015;36:449–56.
8. Jones B, Tuzcu E, Krishnaswamy A, Popovic Z, Mick S, Roselli E, et al. Prognostic significance of mild AR in predicting mortality after TAVR. J Thorac Cardiovasc Surg. 2016;152:783–90.
9. Pibarot P, Hahn RT, Weissman NJ, Monaghan MJ. Assessment of paravalvular regurgitation following TAVR: a proposal of unifying grading scheme. JACC Cardiovasc Imaging. 2015;8:340–60.
10. Reardon MJ, Popma JJ. Residual aortic regurgitation after transcatheter aortic valve replacement under the echocardiographic microscope. J Thorac Cardiovasc Surg. 2016;152:659–60.
11. Herrmann HC, Thourani VH, Kodali SK, Makkar RR, Szeto WY, Anwaruddin S, Desai N, Lim S, Chris Malaisrie S, Kereiakes DJ, Ramee S, Greason KL, Kapadia S, Babaliaros V, Hahn RT, Pibarot P, Weissman NJ, Leipsic J, Whisenant BK, Webb JG, Mack MJ, Leon MB, PARTNER Investigators. One-year clinical outcomes with SAPIEN 3 transcatheter aortic valve replacement in high-risk and inoperable patients with severe aortic stenosis. Circulation. 2016;134:130–40.
12. Hoffmann R, Herpertz R, Lotfipour S, et al. Impact of a new conduction defect after transcatheter aortic valve implantation on left ventricular function. JACC Cardiovasc Interv. 2012;5:1257–63.
13. Tzikas A, van Dalen BM, Van Mieghem NM, et al. Frequency of conduction abnormalities after transcatheter aortic valve implantation with the Medtronic-CoreValve and the effect on left ventricular ejection fraction. Am J Cardiol. 2011;107:285–9.
14. Franzoni I, Latib A, Maisano F, et al. Comparison of incidence and predictors of left bundle branch block after transcatheter aortic valve implantation using the CoreValve versus the Edwards valve. Am J Cardiol. 2013;112:554–9.
15. Urena M, Mok M, Serra V, et al. Predictive factors and long-term clinical consequences of persistent left bundle branch block following transcatheter aortic valve implantation with a balloon-expandable valve. J Am Coll Cardiol. 2012;60:1743–52.
16. Binder RK, Rodés-Cabau J, Wood DA, et al. Transcatheter aortic valve replacement with the SAPIEN 3: a new balloon-expandable transcatheter heart valve. J Am Coll Cardiol Intv. 2013;6:293–300.
17. Webb J, Gerosa G, Lefèvre T, et al. Multicenter evaluation of a next-generation balloon expandable transcatheter aortic valve. J Am Coll Cardiol. 2014;64:2235–43.
18. Tarantini G, Mojoli M, Purita P, et al. Unravelling the (arte)fact of increased pacemaker rate with the Edwards SAPIEN 3 valve. EuroIntervention. 2015;11:343–50.
19. Murray MI, Geis N, Pleger ST, et al. First experience with the new generation Edwards SAPIEN 3 aortic bioprosthesis: procedural results and short term outcome. J Interv Cardiol. 2015;28:109–16.

20. Reardon MJ, Van Mieghem NM, Popma JJ, Kleiman NS, Søndergaard L, Mumtaz M, Adams DH, Deeb GM, Maini B, Gada H, Chetcuti S, Gleason T, Heiser J, Lange R, Merhi W, Oh JK, Olsen PS, Piazza N, Williams M, Windecker S, Yakubov SJ, Grube E, Makkar R, Lee JS, Conte J, Vang E, Nguyen H, Chang Y, Mugglin AS, Serruys PWJC, Kappetein AP, SURTAVI Investigators. Surgical or transcatheter aortic-valve replacement in intermediate-risk patients. N Engl J Med. 2017;376:1321–31.
21. Buellesfeld L, Stortecky S, Heg D, et al. Impact of permanent pacemaker implantation on clinical outcome among patients undergoing transcatheter aortic valve implantation. J Am Coll Cardiol. 2012;60:493–501.
22. Urena M, Webb JG, Tamburino C, et al. Permanent pacemaker implantation following transcatheter aortic valve implantation: impact on late clinical outcomes and left ventricular function. Circulation. 2013;129:1233–43.
23. Chevreul K, Brunn M, Cadier B, et al. Cost of transcatheter aortic valve implantation and factors associated with higher hospital stay cost in patients of the FRANCE (FRench Aortic National CoreValve and Edwards) registry. Arch Cardiovasc Dis. 2013;106:209–19.
24. Tops LF, Schalij MJ, Bax JJ. The effects of right ventricular apical pacing on ventricular function and dyssynchrony: implications for therapy. J Am Coll Cardiol. 2009;54:764–76.
25. Piazza N, de Jaegere P, Schultz C, Becker AE, Serruys PW, Anderson RH. Anatomy of the aortic valvar complex and its implications for transcatheter implantation of the aortic valve. Circ Cardiovasc Interv. 2008;1:74–81.
26. Nazif TM, Williams MR, Hahn RT, Kapadia S, Babaliaros V, Rodés-Cabau J, et al. Clinical implications of new-onset left bundle branch block after transcatheter aortic valve replacement: analysis of the PARTNER experience. Eur Heart J. 2013;35:1599–607.
27. Moreno R, Dobarro D, Lopez de Sa E, Prieto M, Morales C, Calvo Orbe L, Moreno-Gomez I, Filgueiras D, Sanchez-Recalde A, Galeote G, Jimenez-Valero S, Lopez-Sendon JL. Cause of complete atrioventricular block after percutaneous aortic valve implantation: insights from a necropsy study. Circulation. 2009;120:e29–30.
28. Saji M, MuraiT TT, Tabata M, Takanashi S, Takayama M. Autopsy finding of the Sapien XT valve from a patient who died suddenly after transcatheter aortic valve replacement. Cardiovasc Interv Ther. 2013;28:267–71.
29. Roten L, Wenaweser P, Delacrétaz E, et al. Incidence and predictors of atrioventricular conduction impairment after transcatheter aortic valve implantation. Am J Cardiol. 2010;106:1473–80.
30. Siontis GC, Jüni P, Pilgrim T, et al. Predictors of permanent pacemaker implantation in patients with severe aortic stenosis undergoing TAVR: a meta-analysis. J Am Coll Cardiol. 2014;64:129–40.
31. Husser O, Pellegrini C, Kessler T, Burgdorf C, Thaller H, Patrick Mayr N, Kasel AM, Kastrati A, Schunkert H, Hengstenberg C. Predictors of permanent pacemaker implantations and new-onset conduction abnormalities with the SAPIEN 3 balloon-expandable transcatheter heart valve. JACC Cardiovasc Interv. 2016;3:244–54.
32. Kapadia SR, Leon MB, Makkar RR, et al. 5-Year outcomes of transcatheter aortic valve replacement compared with standard treatment for patients with inoperable aortic stenosis (PARTNER 1): a randomised controlled trial. Lancet. 2015;385:2485–91.
33. Joint Task Force on the Management of Valvular Heart Disease of the European Society of Cardiology (ESC) and the European Association for Cardio- Thoracic Surgery (EACTS), Vahanian A, Alfieri O, et al. Guidelines on the management of valvular heart disease (version 2012). Eur J Cardiothorac Surg. 2012;42:S1–44.
34. Smith CR, Leon MB, Mack MJ, et al. Transcatheter versus surgical aortic-valve replacement in high-risk patients. N Engl J Med. 2011;364:2187–98.
35. Adams DH, Popma JJ, Reardon MJ, et al. Transcatheter aortic-valve replacement with a self-expanding prosthesis. N Engl J Med. 2014;370:1790–8.
36. Mack MJ, Leon MB, Smith CR, et al. 5-Year outcomes of transcatheter aortic valve replacement or surgical aortic valve replacement for high surgical risk patients with aortic stenosis (PARTNER 1): a randomised controlled trial. Lancet. 2015;385:2477–84.

37. Thourani VH, Kodali S, Makkar RR, Herrmann HC, Williams M, Babaliaros V, Smalling R, Lim S, Malaisrie SC, Kapadia S, Szeto WY, Greason KL, Kereiakes D, Ailawadi G, Whisenant BK, Devireddy C, Leipsic J, Hahn RT, Pibarot P, Weissman NJ, Jaber WA, Cohen DJ, Suri R, Tuzcu EM, Svensson LG, Webb JG, Moses JW, Mack MJ, Miller DC, Smith CR, Alu MC, Parvataneni R, D'Agostino RB Jr, Leon MB. Transcatheter aortic valve replacement versus surgical valve replacement in intermediate-risk patients: a propensity score analysis. Lancet. 2016;387:2218–25.
38. Dvir D, Eltchaninoff H, Ye J, Kan A, Durand E, Bizios A, Cheung A, Aziz M, Simonato M, Tron C, Arbel Y, Moss R, Leipsic J, Ofek H, Perlman G, Barbanti M, Seidman MA, Blanke P, Yao R, Boone R, Lauck S, Lichtenstein S, Wood D, Cribier A, Webb J. First look at long-term durability of transcatheter heart valves: assessment of valve function up to 10-years after implantation. EuroPCR, Paris, 2016.
39. Eltchaninoff H. Clinical experiences and echo data from Rouen. Chicago: Presented at TVT; 2016.
40. Webb JG, Dvir D. Ten year follow-up of TAVI from Vancouver. Chicago: Presented at TVT; 2016.
41. Johnston DR, Soltesz EG, Vakil N, et al. Longterm durability of bioprosthetic aortic valves: implications from 12,569 implants. Ann Thorac Surg. 2015;99:1239–47.
42. Makkar RR, Fontana G, Jilaihawi H, Chakravarty T, Kofoed KF, de Backer O, Asch FM, Ruiz CE, Olsen NT, Trento A, Friedman J, Berman D, Cheng W, Kashif M, Jelnin V, Kliger CA, Guo H, Pichard AD, Weissman NJ, Kapadia S, Manasse E, Bhatt DL, Leon MB, Søndergaard L. Possible subclinical leaflet thrombosis in bioptostheticaortic valves. N Engl J Med. 2015;373:2015–24. https://doi.org/10.1056/NEJMoa1509233.
43. Holmes DR, Mack MJ. Uncertainty and possible subclinical valve leaflet thrombosis. N Engl J Med. 2015;373:2080–2. https://doi.org/10.1056/NEJMe1511683.
44. De Marchena E, Mesa J, Pomenti S, Marin Y, Kall C, Marincic X, Yahagi K, Ladich E, Kutz R, Aga Y, Ragosta M, Chawla A, Ring ME, Virmani R. Thrombus formation following transcatheter aortic valve replacement. JACC Cardiovasc Interv. 2015;8:728–39. https://doi.org/10.1016/j.jcin.2015.03.005.
45. Tourmousoglou C, Rao V, Lalos S, Dougenis D. What is the best approach in a patient with a failed aortic bioprosthetic valve: transcatheter aortic valve replacement or redo aortic valve replacement? Interact Cardiovasc Thorac Surg. 2015;20:837–43. https://doi.org/10.1093/icvts/ivv037.
46. Leetmaa T, Hansson NC, Leipsic J, Jensen K, Poulsen SH, Andersen HR, Jensen JM, Webb J, Blanke P, Tang M, Norgaard BL. Early aortic transcatheter heart valve thrombosis: diagnostic value of contrast-enhanced multidetector computed tomography. Circ Cardiovasc Interv. 2015;8:e001596. https://doi.org/10.1161/Circinterventions.114.001596.
47. Egbe AC, Pislaru SV, Pellikka PA, Poterucha JT, Schaff HV, Maleszewski JJ, Connolly HM. Bioprosthetic valve thrombosis versus structural failure: clinical and echocardiographic predictors. J Am Coll Cardiol. 2015;66:2285–94. https://doi.org/10.1016/j.jacc.2015.09.022.
48. Córdoba-Soriano JG, Puri R, Amat-Santos I, Ribeiro HB, Abdul-Jawad Altisent O, del Trigo M, Paradis JM, Dumont E, Urena M, Rodés-Cabau J. Valve thrombosis following transcatheter aortic valve implantation: a systematic review. Rev Esp Cardiol (Engl Ed). 2015;68:198–204. https://doi.org/10.1016/j.rec.2014.10.003.
49. Latib A, Messika-Zeitoun D, Maisano F, Himbert D, Agricola E, Brochet E, Alfieri O, Colombo A, Vahanian A. Reversible Edwards Sapien XT dysfunction due to prosthesis thrombosis presenting as early structural deterioration. J Am Coll Cardiol. 2013;61:787–9. https://doi.org/10.1016/j.jacc.2012.10.016.
50. Brown ML, Park SJ, Sundt TM, Schaff HV. Early thrombosis risk in patients with biologic valves in the aortic position. J Thorac Cardiovasc Surg. 2012;144:108–11. https://doi.org/10.1016/j.jtcvs.2011.05.032.
51. Pislaru SV, Hussain I, Pellikka PA, Maleszewski JJ, Hanna RD, Schaff HV, Connolly HM. Misconceptions, diagnostic challenges and treatment opportunities in bioprosthetic valve

thrombosis: lessons from a case series. Eur J Cardiothorac Surg. 2015;47:725–32. https://doi.org/10.1093/ejcts/ezu201.
52. Nkomo VT, Suri RM, Pislaru SV, Greason KL, Sinak LJ, Holmes DR, Mathew V, Rihal CS. Delayed transcatheter heart valve migration and failure. JACC Cardiovasc Imaging. 2014;7:960–2. https://doi.org/10.1016/j.jcmg.2014.02.010.
53. Latib A, Naganuma T, Abdel-Wahab M, Danenberg H, Cota L, Barbanti M, Baumgartner H, Finkelstein A, Legrand V, de Lezo JS, Kefer J, Messika-Zeitoun D, Richardt G, Stabile E, Kaleschke G, Vahanian A, Laborde JC, Leon MB, Webb JG, Panoulas VF, Maisano F, Alfieri O, Colombo A. Treatment and clinical outcomes of transcatheter heart valve thrombosis. Circ Cardiovasc Interv. 2015;8:e001779. https://doi.org/10.1161/CIRCINTERVENTIONS.114.001779.
54. Del Trigo M, Muñoz-Garcia AJ, Wijeysundera HC, Nombela-Franco L, Cheema AN, Gutierrez E, Serra V, Kefer J, Amat-Santos IJ, Benitez LM, Mewa J, Jiménez-Quevedo P, Alnasser S, Garcia Del Blanco B, Dager A, Abdul-Jawad Altisent O, Puri R, Campelo-Parada F, Dahou A, Paradis JM, Dumont E, Pibarot P, Rodés-Cabau J. Incidence, timing, and predictors of valve hemodynamic deterioration after transcatheter aortic valve replacement: multicenter registry. J Am Coll Cardiol. 2016;67:644–55. https://doi.org/10.1016/j.jacc.2015.10.097.
55. Thourani VH, Suri RM, Gunter RL, Sheng S, O'Brien SM, Ailawadi G, Szeto WY, Dewey TM, Guyton RA, Bavaria JE, Babaliaros V, Gammie JS, Svensson L, Williams M, Badhwar V, Mack MJ. Contemporary real-world outcomes of surgical aortic valve replacement in 141,905 low-risk, intermediate-risk, and high-risk patients. Ann Thorac Surg. 2015;99:55–61. https://doi.org/10.1016/j.athoracsur.2014.06.050.
56. Jander N, Sommer H, Pingpoh C, Kienzle RP, Martin G, Zeh W, Pache G, Siepe M, Beyersdorf F, Schumacher M, Neumann FJ, Minners J. The porcine valve type predicts obstructive thrombosis beyond the first three postoperative months in bioprostheses in the aortic position. Int J Cardiol. 2015;199:90–5. https://doi.org/10.1016/j.ijcard.2015.07.022.
57. Vemulapalli S, Dai D, Mack MJ, Holmes DR, Grover F, Makkar R, Thourani VH, Douglas PS; STS/ACC TVT Registry. Incidence and outcomes of valve hemodynamic deterioration in transcatheteraortic valve replacement in U.S. clinical practice: a report from the Society of Thoracic Surgery/American College of Cardiology Transcatheter Valve Therapy Registry. Presented at American College of Cardiology Meeting; April 2–4, 2016; Chicago, IL.
58. Laschinger JC, Wu C, Ibrahim NG, Shuren JE. Reduced leaflet motion in bioprosthetic aortic valves: the FDA perspective. N Engl J Med. 2015;373:1996–8. https://doi.org/10.1056/NEJMp1512264.
59. Giustino G, Sorrentino S, Mehran R, Faggioni M, Dangas G. Cerebral embolic protection during TAVR. A clinical event meta-analysis. J Am Coll Cardiol. 2017;69:463–70.
60. Piazza N, Kalesan B, van Mieghem N, Head S, Wenaweser P, Carrel TP, Bleiziffer S, de Jaegere PP, Gahl B, Anderson RH, Kappetein AP, Lange R, Serruys PW, Windecker S, Jüni P. A 3-center comparison of 1-year mortality outcomes between transcatheter aortic valve implantation and surgical aortic valve replacement on the basis of propensity score matching among intermediate-risk surgical patients. JACC Cardiovasc Interv. 2013;6:443–51.
61. Wenaweser P, Stortecky S, Schwander S, Heg D, Huber C, Pilgrim T, Gloekler S, O'Sullivan CJ, Meier B, Jüni P, Carrel T, Windecker S. Clinical outcomes of patients with estimated low or intermediate surgical risk undergoing transcatheter aortic valve implantation. Eur Heart J. 2013;34:1894–905.
62. Thyregod HG, Steinbruchel DA, Ihlemann N, Nissen H, Kjeldsen BJ, Petursson P, Chang Y, Franzen OW, Engstrøm T, Clemmensen P, Hansen PB, Andersen LW, Olsen PS, Søndergaard L. Transcatheter versus surgical aortic valve replacement in patients with severe aortic valve stenosis: 1-year results from the all-comers NOTION randomized clinical trial. J Am Coll Cardiol. 2015;65:2184–94.

Check for updates

The Impact of Surgical and Trans-Catheter Aortic Valve Replacement on Endothelial Function: New Markers Ahead

25

Fiorella Devito, Marco Moscarelli, Marco Matteo Ciccone, Paola Rizzo, Roberto Ferrari, and Giuseppe Speziale

25.1 Introduction

Aortic stenosis (AS) is a widespread valvular heart disease, especially in Europe and North America due to increased life expectancy. It is estimated a prevalence of 3% particularly in the elderly (over 75 years). The progressive deterioration of the aortic valve has always been considered a degenerative process, however a growing number of studies suggests that degenerative AS represents not a passive process but a biologically active disease, where both proliferative and inflammatory factors play a pivotal role [1]. Moreover, the obstruction of the stenotic valve to the blood flow affects the peripheral vascular integrity by reducing the stroke volume and by the formation of turbulent flow. Surgical aortic valve replacement (AVR) is still considered the gold standard treatment for severe and symptomatic aortic stenosis, however trans-catheter valve implantation (TAVI) techniques are showing comparable results while being less invasive, even in the cohort of patients at intermediate risk for surgery. It may be foreseen, in the light of recent trials, that TAVI will be more frequently offered in relatively younger patients with extended expectation of life, thereby more comprehensive outcomes might be considered in order to compare performance of surgical vs. trans catheter aortic valve replacement.

Marco Moscarelli is a joint first author.

F. Devito • M. Moscarelli (✉) • G. Speziale
GVM Care and Research, Anthea Hospital, Via Camillo Rosalba 35/37, Bari, Italy
e-mail: m.moscarelli@imperial.ac.uk

M.M. Ciccone
Sezione di Malattie dell'Apparato Cardiovascolare, Dipartimento dell'Emergenza e dei Trapianti di Organi, Università degli Studi "Aldo Moro", Bari, Italy

P. Rizzo • R. Ferrari
Department of Cardiology and LTTA Centre, University Hospital of Ferrara and Maria Cecilia Hospital, GVM Care and Research, ES Health Science Foundation, Cotignola, Italy

K. Fattouch et al. (eds.), *Advances in Treatments for Aortic Valve and Root Diseases*, https://doi.org/10.1007/978-3-319-66483-5_25

25.2 Endothelial Function

Aortic stenosis is a form of 'atherosclerotic vascular disease' and it is associated with an increased risk of cardiovascular death; interestingly a limited number of studies have evaluated its effect on vascular integrity and function [2, 3]. Endothelial dysfunction (ED) is a pathological condition characterized by the reduced bioavailability of nitric oxide and represents a precursor of atherosclerotic vascular process. Different studies on patients with coronary artery disease demonstrated that an improvement in endothelial function correlates with a reduced incidence of cardiovascular events. Endothelial function is thereby identified as a prognostic parameter of progression of vascular diseases. Cardiovascular risk factors (arterial hypertension, diabetes, hyperlipidemia, smoking) can impair endothelial integrity by promoting the production of vasoconstrictive substances and reducing the bioavailability of nitric oxide, the most important vasodilatative substance released by endothelium followed by biochemical (acetylcholine, bradykinin) and mechanical (shear wall stress) stimuli [4–6]. This altered balance between the release of vasodilatative and vasoconstrictive substances promotes inflammatory and thrombotic processes, by favoring proliferation and migration of vascular smooth cells, platelet aggregation, production of cytokines, growth factors, monocytes and the consequent expression of adhesion molecules [7, 8].

It is believed that AS has a similar impact on the systemic circulation by impairing the systemic endothelial function. Also, the increase in shear stress that occurs in AS, as a consequence of a reduced cardiac output and a turbulent flow, seems to affect systemic vascular integrity. Several studies have investigated this relationship and have managed to correlate impaired endothelial function and abnormal values of circulating endothelial micro-particles in patients with AS. However, the exact nature of this relation is still under investigation. Poggianti et al. first demonstrated in patient with AS and concomitant coronary artery diseases, the presence of systemic endothelial dysfunction as a precursor of atherosclerosis [9]. Erdogan et al. highlighted that in patients with hypertension, the concomitant presence of AS has a positive predictive value for endothelial dysfunction, hypothesizing the possible role of endothelial dysfunction as a precursor of aortic sclerosis [10].

A quantitative measure of the endothelial function can be obtained with 'macro and micro markers' of endothelial dysfunction.

25.3 Macro-Marker of Endothelial Dysfunction: "Flow-Mediated Vasodilation"

The non-invasive assessment of endothelial function can be performed peripherally at the level of the brachial artery, by measuring changes in artery diameter induced after an increase in the blood flow ("reactive hyperemia"). This technique is conventionally named "flow-mediated vasodilation" (FMD). This process has been validated in clinical research, both in the ischemic and non-ischemic setting [11]. The assessment of FMD is carried out as follow: temperature, food, stress, drugs, and sympathetic stimuli influence the FMD. The study must be performed in a quiet, temperature- controlled room (24 °C), early in the morning. The subjects should not take exciting substances (coffee/tea, chocolate) or play exercise for at least 4–6 h before the exam. In a supine position, the right arm must be immobilized and the right brachial artery must be evaluated in a long axis projection between 5 and 10 cm above the elbow using a 7.0 MHz or higher linear probe. The study should be performed using a high-resolution ultrasonography connected to an image analysis system, for tracing the brachial artery diameter in real time by analyzing B-mode ultrasound images (Figs. 25.1 and 25.2). With the subject in supine position for at least 10 min, the arm is positioned comfortably in order to get clear images of the brachial artery. The selected artery segment to be displayed is above the antecubital fossa in the longitudinal plane. A sphygmomanometer cuff must be placed in the distal site to the artery, on the forearm. After 1 min of flow image baseline acquisition, the artery is occluded by inflating the cuff to a pressure of 200–220 mmHg for 300 s. The cuff deflation induces a short state of high flow (reactive hyperemia) through the brachial artery. The resulting increased shear stress provides the stimulus for dilatation of the brachial artery. The image of the artery is then recorded continuously for 2–3 min after ischemia. The percentage of FMD is calculated as the ratio of the change in diameter (maximal dilatation after deflation baseline) divided by the baseline value × 100. It is expected that in a context of severe aortic stenosis, the FMD is significantly reduced, while after intervention (either surgical or percutaneous) it gradually improves. Figs. 25.1 and 25.2 show FMD values measured before surgery and after 3 months, where an improvement of endothelial function can be seen.

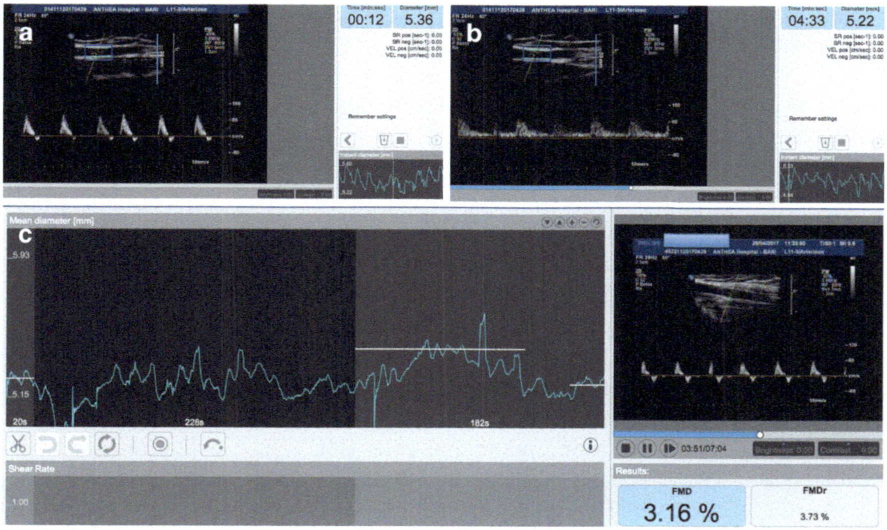

Fig. 25.1 Flow mediated dilation analysis (FMD) day 4 after aortic valve replacement (cardiovascular suite QUIPU www.quipu.eu); (**a**) baseline analysis (before ischemic period); (**b**) after reperfusion; (**c**) final analysis with FMD value of 3.16%. Total length of analysis 420 s (20 s baseline; 240 s of ischemic period; 168 s of reperfusion)

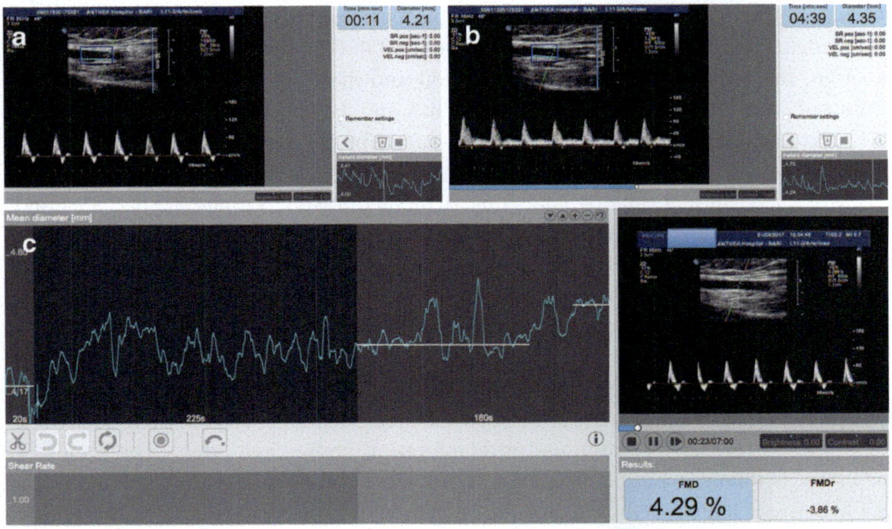

Fig. 25.2 Flow mediated dilation analysis (FMD) day 2 months after aortic valve replacement; (**a**) baseline analysis (before ischemic period); (**b**) after reperfusion; (**c**) final analysis with an improved FMD value of 4.29%. Total length of analysis 420 s (20 s baseline; 240 s of ischemic period; 168 s of reperfusion)

25.4 Micro-Marker of Endothelial Dysfunction: the Role of Circulating Micro-Particles

During the initial stages of AS, lipoprotein deposition and macrophage and T-lymphocyte infiltration in the fibrosa play a key role. The oxidation of low-density lipoproteins and the production of cytokines by activated macrophages and lymphocytes, promotes oxidative stress, inflammation, extracellular matrix remodeling, vavlular interstitial cells pathological differentiation, and finally fibrosis and calcification. Extracellular matrix remodeling is mediated by elevated activity of matrix metalloproteinases and cathepsin S, that contribute to matrix disarray and deposition of disorganized new fibers [12, 13]. In the systemic inflammatory process that occurs during AS, a pivotal role is played by circulating cells.

Valgimigli et al. demonstrated that biochemical substances and circulating factors released in serum in patients affected by coronary disease play a pro-apoptotic role on human umbilical vein endothelial cells (HUVECs), when the serum is incubated with HUVECs and the apoptotic effect is related to the progression of the atherosclerotic plaque and with the number of complex coronary lesions; if similar biochemical scenario happens even in the context of AS need to be deeply investigated [14].

Some studies have shown that increased shear stress in AS stimulates platelet, leukocytes and endothelial cells to micro-particles production (PMPs: CD31(+)/CD61(+), CD62P(+) LMPs: CD11b(+)) and EMPs: CD62E(+) respectively).

Endothelial micro-particles (EMPs) are small phospholipid membrane vesicles (0.1–1 μm) that are released into the systemic circulation following an inflammatory state after apoptosis of endothelial cells. Several studies demonstrated that inflammatory cytokines, reactive oxygen species, thrombin, plasminogen activator inhibitor, C-reactive protein can induce in vitro EMPs production. The production of EMPs has been also demonstrated in inflammatory lesions such as the atherosclerotic plaque, by playing a crucial role in development and progression of atherosclerosis and thrombosis. This pro-atherosclerotic effect on the vascular endothelium is favored in part by the reduced synthesis of nitric oxide, that seems to have a protective function towards EMPs formation and release [15]. Several studies in patients with endothelial dysfunction, investigated the inversely correlation between levels of circulating EMPs and the amplitude of flow-mediated dilatation, establishing the role of circulating EMPs as independent predictors of cardiovascular outcome [16, 17]. Recently Diehl et al. demonstrated that values of EMPs and PMP are abnormal in the serum of patients with severe AS, underlining the crucial role played by inflammation at the level of vascular endothelium during this pathology. Circulating micro-particles are therefore considered prognostic biomarkers of ED and atherosclerotic diseases.

25.5 Aortic Valve Replacement and Endothelial Dysfunction

Surgical aortic valve replacement of a stenotic valve with the aid of cardiopulmonary bypass (CPB) represents the gold standard treatment for symptomatic patients to improve symptoms and prognosis [18]. Some studies demonstrated that degenerative AS compromised endothelial integrity by a decreased output trough a stenotic valve or instability of shear stress, and it is independently associated with endothelial dysfunction. In fact AVR may induce a significant improvement in hemodynamic status and an increase in FMD values in subjects with AS [19, 20].

Morelos et al. studied the role of CPB on systemic endothelial dysfunction in patients undergoing cardiac surgery. They found that patients undergoing AVR experienced an early impairment of peripheral endothelial dysfunction, with the normalization of FMD values after 7 or 10 days [21].

Takata et al. showed that AVR induced an important improvement in endothelial function in as proven by the raising of FMD values after intervention (from 3.1 ± 1.8 to 6.0 ± 2.7%), although the change in brachial artery diameter before and after AVR was not significant (4.0 ± 0.7 mm vs. 3.9 ± 0.6 mm) [19]. On the contrary, Chenevard et al. found no improvement of FMD values after AVR, despite normalization of hemodynamic parameters. These results might suggest that vascular integrity may not be entirely restored after aortic valve replacement.

25.6 Transcatheter Aortic Valve Implantation and Endothelial Dysfunction

Therapeutic decisions regarding AS are based on several criteria, such as operative risk, clinical status and hemodynamic severity [22]. Several studies have proven the advantages of TAVI in patients with contraindications to conventional surgery or at high surgical risk, and recent reports have shown that such percutaneous approach has favorable clinical outcomes at 1 year even in patients considered at intermediate or low risk according to STS risk score [23].

One study in literature assessed endothelial integrity by FMD after TAVI, proving that therapy for severe AS was associated with improved systemic endothelial function and integrity; Horn et al. showed that FMD values measured in the brachial artery increased from 3.2 ± 0.9% before TAVI to 3.6 ± 0.8% after intervention and this change in endothelium response was associated, even if not significantly, with the decrease in mean aortic valve pressure gradient.

On the contraries, different studies have investigated the role of micro-particles in patients undergoing TAVI [24].

The level of EMPs assessed by flow cytometry decreased and there was a close correlation between the fall of EMPs and the increase of FMD, regardless of cardiovascular comorbidities. The wall shear stress (calculated with the formula: 8 × blood viscosity (0.035 dyne × s/cm^2) × flow velocity/diameter) also increased after intervention and it is correlated inversely with levels of EMPs, suggesting that the wall share stress play a crucial role in the cellular survival. The lowering of EMPs levels was also observed 3 months after the procedure.

Jung et al. also observed that after TAVI there was a significant reduction in circulating CD62E+ EMPs at 1, 3 and 6 months of follow-up, but serum concentration of CD31 + /CD42b – EMPs remained unchanged after TAVI procedure and during six months of follow-up. Moreover PMP levels increased significantly after TAVI, assuming a possible predictive role of platelet particles in predicting thrombus formation on cusps of the implanted valve.

However, in a recent report, Marchini et al. have demonstrated that circulating micro-particles levels do not differ significantly 5 days after TAVI, probably because of the unknown MPs half-life and intense stress correlated to the procedure itself. They hypothesized that a longer time is needed to restore endothelial integrity and function [25, 26].

25.7 Perspectives

Aortic stenosis is associated with endothelial dysfunction. There are probably two mechanisms that might explain this condition. First: the same 'inflammatory vascular process' that affects the aortic valve simultaneously interferes with the peripheral arterial vessels. Second: once the aortic valve becomes stenotic, the reduction of the stroke volume, the blood flow turbulence and the variation of the wall share stress maintain and implement the state of endothelial dysfunction. Aortic valve replacement and TAVI may both improve the endothelial performance by relieving the stenosis. Endothelial function can be assessed and quantitative measured with macro-marker (flow mediated dilation) and micro-marker (e.g. circulating endothelium derived micro-particles). Evaluating endothelial function before and most importantly after AVR and TAVI could represent a predictive factor particularly to identify the best therapeutic choice in patients at intermediate surgical risk who could benefit from both therapeutic options. However, more studies are needed to validate the role of flow these markers in such a context.

Conflict of Interest None declared.

References

1. Manning WJ. Asymptomatic aortic stenosis in the elderly: a clinical review. JAMA. 2013;310:1490–7.
2. Stewart BF, Siscovick D, Lind BK, Gardin JM, Gottdiener JS, Smith VE, Kitzman DW, Otto CM. Clinical factors associated with calcific aortic valve disease. Cardiovascular health study. J Am Coll Cardiol. 1997;29:630–4.
3. Thanassoulis G, Massaro JM, Cury R, Manders E, Benjamin EJ, Vasan RS, Cupple LA, Hoffmann U, O'Donnell CJ, Kathiresan S. Associations of long-term and early adult atherosclerosis risk factors with aortic and mitral valve calcium. J Am Coll Cardiol. 2010;55: 2491–8.
4. Chatzizisis YS, Coskun AU, Jonas M, Edelman ER, Feldman CL, Stone PH. Role of endothelial shear stress in the natural history of coronary atherosclerosis and vascular remodeling: molecular, cellular, and vascular behavior. J Am Coll Cardiol. 2007;49:2379–93.
5. Furchgott RF, Zawadzki JV. The obligatory role of endothelial cells in the relaxation of arterial smooth muscle by acetylcholine. Nature. 1980;288:373–6.
6. Bonetti PO, Lerman LO, Lerman A. Endothelial dysfunction: a marker of atherosclerotic risk. Arterioscler Thromb Vasc Biol. 2003;23:168–75.
7. Mizia-Stec K, Gasior Z, Mizia M, Haberka M, Holecki M, Zwolinska W, Katarzyna K, Skowerski M. Flow-mediated dilation and gender in patients with coronary artery disease: arterial size influences gender differences in flow-mediated dilation. Echocardiography. 2007;24:1051–7.
8. Gutierrez E, Flammer AJ, Lerman LO, Elizaga J, Lerman A, Fernandez-Aviles F. Endothelial dysfunction over the course of coronary artery disease. Eur Heart J. 2013;34:3175–81.
9. Poggianti E, Venneri L, Chubuchny V, Jambrik Z, Baroncini LA, Picano E. Aortic valve sclerosis is associated with systemic endothelial dysfunction. J Am Coll Cardiol. 2003;41:136–41.
10. Erdogan T, Cetin M, Kocaman SA, Durakoglugil ME, Ergul E, Canga A. Aortic valve sclerosis is a high predictive marker of systemic endothelial dysfunction in hypertensive patients. Herz. 2013;38:915–21.
11. Diehl P, Nagy F, Sossong V, Helbing T, Beyersdorf F, Olschewski M, Bode C, Moser M. Increased levels of circulating microparticles in patients with severe aortic valve stenosis. Thromb Haemost. 2008;99:711–9.
12. Kaden JJ, Vocke DC, Fischer CS, Grobholz R, Brueckmann M, Vahl CF, Hagl S, Haase KK, Dempfle CE, Borggrefe M. Expression and activity of matrix metalloproteinase-2 in calcific aortic stenosis. Z Kardiol. 2004;93:124–30.
13. Helske S, Syvaranta S, Lindstedt KA, Lappalainen J, Oorni K, Mayranpaa MI, Lommi J, Turto H, Werkkala K, Kupari M, Kovanen PT. Increased expression of elastolytic cathepsins s, k, and v and their inhibitor cystatin c in stenotic aortic valves. Arterioscler Thromb Vasc Biol. 2006;26:1791–8.

14. Valgimigli M, Agnoletti L, Curello S, Comini L, Francolini G, Mastrorilli F, Merli E, Pirani R, Guardigli G, Grigolato PG, Ferrari R. Serum from patients with acute coronary syndromes displays a proapoptotic effect on human endothelial cells: a possible link to pan-coronary syndromes. Circulation. 2003;107:264–70.
15. Wang JM, Wang Y, Huang JY, Yang Z, Chen L, Wang LC, Tang AL, Lou ZF, Tao J. C-reactive protein-induced endothelial microparticle generation in huvecs is related to bh4-dependent no formation. J Vasc Res. 2007;44:241–8.
16. Nozaki T, Sugiyama S, Koga H, Sugamura K, Ohba K, Matsuzawa Y, Sumida H, Matsui K, Jinnouchi H, Ogawa H. Significance of a multiple biomarkers strategy including endothelial dysfunction to improve risk stratification for cardiovascular events in patients at high risk for coronary heart disease. J Am Coll Cardiol. 2009;54:601–8.
17. Leroyer AS, Isobe H, Leseche G, Castier Y, Wassef M, Mallat Z, Binder BR, Tedgui A, Boulanger CM. Cellular origins and thrombogenic activity of microparticles isolated from human atherosclerotic plaques. J Am Coll Cardiol. 2007;49:772–7.
18. Castrovinci S, Emmanuel S, Moscarelli M, Murana G, Caccamo G, Bertolino EC, Nasso G, Speziale G, Fattouch K. Minimally invasive aortic valve surgery. J Geriatr Cardiol. 2016;13:499–503.
19. Takata M, Amiya E, Watanabe M, Ozeki A, Watanabe A, Kawarasaki S, Nakao T, Hosoya Y, Uno K, Saito A, Murasawa T, Ono M, Nagai R, Komuro I. Brachial artery diameter has a predictive value in the improvement of flow-mediated dilation after aortic valve replacement for aortic stenosis. Heart Vessel. 2015;30:218–26.
20. Chenevard R, Bechir M, Hurlimann D, Ruschitzka F, Turina J, Luscher TF, Noll G. Persistent endothelial dysfunction in calcified aortic stenosis beyond valve replacement surgery. Heart. 2006;92:1862–3.
21. Morelos M, Amyot R, Picano E, Rodriguez O, Mazzone AM, Glauber M, Biagini A. Effect of coronary bypass and cardiac valve surgery on systemic endothelial function. Am J Cardiol. 2001;87:364–6. A310
22. Mylotte D, Sharif F, Piazza N, Moscarelli M, Fattouch K, Modine T. Transcatheter aortic valve implantation in 2015. J Geriatr Cardiol. 2016;13:511–3.
23. Amabile N, Boulanger CM, Caussin C. Unexpected benefits of TAVI: a therapy for the heart and the vessels. EuroIntervention. 2015;10:1375–7.
24. Horn P, Stern D, Veulemans V, Heiss C, Zeus T, Merx MW, Kelm M, Westenfeld R. Improved endothelial function and decreased levels of endothelium-derived microparticles after transcatheter aortic valve implantation. EuroIntervention. 2015;10:1456–63.
25. Marchini JF, Miyakawa AA, Tarasoutchi F, Krieger JE, Lemos P, Croce K. Endothelial, platelet, and macrophage microparticle levels do not change acutely following transcatheter aortic valve replacement. J Negat Results Biomed. 2016;15:7.
26. Jung C, Lichtenauer M, Figulla HR, Wernly B, Goebel B, Foerster M, Edlinger C, Lauten A. Microparticles in patients undergoing transcatheter aortic valve implantation (TAVI). Heart Vessel. 2017;32:458–66.

26 Risk Assessment

Ettore Augugliaro

Every year millions of patients who suffer from valvular heart disease (VHD) undergo a heart surgery. The comorbidity, prior clinical conditions, but also surgery, anesthesia, an intensive post-operative care, so all the perioperative and post-operative procedures have an important prognostic effect on patient morbidity and mortality.

Therefore, the main goal is to assess and reduce the risk.

Hence, an accurate VHD evaluation and staging to undergo a heart surgery is the basis of the surgical success meant as quality and patient life expectancy.

It is necessary to evaluate it from an ethical point of view, taking into account the high cost and the difficult therapeutic act regarding elderly patients; this is why the multidisciplinary, the *heart team,* personal medicine with a stratification of the individual risk was born.

Guidelines, consensus papers and experts recommendations help the specialist to choose the best strategy for each patient taking into account not just the effect on the outcome but also the healthy-risk relation linked to a particular both medical and surgical therapeutic procedure.

The improvement of surgical techniques and the development of anesthesiology and ICU have allowed over the years to plan effective strategies which are standardized with a wider range of helpful-therapeutic options.

As a matter of fact, the development of less invasive surgical techniques, the spread of hybrid procedures, device and latest generation monitoring systems, an advanced patient management and risk scores allow on the one hand to evaluate the patient in a better way with a reduction of mortality and morbidity rates; on the other hand these are a way forward the decision-making of valvular abnormalities.

E. Augugliaro, MD
Maria Eleonora Hospital, Palermo-GVM-Care and Research, Palermo, Italy
e-mail: ettore.augugliaro@gmail.com

K. Fattouch et al. (eds.), *Advances in Treatments for Aortic Valve and Root Diseases*, https://doi.org/10.1007/978-3-319-66483-5_26

26.1 Epidemiology

The annual report 'World Health Statistics' (June 2016) by the World Health Organization (WHO) gives us some directions about health conditions of 194 countries' population:

The report underlines that life expectancy for children born in 2015 is 71.4 years (73.8 for females and 69.1 for males) with an outstanding gap between countries with a high and low income. Indeed, life expectancy for children born in the 29 industrialized and high-income countries reach 80 years old while for those born in the 22 countries of Sub-Saharan Africa life expectancy is less than 60 years old. The 'World Health Statistics' of 2017 points out how the quality of health data has been considerably improving in recent years. However, a lot of countries don't regularly collect data with the suitable quality to control SDG (Sustainable Development Goals) index linked to health. Almost half of deaths at a global level are not wrote down with a clearly defined cause. Dr. Marie-Paule Kieny, the WHO Assistant Director-General for Health Systems and Innovation, has declared that "if countries don't know what makes people get sick and die, it's a lot harder to know what to do about it."

The increase of life expectancy and the reduction of birth rates in the North's industrialized countries set up a specific risk factor represented by geriatric age which has a higher risk of comorbidity, mortality and perioperative complications.

Indeed, thinking that age is a specific risk factor which is important for the prognostic stratification of the patient who suffer from VHD is something agreed by everyone and even literature talks about it.

Diversification of this population for age groups has been experienced, identifying an adequate terminology [1].

In the lowest part of the risk scale there are the so-called 'young old' from 65 to 75 who are not seen from adults on a clinical and biological level.

In the medium part of the scale there are patients aged between 75 and 85 years old (the so-called 'old old').

At the top of the pyramid the so-called 'oldest old' (>85) are considered as a high risk category because of a higher level of disability and comorbidity.

However, this system can't be enough for the staging of the patient's risk because it doesn't give us information about the patient's biological age meant as a picture of the capability and functional reserve of organs and apparatus which are involved in the patient's surgical path.

Indeed, decline and vulnerability of physiological mechanisms to harmful stimulus help us to identify a weak patient, not necessarily old.

Scores of surgical risk which are validated and used in the clinical practice don't help us so much. Something more comes from scores which evaluate patient's weakness, with an evaluation of the old patient's resilience with a functional reserve impairment. Another important role can be made by some scores which are able to evaluate post-operative risks, in particular as regards old and weak patients.

Unfortunately, there are a lot of valuable studies that come from literature, but their outcomes seem to be fragmented, not univocal and with a medical communities place and will in validating them inside the clinical practice. Possibly, the integration of the fragility within risks' assessment models of today will move towards a more appropriate treatment. There is a urgent need for a more accurate method of risks stratification which includes weakness, especially for older patients.

26.2 Guidelines

Both European and American guidelines (2012 ESC/EACTS Guidelines on the management of valvular heart disease and 2014 AHA/ACC Guideline for the Management of Patients With Valvular Heart Disease—2017 AHA/ACC Focused Update of the 2014 AHA/ACC Guideline for the Management of Patients With Valvular Disease) show that together with the objective examination, ECG and chest X-ray, symptoms and clinical conditions, the echocardiography is the main method for a diagnosis and a prognosis of valvulopathy [2–4]. However, important and additional information will be given by the experience and expertise of stress echocardiography, magnetic resonance imaging and computed tomography which has a pivotal role in the evaluation of patients being submitted to undergo a transcatheter aortic valve implantation (TAVI) [5, 6].

The stratification of operating risks, based mainly on the EuroSCORE and STS *score* estimates is compulsory even if these methods are quite imperfect and overestimate the risks. Furthermore, *scores* in place don't take into account factors that are difficult to define such as patients frailty or high impact anatomic conditions over the risk such as porcelain aorta. In the light of the above, it is advisable that the evaluation with a digital score goes hand-in-hand with the *heart team* clinical opinion [7].

The panel assessment will have to investigate functional status (ADL, IADL, MNA, BARTHEL INDEX, etc) as well as psychic and mental conditions (MMSE—SPMSQ, GDS, CAM—NEECHAM, BARS, etc) and social and environmental conditions (housing, economic conditions and social network), besides health conditions, so objective examination, asking patients about any medicinal products they take and comorbidity and instrumental diagnostic testing, stratifying the risk in a completely specific and individual way.

This approach of 'heart team' is particularly advisable for the management of high-risk patients and it is also important for other sub-groups such as asymptomatic patients whose evaluation of valve repairability is a key element for the decision-making process.

Usually, before surgery this kind of procedure has to be granted: the Cardiologist gives guidance about surgery, the Cardiothoracic surgeon rules on its executability and the Anesthesiologist evaluates the anesthesiology risk. Besides the Cardiologist, the Cardiothoracic surgeon and the Anesthesiologist, other professionals have to be part of the panel.

It is also necessary to assess general conditions which can make surgery possible and if it can get the prior extracardiac pathology worse. The Specialist will have to aim to maximize the treatment and evaluate if, delaying surgery (e.g. for respiratory disease), the patient could take a minor risk and make it through reducing possible post-operative complications.

The general clinical condition will be assessed by the Gerontologist who will give his advice about patient possibility to come out of surgery. The Neurologist, the Nephrologist and the Pulmonologist are the most frequently involved specialists;

Medical panel has always to take into account if surgery is quoad vitam or quoad valetudinem, especially in case of malignant disease [7].

Therefore, post-procedure quality and life expectancy have to be assessed. It is important not to neglect if the patient has adequate arguments and is aware of surgery risks and post-operative efforts.

Decision-making process can be summed up according to the approach mentioned in Table 26.1 below [2].

In the procedural timing the relation between risks and benefits with long term consequences of the surgery has to be always clear, as we have already mentioned, patients comorbidity and frailty particularly in old age. According to the AHA/ACC A risk-assessment scheme combining these factors is presented in Table 26.2 procedure-specific impediments must be taken into consideration. A number of mechanisms to evaluate frailty assess the ability to perform activities of daily living (independence in feeding, bathing, dressing, transferring, toileting, urinary continence, etc.) and measurements of gait speed, grip strength, and muscle mass. Published frailty scores are available, but a limited evaluation may use the following: no frailty (able to perform all activities of daily living and perform a 5-m walk in <6 s), mild degree of frailty (unable to performactivity of one activity daily living or unable to perform a 5-m walk in <6 s), and moderate-to-severe degree of frailty (unable to perform ≥2 activities of daily living). Further research is required to enhance the predictive accuracy of current risk scores, particularly in patients undergoing transcatheter therapy. The overall risks versus benefits should then be discussed with the patient and family using a shared decision-making process. In addition to the risk classification in Table 26.2, it is appropriate to defer any type of intervention in patients who will not benefit in terms of symptoms or improved life span from the procedure. This group of patients in whom surgical or transcatheter intervention for severe VHD is futile are those with (1) a life expectancy of <1 year, even with a successful procedure, and (2) those who have a chance of "survival with benefit" of <25% at 2 years. Survival with benefit means survival with improvement by at least one New York Heart Association (NYHA) or Canadian Cardiovascular Society class in heart failure (HF) or angina symptoms, improvement in quality of life, or improvement in life expectancy. Those patients with severe frailty may fall into this category (Nishimura et al. 2014 ACC/AHA) [3, 4].

26.3 Risk Score

There are multiple risks from VHD which has a variable percentage impact from patient to patient. A lot of these effects have led to the construction and the development of multiple predictive systems whose prerogative consists of identifying

Table 26.1 Essential questions in the evaluation of a patient for valvular intervention

- Is valvular heart diseases severe?
- Does the patient have symptoms?
- Are symptoms related to valvular disease?
- What are patient life expectancy' and expected quality of life?
- Do the expected benefits of intervention (vs. spontaneous outcome) outweigh its risks?
- What are the patient's wishes?
- Are local resources optimal for planned intervention?

Guidelines on the management of valvular heart disease (version 2012)

Table 26.2 Risk assessment combining STS risk estimate, frailty, major organ system dysfunction, and procedure-specific impediments

	Low risk (must meet ALL criteria in this column)	Intermediate risk (any 1 criterion in this column)	High risk (any 1 criterion in this column)	Prohibitive risk (any 1 criterion in this column)
STS PROM*	<4% **AND**	4 to 8% **OR**	>8% **OR**	Predicted risk with surgery of death or major morbidity (all-cause) >50% at 1 year **OR**
Frailty†	None **AND**	1 Index (mild) **OR**	>2 Indices (moderate to severe) **OR**	
Major organ system compromise not to be improved postoperatively‡	None **AND**	1 Organ system **OR**	No more than 2 organ systems **OR**	>3 Organ systems **OR**
Procedure-specific impediment§	None	Possible procedure-specific impediment	Possible procedure-specific impediment	Severe procedure-specific impediment

*Use of the STS PROM to predict risk in a given institution with reasonable reliability is appropriate only if institutional outcomes are within 1 standard deviation of STS average observed/expected ratio for the procedure in question.

†Seven frailty indices: Katz Activities of Daily Living (independence in feeding, bathing, dressing, transferring, toileting, and urinary continence) and independence in ambulation (no walking aid or assist required or 5-meter walk in <6 s). Other scoring systems can be applied to calculate no, mild-, or moderate-to-severe frailty.

‡Examples of major organ system compromise: Cardiac—severe LV systolic or diastolic dysfunction or RV dysfunction, fixed pulmonary hyperte nsion; CKD stage 3 or worse; pulmonary dysfunction with FEV1 <50% or DLCO2 <50% of predicted; CNS dysfunction (dementia, Alzheimer's disease, Parkinson's disease, CVA with persistent physical limitation); GI dysfunction—Crohn's disease, ulcerative colitis, nutritional impairment, or serum albumin <3.0; cancer—active malignancy; and liver—any history of cirrhosis, variceal bleeding, or elevated INR in the absence of VKA therapy.[page23image24184]

§Examples: tracheostomy present, heavily calcified ascending aorta, chest malformation, arterial coronary graft adherent to posterior chest wall, or radiation damage.

CKD indicates chronic kidney disease; CNS, central nervous system; CVA, stroke; DLCO2, diffusion capacity for carbon dioxide; FEV1, forced expiratory volume in 1 s; GI, gastrointestinal; INR, international normalized ratio; LV, left ventricular; PROM, predicted risk of mortality; RV, right ventricular; STS, Society of Thoracic Surgeons; and VKA, vitamin K antagonist

clinical variables which outline organ dysfunctions that cumulatively represent a personal risk for complications or death.

Uses and goals of the scores as well as database construction have to be improving the type of patient care without ever fall into the temptation and or deceit of selection.

Today, the most commonly used scores in heart surgery are the Euroscore II (European System for Cardiac Operative Risk Evaluation II), the STS (Surgeon Thoracic Surgery), Risk Calculator and the ACEF score.

Both of them are essential decision-making instruments even if their accuracy is lacking to some extent.

They have definitely overcome older scores made for younger populations such as the Initial Parsonnet score, the Cleveland Clinic score, the French score and many others (Figs. 26.1, 26.2, and 26.3) [9, 10].

26.4 EuroSCORE

EuroSCORE II (Fig. 26.4) has involved for its validation about 20,000 patients coming from 128 centres of eight European countries including 68 pre-operative risk factors and 29 related to surgery. There have been included 18 parameters of

	Initial Parsonnet score	Cleveland Clinic score	French score	Euro score	Pons score	Ontario Province Risk score
Patient data						
Age	✓	✓	✓	✓	✓	✓
Gender	✓			✓		✓
Body weight	✓	✓				
Cardiac						
Unstable agina				✓		
Aortic stenosis	✓	✓				
Active endocarditis				✓		
Congenital heart defect	✓					
Hypertension, arterial	✓					
Hypertension, pulmonary	✓			✓		
LV aneurysm	✓				✓	
LV ejection fraction	✓	✓	✓	✓		✓
Mitral insufficiency		✓				
Myocardial infarction (MI)			✓	✓	✓	
NYHA					✓	
Post MI VSD			✓	✓		
Ventricular tachycardia/fibrillation			✓	✓		
Pulmonary						
Asthma	✓			✓		
COPD		✓		✓		
Renal						
Dialysis	✓		✓			
Creatinine		✓	✓	✓	✓	
Acute renal failure	✓			✓		
Other						
Anemia		✓				
Diabetes	✓	✓				
Liver disease					✓	
History of TIA, stroke		✓		✓		
Paraplegia	✓					
Pacemaker	✓					
Vascular						
Aortic dissection, acute			✓			
Peripheral arterial disease				✓		
History of vascular surgery		✓		✓		
Preoperation						
Ventilation			✓	✓	✓	
IABP	✓			✓		
Inotropes				✓		
Resuscitation				✓		
Cardiogenic shock	✓				✓	
Operation						
Combined surgery	✓		✓	✓	✓	✓
Urgent/emergency	✓	✓		✓	✓	✓
Reoperation	✓	✓	✓	✓	✓	✓

Fig. 26.1 The items of the older scores

Design of selected risk scores

	Developed to predict	Center	Score development	Score validation	Statistics
Initial Parsonnet score 1989	Mortality	Single center/ USA	Retrospective: 3500 patients	Prospective: 1332 patients	Univariate and logistic regression analysis
Cleveland Clinic score 1992	Mortality/ morbidity	Single center/ USA	Retrospective: 5051 patients	Prospective: 4069 patients	Univariate and logistic regression analysis
French score 1995	Mortality/ morbidity	Multicenter/ France	Prospective: 7181 patients	–	Univariate and logistic regression analysis
Euro score 1999	Mortality	Multicenter/ Europe	Prospective: 19 030 patients	–	Univariate and logistic regression analysis
Pons score 1996	Mortality	Multicenter/ Spain	Prospective: 916 patients	Prospective: 392 patients	Univariate and logistic regression analysis
Ontario Province Risk score 1995	Mortality/ morbidity	Multicenter/ Canada	Retrospective: 6213 patients	Retrospective: 6885 patients	Univariate and logistic regression analysis

Fig. 26.2 Design of selected risk scores

TABLE 1.A SUMMARY OF CARDIAC SURGERY RISK-STRATIFICATION MODELS[4,31] (WITH PERMISSION)

Model	*Region*	*Year of data collection*	*Year of publication*	*Number of patients (centres)*	*Risk variables*
Amphiascore	Netherlands	1997-2001	2003	7 282 (1)	8
Cabdeal	Finland	1990-1991	1996	386 (1)	7
Cleveland Clinic	USA	1986-1988	1992	5 051 (1)	13
EuroSCORE (additive)	Europe	1995	1999	13 302 (128)	17
EuroSCORE (logistic)	Europe	1995	1999	13 302 (128)	17
French score	France	1993	1995	7 181 (42)	13
Magovern	USA	1991-1992	1996	1 567 (1)	18
NYS	USA	1998	2001	18 814 (33)	14
NNE	USA	1996-1998	1999	7 290 (N/A)	8
Ontario	Canada	1991-1993	1995	6 213 (9)	6
Parsonnet	USA	1982-1987	1989	3 500 (1)	16
Parsonnet (modified)	France	1992-1993	1997	6 649 (42)	41
Pons	Spain	1994	1997	1 309 (7)	11
STS risk calculator*	USA	2002-2006	2007		
isolated CABG				774 881 (819)	49
valve procedures				109 759	50
CABG and valve				101 661	50
Toronto	Canada	1993-1996	1999	7 491 (2)	9
Toronto (modified)	Canada	1996-1997	2000	1 904 (1)	9
Tremblay	Canada	1989-1990	1993	2 029 (1)	8
Tuman	USA	N/A	1992	3 156 (1)	10
UK national score	UK	1995-1996	1998	1 774 (2)	19
Veterans Affairs	USA	1987-1990	1993	12 712 (43)	10

USA = United States of America, EuroSCORE = European System for Cardiac Operative Risk Evaluation, NYS = New York State, NNE = Northern New England, STS = Society of Thoracic Surgeons, CABG = cornary artery bypass graft surgery, UK = United Kingdom.
* The STS risk calculator consists of seven risk-prediction models in three main catagories, namely isolates CABG, valve procedures, and combined CABG and valve procedures. Data represented for the STS risk calculator reflect the number of patient and risk variables captures in the database used for the latest models developed (version 2.61).

Fig. 26.3 A summary of cardiac surgery risk-stratification models [4, 8] (with permission)

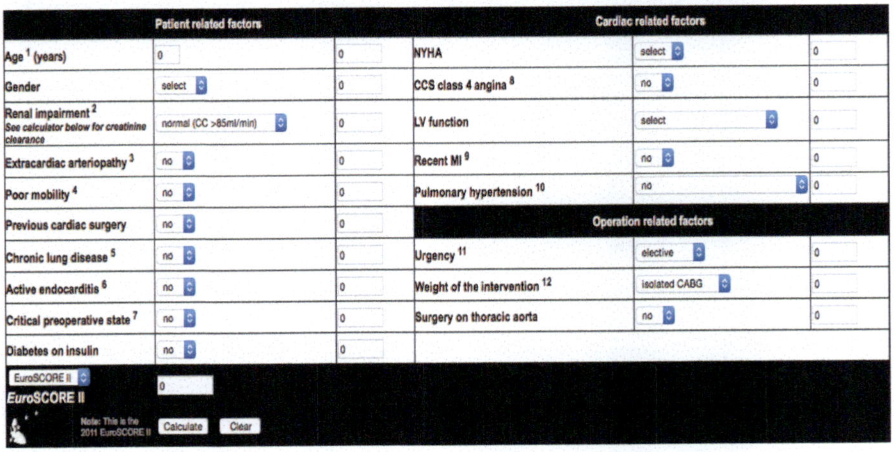

Patient related factors			Cardiac related factors		
Age [1] (years)	0	0	NYHA	select	0
Gender	select	0	CCS class 4 angina [8]	no	0
Renal impairment [2] See calculator below for creatinine clearance	normal (CC >85ml/min)	0	LV function	select	0
Extracardiac arteriopathy [3]	no	0	Recent MI [9]	no	0
Poor mobility [4]	no	0	Pulmonary hypertension [10]	no	0
Previous cardiac surgery	no	0	**Operation related factors**		
Chronic lung disease [5]	no	0	Urgency [11]	elective	0
Active endocarditis [6]	no	0	Weight of the intervention [12]	isolated CABG	0
Critical preoperative state [7]	no	0	Surgery on thoracic aorta	no	0
Diabetes on insulin	no	0			
EuroSCORE II	0				
Note: This is the 2011 EuroSCORE II	Calculate	Clear			

Fig. 26.4 Euroscore II

these in three sub-groups, through a univariate analysis and a logistic regression, each one with its ‘relative weight’ (Fig. 26.4). Apart from giving a mortality risk encoded in percentage, literature has shown that the percentage coming from the calculation that allows us dividing patients into low, high and medium risk indirectly results also in post-operative complications. Consequently, the increase of the value in percentage and the increase of the risk will be connected to a more long lasting mechanical ventilation, hospitalization in I.C.U., post-operative AKI, neurological complications [11–13].

26.5 STS

STS (Surgeon Thoracic Surgery) Risk Calculator has recruited about 5,800,000 patients until September the 20th of 2016, 1119 operators, 50 US and Canada centres (1071 operators through the participation of almost 90%), 62 ICU, 19 international centre (Argentina, Singapore, Australia, Brazil, Israel, United Arab Emirates); Parameters which have been taken into account are more than double compared to EUROSCORE II; it has 12 supporting hospitals, elaboration and statistical checking of the Duke University with a biannual report with surgery activity and risk indicators. In addition to a mortality risk encoded in percentage, it directly calculates morbidity and the time course of hospitalization, neurological complications such as the stroke, longer ventilation, deep sternal wound infection (DSWI), renal impairment, and reoperation.

There are seven types of surgeries taken into account (Fig. 26.5):

1. CABG only
2. aortic valve replacement
3. mitral valve replacement
4. mitral valve repair

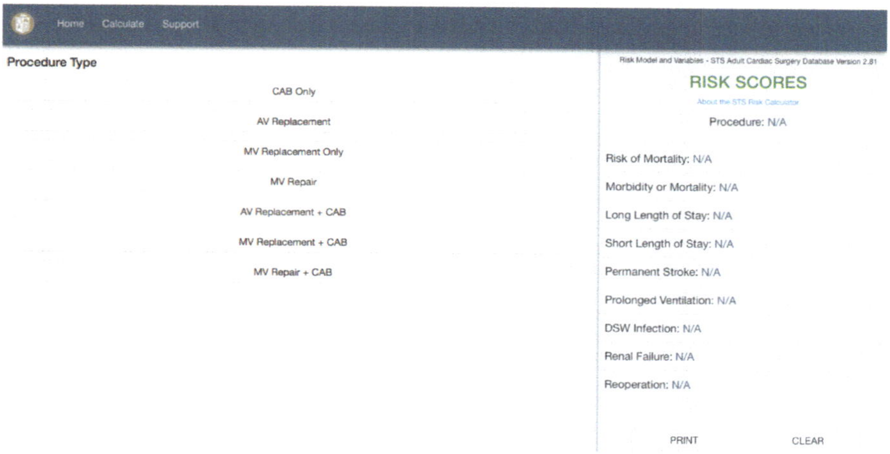

Fig. 26.5 STS Risk Score

5. BPAC + aortic valve replacement
6. BPAC + mitral valve replacement
7. BPAC + mitral valve repair

Both scores are not good for old patients (their clinical experiences mainly concern younger patients) and they don't still include important variables (porcelain aorta, chest radiotherapy, hepatic disease, efficient CABG, frailty)

These restrictions have lead the cardiological and cardiothoracic surgery communities to recognize the importance of a score for the sub-group of old patients with greater attention to the life expectancy [14–17].

26.6 ACEF

Another score which has to be mentioned is ACEF score (Fig. 26.6), validated on 4091 patients of 4557 enrolled patients. It has been compared to five different scores (Cleveland clinic, Northern New England Score, Parsonnet and Euroscore, logistic and standard) [18]. Great prior outcomes on ACEF's calibration and discrimination, similar or even greater than other scores. ACEF takes into account only three parameters (age, serum creatinine and EF (%).

Tested and compared to EUROSCORE, subsequently to its output in 2011 by Ranucci et al. in J Thorac Cardiovasc Surg: in other 29,659 in elective heart surgery, it showed its strengths [19]:

- The 3 factors are numbers, not conditions (no subjective interpretation is possible)
- Complex models suffer from multicollinearity (same concept expressed by different variables)

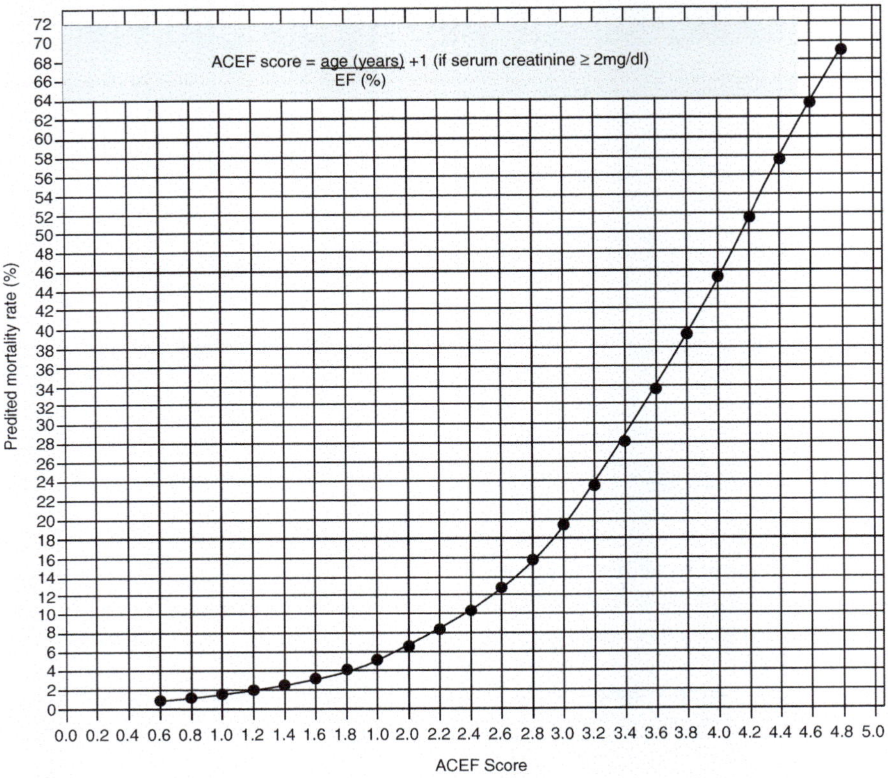

Fig. 26.6 ACEF Score

- Complex models pretend to fit very low and very high risk conditions
- Complex models require complex calculations
- Complex models may suffer from overfitting, when applied to small/medium-activity centers

'……Sometimes a simple model could overcome a more complex model. Nevertheless,…deliberately limiting the complexity of the model is not fruitful when the problem is evidently complex.

Conversely,… the appropriate response is to define a different complex model that captures whatever aspect of the problem led to the simple model performing well'

ACEF has recently been included in the European Guidelines on Myocardial Revascularization for mortality risk assessment even in patients undergoing a percutaneous coronary intervention. Recently, Ranucci et al., published ACEF II that included the emergency patient and, through are-modulation of the coefficients and the inclusion of anaemia, appears more adequate to the present cardiac surgery scenario [20].

Recent validation and comparison of these scores in VHD can be seen through a range of studies published in literature:

The first of the greatest works dates back to 2009 *-ATS (PART 1-2-3-), Shanian et al.:*

In 'PART-2' i.e. the study of 109,759 patients who underwent a isolated aortic valve replacement and in 'PART 3', 101,661 patients submitted to a combined heart surgery – valve + CABG, it's showed how STS presents a good discrimination but a limited calibration in high-risk patients [21].

Other data from literature come from *E.J.C.Surg.—2012 Nashef et al.—*:

Taking just 10,353 from 22,381 patients who undergo isolated valve procedures in 154 hospitals, 43 countries and 12 weeks (May–July 2010) it follows a good Euroscore II discrimination and calibration with the reliable O/E ratio.

In *EHJ-2013-Barili et al.* 12,325 patients enrolled in 6 years (from 2006 to 2011) in three centres and 8187 of them were submitted to isolated valvular surgery with an emphasis of low calibration for high-risk patients and percutaneous procedures are not included in this survey.

It is interesting reading authors' remarks:'*..As both additive and logistic EuroSCORE risk models have been developed for quite sometime now, it is expected that they may not reflect accurately the current cardiac surgical practice that has changed over the years due to improved surgical techniques and postoperative patient management advances.....'*

'*.....Recently, the limitations of EuroSCORE original models' performances were also highlighted by the comparison with the STS score, which predicts more accurately the observed mortality, especially in the highest risk patients. In fact, the STS score is derived from a larger data set of patients operated in a more current era, and risk models were separately developed into three different surgical categories (CABG, valves, and CABG plus valves) and included more covariates...'* [22].

In *AM. J. Cardiol.—2013—Durand et al. show*:

- Euro SCORE II and the STS score are better calibrated than the logistic EuroSCORE but have moderate discrimination for predicting 30-day mortality after TAVR [23].

The increasing demand of less invasive procedures, such as the percutaneous ones, and low impact procedures with regard to high-risk patient outcome made the validation of prerogative scores of heart surgery.

Cardiology 2013. Stähli B et al., show that l'Euroscore II provided better discrimination and calibration and that l'STS underestimated mortality [24].

In *Euro J Cardiothorac Surg. 2013 Haensig et al.,* authors assess in depth only TA-TAVI procedures from February 2006 to May 2011, including 360 high-risk patients. The outcome is that STS discriminates and calibrates better than EuroSCORE II [25].

In *E. J. of Cardio-Thoracic Surgery (2014). R. L.* Osnabrugge et al., show that EuroSCORE II and the STS-PROM on 50,588 patients from a multi-institutional statewide database of all cardiac surgeries performed since 2003. Model performance was assessed using the area under the receiver operator curve (AUC), observed vs. expected (O:E) ratios and calibration plots.

Nevertheless, it should be considered that of 50,588 patients only 9717 of them were VHD or VHD + CAD patients.

EuroSCORE II may be more accurate in AVR (O:E = 0.96 vs. STS-PROM: 0.76). Performance of both models improved when only recent cases (after 1 January 2008) were used. Ongoing TAVI trials aimed at patients with an estimated 4–10% risk of mortality are enrolling patients with mean estimated risks of 6.2% (EuroSCORE II) or 6.0% (STS-PROM), and an actual mortality rate of 4.6% (EuroSCORE II) or 4.8% (STS-PROM) [26].

In J Cardiothorac Vasc Anesth. 2014. Biancari et al.

In an important meta-analysis they collect more than ten great works published in literature about aortic valve with a traditional surgical approach or TAVI with different approaches, with these results (Fig. 26.7, 26.8, and 26.9) [27].

'*.... the ESII and STS scores seemed to predict accurately the operative mortality risk.....*

..... underpredicted mortality in TAVR patients and somewhat overpredicted mortality in SAVR patient:

In particular, the ESII seemed to be accurate in patients with low operative risk

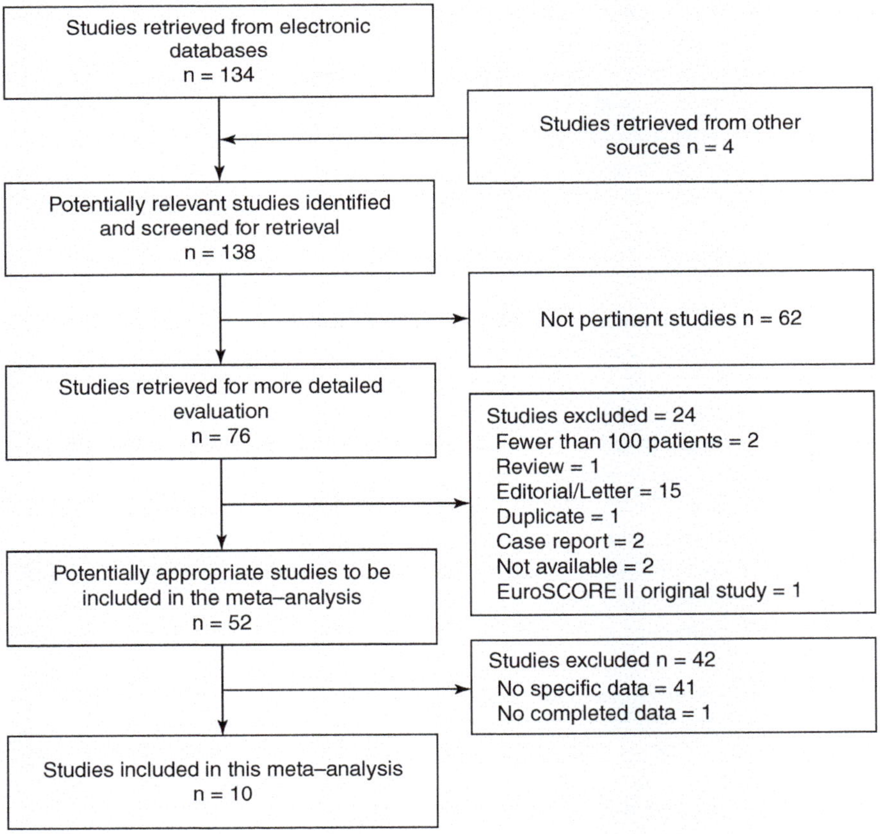

Fig. 26.7 Literature search flow chart

Author	Year	Study Interval	Country	Type of Study	Procedure	No. of Patients	Operative Mortality (%)	Mean ESII Score (%)	ESII Score AUC	Mean STS Score (%)	STS Score AUC
Barili	2013	2006–2012	Italy	Multicenter	Isolated AVR	1,758	1.4	1.9	0.81	2.0	0.85
Durand	2013	2006–2011	France	Institutional	TAVR	250	7.6	7.7	0.66	7.3	0.58
Haensig	2013	2006–2011	Germany	Institutional	TAVR	360	11.4	6.7	0.49	11.7	0.65
Laurent	2013	2006–2011	France	Institutional	Isolated AVR and AVR+CABG	314	5.7	2.3	0.77	2.8	0.73
Sedaghat	2013	2008–2012	Germany	Institutional	TAVR	206	6.8	9.2	0.71	9.5	0.69
Stähli	2013	–	Switzerland	Institutional	TAVR	350	9.1	8.0	0.70	6.5	0.59
Wang	2013	2005–2012	Australia	Institutional	Isolated AVR	620	2.9	3.8	0.71	2.8	0.72
Watanabe	2013	2006–2011	France	Institutional	TAVR	453	12.6	8.1	0.68	8.1	0.60
Wendt	2013	1999–2012	Germany	Institutional	Isolated AVR	1512	4.2	3.2	0.72	4.8	0.73
Wendt	2013	1999–2012	Germany	Institutional	Transfemoral TAVR	291	11.7	6.4	0.55	6.1	0.63
Wendt	2013	1999–2012	Germany	Institutional	Transfemoral TAVR	155	7.7	8.4	0.84	10.5	0.79
Osnabrugge	2014	2003–2012	USA	Multicenter	Isolated AVR	4107	2.9	3.0	0.71	3.8	0.74
Osnabrugge	2014	2003–2012	USA	Multicenter	AVR+CABG	3480	4.1	5.4	0.72	5.9	0.74

Abbreviations: AUS, area under the receiver operating characteristics curve; AVR, surgical valve replacement; CABG, coronary artery bypass graft; ESII, EuroSCORE II score; STS, Society of Thoracic Surgeons score; TAVR, transcatheter aortic valve replacement.

Fig. 26.8 Characteristics of studies evaluating the performance of EuroSCORE II and society of thoracic surgeons scores in predicating operative morality in patients who underwent surgical aortic valve replacement and trans catheter aortic valve replacement

Fig. 26.9 Mortality in aortic valve procedures

	Mortality (%)	Mean Predicted Mortality (%) ESII	STS
All aortic valve procedures (10 studies)	6.1	5.1 (4.0–6.2)	6.3 (4.5–7.5)
TAVR (6 studies)	9.6	7.8 (7.2–8.3)	8.5 (7.3–9.6)
SAVR (5 studies)	3.1	3.3 (2.1–4.4)	3.7 (2.4–5.0)

We can find the same result in Euroscore II, for low-risk patients, in The Journal of Thoracic and Cardiovascular Surgery—December 2014. Performance of the European System for Cardiac Operative Risk Evaluation II: A meta-analysis of 22 studies involving 145,592 cardiac surgery procedures [27, 28].

In this survey too a lower discrimination for high-risk patients comes up.

In a ceaseless and necessary increase of specific scores, other surveys have to be mentioned:

In Am J Cardiol 2015—Philippe Debonnaire, et al.

They evaluate TAVI2-SCORe, new- generation scores for TAVI

One-year mortality was 17.0% (n (80 of 471). Porcelain thoracic aorta (hazard ratio (HR) 2.56), anemia (HR 2.03), left ventricular dysfunction (HR 1.98), recent myocardial infarction (HR 3.78), male sex (HR 1.81), critical aortic valve stenosis (HR 2.46), old age (HR 1.68), and renal dysfunction (HR 1.76) formed the TAVI2-SCORe (all $p < 0.05$). According to the number of points assigned (1 for each variable and 2 for infarction), patients were stratified into five risk categories. TAVI2-SCORe showed better discrimination ability *vs.* LES-I, LES-II, and STS score (0.609, 0.633, and 0.50, respectively). Cumulative 1-year survival rate was 54% vs. 88% for patients with TAVI2-SCORE. Contrary to surgical risk scores, there was no significant difference between observed and expected 1-year mortality for all TAVI2-SCORe risk strata (all p > 0.05, Hosmer-Lemeshow statistic 0.304), suggesting superior calibration performance. In conclusion, the TAVI2-SCORe is an accurate, simple, and bedside-available score predicting 1-year mortality post-TAVI, outperforming conventional surgical risk scores for this end point [8].

In Cardiology Journal 2016, Karol Zbroński et al. in a comparing survey of risk models in TAVI, EuroSCORE I, EuroSCORE II, STS, ACEF, Ambler's, OBSERVANT and SURTAVI scores [29].

They notice a little distinction capacity of some random studied models, regardless of the specific project for TAVI or traditional surgery. It could be explained by the lack of potentially important clinical conditions (anaemia, hypoalbuminemia, hepatic impairment, etc) and anatomic (porcelain aorta, calcium distribution on native valve, delivery route morphology, etc). It is suggested that these clinical factors reflect an impaired health condition that can affect the early physical therapy process.

Furthermore, in J Cardiovasc Med 2013 Dec; D'Ascenzo F et al. In TAVI patients, study how ACEF score, STS score and Logistic Euroscore provided only a moderate correlation and a low accuracy both for 30-day and medium-term outcomes [30].

Finally, in a wide systematic review and meta-analysis of 22 surveys, in Am J Cardiology, 2016, Sullivan et al. they show that EuroScore II and STS Score outperform the ACEF score on discrimination [31].

But it has to be considered how an objective analysis which emphasizes how the author supported key points and their use with reasonable and implementable arguments based on evidence it has been partly weak as underlined by Ranucci himself in The hidden Traps of Meta-Analyses on Cardiac Surgery Mortality Risk Scores Am J of Cardiology, 2017 [32].

26.7 Risk Scores Implementation

The concept of risk stratification of cardiac surgical patients is developed, with an intention to identify high-risk patients and to improve the outcome by appropriately modifying it when possible. Perioperative morbidity and mortality result from multiple factors and these have been studied to stratify the risk. Many systems such this have been formulated to assess the risk. Several newer scores have been produced claiming benefit over the preexisting ones. It is time that the cardiac surgical teams give a fresh look at ameliorating the morbidities and mortality by modifying the perioperative risk factors and improve the outcome.

Hence, there is not just the straightened need to change all factors that can be responsible for perioperative complications, but also to implement risk scores validated by guidelines.

First of all, cardiac anesthesiologists and cardiac surgeons have to consider an aware and meticulous approach by pre-operative onwards allowing the intervention over variables and adjustable risk factors (LV dysfunction and congestive heart failure, control of diabetes, control of hypertension, alleviation of renal dysfunction, managing of atherosclerosis, smoking cessation, dental assestment, anemia, maneuvers to decrease stroke, nutritional assessment for management of obesity etc.) [33].

The contemporary setup of an outpatient preoperative evaluation in nonemergency clinical situations has demonstrated effectiveness, cost reduction, and enhanced patient comfort. In recent years, the role of outpatient management has been reinvented and expanded into a comprehensive concept of perioperative anesthesia/surgical home (PASH) [34].

The multi-year experience and prevalent practice in North America and Canada with an organized work system improved outcomes. The establishment of highly functional and efficient outpatient PEC for nonemergency cardiovascular day of admission surgery (DAS) will reduce the rate of complications.

In the VHD patient's anesthesiological assessment the first step is simple and non-specific ASA (American Society of Anesthesiologist) Score:

It includes five classes:

1. patient is completely healty
2. patient has a mild systemic disease
3. patient has a severe systemic disease that is not incapaciting
4. patient has an incapaciting disease is a constant threat to life
5. A moribund patient who is not expected to live 24 h with or whitout surgery

However, ASA does not exactly access the perioperative conditions, it does not consider most variabilities. Also the definition of systematics disease makes a lot of confusion in practice. Therefore, the new seven-grade classification has been suggested [35].

1. no risk to life

   1.5) almost no risk to life

2. light risk to life

   2.5) middle risk to life

   There are no changes in other three grades,

3. heavy risk to life
4. very dangerous risk to life
5. almost death risk to life

The Cardiac Anesthesia Risk Evaluation (CARE) Score was created to develop a simple risk classification tool to predict mortality and morbidity after cardiac surgery [36].

Shows similar accuracy to more complex cardiac anesthesia risk assessment schematics.

Does not account for age and left ventricular (LV) function. The score contains only 6 variables (compared to EuroSCORE, which contains 18 variables) but shows similar accuracy.

Quickly risk-stratifies patients undergoing cardiac surgery in the clinical setting.

Requires fewer variables and data, including those that may be hard to obtain on the day of surgery.

The Cardiac Anesthesia Risk Evaluation (CARE) score

Score	Score definition
1.	Patient with stable cardiac disease and no other medical problem. A non-complex surgery is undertaken
2.	Patient with stable cardiac disease and one or more controlled medical problems[a] A non-complex surgery is undertaken
3.	Patient with any uncontrolled medical problem[b] OR patient in whom a complex surgery is undertaken[c]
4.	Patient with any uncontrolled medical problem[b] AND in whom a complex surgery is undertaken[c]
5.	Patient with chronic or advanced cardiac disease for whom cardiac surgery is undertaken as a last hope to save or improve life
E.	For emergency surgery undertaken as soon as diagnosis is made and operating room is available, E is added to the score (applicable only to scores 3, 4 and 5)

[a]Examples: controlled hypertension; diabetes mellitus; peripheral vascular disease; chronic obstructive pulmonary disease; controlled systemic diseases; others as by clinical judgment

[b]Examples: unstable angina on intravenous heparin or nitroglycerin; preoperative intra-aortic balloon pump; heart failure with pulmonary or peripheral edema; uncontrolled hypertension; renal insufficiency (creatinine level >140 μmoL/L); debilitating systemic diseases; others as by clinical judgment

[c]Examples: reoperation; combined valve and coronary artery surgery; multiple valve surgery; left ventricular aneurysmectomy; repair of ventricular septal defect after myocardial infarction; coronary artery bypass of diffuse and/or heavily calcified vessels requiring multiple endarterectomy or stentectomy; others as by clinical judgment

Recently, using the American College of Surgeons National Surgical Quality Improvement Program (NSQUIP) database, a new predictive model has been developed to assess the risk of intraoperative/postoperative myocardial infarction or cardiac arrest. Is based on five predictors of perioperative myocardial infarction/cardiac arrest (functional status, elevated creatinine, ASA class, age, type of surgery [37, 38].

The risk calculator uses 20 patient predictors (e.g., age, ASA class, BMI, HTN) and the planned procedure (CPT code) to predict the chance that patients will have any of 15 different outcomes within 30-days following surgery. The outcomes include:

- Serious complication (death, cardiac arrest, myocardial infarction, pneumonia, progressive renal insufficiency, acute renal failure, PE, DVT, return to the operating room, deep incisional SSI, organ space SSI, systemic sepsis, unplanned intubation, UTI, wound disruption)
- Any complication (superficial incisional SSI, deep incisional SSI, organ space SSI, wound disruption, pneumonia, unplanned intubation, PE, ventilator >48 h,

progressive renal insufficiency, acute renal failure, UTI, stroke, cardiac arrest, myocardial infarction, DVT, systemic sepsis)
- Pneumonia
- Cardiac Complication (cardiac arrest or MI)
- Surgical Site Infection (SSI)
- Urinary Tract Infection (UTI)
- Venous Thromboembolism (VTE)
- Renal Failure (progressive renal insufficiency or acute renal failure)
- Colon Ileus (Conditionally displayed based on the selected Procedure)
- Colon Anastomotic Leak (Conditionally displayed based on the selected Procedure)
- Readmission
- Return to OR
- Death
- Discharge to Nursing or Rehab Facility
- Predicted Length of Hospital Stay

The risk calculator was built using data collected from >2.7 million operations from 586 hospitals participating in ACS NSQIP from 2010–14. Entering the most complete and accurate patient information will provide the most precise risk information. However, the estimates can still be calculated if some of the patient information is unknown [39].

The results show if the patient is having a risk to develop any of nine different complications within the first 30-days following surgery. The predicted risk can be adjusted by using the Surgeon Adjustment of Risk button, and it should be used if the surgeon feels that the patient has significant risk factors for surgery that have not been previously listed. Development and implementation of NSQUIP models have resulted in morbidity and mortality reduction, reduced number of hospital days and reduced hospital costs.

In light of recently published ESC/ESA guidelines, even in non cardiac surgery, use of clinical risk indices for perioperative risk stratification is strongly recommended, and between them, the NSQIP model or the Lee risk index is recommended for cardiac perioperative risk stratification (Class of recommendation Ia/Level of evidence B).

The Charlston Comorbidity Index (CCI) calculator predict inpatient mortality and cardiac and renal morbidity by using Hospital administrative data such as: COPD, patient's age, myocardial infarction, congestive heart failure, peripheral vascular disease, cerebrovascular disease, diabetes mellitus, chronic kidney disease, hemiplegia, leukemia, solid tumor, AIDS, malignant liymphoma, liver disease, connective tissue disease, dementia, peptic ulcer disease.

Beyond risk scores which cover a wide area of implementation as regards non-cardiac surgery too, efforts made to implement risks in cardiac surgery, in particular the post-operative one, cannot be neglected, instead they are the backbone of an increasingly integrated and multidisciplinary approach [40].

As it has already happened in the implementation of scores in the myocardial revascularization (Post Cardiac Surgery Prognostic Score—POCAS), in PLoS One—2010, Ranucci M et al. for example, with the inclusion of the HR >120 beats per minute and BL >4 mmol/L. in the assessment of the severity of clinical conditions after cardiac surgery, increased the AUC of the logistic EuroSCORE by 0.88 and that of the ACEF by 0.86, without relevant changes in calibration for both models [41, 42].

Reliability and accuracy of E-PASS (Estimation of Physiologic Ability and Surgical Stress) in predicting post-operative risks in cardiac surgery which show a good calibration and discrimination if compared to Euroscore II and Ontario province Risk Score have been validated [43].

Finally, several surveys assess the non-superiority versus risk scores for cardiothoracic surgery of (Simplified Acute Physiology Score (SAP II), Sepsis-related Organ Failure Assessment (SOFA), Acute Physiology and Chronic Health Evaluation (APACHE II)

Interesting are also the scores for the Readmissions or "bounce back" to the intensive care unit (ICU) following cardiac surgery. It's associated with an increased risk of morbidity and mortality.

The Bounce Back After Transfer (BATS) prediction score [44].

A predictive model (BATS) can determine the risk of a bounce back to the ICU after transfer to the floor. The risk of bounce back increased postoperative morbidity, mortality, and cost of care. Independent predictors for bounce back included female sex, NYHA class III/IV, urgent or emergent operative status and postoperative renal failure.

26.8 Frailty

Finally, an important role of risk score in VHD implementation comes from frailty evaluation [45]. Increasing life expectancy comes from a corresponding rise of the average age of patients presenting cardiovascular diseases (CVDs). It represents an important and too wide chapter always turmoiling and in evolution. Therefore we have to pay attention to the key concepts, important surveys and the latest data in literature [33].

In BMJ 2017—Rebecca Rowe et al. show how apoptosis, senescence, repair, inflammation and immune activation have all been implicated as pathways responsible for this decline (Fig. 26.10). Biological age' is often taken as a crude index of frailty, while chronological age is a poor correlate. Indeed up to 75% of patients over the age of 85 years are not frail [46].

A number of frailty scores have been designed by geriatricians comprising a combination of functional tests, laboratory tests, questionnaires, descriptive scales, disability assessments and comorbidity assessments. High scores in these are associated with adverse outcomes in elderly patient populations and may aid clinical management. However, it is complex and takes 10–20 min to perform. The practicality of incorporating it into routine pre-operative cardiac assessment would be challenging. Gait speed was measured prior to discharge. Although this is useful to allow prediction of future events, it is not helpful at presentation. Therefore, for frailty to be incorporated into preprocedural risk assessment, a different form of assessment is required. We and others have found that Canadian Study of Health and Ageing score is an easy and reliable tool to assess frailty.

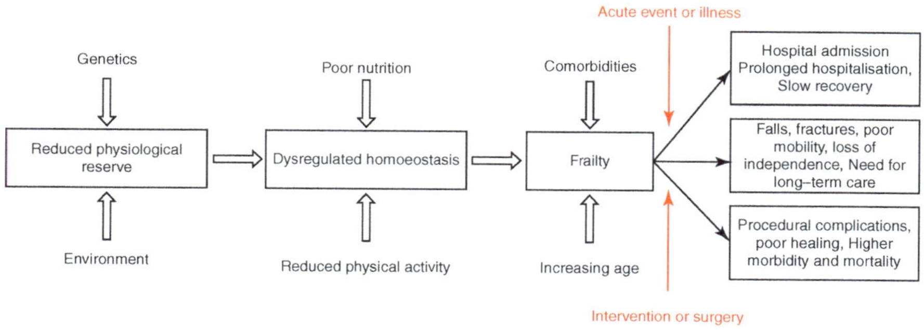

Fig. 26.10 Decline and Frailty

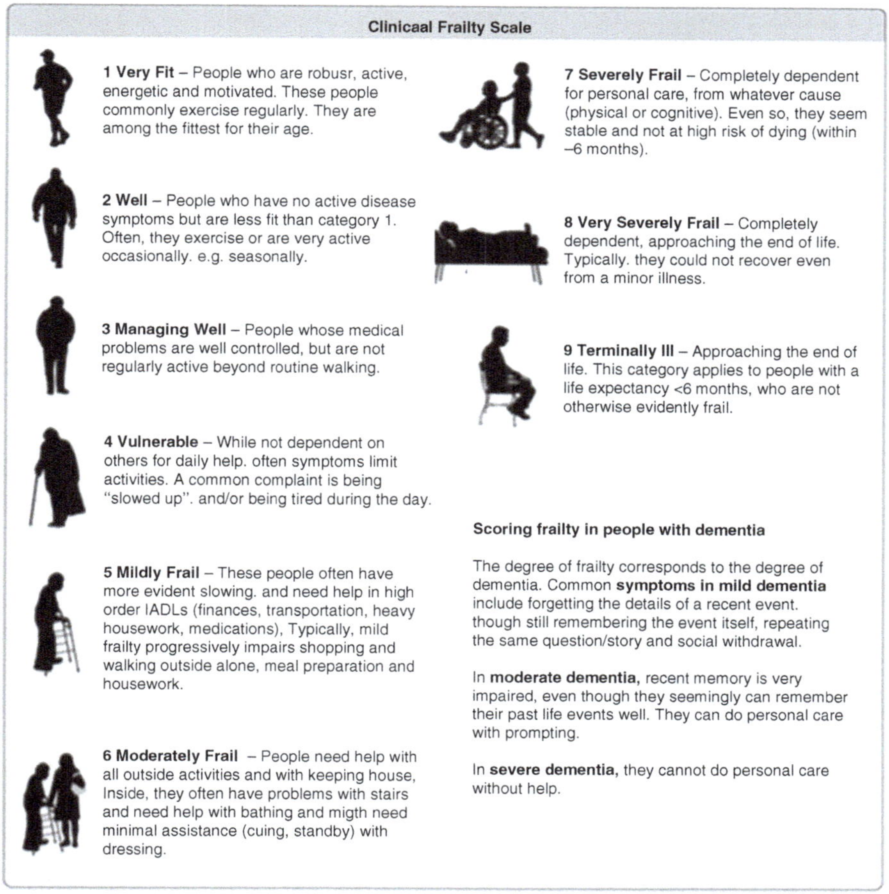

The importance of frailty has been acknowledged by the American Heart Association (AHA) which has called for a better under-standing of frailty in cardiac care. They have suggested that trials should include improved characterisation of the elderly population and the evaluation of the influence of frailty and cognitive decline on outcomes.

In Thorac Cardiovasc Sur. 2013—Mack. M Frailty is formally defined as a clinical syndrome of multi system impairment that results in a decreased physiologic reserve and an increased vulnerability to stressors. Although risk increases with chronologic age and comorbidity but these factors alone are insufficient to predict outcomes and benefit [47].

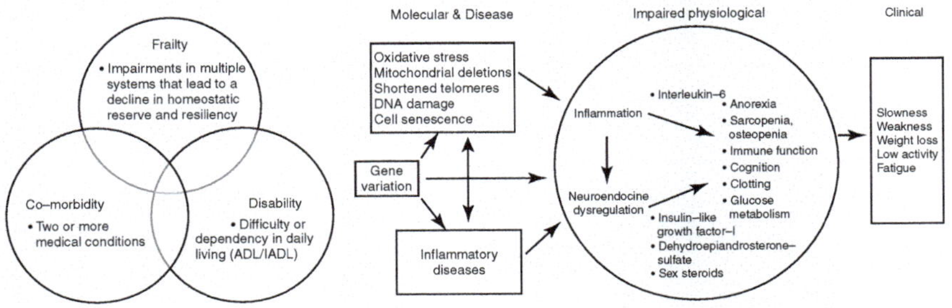

A further complete and organized model comes from Afilalo:

In *Circulation* 2012; Afilalo et al. underscore that ' *There is an unmet need to combine established cardiac surgery risk scores with measures of frailty and disability to provide a more complete model for risk prediction in elderly patients undergoing cardiac surgery.'*

'One out of two patients with advanced cardiovascular disease exhibits signs of frailty or cognitive impairment. Identification of frailty or cognitive impairment, when objectified with a validated instrument, confers a negative effect on prognosis and may be an important clue that the patient with advanced cardiovascular disease is entering the end-of-life phase' (Fig. 26.11) [48, 49].

Risk Scores in this study included

- the Society of Thoracic Surgeons Predicted Risk of Mortality (STS-PROM)
- the Society of Thoracic Surgeons Predicted Risk of Mortality or Major Morbidity (STS-PROMM)
- the logistic EuroSCORE
- the revised Parsonnet score
- Age-Creatinine-Ejection Fraction (ACEF) score.

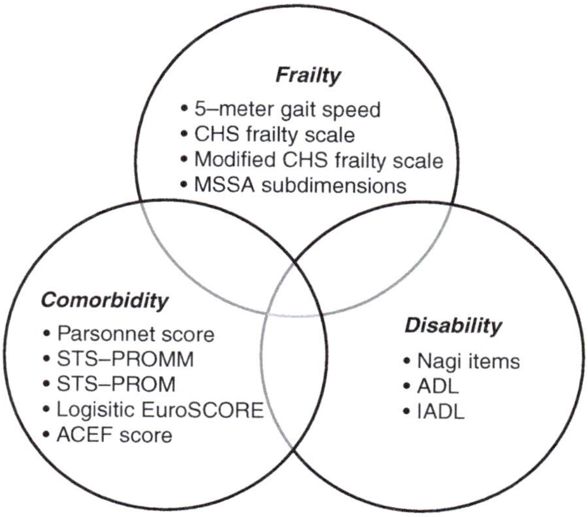

Fig. 26.11 Various scales to measure frailty, disability, and comorbidity/cardiac surgery risk. CHS indicates Cardiovascular Health Study; *MSSA* MacArthur Study of Successful Aging, *STS-PROMM* Society of Thoracic Surgeons Predicted Risk of Mortality or Major Morbidity, *STS-PROM* Society of Thoracic Surgeons Predicted Risk of Mortality, *ACEF* age creatinine ejection fraction, *ADL* activities of daily living, *IADL* instrumental activities of daily living

Disability Scales in this study included

- the 6-item Katz Activities of Daily Living (ADL) scale (going to the toilet, bathing, dressing, eating, moving around, controlling bladder/ bowel)
- the 7-item Older Americans Research and Services Instrumental Activities of Daily Living (IADL) scale (doing house- work, going shopping, preparing meals, handling money, taking medicine, using telephone, getting to places)
- the 7-item Nagi scale

Frailty Scales in this study included

- the 5-item Cardiovascular Health Study (CHS) frailty scale (gait speed, handgrip strength, inactivity, exhaustion, weight loss)
- the 7-item expanded CHS frailty scale (CHS scale cognitive impairment and depressed mood)
- the 4-item MacArthur Study of Successful Aging (MSSA) frailty scale subdimensions (gait speed, handgrip strength, inactivity, cognitive impairment)
- gait speed alone—with frailty defined as 6 s required to walk 5 m (Table 26.3 for a detailed description of the gait speed test).

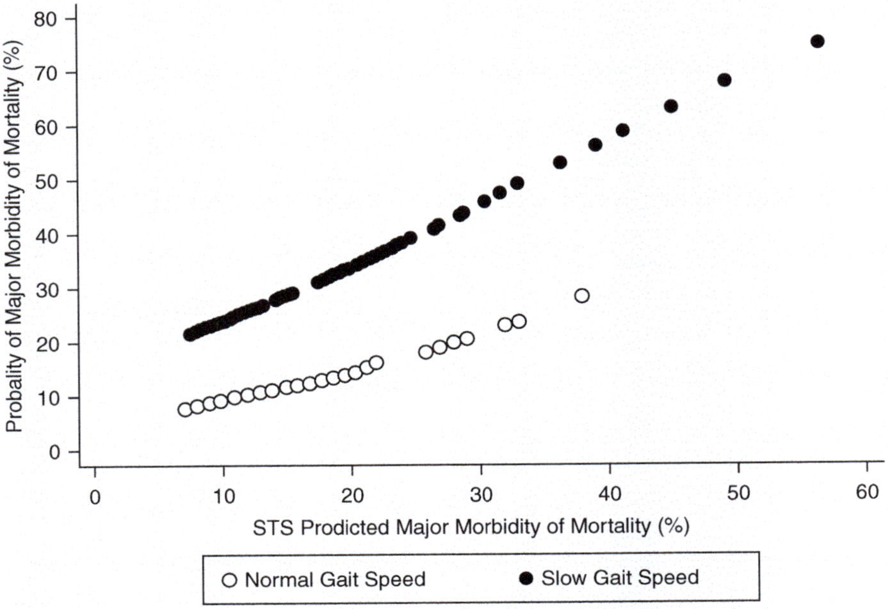

Table 26.3 Five-meter gait speed test

Instruct to "Walk at your comfortable pace" until a few steps past the 5-m mark (should not start to slow down before)
Begin each trial on the word "Go"
Start the timer with the final footfall after the 0-m line
Stop the timer with the first footfall after the 5-m line
Repeat three times and record average, allowing sufficient time for recuperation between trials
Frailty is defined as an average time taken to walk the 5-m course ≥6 s

In Clin Interv Aging 2014 Xujiao C et al. Two major frailty models have been described in the literature. The frailty phenotype defines frailty as a distinct clinical syndrome meeting three or more of five phenotypic criteria: weakness, slowness, low level of physical activity, self-reported exhaustion, and unintentional weight loss [49]. The frailty index defines frailty as cumulative deficits identified in a comprehensive geriatric assessment. Chronic inflammation is likely a key pathophysiologic process that contributes to the frailty syndrome directly and indirectly through other intermediate physiologic systems, such as the musculoskeletal, endocrine, and hematologic systems. The complex multifactorial etiologies of frailty also include obesity and specific diseases (Table 26.4).

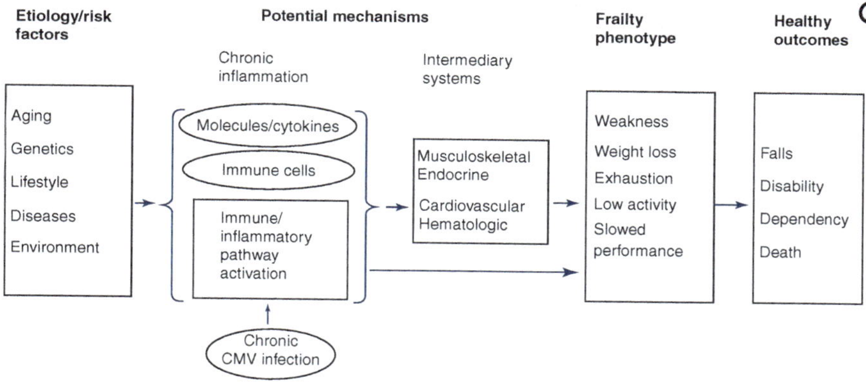

Pathogenesis of the frailty syndrome: current understanding of potential underlying mechanisms and hypothetical modal pathways leading to frailty

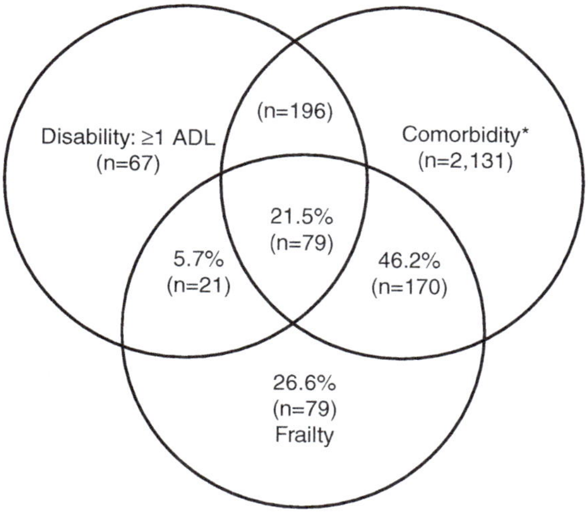

Table 26.4 The frailty phenotype (FP)

FP criteria	Measurement
Weakness	Grip strength: lowest 20% (by sex, body mass index)
Slowness	Walking time/15 ft: slowest 20% (by sex, height)
Low level of physical activity	Kcal/week: lowest 20% Males: 383 Kcal/week Females: 270 Kcal/week
Exhaustion; poor endurance	"Exhaustion" (self-report)
Weight loss	>10 lb lost unintentionally in prior year

Note: Adapted from Fried LP, Tangen C, Walston J, et al. Frailty in older adults: evidence for a phenotype. J Gerontol A Biol Sci Med Sci. 2001;56A:M1–M11, by permission of Oxford University Press.5

In a systematic review in J Thorac Cardiovasc Surg. 2014, Aresh Sepehri et al. and in Gen Thorac Cardiovasc Surg (2015) Hiroshi Furukawa et al., underscore that. Frailty predicts postoperative outcomes independent of existing cardiac preoperative risk scores and It has been estimated that the prevalence of frailty in the cardiovascular disease population is considerably increasing [33, 50].

Conclusion

It has to be clear that scores' use and implementation don't replace our responsibility to frame and deepen the individual case. The panel approach in heart team has to push us towards a individual medicine. All measures that can improve patients' hospital stay have to be implemented remembering that maths objectivity and reproducibility, as opposed to the subjectivity and variability of clinical evaluation, do not have to give us an illusive presumption ofdo certainty.

References

1. Garfein AJ, Herzog AR. Robust aging among the young-old, old-old, and oldest-old. J Gerontol B Psychol Sci Soc Sci. 1995;50((2):S77–87.
2. The Joint Task Force on the Management of Valvular Heart Disease of the European Society of Cardiology (ESC), European Association for Cardio-Thoracic Surgery (EACTS), Vahanian A, Alfieri O, Andreotti F, Antunes MJ, Barón-Esquivias G, Baumgartner H, Borger MA, Carrel TP, De Bonis M, Evangelista A, Falk V, Iung B, Lancellotti P, Pierard L, Price S, Schäfers HJ, Schuler G, Stepinska J, Swedberg K, Takkenberg J, Von Oppell UO, Windecker S, Zamorano JL, Zembala M. Guidelines on the management of valvular heart disease (version 2012). Eur Heart J. 2012;33:2451–96.
3. Nishimura RA, Otto CM, Bonow RO, Carabello BA, Erwin JP III, Guyton RA, O'Gara PT, Ruiz CE, Skubas NJ, Sorajja P, Sundt TM III, Thomas JD. 2014 AHA/ACC Guideline for the management of patients with valvular heart disease a report of the American College of Cardiology/American Heart Association Task Force on Practice Guidelines. Circulation. 2014;129(23):2440–92.
4. Nishimura RA, Otto CM, Bonow RO, Carabello BA, Erwin JPIII, Fleisher LA, Jneid H, Mack MJ, McLeod CJ, O'Gara PT, Rigolin VH, Sundt TMIII, Thompson A. AHA/ACC Focused update of the 2014 AHA/ACC guideline for the management of patients with valvular heart disease a report of the American College of Cardiology/American Heart Association Task Force on Clinical Practice Guidelines. Circulation. 2017.; https://doi.org/10.1161/CIR.0000000000000503
5. Baumgartner H, Hung J, Bermejo J, et al. Echocardiographic assessment of valve stenosis: EAE/ASE recommendations for clinical practice. Eur J Echocardiogr. 2009;10:1–25.
6. Lancellotti P, Tribouilloy C, Hagendorff A, Moura L, Popescu BA, Agricola E, Monin JL, Pierard LA, Badano L, Zamorano JL, European Association of Echocardiography. European Association of Echocardiography recommendations for the assessment of valvular regurgitation. Part 1. Aortic and pulmonary regurgitation (native valve disease). Eur J Echocardiogr. 2010;11:223–44.
7. Rosenhek R, Iung B, Tornos P, et al. ESC Working group on valvular heart disease position paper: assessing the risk of interventions in patients with valvular heart disease. Eur Heart J. 2012;33:822–8.
8. Debonnaire P, et al. Value of the "TAVI2-SCORe" versus surgical risk scores for prediction of one year mortality in 511 patients who underwent transcatheter aortic valve implantation. Am J Cardiol. 2015;115(2):234–42.

9. Geissler HJ, Holzl P, Marohl S, Kuhn-Regnier F, Mehlhorn U, Südkamp M, Rainer de Vivie E. Risk stratification in heart surgery: comparison of six score systems. Eur J Cardiothorac Surg. 2000;17(4):400–6.
10. Prins C, Jonker DV, Botes L, Smit FE. Cardiac surgery risk-stratification models. Cardiovasc J Afr. 2012;23(3):160–4.
11. Nashef SAM, Roques F, Sharples LD, Nilsson J, Smith C, Goldstone AR. EuroSCORE II. Eur J Cardiothorac Surg. 2012;41:734–45.
12. Noyez L, Kievit PC, van Swieten HA, de Boer M-J. Cardiac operative risk evaluation: the EuroSCORE II, does it make a real difference? Neth Heart J. 2012;20:494–8.
13. Roques F, Michel P, Goldstone AR, Nashef SA. The logistic EuroSCORE. Eur Heart J. 2003;24(9):882–3.
14. Clark RE. The STS national database: alive, well, and growing. Ann Thorac Surg. 1991;52(1):5.
15. Clark RE. The Society of Thoracic Surgeons National Database status report. Ann Thorac Surg. 1994;57(1):20–6.
16. Welke KF, Ferguson TB, Coombs LP, Dokholyan RS, Murray CJ, Schrader MA, Peterson ED. Validity of the society of thoracic surgeons National Adult Cardiac Surgery Database. Ann Thorac Surg. 2004;77(4):1137–9.
17. Brown JM, Wu C, Sikora JH, Griffith BP, Gammie JS. Isolated aortic valve replacement in North America comprising 108,687 patients in 10 years: changes in risks, valve types, and outcomes in the Society of Thoracic Surgeons National Database. J Thorac Cardiovasc Surg. 2009;137:82–90.
18. Ranucci M, Castelvecchio S, Menicanti L, Frigiola A, Pelissero G. Risk of assessing mortality risk in elective cardiac operations age, creatinine, ejection fraction, and the law of parsimony. Circulation. 2009;119:3053–61.
19. Ranucci M, Castelvecchio S, Conte M, Megliola G, Speziale G, Fiore F, Guarracino F, Scolletta S, Escobar RM, Falco M, Bignami E, Landoni G. The easier, the better: age, creatinine, ejection fraction score for operative mortality risk stratification in a series of 29,659 patients undergoing elective cardiac surgery. J Thorac Cardiovasc Surg. 2011;142(3):581–6. Epub 2011 Jun 24.
20. Ranucci M, Pistuddi V, Scolletta S, de Vincentiis C, Menicanti L. The ACEF II Risk Score for cardiac surgery: updated but still parsimonious. Eur Heart J. 2017.; https://doi.org/10.1093/eurheartj/ehx228
21. Shahian DM, et al. The society of thoracic surgeons risk model for operative mortality after multiple valve surgery (Part 1-2-3). Eur J Cardiothorac Surg. 2013;95(4):1484–90.
22. Barili F, et al. Does Euroscore II perform better than its original version? A multicentre validation study. Eur Heart J. 2013;34(1):22–9.
23. Durand E, et al. Performance analysis of Euroscore II compared to the original logistic EuroSCORE and STS scores for predicting 30-day mortality after TAVI. Am J Cardiol. 2013;111(6):891–7.
24. Stähli B, et al. Early and late mortality in patients undergoing transcatheter aortic valve implantation: comparison of the novel EuroScore II with established risk scores. Cardiology. 2013;126(1):15–23.
25. Haensig M, et al. Is the new EuroSCORE II a better predictor for transapical aortic valve implantation? Eur J Cardiothorac Surg. 2013;44(2):302–8.
26. Osnabrugge RL, et al. Performance of EuroSCORE II in a large US database: implications for transcatheter aortic valve implantation. Eur J Cardiothorac Surg. 2014;46(3):400–8.
27. Biancari F, et al. Meta-analysis on the performance of the EuroSCORE II and the Society of Thoracic Surgeons Scores in patients undergoing aortic valve replacement. J Cardiothorac Vasc Anesth. 2014;28(6):1533–9.
28. Guida P, Mastro F, Scrascia G, Whitlock R, Paparella D. Performance of the European system for cardiac operative risk evaluation II: a meta-analysis of 22 studies involving 145,592 cardiac surgery procedures. J Thorac Cardiovasc Surg. 2014;148(6):3049–57.e1.
29. Zbroński K, Huczek Z, Puchta D, Paczwa K, Kochman J, Wilimski R, Scisło P, Rymuza B, Filipiak KJ, Opolski G. Outcome prediction following transcatheter aortic valve implantation: multiple risk scores comparison. Cardiol J. 2016;23(2):169–77.

30. D'Ascenzo F, Ballocca F, Moretti C, Barbanti M, Gasparetto V, Mennuni M, D'Amico M, Conrotto F, Salizzoni S, Omedè P, Colaci C, Zoccai GB, Lupo M, Tarantini G, Napodanno M, Presbitero P, Sheiban I, Tamburino C, Marra S, Gaita F. Inaccuracy of available surgical risk scores to predict outcomes after transcatheter aortic valve replacement. J Cardiovasc Med (Hagerstown). 2013;14(12):894–8.
31. Sullivan PG, Wallach JD, Ioannidis JPA. Meta-analysis comparing established risk prediction models (EuroSCORE II, STS Score, And ACEF Score) for perioperative mortality during cardiac surgery. Am J Cardiol. 2016;118(10):1574–82.
32. Ranucci M. The hidden traps of meta-analyses on cardiac surgery mortality risk scores. Am J Cardiol. 2017;120:337–8.
33. Tanemoto HFK. Frailty in cardiothoracic surgery: systematic review of the literature. Gen Thorac Cardiovasc Surg. 2015;63:425–33.
34. Silvay G, Zafirova Z. Ten years experiences with preoperative evaluation clinic for day admission cardiac and major vascular surgical patients: model for "perioperative anesthesia and surgical home". Semin Cardiothorac Vasc Anesth. 2016;20(2):120–32.
35. Daabiss M. American society of Anesthesiologists physical status classification. Indian J Anaesth. 2011;55:111–5.
36. Dupuis J-Y, Wang F, Nathan H, Lam M, Grimes S, Bourke M. The cardiac anesthesia riskevaluation score a clinically useful predictor of mortality and morbidity after cardiac surgery. Anesthesiology. 2001;94:194–204.
37. Visser A, Geboers B, Gouma DJ, Goslings JC, Ubbinik DT. Predictors of surgical complications: a systematic review. Surgery. 2015;158:58–65.
38. Cohen ME, Liu Y, Ko CY, Hall BL. An examination of American College of Surgeons NSQIP surgical risk calculator accuracy. J Am Coll Surg. 2017;224(5):787–795.e1.
39. Bilimoria KY, Liu Y, Paruch JL, Kmiecik TE, Ko CY, Cohen ME. Development and evaluation of the universal ACS NSQIP surgical risk calculator: a decision aid and informed consent tool for patients and surgeons. J Am Coll Surg. 2013;217(5):833–842.e3.
40. Charlson M, Szatrowski TP, Peterson J, Gold J. Validation of a combined comorbidity index. J Clin Epidemiol. 1994;47(11):1245–51.
41. Tamayo E, Fierro I, Bustamante-Munguira J, Heredia-Rodríguez M, Jorge-Monjas P, Maroto L, Gómez-Sánchez E, Bermejo-Martín FJ, Álvarez FJ, Gómez-Herreras J. Development of the post cardiac surgery (POCAS) prognostic score. Crit Care. 2013;17:R209.
42. Ranucci M, Ballotta A, Castelvecchio S, Baryshnikova E, Brozzi S, Boncilli A, for the Surgical and Clinical Outcome Research (SCORE) Group. Intensive care unit admission parameters improve the accuracy of operative mortality predictive models in cardiac surgery. PLoS One. 2010;5(10):e13551.
43. Kotera A, Haga Y, Kei J, Okamoto M, Seo K. Evaluation of estimation of physiologic ability and surgical stress to predict in-hospital mortality in cardiac surgery. J Anesth. 2011;25(4):481–91.
44. Magruder JT. A predictive model and risk score for unplanned cardiac surgery intensive care unit readmissions. J Card Surg. 2015;30(9):685–90.
45. Bagnall NM, Faiz O, Darzi A, Athanasiou T. What is the utility of preoperative frailty assessment for risk stratification in cardiac surgery? Interact Cardiovasc Thorac Surg. 2013;17(2):398–402.
46. Rowe R, Iqbal J, Murali-krishnan R, Sultan A, Orme R, Briffa N, Denvir M, Gunn J. Role of frailty assessment in patients undergoing cardiac interventions. BMJ. 2017;1:e000033.
47. Mack M. Frailty and aortic valve disease. J Thorac Cardiovasc Surg. 2013;145(3 Suppl):S7–10.
48. Afilalo J, Mottillo S, Eisenberg MJ, Alexander KP, Noiseux N, Perrault LP, Morin J-F, Langlois Y, Ohayon SM, Monette J, Boivin J-F, Shahian DM, Bergman H. Addition of frailty and disability to cardiac surgery risk scores identifies elderly patients at high risk of mortality or major morbidity. Circ Cardiovasc Qual Outcomes. 2012;5:222–8.
49. Chen X, Mao G, Leng SX. Frailty syndrome: an overview. Clin Interv Aging. 2014;9:433–41.
50. Sepehri A, Beggs T, Hassan A, Rigatto C, Shaw-Daigle C, Tangri N, Arora RC. The impact of frailty on outcomes after cardiac surgery: a systematic review. J Thorac Cardiovasc Surg. 2014;148(6):3110–7.

Part VII

Heart Valve Clinic

The Heart Valve Centre

27

John B. Chambers and Patrizio Lancellotti

27.1 Introduction

Specialist valve clinics are best practice for the care of patients with valve disease [1]. In hospitals of sufficient size their remit extends beyond the outpatient clinic to include specialist inpatient care including infective endocarditis [2]. Valve clinics are also the focus for training and education, raising awareness of valve disease and implementing plans to improve detection particularly in the community [3]. In parallel, specialist MDTs were established for developing TAVI programmes and mitral valve repair. The most recent international guidelines in valve disease [3, 4] extended these developments further with the idea of a 'surgical center of excellence'. These are essential if clinically aggressive recommendations for prophylactic repair of degenerative mitral disease are to be effective and not result in premature mitral valve replacement. Standards defining such centers of excellence have now been agreed in international consensus documents [5, 6].

Thus the concept of specialist valve care has evolved from more than one root and the purpose of this chapter is to draw these strands together (Fig. 27.1) to describe the standards required of a specialist surgical center and how it relates to community-based and national valve care programmes (Table 27.1).

J.B. Chambers, M.D. (✉)
Cardiothoracic Centre, Guy's and St Thomas' Hospitals, London, UK
e-mail: jboydchambers@aol.com

P. Lancellotti, M.D., Ph.D.
Department of Cardiology, University of Liège Hospital, GIGA Cardiovascular Sciences, Heart Valve Clinic, CHU Sart Tilman, Liège, Belgium

GVM Care and Research, E.S. Health Science Foundation, Lugo, RA, Italy

K. Fattouch et al. (eds.), *Advances in Treatments for Aortic Valve and Root Diseases*, https://doi.org/10.1007/978-3-319-66483-5_27

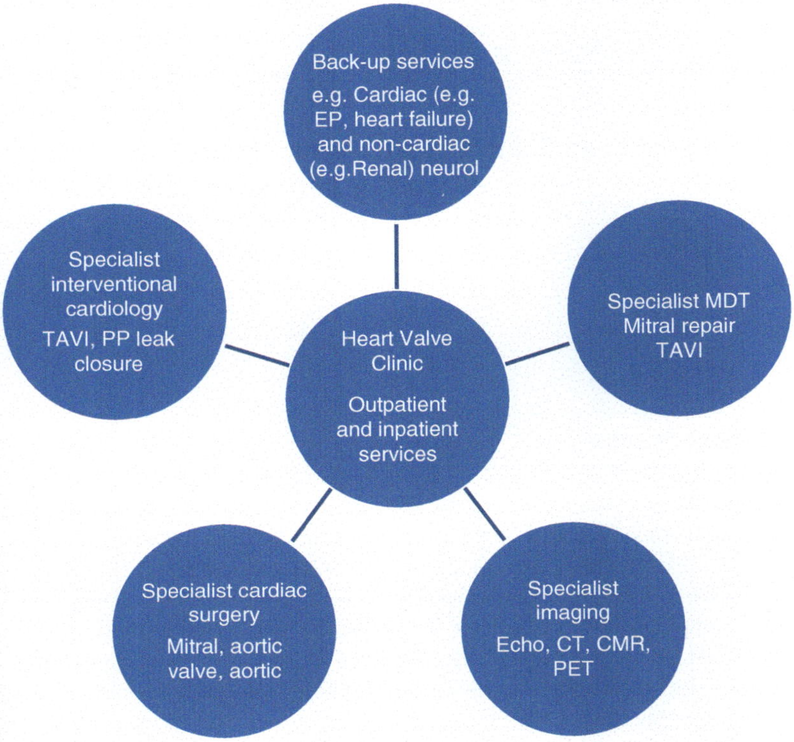

Fig. 27.1 Components of a heart valve centre

Table 27.1 The roles of different locations or levels in the care of heart valve disease

Location or level	Roles
Heart valve center	Cardiac surgery including mitral valve repair, interventional valve procedures, specialist inpatient opinions including a specialist endocarditis service, specialist outpatient valve clinic, training and education, communication with referring hospitals and community, regular audit
Referring hospital	Outpatient clinic, inpatient opinions, expert echocardiography
Community	Detection programmes, dental surveillance, patient interest groups
National and regulatory bodies	National and international guidance documents, professional bodies overseeing medical training and validation and standards, accreditation of imaging labs, monitoring for early prosthetic valve failures
Commercial organisations	Proctorship for new techniques

27.2 Why Is a Heart Valve Center Necessary?

Patients with valve disease are often cared for by general cardiologists or general physicians who may be less skilled than a specialist in making a diagnostic formulation [7, 8]. A reduced LV ejection fraction in severe aortic stenosis may still be seen as a contraindication to surgery [9] while a LV ejection fraction of 55% in a patient with severe mitral regurgitation may be mistaken for normal function. Accepted management guidelines tend not to be followed adequately [10] and advances in practice, for example changes in thresholds for repair, are less likely to be assimilated by a generalist than by a cardiologist who undertakes specialist continuing education. Furthermore applying accepted guidelines requires specialist experience especially in determining that a patient is genuinely asymptomatic. The absence of specialisation may result in patients being referred for surgery too late or not at all. In the EuroHeart Survey [9], around one half with valve disease were in NYHA Class III or IV at the time of surgery. Around a third with severe aortic stenosis aged 75 or more, were not referred at all [11]. The main reasons cited were age or LV ejection fraction reduced to 35–50% rather than a significant co-morbidity suggesting that the majority were denied surgery inappropriately. Patients may also be referred to a surgeon at the correct time but receive suboptimal surgery. The EuroHeart Survey [9] found that 50% of patients with mitral regurgitation received a replacement valve rather than repair and, in the USA, just over a third of operations for mitral regurgitation in the year 2000 were repairs [12].

27.3 Basic Standards of the Heart Valve Center

There are basic minimum requirements for all heart valve centers (Table 27.2) including a heart valve clinic (Sect. 27.4) and expert imaging (Sect. 27.5). The minimum interventional services available must be: replacement of valves in all 4 positions; mitral valve repair; tricuspid annuloplasty and repair; ancillary procedures, left atrial appendage closure, AF ablation; percutaneous balloon mitral valvotomy; TAVI; percutaneous repair of paraprosthetic regurgitation; aortic replacement. Aortic valve repair, transcatheter mitral and tricuspid procedures, and the Ross procedure are highly specialised and cannot be available at every center but there should be the ability to transfer to centers offering these procedures if required.

There should be 24 h, 7-day cover for all aspects of the service. Cross-cover should be feasible for leave and sickness and is particularly important for highly-specialised procedures like mitral valve repair or balloon mitral valvotomy.

There should be sufficient beds to allow uninterrupted transfer of patients from peripheral hospitals and sufficient ITU capacity to allow urgent surgery when clinically indicated. Operating schedules should allow urgent or emergent operations (e.g. for endocarditis).

A comprehensive valve service requires immediate access to opinions from cardiologists specialising in heart failure and electrophysiology. Extra-cardiac specialties include intensive care, vascular surgery, general surgery (especially gastrointestinal), neurology, renal, infection, stroke and elderly care medicine, psychology, and dental surgery. Geneticists should be available for selected patients with mitral prolapse or aortic dilatation.

There must be robust internal audit processes [16, 17] including rates of repair, outcome of operations (including echocardiographic assessment), complications, durability of repair and rates of reoperation. The results must be available for

Table 27.2 Minimum requirements of a Heart Valve Center

• Specialist valve clinic [1] as a hub between community, other hospitals and extracardiac departments, and between non-invasive cardiologists, surgeons and interventional cardiologists
• Expert imaging with accredited operators and departments [13, 14]: - Expert echocardiography including 3D and stress echocardiography and perioperative transoesophageal echocardiography [15]. - Cardiac CT, magnetic resonance and PET
• Multidisciplinary teams with competencies in mitral valve repair, aortic valve repair, and transcatheter aortic and mitral valve techniques - Named cardiac surgeons and cardiologists with special interest in valve disease - Named imaging specialists, cardiac anaesthetists and interventional cardiologists specialising in transcatheter procedures - Regular case discussions - Systematic approach to reduce medical and surgical risks
• Back-up services - Other specialist cardiologists including heart failure and arrhythmia - Extracardiac specialties e.g., intensive care, vascular surgery, general surgery, experts in gastrointestinal, neurology, renal, stroke and elderly care medicine, psychology, and dental surgery
• Basic cardiac surgical procedures and volumes - Replacement of all valves, mitral and tricuspid repair, AF ablation - Percutaneous: Mitral balloon valvotomy, TAVI, closure techniques for paraprosthetic regurgitation - Aortic replacement
• Data review: - Internal audit processes including rates of repair and hemodynamic results on, complications, durability of repair and rates of reoperation - Results available for internally and external review - Involvement in national databases

Table 27.3 Data for collection in repair and replacement for organic mitral or aortic valve disease

Grading of the valve lesion
Preoperative risk assessment and stratification
Preoperative multidisciplinary team classification for repair as 'likely', 'unlikely' or 'not feasible'
Operative mortality and morbidity at 30 days
Early postoperative hemodynamic function: Transvalvular velocity and mean gradient (all positions) and effective orifice area (aortic position) of replacement or transcatheter valves Presence and grade of paraprosthetic regurgitation Residual regurgitation and new obstruction after repair or systolic anterior motion of the anterior mitral leaflet
Follow-up: Durability of repair based on echocardiography Requirement for redo procedure

internal and external review. Examples of surgical data for collection are suggested in Table 27.3 and example targets for mitral valve repair in Table 27.4. Universal recording of all surgical valve procedures in national databases should be required, as is the case for transcatheter devices in the US [22, 23]. There should be a

Table 27.4 Example targets for surgical outcomes in repair of mitral valve prolapse

	Rate
Mortality	<1% [18, 19]
Major complication	<2% [19]
Repair for P2 prolapse	≥90% [16]
Significant residual mitral regurgitation	≤5% at 5 years [18]
Reoperation rate	
Posterior repair	≤1% per year [20]
Anterior repair	≤2% per year [20, 21]

systematic approach to safety [17] including the use of WHO checklists and regular audit meetings with effective feedback of results.

27.4 The 'Heart Valve Clinic

This acts as a hub between community, other hospitals and extracardiac departments [1]. It is the site for assessing new outpatient referrals and conducting the surveillance of asymptomatic moderate and severe valve disease. It determines the correct timing of surgery and referral to an appropriately qualified and experienced surgeon or interventional cardiologist (Table 27.3). The clinics will supervise training in valve disease and will set standards and promote internal audit.

The composition of the staff at Heart Valve Clinics will vary according to local requirements. A cardiologist specialising in valve disease is the core at every clinic and a surgeon should ideally be present. In the UK, consultant scientists may deliver surveillance echocardiography and specialist nurses may see patients after uncomplicated valve replacement under the auspices of a cardiologist [24–26]. Delegating surveillance in this way allows the cardiologist to spend more time with patients in whom clinical decisions are required. However some 10–15% of cases require cardiological assessment and a further 20% of patients within a nurse-led clinic [27] may require medical advice to guide the nurse at the index visit. Therefore, a cardiologist should always be present, but, if not, there should be a clear action plan for dealing with urgent or non-urgent enquiries.

A heart valve specialist can be defined by [2]: (1) a record of training within a centre with recognised expertise in valve disease; (2) valve-related programmed activity e.g. valve clinics, inpatient care, involvement with valve-specific multidisciplinary team meetings, complex echocardiograms to assess valve disease, research; (3) continuous medical education (CME); (4) registration of interest with membership of a recognised national body (including the European Society of Cardiology Council on Valvular Heart Disease, British Heart Valve Society, Heart Valve Society, or European Society for Cardiothoracic Surgery).

Clinicians running the clinic are also responsible for inpatient care of patients with heart valve disease and educating and will also be an integral part, often the leader, of all MDT. There should be regular case discussions to plan the timing and details of surgery, to decide between conventional and transcatheter intervention and to review results. For patients that need emergent treatment a multidisciplinary meeting might not always be possible. The details of multidisciplinary teams are discussed in Sects. 27.6, 27.7 and 27.8.

Heart valve clinics may be established at non-specialist peripheral hospitals but should have links with the valve clinic at a cardiac center to allow review of imaging and other data, and second opinion consultations. There may also be virtual links with MDT meetings at the centre. In a 2014 UK survey, only 11% of peripheral hospitals and 60% of cardiac centers had heart valve clinics [28].

27.5 Expert Imaging

Echocardiography is the mainstay for the detection and assessment of valve disease. However, other modalities, notably cardiac magnetic resonance (CMR) and computed tomography (CT) are used if echocardiographic imaging is suboptimal and can provide complementary information, particularly to aid risk assessment.

Operators and departments need to be accredited by national or international systems [13, 14]. 3D and stress echocardiography needs to be available. There must be provision for out of hours studies and perioperative transesophageal echocardiography [15].

Cardiac CT and CMR need to be deployed with a coherent multimodality approach. These techniques should be used to provide basic anatomical and functional information if echocardiographic imaging is suboptimal but also to give complementary information (e.g. aortic valve calcification).

PET is increasingly used in suspected prosthetic valve or pacemaker endocarditis [29] and should also be available.

27.6 Mitral Valve Multidisciplinary Teams

The team must include at minimum a surgeon with special expertise in mitral valve repair, a cardiologist specialising in echocardiography and an interventional cardiologist.

Surgeons performing mitral valve repair surgery should undergo training in mitral repair, atrial fibrillation ablation [18], and tricuspid annuloplasty [16] as part of their national board certified surgical training. Surgeons should also be mentored through new repair techniques and in the implantation of new types of heart valve replacement to minimise the effects of the 'learning curve' on adverse results [18, 30, 31]. There is a tendency for new products to require increasingly technique-sensitive implantation procedures and regulatory bodies have insisted that manufacturers implement training and accreditation programmes where this is necessary to reduce procedural risk (ISO). The International Standard for transcatheter valves (ISO) requires manufacturers to "establish a structured training program for the physician and staff who will be involved in the peri-procedural care of the patient". This principle should be seen as the rule rather than the exception. Effective training can occur by collaborative working within units, visits to other units, or by inviting external experts.

27.6.1 Assignment for Mitral Valve Repair

Repairable primary disease should be operated on by surgeons with special expertise in valve repair [16, 18] and acceptable results (Table 27.3). Some types of P2 repair in degenerative disease may be relatively straightforward, but it is not always possible to guarantee this during preoperative assessment. A surgeon without specialist expertise might then find him or herself forced to implant a replacement valve while a more specialised surgeon might have successfully repaired it.

Implantion of annuloplasty rings are a part of the regular work of all cardiac surgeons, Repair procedures for functional mitral regurgitation should therefore be performed under the auspices of a surgeon with specialised training and interest in valve repair.

27.6.2 Surgeon and Hospital Volumes

The relationship between case volume and outcomes for surgery and transcatheter interventions is complex, but volume recommendations already exist or are being discussed for percutaneous coronary intervention [32], vascular surgery [33] and percutaneous valve techniques [22, 23]. What constitutes sufficiently high individual surgeon or hospital volumes to maintain good results for repair of mitral valve prolapse is controversial. A large retrospective review showed that mitral repair rates were higher and mortality rates lower in large volume hospitals. A high hospital volume partly reflects high individual surgeon volumes [31, 34] but may also be a surrogate for excellent facilities and processes.

Annual thresholds of 20–40 mitral valve repair procedures for individual surgeons [18, 34, 35] have been suggested based on expert consensus or the observation from retrospective analyses that repair rates are on average higher among higher volume surgeons. Similarly, hospital volumes of >50 per year have been suggested [18], although studies in the US [35] have not confirmed that center volume alone reliably predicts outcome.

For mitral valve replacement, no individual surgeon thresholds have been identified. Lower mortality rates are shown in higher volume centres [36], including one study with centre volumes >80 per year for repair and replacement [37].

These few studies are all retrospective making it difficult to control for the characteristics of individual patients or surgeons and repair rates were not matched with the preoperative likelihood of repair. Within the populations there were low-volume surgeons with high repair rates and high volume surgeons with low repair rates [34, 35]. Furthermore, these publications did not record non-fatal complications including stroke and bleeding, rates of residual mitral regurgitation or need for redo surgery. In view of these limitations, the ability to demonstrate good results (Table 27.4) is a more important standard than the attainment of volume targets but it is likely these will not be attained without an annual minimum of 40 mitral repairs per surgeon and an annual center volume of >80 mitral repairs and replacements.

27.7 Aortic Valve Multidisciplinary Teams

Multidisciplinary meetings are not required for straightforward decisions (e.g. symptomatic severe aortic stenosis for patients suitable for conventional surgery). However, in patients with comorbidities, that may also contribute to symptoms and increase the risk of cardiac surgery, MDT discussion is mandatory. There is also increasing focus on surgical issues such as prosthesis selection [38] particularly in younger patients in whom the possibility of future valve-in-valve procedures should be considered.

Team discussions are already established for severely symptomatic patients being considered for TAVI. The team includes a surgeon, interventional cardiologist, cardiologist specialising in echocardiography and other relevant specialists as appropriate (e.g. elderly care or renal physicians). Team discussions are often necessary for other patients with aortic stenosis: asymptomatic severe aortic stenosis; low-flow low gradient aortic stenosis; patients with symptoms despite apparently moderate aortic stenosis. Decisions about surgery for coexistent mitral regurgitation [39] or the advisability of replacing a valve with moderate stenosis at the time of coronary bypass grafting are also frequently difficult [4, 40].

Conventional aortic valve replacement is part of the basic surgical training. However, as for the mitral position, new designs of valves with different implantation techniques should be introduced with the help of a proctor to minimise the learning curve. The Ross operation is another example of a complex operation that must be learned at a centre with a large experience in this type of operation.

Repair techniques are feasible in bicuspid or prolapsing aortic valves but remain underutilised. Approximately 60% of regurgitant aortic valves may be repaired at a specialist centre [41, 42]. Aortic root remodelling might be part of these repair procedures. Experience and expertise is needed for the whole team since careful preoperative assessment and intraoperative imaging are essential [42, 43].

27.7.1 Volumes

The effect of procedural volume has been observed for aortic valve replacement [36] with a mortality rate of 9.1% for surgeons with annual volumes of less than 22 cases compared with a rate of 6.5% for those with annual volumes exceeding 42 cases. No volume data are available for aortic valve repair. Individual surgeon and hospital volumes are unlikely to be perfect surrogates for outcome data and the ability to demonstrate good results is more important than working to volume targets.

27.8 Endocarditis Multidisciplinary Team Approach

A multidisciplinary team approach is regarded essential for optimal treatment of patients with endocarditis [2, 44, 45] and has been shown to reduce 1 year mortality from 18.5 to 8.2% [44]. The team should include cardiologists with specialist competencies in valve disease, echocardiographers, surgeons with expertise in complex valve surgery, specialist in infectious diseases and/or medical microbiology (depending on the local model of service delivery). Other experts must be available: a specialist in spinal conditions; an electrophysiologist specialized in extraction of pacemakers and ICDs [46]; a specialist in adult congenital heart disease; a neurologist and neurosurgeon to advise on the management of cerebral complications; a renal physician.

All cases of possible endocarditis identified on cultures, signs and symptoms, including intracardiac device (CIED) infections, should be referred to the specialist team who should then assume or direct the management of those with confirmed IE. The patient should be nursed in a specialist area by staff with the competencies required to recognise deteriorating valve function and other complications.

All cases should be discussed immediately on transfer or admission by the specialist cardiologist, the infection specialist and cardiac surgeon. If surgery appears likely, the cardiac surgeon should be actively involved to discuss timing and schedule the operation. The team should have regular MDT meetings to follow the progress of inpatients and referrals, make decisions about their management. The need for a formal MDT discussion should never delay emergent surgery.

The mortality is worse if this is delayed, but may be approximately halved [47] when performed as soon as clinically indicated. Operating schedules should allow for urgent or emergent surgery in patients with endocarditis.

Much aortic and mitral valve endocarditis surgery should be within the remit of an appropriately trained consultant surgeon. However, certain situations might call for additional expertise such as aortic root abscess and where there is a chance of valve repair. The relative merit of immediate surgery (with a lower chance of repair) as against elective surgery (with a higher chance of repair [48] but also of heart failure and irreversible myocardial damage) requires fine judgement. Joint consultant operating should be considered for challenging cases.

27.9 Community and Extracardiac Clinics

The cardiologist running the valve clinic is usually also instrumental in initiating improvement programmes in the community. However there are local differences and some community physicians are in charge of programmes. The key aspects of community outreach are: improving detection of valve disease; optimising referral to a heart valve center of excellence; educating patients.

27.9.1 Improving Detection

Valve disease is under detected [49]. A murmur at auscultation is a good cue but only about a third are associated with significant valve disease and auscultation also has limited sensitivity [50] particularly when performed by generalists [8]. Echocardiography is known to maximise detection [51] but for population screening has rarely been deployed beyond local research projects. Furthermore this would involve major resources and may not be appropriate economically, medically or because of the real risks of medicalising normal people [52, 53].

However echocardiography is not yet fully used for groups known to be at the highest risk of valve disease [54] including those with a potentially cardiac symptom or AF (Table 27.5). In an analysis of community-based echo, the yield of valve disease doubled if a symptom, abnormal ECG were added to murmur as indications for echo [55]. First degree relatives of probands with bicuspid aortic valves have approximately a 10% chance of aortic valve or aortic pathology [56] and should also be offered screening [57]. Patients who have lived during childhood and adolescence in countries with a high population prevalence of rheumatic disease [58] could also be offered screening particularly before non-cardiac surgery or during pregnancy.

It may be reasonable to auscultate patients aged over 75 years at well-person or flu-vaccination clinics or since they have a 10–15% chance of moderate or severe valve disease [49, 59, 60]. It is likely that a particularly high risk subgroup can be defined by the presence of risk factors like hypertension, diabetes, obesity, hypercholesterolemia, renal disease, or coronary artery disease [61]. Community based echocardiography needs to be delivered to a high-standard and must be integrated in the whole network of valve care (Table 27.6)

Table 27.5 Indications for community echocardiography

Established indications
Cardiac symptoms (exertional breathlessness, chest pain, syncope, unexplained decrease in exercise tolerance)
Atrial fibrillation without previous echocardiography
Abnormal resting 12 lead ECG
Clinically obvious systolic murmur
Any diastolic murmur
Relative of patients with bicuspid aortic valve
Additional indications
Patients from areas with a high population prevalence of rheumatic disease
Age over 75 years, particularly in patients with risk factors e.g. hypertension, diabetes, obesity, hypercholesterolemia, renal disease, or coronary artery disease

Table 27.6 Properties of community echocardiography for valve disease

Availability of echocardiography within 2 weeks for patients with chronic cardiac symptoms[a]
Availability of echocardiography within 1 month for patients with an asymptomatic murmur[b]
Automatic referral of patients found to have moderate or severe valve disease to a valve clinic
Links with a cardiothoracic centre in a hub and spoke arrangement either via a specialist valve clinic at a local hospital or run by a general practitioner with specialist cardiovascular interests
Provision for structured surveillance of patients with mild native disease or normally-functioning replacement valves
Shared archiving between community and hospital
Training of general practitioners and education of patients
Community echocardiography by accredited operators within high-quality accredited departments including quality assurance, expert back-up, and clinical links

[a]Processes for urgent or emergency assessment of patients with acute or severe symptoms must exist

[b]Although not clinically urgent there is evidence that waiting too long for echocardiography induces anxiety which is not then dispelled by a normal echocardiogram

27.9.2 Improving Referral

There is lack of awareness of the relative safety of modern surgery and a proportion of elderly people are not referred appropriately despite having symptomatic severe aortic stenosis and reasonable general health. The establishment of a TAVI programme leads to a surge in referrals many of whom are suitable for conventional surgery [62, 63]. There need to be local, national and international educational programmes to encourage general practitioners and hospital based non-cardiologists to refer patients with possible valve disease to specialist valve clinics [1].

The significance of echocardiography reports may be underappreciated by non-cardiologists and significant valve disease not recognised so it is vital that diagnostic echocardiography occurs within a comprehensive clinical framework including cardiology oversight. The clinical lead for valve disease in the area either based at the local hospital or a general practitioner with a special interest in cardiovascular and valve disease should ensure that echocardiography leads to:

(a) referral of patients found to have moderate or severe valve disease to a specialist valve clinic
(b) appropriate surveillance of patients with mild disease e.g. return to community-based clinic, call-back for serial open access studies
(c) appropriate referral back to the general practitioner of patients with normal echocardiograms to ensure exclusion of other diseases e.g. angina, chronic lung disease

The need for surveillance and timely referral for surgery may not be sufficiently recognised leading to patients being referred late once significant symptoms develop. The presence of a valve clinic acts as a beacon for referral. However in addition the lead cardiologist should ensure that education about significant advances is disseminated to the community.

Endocarditis is a rare disease and easily missed. Community physicians should be trained to think of the diagnosis if fever fails to resolve in a patient with structural heart disease especially with a replacement valve or prior endocarditis. Since prior antibiotic therapy is the most common cause of culture negative endocarditis it is important to take blood cultures before starting antibiotics if endocarditis is possible. Community physicians need to be updated on the need for antibiotic prophylaxis before invasive dental procedures.

27.9.3 Patient Education

The valve clinic is a focus for educating about the symptoms of valve disease and other indications for surgery. Discussions about the type of valve replacement can begin well before surgery becomes necessary, Other important components include the need for dental surveillance.

Patients need to be provided with information and be guided to reliable websites since much information available is unreliable. A guidance report ‘UK heart surgery today: accessible information for patients’ [62, 63] might allow patients to make better-informed decisions about their surgery. Patient self-help groups may also be helpful in improving awareness and knowledge about valve disease.

27.10 National Organisation

Ideally universal entry onto national databases should be required. In the UK, outcome data adjusted for case-mix and compared against a contemporary peer-group standard are published for hospitals and individual surgeons [62, 63]. There is a quality assurance ‘Governance Toolkit’ allowing surgeons to monitor their own performance, an approach which has been shown to reduce procedural deaths for coronary intervention in programmes run in some US states [64].

Universal recording of all surgical valve procedures in national databases should be required, as is the case for transcatheter devices in the USA [22, 23]. These would generate early warning of generic problems and also facilitate the evaluation of new techniques and help determine the feasibility of wider dissemination. In the past, however, design problems with heart valves have first been identified, not through registries, but through the vigilance of clinicians who reported their concerns to their national regulatory authorities. Clinicians should therefore make use of established reporting systems for adverse incidents related to all medical devices.

National cardiovascular professional societies should establish, coordinate and monitor specialist training for all members of heart valve multidisciplinary teams including surgeons, interventional cardiologists and cardiologists, anaesthesiologists and scientists specialising in imaging. It would also be ideal to have a pathology laboratory, independent of valve manufacturers, examining explanted valves to determine mechanisms of failure.

27.11 Evidence for Effectiveness of Specialist Services

There is no RCT comparing results from a specialist valve service against usual care and it is doubtful whether such a study is feasible or even necessary. There is much indirect evidence. The retrospective data on surgical and center volumes for both mitral repair and aortic valve surgery show that results are, in general, better for high volume surgeons in high-volume centers. Studies [65] showing that watchful waiting in severe degenerative MR is safe already mandate careful follow-up by experts which effectively endorses the concept of the clinic. Recently a case-control study has shown that patients with aortic stenosis have shorter delays between symptom-onset and presentation and also less severe symptoms compared with patients in non-specialist clinics [66].

Numerous studies show that valve clinics improve adherence to guidelines [10] and reduce the number of inappropriate echocardiograms [10, 67, 68] mostly those performed unnecessarily for normally-functioning mechanical valves. Reducing inappropriate echocardiograms could save €45–105 per 1000 population per year

[68, 69]. A cost-effectiveness simulation showed that the UK model of devolved surveillance saves about €70,000 per 1000 patients [24].

Referral patterns to a national center of excellence will be subject to individual national organisation. Potentially no cardiac surgery other than that required in trauma centers should occur outside cardiac centers of excellence. An interim stage must involve demonstrating unequivocally through the accumulation of prospective data that specialist centers of excellence attain better results matched by case mix and the preoperative characteristics of the valve.

Conclusion

Broad consensus favours organisation into multidisciplinary teams with specialisations appropriate to the case-mix and type of intervention being offered. There should be structured training programs for the physicians and staff involved in the peri-procedural care of the patient and these should be overseen by national professional societies. Whilst it is recognised that good results are usually associated with relatively high individual and center volumes, this relationship is complex. Results of surgery need to include detailed information about acute and longer-term hemodynamic results and adverse events including the need for redo surgery matched to the preoperative pathology and risk. These results should be readily available to patients, referrers and government agencies.

MCQ

1. **Which statement about surgical volumes is correct?**
   (a) There is a close relationship between center volume and mitral repair rates
   (b) In general mitral repair rates are highest for high volume surgeons in high volume centers
   (c) There is no relationship between aortic surgery mortality and individual surgeon volumes
   (d) There is no relationship between center volumes and mortality for mitral replacement
2. **Which statement about valve disease is correct?**
   (a) Valve disease is rarely missed
   (b) The incidence of valve disease is increased if atrial fibrillation, cardiac symptom or cardiac history is added to murmur as indications for echocardiography
   (c) The incidence of valve disease in the West is falling
   (d) A murmur is a reliable indicator of valve disease
3. **Which statement is correct?**
   (a) Problems with valve designs are usually detected by national monitoring agencies
   (b) In the Euro Heart Valve surgery approximately one half had surgery in NYHA III or IV
   (c) Rheumatic fever is still the most common cause of valve disease in industrialised countries
   (d) Patient education is not a role for the valve clinic–

References

1. Lancellotti P, Rosenhek R, Pibarot P, Iung B, Otto CM, Tornos P, et al. Heart valve clinics: organisation, structure and experiences. Eur Heart J. 2013;34:1597–606.
2. Chambers J, Sandoe J, Ray S, Prendergast B, Taggart D, Westaby S, et al. The infective endocarditis team: recommendations from an international working group. Heart. 2014;100:524–7.
3. Arden C, Chambers J, Ray S, Prendergast B, Taggart D, Westaby S, Grothier L, Wilson J, Campbell B, Sandoe J, Gohlke-Bärwolf C, Mestres C, Rosenhek R, Pibarot P, Otto C. Can we improve the detection of heart valve disease? Heart. 2014;100:271–3.
4. Nishimura RA, Otto CM, Bonow RO, Carabello BA, Erwin JP, Guyton RA, et al. AHA/ACC Guideline for the management of patients with valvular heart disease. J Am Coll Cardiol. 2014. https://doi.org/10.1016/j.jacc.2014.02.536.
5. Chambers J, Ray S, Prendergast B, Graham T, Campbell B, Greenhalgh D, Petrou M, Tinkler J, Gohlke-Bärwolf C, Mestres C, Rosenhek R, Pibarot P, Otto C, Sundt T. Standards for heart valve surgery in a 'Heart Valve Centre of Excellence'. Open Heart. 2015b;2(1):e000216.
6. Chambers J, Prendergast B, Iung B, Rosenhe R, Zamoran JL, Piérard LA, Modine T, Falk V, Kappetein AP, Pibarot P, Sundt T, Baumgartner H, Bax JJ, Lancellotti P. Standards defining a "Heart Valve Centre": ESC Working Group on Valvular Heart Disease and European Association for Cardiothoracic Surgery Viewpoint. Euro Heart J. 2017;38:2177–83; and Eur J Cardiothorac Surg 2017;52:418–24
7. Fink JC, Schmid CH, Selker HP. A decision aid for referring patients with systolic murmurs for echocardiography. J Gen Int Med. 1994;9:479–84.
8. Mangione S, Nieman LZ. Cardiac auscultatory skills of internal medicine and family practice trainees. A comparison of diagnostic proficiency. JAMA. 1997;278:717–22.
9. Iung B, Baron G, Butchart EG, Delahaye F, Gohlke-Barwolf C, Levang OW, Tornos P, Vanoverschelde J-L, Vermeer F, Boersma E, Ravaud P, Vahanian A. A prospective survey of patients with valvular heart disease in Europe: The Euro Heart Survey on valvular heart disease. Eur Heart J. 2003;24:1231–43.
10. Taggu W, Topham A, Hart L, Carr-White G, Sulke N, Patel NR, Lloyd G. A cardiac sonographer led follow up clinic for heart valve disease. Int J Cardiol. 2009;132:240–3.
11. Iung B. Management of the elderly patient with aortic stenosis. Heart. 2008;94:519–24.
12. Savage EB, Ferguson TB, DeSesa VJ. Use of mitral valve repair: analysis of contemporary United States experience reported by the society of thoracic surgeons national cardiac database. Ann Thorac Surg. 2003;75:820–5.
13. Nihoyannopoulos P, Fox K, Fraser A, Pinto F. EAE laboratory standards and accreditation. Eur J Echo. 2007;8:80–7.
14. Picard MH, Adams D, Bierig SM, et al. American Society of Echocardiography recommendations for quality echocardiography laboratory operations. J Am Soc Echo. 2011;24(1):1–10. https://doi.org/10.1016/j.echo.2010.11.006.
15. Van Dyck MJ, Watremez C, Boodwhani M, Vanoverschelde J-L, El Khoury G. Transesophageal echocardiographic evaluation during aortic valve repair surgery. Anesth Analg. 2010;111:59–70.
16. McCarthy PM. When is your surgeon good enough? When do you need a 'referent surgeon'? Curr Cardiol Rep. 2009;11:107–13.
17. Vincent C, Moorthy K, Sarker SK, Chang A, Darzi AW. Systems approaches to surgical quality and safety. From concept to measurement. Ann Surg. 2004;239:475–82.
18. Bridgewater B, Hooper T, Munsch C, et al. Mitral repair best practice: proposed standards. Heart. 2006;92:939–44.
19. Fedak PW, McCarthy PM, Bonow RO. Evolving concepts and technologies in mitral valve repair. Circulation. 2008;117:963–74.
20. David TE, Ivanov J, Armstrong S. Late outcomes of mitral valve repair for floppy valves: implications for asymptomatic patients. J Thorac Cardiovasc Surg. 2003;125:1143–52.
21. Braunberger E, Deloche A, Berrebi F, Abdallah F, Celestin JA, Meimoun P, Chatellier G, Chavaud S, Fabiani JN, Carpentier A. Very long-term results (more than 20 years) of valve

repair with Carpentier's techniques with non rheumatic mitral valve insufficiency. Circulation. 2001;104(12 Suppl 1):I8–11.
22. Tomasso CL, Bolman RM, Feldman T, et al. Multisociety (AATS, ACCF, SCAI, and STS) expert consensus statement: operator and institutional requirements for transcatheter valve repair and replacement, part 1: transcatheter aortic valve replacement. J Am Coll Cardiol. 2012;59:2028–42.
23. Tommaso CL, Fullerton DA, Feldman T, et al. SCAI/AATS/ACC/STS operator and institutional requirements for transcatheter valve repair and replacement. Part II mitral valve. J Am Coll Cardiol. 2014;64:1515–26.
24. Ionescu A, McKenzie C, Chambers J. Are valve clinics a sound investment for the health service? A cost-effectiveness model and an automated tool for cost estimation. Open Heart. 2015;2:e000275. https://doi.org/10.1136/openhrt-2015-000275.
25. Parkin D, Chambers J. Routine follow-up for patients with prosthetic valves: the value of a nurse-led valve clinic. Br J Cardiol. 2012;19:204–6.
26. Parkin D, Chambers J. What is the value of a nurse-led clinic for patients with replacement heart valves? Br J Cardiac Nurs. 2015;10:145–9.
27. Chambers JB, Lloyd G, Rimington HM, Parkin D, Hates AM, Baldrock-Apps G, Topham A. Multidisciplinary valve clinics with devolved surveillance: a 2 year audit. Br J Cardiol. 2011;18:231–2.
28. Bhattacharyya S, Pavitt C, Lloyd G, Chambers JB. Provision, organisation and models of heart valve clinics within the United Kingdom. Q J Med. 2015;108:113–7. https://doi.org/10.1093/qjmed/hcu164. First published online: 6 Aug 2014.
29. Bruun NE, Habib G, Thuny F, Sogaard P. Cardiac imaging in infectious endocarditis. Eur Heart J. 2014;35:624–32.
30. Holzhey DM, Seeburger J, Misfeld M, Borger MA, Mohr FW. Learning minimally-invasive mitral valve surgery: a cumulative sum sequential probability analysis of 3895 operations from a single high volume center. Circulation. 2013;128:483–91.
31. Kilic A, Shah AS, Conte JV, Baumgartner WA, Yuh DD. Operative outcomes in mitral valve surgery: combined effects of surgeon and hospital volume in a population-based analysis. J Thorac Cardiovasc Surg. 2013;146:638–46.
32. Levine GN, Bates ER, Blankenship JC, Bailey SR, Bittl JA, Cercek B, et al. 2011 ACCF/AHA/SCAI guideline for percutaneous coronary intervention: a report of the American College of Cardiology foundation/American Heart Association task force on practice guidelines and the Society for Cardiovascular Angiography and Interventions. Circulation. 2011;124:e574–651.
33. Karthikesingam A, Hinchcliffe RJ, Loftus IM, Thompson MM, Holt PJ. Volume-outcome relationships in vascular surgery: the current status. J Endovasc Ther. 2010;17:356–65.
34. Bolling SF, Li S, O'Brien SM, Brennan JM, Prager RL, Gammie JS. Predictors of mitral valve repair: clinical and surgeon factors. Ann Thorac Surg. 2010;90:1904–11.
35. Gammie JS, O'Brien SM, Griffith BP, Ferguson TB, Peterson ED. Influence of hospital procedural volume on care process and mortality for patients undergoing elective surgery for mitral regurgitation. Circulation. 2007;115:881–7.
36. Birkmeyer JD, Siewers AE, Finlayson EVA, Stukel TA, Lucas FL, Batista I, et al. Hospital volume and surgical mortality in the United States. N Engl J Med. 2002;346:1128–37.
37. Vassileva CM, Boley T, Markwell S, Hazelrigg S. Impact of hospital annual mitral procedural volume on mitral valve repair rates and mortality. J Heart Valve Dis. 2012;21:41–7.
38. Rahimtoola SH. Choice of prosthetic heart valve in adults. J Am Coll Cardiol. 2010;55:2413–26.
39. Unger P, Dedobbeleer C, van Camp G, Plein D, Cosyns B, Lancellotti P. Mitral regurgitation in patients with aortic stenosis undergoing valve replacement. Heart. 2010;96:9–14.
40. Vahanian A, Alfieri O, Andreotti F, Antunes MJ, Baron-Esquivias G, Baumgartner H, et al. Guidelines on the management of valvular heart disease (version 2012). Eur Heart J. 2012;33:2451–96.
41. Aicher D, Fries R, Rodionycheva S, Schmidt K, Langer F, Schaefers HJ. Aortic valve repair leads to a low incidence of valve-related complications. Eur J Cardiothorac Surg. 2010;37:127–32.

42. Langer F, Aicher D, Kissinger A, Wendler O, Lausberg H, Fries R, Schaefers H-J. Aortic valve repair using a differentiated surgical strategy. Circulation. 2004;110(Suppl II):II-67–73.
43. le Polain de Waroux JB, Pouleur AC, Robert A, Pasquet A, Gerber BL, Noirhomme P, El Khoury G, Vanoverschelde JL. Mechanisms of recurrent aortic regurgitation after aortic valve repair. J Am Coll Cardiol Cardiovasc Imaging. 2009;2:931–9.
44. Botelho-Nevers E, Thuny F, Casalta JP, et al. Dramatic reduction in infective endocarditis-related mortality with a management-based approach. Arch Intern Med. 2009;169:1290–8.
45. Tornos P, Iung B, Permanyer-Miralda G, Baron G, Delahaye F, Gohlke-Bärwolf C, Butchart EG, Ravaud P, Vahanian A. Infective endocarditis in Europe: lessons from the Euro heart survey. Heart. 2005;91(5):571.
46. Ruttmann E, Hangler HB, Kilo J, Hőfer D, Műller LC, Hintringer F, Műller S, Laufer G, Antretter H. Transvenous pacemaker lead removal is safe and effective even in large vegetations: an analysis of 53 cases of pacemaker lead endocarditis. Pacing Clin Electrophysiol. 2006;29:231–6.
47. Thuny F, Beurtheret S, Mancini J, et al. The timing of surgery influences mortality and morbidity in adults with severe complicated endocarditis: a propensity analysis. Eur Heart J. 2011;32:2027–33.
48. Iung B, Rousseau-Paziaud J, Cormier B, Garbarz E, Fondard O, Brochet E, Acar C, Couëtil J-P, Hvass U, Vahanian A. Contemporary results of mitral valve repair for infective endocarditis. J Am Coll Cardiol. 2004;43:386–92.
49. d'Arcy JL, Coffey S, Loudon M, Kennedy A, Pearson-Stuttard J, Birks J, Frangou E, Farmer AJ, Mant D, Wilson J, Myerson SG, Prendergast BD. Large-scale community echocardiographic screening reveals a major burden of undiagnosed valvular heart disease in older people: The OxVALVE Population Cohort Study. Eur Heart J. 2016;37(47):3515–22. https://doi.org/10.1093/eurheartj/ehw229.
50. Roldan CA, Shively BK, Crawford MH. Value of cardiovascular physical examination for detecting valvular heart disease in asymptomatic subjects. Am J Cardiol. 1996;77:1327–31.
51. Marijon E, Ou P, Celermajer S, et al. Prevalence of rheumatic heart disease detected by echocardiographic screening. N Engl J Med. 2007;357:470–6.
52. McDonald, Daly, Jelinek, et al. Opening Pandora's box: the unpredictability of reassurance by a normal test result. Br Med J. 1996;313:329–32.
53. Stoate HG. Can health screening damage your health? JR Coll Gen Pract. 1989;39:193–5.
54. Douglas PS, Garcia MJ, Haines DE, et al. ACCF/ASE/AHA/ASNC/HFSA/HRS/SCAI/SCCM/SCCT/SCMR 2011. Appropriate use criteria for echocardiography. JACC. 2011;57:1126–66.
55. Chambers JB, Kabir S, Cajeat E. The detection of heart disease by open access echocardiography: a retrospective analysis. Br J Gen Pract. 2014;64:86–7.
56. McBride KL, Garg V. Heredity of bicuspid aortic valve: is family screening indicated? Heart. 2011;97:1193–5.
57. Warnes CA, Williams RG, Bashore TM, et al. 2008 guidelines for the management of adults with congenital heart disease. JACC. 2008;52:e1–e121.
58. Carapetis JR, Steer AC, Mulholland EK, Weber M. The global burden of group A streptococcal diseases. Lancet Infect Dis. 2005;5:685–94.
59. Eveborn GW, Schirmer H, Heggelund G, et al. The evolving epidemiology of valvular aortic stenosis. The Tromso Study. Heart. 2012;99(6):396–400. https://doi.org/10.1136/heartjnl-2012-302265.
60. Lindroos M, Kupari M, Heikkila J, et al. Prevalence of aortic valve abnormalities in the elderly: an echocardiographic study of a random population sample. J Am Coll Cardiol. 1993;21:1220–5.
61. Stewart BF, Siscovick D, Lind BK, et al. Clinical factors associated with calcific aortic valve disease. JACC. 1997;29:630–4.
62. Grant SW, Devbhandari MP, Grayson AD, et al. What is the impact of providing a Transcatheter Aortic Valve Implantation (TAVI) service on conventional aortic valve surgical activity, patient risk factors and outcomes in the first two years? Heart. 2012;96:1633–7.

63. Grant SW, Hickey GL, Cosgriff R, Cooper G, Deanfield J, Roxburgh J, Bridgewater B. Creating transparency in UK adult cardiac surgery data. Heart. 2013;99:1067–8.
64. Wijns W, Kolh PH. Experience with revascularization procedures does matter: low volume means worse outcome. Eur Heart J. 2010;31(16):1954–7. https://doi.org/10.1093/eurheart/ehq172.
65. Rosenhek R, Rader F, Klaar U, et al. Outcome of watchful waiting in asymptomatic severe mitral regurgitation. Circulation. 2006;113:2238–44.
66. Zilbersak R, Gabriel H, Maurer G, Rosenhek R. Optimized timing of surgery in aortic stenosis: impact of a valve clinic program
67. Gurzun MM, Ionescu A. Appropriateness of use criteria for transthoracic echocardiography: are they relevant outside the USA? Eur Heart J Cardiovasc Imaging. 2014;15:450–5.
68. Zaidi A, Ionescu A, Sharma R, et al. Echocardiographic surveillance of aortic valve stenosis: towards a standardized approach. J Heart Valve Dis. 2012;21:707–13.
69. Turpie D, Maycock M, Crawford C, et al. Establishing an aortic surveillance clinic. Br J Cardiol. 2010;17(6):286–9.

Index

K. Fattouch et al. (eds.), *Advances in Treatments for Aortic Valve and Root Diseases*, https://doi.org/10.1007/978-3-319-66483-5